Emergency care

For our children
Thomas and Owen Greaves
Matthew, James
and Sarah Porter
and
Jack Hodgetts

For WB Saunders:

Commissioning Editor: Susan Young
Project Development Manager: Catherine Jackson
Project Manager: Cheryl Brant
Design Direction: Judith Wright

emergency care

emergency care:

A TEXTBOOK FOR PARAMEDICS
Second Edition

Edited by

Ian Greaves

OStJ FRCP FFAEM FIMC RCS(Ed) DTM&H DMCC DipMedEd RAMC
Visiting Professor of Emergency Medicine, University of Teesside
Consultant in Emergency Medicine, British Army

Keith Porter

FRCS FRCSEd(Hon) DipIMC RCS(Ed)
Consultant Trauma Surgeon, Selly Oak Hospital, Birmingham

Tim Hodgetts

QHP OstJ FRCP FRCSEd(Hon) FFAEM FIMC RCSEd MMedEd RAMC
Visiting Professor of Emergency Medicine, University of Birmingham
Consultant in Emergency Medicine, British Army

and

Malcolm Woollard

MPH, MBA, MA(Ed), DipIMC(RCSEd), PGCE, RN, SRPara, FASI, ILTM
Visiting Professor in Prehospital Emergency Care and
Director, Faculty of Prehospital Care Research Unit,
University of Teesside

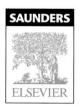

SAUNDERS

ELSEVIER

EDINBURGH LONDON OXFORD PHILADELPHIA ST LOUIS SYDNEY TORONTO 2006

SAUNDERS

ELSEVIER

An imprint of Elsevier Limited

First edition 1997
Second edition 2006

ISBN 0 7020 2586 0
EAN 9780702025860

British Library Cataloguing in Publication Data
A catalogue record for this book is available from the British Library

Library of Congress Cataloging in Publication Data
A catalog record for this book is available from the Library of Congress

Note
Medical knowledge is constantly changing. As new information becomes available, changes
in treatment, procedures, equipment and the use of drugs become necessary. The author and
the publishers have taken care to ensure that the information given in this text is accurate and
up to date. However, readers are strongly advised to confirm that the information, especially
with regard to drug usage, complies with the latest legislation and standards of practice.

Printed in Italy

The
Publisher's
policy is to use
**paper manufactured
from sustainable forests**

Working together to grow
libraries in developing countries

www.elsevier.com | www.bookaid.org | www.sabre.org

ELSEVIER   BOOK AID International   Sabre Foundation

Contents

Contributors

Bruce Armstrong RGN, RMN
Consultant Nurse, Basingstoke Hospital

Peter Baskett FRCA, MRCP
Formerly Consultant Anaesthetist, Frenchay Hospital,
Bristol

James Briscoe MRCPsych
Honorary Clinical Lecturer, Department of Psychiatry,
University of Birmingham, Birmingham

Christopher Carney DipIMC.RCS(Ed)
Chief Executive, East Anglia Ambulance Service Trust,
Norwich

Timothy Coats FRCS
Professor of Accident & Emergency Medicine,
Leicester Royal Infirmary

Peter Driscoll MD, FRCS, FFAEM
Consultant and Senior Lecturer, Department of Emergency
Medicine, Hope Hospital, Salford

Peter Dyer FRCS(Ed), FFD.RCSI
Consultant in Maxillofacial Surgery, Royal Lancaster
Infirmary

Judith Fisher FRCGP
Formerly Consultant in Primary Care,
Royal London Hospital, London

Ian Greaves OStJ, MB ChB, FRCP, FFAEM, DTM&H, FIMC.RCS(Ed)
DMCC, DipMedEd, RAMC
Professor of Emergency Medicine, University of Teesside,
Consultant in Emergency Medicine British Army

Carl Gwinnutt FRCA
Consultant Anaesthetist, Hope Hospital, Salford

Jacqueline Hanson FRCS, FFAEM
Consultant in Accident & Emergency Medicine,
Preston Royal Infirmary, Preston

Tim Hodgetts QHP, OStJ, MB BS(Hons), FRCP, FFAEM, MmedEd,
FIMC.RCS(Ed), RAMC
Professor of Emergency Medicine, University of
Birmingham, Consultant in Emergency Medicine,
British Army

Graham Johnson FRCS, FFAEM
Consultant in Emergency Medicine,
St James University Hospital, Leeds

Jason Kendall MRCP(UK), DipIMC.RCS(Ed), MD
Consultant in Accident & Emergency Medicine,
Frenchay Hospital, Bristol

Alastair Main MD, FRCP
Consultant in Geriatric Medicine, Queen Elizabeth
Hospital, Birmingham

David Morgan-Jones
General Practitioner, Royal Army Medical Corps

Gordon J A Morris MRCGP, AFOM, DRCOG
Senior Medical Officer, Occupational Health Care
Services, Glasgow

Julie Nancarrow MB, ChB, DipIMC, FRCSEd, MRCGP, FFAEM
Consultant in Emergency Medicine
Warwick University

Jerry Nolan FRCA
Department of Anaesthesia, Royal United Hospital, Bath

Mike Parr FRCA
Intensive Care Unit, Royal North Shore Hospital, Sydney,
Australia

Gavin Perkins MRCP
SpR in Respiratory Medicine
University Hospital, Birmingham

Keith Porter MB BS, FRCS, DipIMC.RCS(Ed), FRCSEd(Hon), FRCS(Ed),
FRCS(Eng), FINCRCS(Ed)
Consultant Surgeon, Selly Oak Hospital, Birmingham

James Ryan MCh, FRCS
Leonard Cheshire Professor of Post Conflict Recovery,
University College London

John Scott DipIMC.RCS(Ed), DA
General Practitioner, Cambridge

Jason Smith MRCP(UK), RN
Consultant in Emergency Medicine, Royal Navy

Andrew Thurgood MSc, RGN, DIMC RSC Ed, Dip HS, SRPara
Immediate Care Practitioner & Nurse Consultant,
Birmingham

Ian Todd LLB(Hons), DipIMC.RCS(Ed), SRPara
Paramedic Officer, Warwickshire Ambulance Service NHS
Trust; Visiting Research Fellow, University of Warwick

Lee Wallis MRCP(UK), RN
Consultant in Emergency Medicine, Royal Navy,
Johannesburg, South Africa

Malcolm Woollard MPH, MBA, DipIMC(RCSEd). PGCE, SRPara,
RN, FASI, ILTM
Visiting Professor in Prehospital Emergency Care and
Director, Faculty of Prehospital Care Research Unit,
University of Teesside

Preface to the second edition

The first edition of *Emergency Care* was published in 1997 and very rapidly established itself as a standard textbook for paramedics and others working in the field of pre-hospital medicine. However this is a very rapidly developing area and it is now time for a revised version.

This second edition has been completely revised in the light of current best practice and the developing trends in prehospital care. Every chapter has been revised, many have been rewritten, and four new chapters have been added. We hope that this edition will continue to be a relevant and accessible resource for all those who work in this challenging field.

Once again we are grateful to our contributors, especially to the somewhat smaller band who have contributed to the new edition, but also to those whose contributions to the first edition were so much appreciated. Nevertheless, as always our greatest debt is to our families without whose support yet another project would never have been completed.

IG
KP
TJH
MW
Teeside 2004

Preface to the first edition

The role of the ambulance service paramedic in the pre-hospital management of the acutely ill and injured has been increasingly recognized during the last few years. Along with the development of this role has come a general acceptance of the need for consistent and rational education for the paramedical profession. As this book goes to press, the first degree courses for paramedics in the UK are in preparation.

The time is right for a paramedic textbook that offers guidelines for safe practice against a background of sound scientific information. We hope that this book will fill this role. *Emergency Care: A Textbook for Paramedics* is the first comprehensive British textbook for paramedics – and importantly, the first book based on British practice.

As there are variations in practice between ambulance services in different parts of the UK, there may be occasional discrepancies between the text and readers' local guidelines. An editorial path has been taken which corresponds (we hope) with the practice in a majority of services. Additionally, we have described a number of procedures which we believe are likely to be added to the paramedic role in the not too distant future.

This book is intended to be a comprehensive textbook for paramedics from basic training to an advanced level of practice, and we have not therefore provided extensive references.

Suggestions for further reading are given at the end of individual chapters for those who wish to study particular subjects in greater detail.

Because of the size of the book, we suspect that most readers will read individual chapters as the need arises. For this reason, chapters need to be able to stand alone and we make no apology for any repetition of important material that this entails.

Those who wish to assess their knowledge may find the companion book *Emergency Care: A Self-assessment Guide* useful.

This book is written primarily for ambulance service paramedics, but we believe that it will also be useful to doctors (especially those involved in immediate care), members of the emergency and rescue services, first-aiders, and medical students.

We hope that this text will prove popular with paramedics, and will go some way to establishing a consistent national standard for practice. We would welcome any comments, suggestions or criticisms from readers.

Ian Greaves
Tim Hodgetts
Keith Porter

Acknowledgements

The editors would like to thank all those who have contributed to this or the previous edition of *Emergency Care*: without them, this project would not exist. We would like once again to take this opportunity to express our particular thanks to all those who contributed to the first edition: Bruce Armstrong, Harry Baker, Peter Baskett, James Briscoe, Terry Brown, Christopher Carney, Timothy Coats, Michael Colquhoun, Gareth Davies, Corah Dempsey, Peter Driscoll, Peter Dyer, Judith Fisher, Alasdair Gray, Ian Greaves, Marcus Green, Paul Grout, Carl Gwinnutt, Jacqueline Hanson, Kenneth Hines, Tim Hodgetts, Peter Holden, John Hopper, Phil Hormbrey, Jason Kendall, Juergen Klein, Colville Laird, Richard Lewis, Kevin Mackway-Jones, Alastair Main, Alastair McGowan, Ian McNeil, Gordon J A Morris, Chris Moulton, Julie Nancarrow, Jerry Nolan, Mike Parr, Keith Porter, Brian Robertson, Colin Robertson, Jim Ryan, John Scott, Howard Sherriff, Sean Walsh, Alastair Wilson, Malcolm Woollard. We are grateful for their expertise and their patience. We would also like to thank all those who have given us permission to reproduce copyright material.

Once again, however, our chief debt is to our families for putting up with yet another "final project".

DRUG DOSES

We believe the drug doses and regimens in this book to be correct. However, we recommend that if you are using a drug with which you are not familiar you should consult the *British National Formulary* and the current edition of the *Joint Royal Colleges Ambulance Liaison Committee Clinical Practice Guidelines for use in UK Ambulance Services* first.

Section **1**

SETTING THE SCENE

Chapter 1

Scene approach and assessment

CHAPTER CONTENTS

APPROACHING THE SCENE

DRIVING TO THE SCENE

When driving an emergency vehicle to the scene of an accident or medical emergency the priority is safety, not speed – safety of oneself and of other road users. If expeditious transport is required from the scene to the hospital, then the safety of the patient is an additional concern.

> When driving an emergency vehicle the priority is safety, not speed

Consider this: a vehicle driven 3 miles on urban roads at an average of 60 miles per hour will take 3 minutes to travel the distance, whereas a vehicle driven at an average of 40 miles per hour will take 4½ minutes – a difference of only 1½ minutes. It might be argued that such a time saving may be critical if the patient is in ventricular fibrillation following myocardial infarction or has an obstructed airway following head injury, but this will not be true in the majority of cases. The likelihood of an accident en route (involving the emergency vehicle or road users trying to avoid the emergency vehicle, or both) will increase as the driving speed increases. The driver of an emergency vehicle therefore has a responsibility to balance safe driving with an acceptable response time.

> An emergency vehicle driver must balance safe driving with an acceptable response time

The quality of the despatch information may influence, consciously or subconsciously, how the emergency vehicle driver responds to the scene. The following are three examples of despatch information to the same incident, which illustrate the importance of high-quality information. What should the response be in each case?

> 1. *Seventy-year-old woman collapsed in East Street outside Lloyds Bank.*
> 2. *Seventy-year-old woman collapsed, not breathing, no pulse in East Street outside Lloyds Bank.*
> 3. *Seventy-year-old woman collapsed, now fully alert but injured right wrist in fall, in East Street outside Lloyds Bank.*

The advanced driving techniques taught to emergency service personnel are often referred to as *defensive driving*. These techniques are described in detail in *Roadcraft: the police driver's handbook* (see Further reading). The fundamental principle is to provide an appropriate attitude to driving, particularly towards speed and risk taking. In the heat of battle soldiers may become blind to everything other than their immediate objective: this "red mist" may also engulf the emergency service driver, who will ignore road conditions and threaten the safety of other road users in an attempt to reach the scene as quickly as possible. This "red mist" can be minimized by concentration on the driving, rather than concentration on anticipated problems and tasks at the scene.

In the UK an emergency service vehicle has no legal right of way when using visual and audible warnings: the ambulance driver must rely on the courtesy of other road users to give way. Defensive driving techniques recognize the need for continuous caution in case other vehicles do not give way, whilst teaching the driver how best to use the available road. Figure 1.1 shows how an ambulance can position itself on a rural road to get the best view of oncoming traffic and to anticipate oncoming hazards; Figure 1.2 explains the "arrowhead" principle.

The public road user may react in a variety of ways to an approaching ambulance:

- sudden braking
- sudden changing of lane
- failure to give way.

It is important that the emergency vehicle is not driven aggressively. If the ambulance is too close to the vehicle in front there may be a collision if the other vehicle suddenly brakes. Alternatively, other vehicle drivers may be panicked into an erratic move which is dangerous to themselves or to others. Where a driver makes a special effort to give way this should be acknowledged: the same driver will then be disposed to give way the next time.

There should be a 2-second gap between your vehicle and the vehicle in front. A roadside marker such as a lamp-post should be identified, and as the vehicle in front passes the marker the sentence:

> **"Only a fool breaks the 2-second rule"**

should be said. It should be possible to complete this sentence before the ambulance passes the marker.

The ambulance driver should be aware of the limitations of the ambulance's visual and audible warnings. Strobe lights are generally of higher intensity than rotating halogen lights, but tend to be unidirectional: additional strobe lights

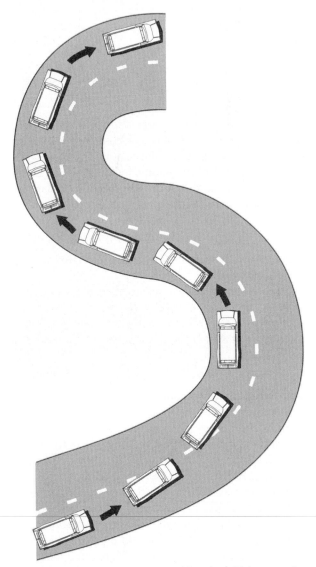

Figure 1.1 Driving on a rural road: position the vehicle to get the best view of the road ahead

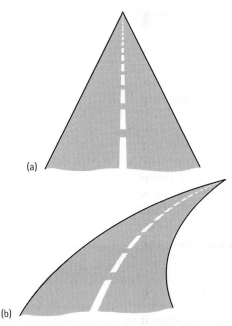

Figure 1.2 The arrowhead principle. The verges of the road form an "arrowhead" on the horizon; when the arrowhead is moving (a), accelerate; when the arrowhead is stationary (b), maintain speed or decelerate until it starts to move again

---

Box 1.1 Advanced safe driving tips

- Devote your concentration to driving, not to how you will respond on arrival at the scene (beware of "red mist")
- Always ensure you can stop within the distance you can see
- Keep a safe distance from the vehicle in front (remember the 2-second rule)

must be mounted on the side of the vehicle or on the end of a light-bar for all-round visibility. Roof-mounted lights may not be seen if the ambulance is very close to the vehicle in front and its driver may simply think he or she is being followed by an angry van driver. Strobe lights mounted on the ambulance's grille or dashboard will identify the vehicle in this situation.

Sirens tend to be non-directional and vehicles approaching a junction at right angles to the ambulance may not hear the ambulance's siren. Even when the siren is heard, it can be difficult to determine from which direction the ambulance is coming. When travelling at high speed, as on a motorway, a siren will provide very little advance warning: far more effective here is the use of alternating dipped and full-beam headlights.

The biggest limitation of lights and sirens is that they provide no legal protection in the event of an accident. An ambulance driver who causes an accident can expect to be charged with dangerous driving at the very least.

> Lights and sirens provide no legal protection in the event of an accident

It has been popular to request a police escort for an ambulance, especially for the seriously ill or injured patient who is transferred between hospitals. Such a decision should be considered carefully. A police escort is effective if the police vehicle moves ahead of the ambulance to clear a route (e.g. to stop traffic at a junction) and then allows the ambulance to pass. This would be useful in city traffic and may best be performed by two police cars or motorcyclists alternately moving ahead of the ambulance. The danger of a police escort is that it may become a race to keep up with the more powerful car; worse, other road users may only identify the first emergency vehicle and turn back into the path of the ambulance (the incidence of ambulance accidents is increased when a police escort is used).

PARKING AT THE SCENE

On a residential street it may be possible to extinguish all warning lights; on a commercial street in the day double-parking may be unavoidable, which may obstruct the flow of traffic – hazard lights or beacons are then used at the driver's discretion. When an ambulance is the first or only emergency vehicle to arrive at the scene of a road traffic accident the vehicle is parked in the *fend-off* or *on-line* position (Figure 1.3) to protect the incident. In the fend-off position beacons may be less visible to approaching traffic and headlights may distract traffic in the opposite carriageway but if a vehicle shunts an ambulance in the on-line position the ambulance may be pushed forward onto the casualties and rescuers. The parking position for a combined emergency service response to a road traffic accident entrapment is shown in Figure 1.4.

If the ambulance is left unattended it should be locked. This is going to become an even more important precaution now that UK ambulance services have begun to carry morphine following a recent change in guidelines. Even if

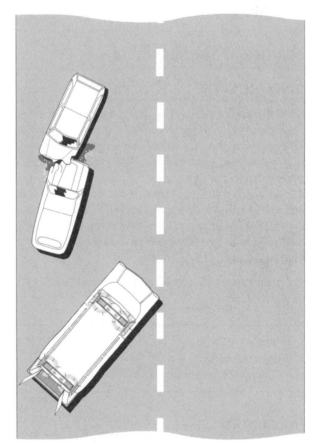

Figure 1.3 The fend-off position

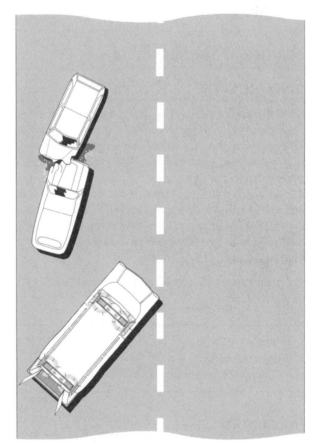

Figure 1.4 Combined emergency services parking at a motorway accident

morphine is not carried for use by ambulance personnel, opportunist thieves may look for such drugs or take other items of valuable equipment. If the police are controlling an incident the keys should be left in the ignition so that a vehicle can be moved if necessary.

IMMEDIATE-CARE DOCTORS

Immediate-care doctors may be requested to attend the scene by the ambulance service, where a British Association for Immediate Care (BASICS) scheme exists. A green beacon identifies a registered medical practitioner – sirens can only be used by doctors with the approval of the county's Chief Police Officer. The doctor will park as directed by the police; the accepted position is in front of the ambulance, beacons should be extinguished and keys left in the ignition.

PRIORITIES AT THE SCENE

SETTING THE SCENE

It is 1600 hours on Monday and you have arrived at the scene of a pedestrian road traffic accident. A member of the public dialled 999, asked for the ambulance service and simply said a child had been hit by a car when crossing the road at the busy corner of North and East Streets in Townsville. There is a crowd of 15 people. Traffic is at a standstill behind the incident and is moving very slowly in the opposite direction, which is the direction from which you approach. The child is lying unconscious but breathing on the road. A woman is cradling the child's head. What do you do?

The priorities at the scene can be remembered as CONTROL then ACT.

A >	Assess
C >	Communicate
T >	Triage, treat and transport

SCENE CONTROL

The first priority is to control the scene after approaching and parking in the carriageway that is free beyond the incident. The incident is now protected in both directions. Beacons should be left switched on. Members of the public should be cleared from obstructing the road and the engine of the vehicle involved in the accident turned off.

Scene control is a responsibility of the police, who will be required at this incident for traffic control. In a protracted incident, such as a vehicle entrapment, the police will establish and maintain a cordon to protect the rescuers and will determine the approach routes for emergency service vehicles.

Safety is of paramount concern. Always think of your own safety first, then the safety of other rescuers and bystanders

---

Box 1.2 The 1–2–3 of safety

1 > Self
2 > The scene (bystanders, rescuers)
3 > The casualties

Box 1.3 Ambulance officer's personal protective equipment (Figure 1.5)

- Hard hat with chin strap
- Eye protection (goggles, glasses or visor)
- Ear protection
- High-visibility jacket, with identifying markings
- Heavy-duty gloves
- Patient treatment gloves
- Robust footwear

---

and finally the safety of the casualties. This is the 1-2-3 of safety.

Protecting oneself

Individual emergency service personnel must be responsible for their own safety. In this situation at least a high-visibility vest marked with the level of training ("Ambulance" for general duties personnel, "Technician" or "Paramedic") must be worn. Where there is a hazard from glass or sharp metal a jacket with full-length sleeves should be worn, again appropriately marked, together with a helmet with integral visor. Helmets must be fitted with a secure chin strap, otherwise the temptation will be to discard one that falls off when the officer bends forward to treat a patient. A high-visibility jacket is mandatory at all road traffic collisions. All patients should be assumed to be infectious in terms of communicable diseases such as hepatitis B and C or acquired immune deficiency syndrome (AIDS). Protective gloves must be worn when treating patients and where there is contact with blood, eye protection is also recommended – this may be the visor of a helmet, goggles or protective glasses (the latter being the most suitable for general daily use).

If a chemical hazard is identified, the scene must not be entered until it is declared safe to do so by the fire service. It is the fire service's responsibility to identify the nature of a chemical hazard, which is done from the United Nations product number displayed on the hazard plate (see Chapter 44). The fire service control centre will have computerized access to information on the chemical or chemicals, including first-aid action and specific antidotes, and this information can be made available through the CHEMDATA system on the pumping appliances. Extreme caution must also be exercised when attending other specific incidents, as described below.

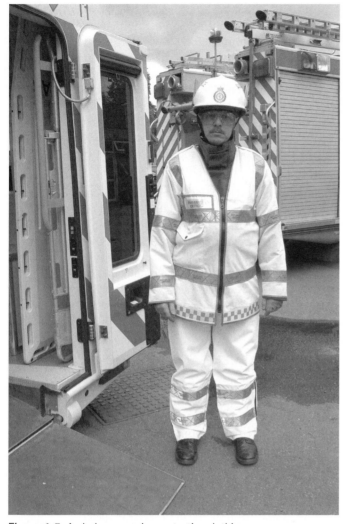

Figure 1.5 Ambulance service protective clothing

Shooting

Is there still a threat from the assailant? Is the patient also carrying a weapon? Is police support needed before proceeding?

Bomb

Unexploded bomb: can the suspect device be seen? If it can, you are in the wrong place! *Exploded bomb* (Figure 1.6): have the police searched for secondary devices? Radios should not be used until this search has been made (they may detonate a radio-controlled device).

Electric cable down

Power may be restored without investigation of the cause. The power company should be notified.

Rail

Has power to overhead cables or the live rail been isolated? Diesel trains can still run.

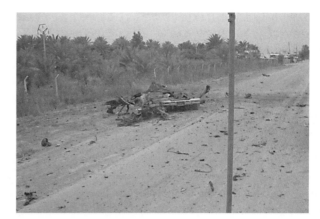

Figure 1.6 The aftermath of a terrorist explosion. A vehicle-borne improvised explosive device (VBIED) has just exploded

Protecting bystanders

Bystanders must be protected from becoming part of the incident and approaching vehicles (for example, on a motorway) must have adequate warning to slow down safely.

Protecting casualties

The safety of the casualties is ensured by protecting the scene with the emergency service vehicles and a cordon. A *snatch rescue* may be appropriate when the patient's life is in immediate danger, for example from fire or toxic chemical. In the UK it is the responsibility of the fire service to rescue casualties from a hazardous environment. It would be unwise for an ambulance officer to attempt such a rescue without adequate personal protective equipment. During a snatch rescue every reasonable attempt should be made to extricate the patient safely, but spinal immobilization in particular may have to be compromised in order to save life.

SCENE ASSESSMENT (ACT)

After taking control of an incident the next priority is to assess the scene. There are three important elements to the scene assessment:

- assessment of hazards, both present and potential
- reading the scene
- rapid assessment of the number and severity of casualties.

An *assessment of hazards* will be made during the approach to the incident, but further hazards, which may not have been initially evident, are evaluated during the scene assessment. Hazards at a road traffic accident can be actual (fire, chemical spillage) or potential (fire due to ignition of petrol on the road). Electricity supply through overhead cables is commonly interrupted as a result of "bird strike" and it is therefore usual for power to be restored without the reason being investigated. Emergency service personnel should not approach an incident involving a fallen electricity cable unless the power company has been contacted and the supply isolated. It is not necessary to touch a cable to be electrocuted – electricity can arc several metres.

An assessment of hazards is not restricted to the scene of a road traffic accident. For example, electricity could also be a hazard when a gardener has run over a lawnmower cable or a child is still holding a fork that has been pushed into a mains adaptor.

It is important to take time to *read the scene*. At a road traffic accident this involves "reading the wreckage", where observation of the nature of deformation of a vehicle and its position may help to identify the injuries the patient has sustained. This is discussed in detail later in this chapter. Additionally, reading the scene may give vital clues to the nature of a medical illness: a young woman found unconscious at home with an empty bottle of pills is likely to have taken an overdose and a sweaty, unresponsive man with a Medic-Alert bracelet which says *"I am an insulin-dependent diabetic"* has a high probability of being unresponsive because of hypoglycaemia.

> Read the scene for clues to injuries following trauma or to the reason for medical illness

Assessment of the scene also involves an assessment of the *number and severity of casualties*. At this stage the need is to establish what resources are immediately required at the scene. A detailed examination of each patient is not necessary but a rapid assessment of each patient's airway, breathing and circulation should be done (see Chapter 2).

COMMUNICATE (A*C*T)

Prehospital care requires teamwork and good teamwork demands good communication. There are several levels of communication to consider:

- communication with the patient
- communication between ambulance crew members
- communication with ambulance control
- communication with other emergency services at the scene
- communication with the hospital.

> Good communication is central to effective emergency service teamwork

When assistance is required at an incident scene it is useful to remember the mnemonic ETHANE when communicating with ambulance control.

E	Exact location
T	Type of incident
H	Hazards, present and potential
A	Access
N	Number, severity and type of casualties
E	Emergency services, present and required

Information is usually passed to the hospital indirectly via the ambulance control. Some ambulance services allow direct radio communication between hospital and the crew but this "talk through" must be requested through ambulance control. The value of advance warning is that appropriate staff can be summoned to assemble in the accident and emergency department to receive the patient, which is particularly important in cases of severe trauma and cardiac arrest.

The essential information the hospital will require to be able to assemble the appropriate staff and prepare equipment is:

- *age of the patient* (adult or child is adequate, but knowing the age of a child allows the preparation of equipment such as endotracheal tubes and the calculation of drug doses)
- *nature of the priority call* (trauma or cardiac arrest)
- *abnormal vital signs* (a head-injured patient with a Glasgow Coma Scale score below 9 requires intubation, if not already performed; the senior duty surgeon should be informed if there is an adult with hypotension of below 90 mmHg following trauma).

TRIAGE, TREATMENT AND TRANSPORT (AC*T*)

Triage is the sorting of patients into priorities for treatment and is discussed in detail in Chapter 58. Where there is only one injured victim, then the patient's injuries are prioritized. The systematic approach to the individual patient assessment and treatment is discussed in Chapter 2. This is the ABC system.

A	>	Airway (with control of the cervical spine)
B	>	Breathing (with oxygen)
C	>	Circulation (with control of external bleeding)

Transport to hospital should not be delayed for treatment that is not essential to saving life, reducing suffering or reducing long-term morbidity. The *golden hour* is the time from injury to the time of definitive treatment (emergency operation) and following trauma, every attempt should be made to deliver the patient well inside this golden hour. If the patient is trapped in a vehicle, this hour can easily slip by at the scene. After every 10 minutes spent at the scene, ask yourself, *"Why am I still here?"*. It is more appropriate in prehospital care, therefore, to think in terms of a *platinum 10 minutes* to rapidly assess and stabilize the patient before transport.

> The golden hour does not start when the ambulance arrives on scene but when the incident occurs

Packaging for transport (treatment and monitoring) and the selection of the best method of transport are discussed later in this book.

Box 1.4 Patterns of injury with front and side vehicle impact

Front impact
Facial injuries/airway compromise (windscreen)
Head injury (facial impact)
Cervical spine injury (flexion on deceleration; extension on facial impact)
Clavicle, sternum and rib fractures (and underlying organ injury) from seatbelt
Chest injury (steering wheel)
Abdominal visceral injury (seatbelt/steering wheel)
Patella and femoral fracture, posterior dislocation of hip (dashboard intrusion)
Lower leg fractures and dislocations (engine intrusion/pedals)

Side impact
Lateral flexion injury of cervical spine
Ipsilateral chest injury
Ipsilateral pelvis injury; central dislocation of the hip
Ipsilateral limb injuries
Ipsilateral abdominal visceral injury

READING THE WRECKAGE

Relating the deformation of a vehicle involved in an accident to the occupants' potential injuries is known as *reading the wreckage*. Metal is stronger than tissue and bone so if there is significant deformation of the vehicle involving the passenger compartment, the ambulance officer should anticipate a greater deformity of the human body, even if this was only temporary at the time of impact. Reading the wreckage enables the ambulance officer to actively seek a pattern of injuries, even if the patient is unaware of them all (pain in one body region can distract the patient from injuries elsewhere).

> Reading the wreckage allows the ambulance officer to anticipate a pattern of injuries

The pattern of injuries will depend on the type of impact. Box 1.4 lists the injuries that should be anticipated from a front or side impact.

Entrapment may be relative or absolute. *Relative entrapment* is when the occupant is unable to get out of the vehicle unassisted – for example, is unable to open the car door because of a broken arm. An *absolute entrapment* is when the occupant is physically restrained by the deformed wreckage.

> Vehicle entrapment may be relative or absolute

FURTHER READING

Calland V 2000 Safety at scene. Mosby, London
HMSO 1994 Roadcraft: the police driver's handbook. HMSO, London
Hodgetts T, Mackway-Jones K (eds) 2002 Major incident medical management and support. BMJ Books, London

Chapter 2

Approach to the patient

The approach to the patient follows scene safety and scene assessment. In trauma cases you will already have information about the patient's likely injuries after "reading the wreckage" or understanding the nature of the accident. In medical cases important clues will be gained on approach – the salbutamol inhaler by the bedside, the oxygen cylinder in the corner of the room or the box of assorted medications on the table (Figure 2.1). Assessment of the scene and assessment of the patient are vital and complementary parts of the same process.

Remember when dealing with a trauma case that certain mechanisms predict serious injuries whatever the apparent state of the patient.

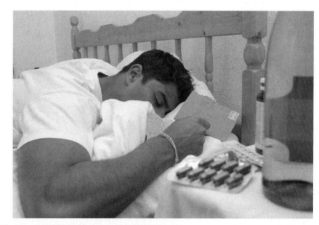

Figure 2.1 Clues in a patient's bedroom

- Patient falling from a height greater than 5 metres
- Road traffic accident (Figure 2.2) with an extrication time greater than 20 minutes
- Patient ejected from a vehicle
- Loss of life in the same vehicle
- Child (less than 12 years old) pedestrian or cyclist struck by a vehicle
- Pedestrian struck by a vehicle and thrown
- Vehicle intrusion greater than 30 cm

All such patients must be taken to hospital whatever their apparent injuries.

When dealing with an incident involving multiple casualties it will be necessary to carry out the process of triage;

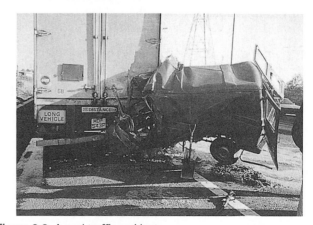

Figure 2.2 A road traffic accident

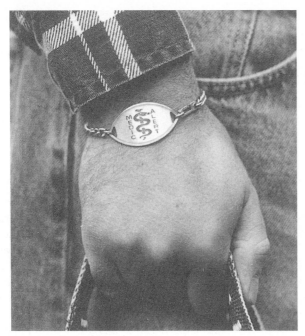

Figure 2.3 A Medic–Alert bracelet

that is, to sort casualties into priorities for treatment and to "do the most for the most" (Chapter 58).

During the course of examining a patient, any Medic-Alert bracelet or card (Figure 2.3) should be identified. Wherever possible, relevant medical history, current medication and allergies should be established. These points can be remembered using the mnemonic AMPLE.

A	>	Allergies
M	>	Medication
P	>	Past history
L	>	Last meal
E	>	Event (i.e. current problem)

This information is just as important in a trauma case as in a medical case: why did the patient crash the car on a straight road in good visibility? Does the patient suffer from diabetes mellitus or epilepsy? Did a hypoglycaemic episode or a myocardial infarction *cause* the accident?

PRIMARY AND SECONDARY SURVEYS

The patients seen by ambulance personnel may be divided broadly into two groups:

- medical patients
- trauma patients.

The initial approach to these two groups is *identical*. The components of the systematic approach are:

- primary survey
- resuscitation

- secondary survey
- definitive care.

The role of the *primary survey* is to identify any life-threatening problems or injuries.

> **The primary survey identifies life-threatening problems**

Whenever possible, treatment of any life-threatening problem is carried out as soon as that problem is identified.

> **Primary survey and resuscitation take place simultaneously**

The primary survey is a rapid process ideally taking only a minute or two. In critical trauma (and in some medical conditions) only the primary survey and resuscitation should be undertaken by the paramedic. The secondary survey (which identifies non-life-threatening problems) and definitive treatment are most appropriately carried out en route to hospital or after arrival there.

> **The *secondary survey* identifies non–life–threatening problems**

THE PRIMARY SURVEY

The primary survey follows the simple system of ABCDE.

A	>	Airway with cervical spine control
B	>	Breathing with adequate ventilation/oxygenation
C	>	Circulation with control of external haemorrhage
D	>	Disability and neurological examination
E	>	Exposure and evaluation

The philosophy of this approach is to deal with life-threatening problems in order of priority. Rigorous application of this approach is the basis of good paramedical practice.

Importantly, if the patient's condition deteriorates one must *always* revert to the ABCs. It can be said that *the most important examination is the re-examination.*

In time-critical trauma cases (where the patient is not entrapped) the principle should be establishment of airway and breathing on scene, with consideration of vascular access en route to hospital. Unnecessary delay at the scene may well jeopardize patient outcome.

Although this system was originally designed for use in trauma, it is equally relevant to the management of life-threatening medical conditions.

> **Unnecessary delay at the scene may well jeopardize patient outcome**

> **Box 2.1 Causes of airway obstruction**
>
> - Tongue
> - Blood
> - Vomitus
> - Broken dentures
> - Teeth and debris
> - Foreign bodies
> - Laryngotracheal injuries
> - Swelling from burns or allergies

"A" – AIRWAY WITH CERVICAL SPINE CONTROL

A clear airway free from obstruction or potential obstruction is essential. Causes of airway obstruction are given in Box 2.1.

In medical emergencies a clear airway is obtained by using a combination of head tilt and chin lift. In trauma patients, however, it is important to prevent cervical movement so only a chin lift or a jaw thrust manoeuvre is used. In-line cervical immobilization should be maintained during all airway manoeuvres. Cervical immobilization means in-line stabilization, *not* traction, which may produce or exacerbate spinal cord injury.

Well-fitting dentures should be retained. Visible foreign bodies and debris should be removed using a finger sweep or suction. A blind finger sweep is not recommended, as this may further impact a foreign body.

Once opened and cleared, the airway should be secured; this may involve the use of an appropriately sized oropharyngeal or nasopharyngeal airway and in some cases orotracheal intubation. It is important to remember that opening an airway has priority over cervical spine protection and in a difficult situation it may be necessary to accept some cervical spine movement.

> The airway has priority over the cervical spine

Approximately 5% of unconscious trauma patients have a cervical spine injury. It is imperative to have a high index of suspicion and anyone who is unconscious, has an altered level of consciousness or has evidence of blunt injury above the clavicle should be regarded as having a cervical spinal injury until it is proved otherwise. Once the airway has been opened, cleared and secured, an appropriately sized semi-rigid collar is fitted and manual immobilization is maintained.

Failure to obtain a clear airway may demand specialized interventions with appropriate assistance (Chapter 7). It may be possible to achieve some assisted ventilation in the case of partial airway obstruction, in which case the patient should be transferred to hospital urgently. Where the patient is trapped, skilled medical assistance may be available from a hospital "flying squad" or an immediate-care (BASICS) doctor.

Cervical spine injury may also complicate medical problems if, for example, a fit has caused a fall or a patient with severe rheumatoid arthritis has a relatively minor car accident.

"B" – BREATHING

Look, feel and listen for 5 seconds to ascertain whether the patient is breathing. It is important to recognize patients in whom there is *no* spontaneous respiration or who are hypoventilating (Greek *hypo*, under), as hypoxia is rapidly life threatening.

The respiratory rate should be determined by counting for 15 seconds and multiplying by 4 to give an approximate minute rate. During the secondary survey a more accurate rate may be determined, by counting for a whole minute.

The normal respiratory rate in adults is between 12 and 18 breaths per minute. All patients with a reduced (less than 12) or increased (greater than 18) respiratory rate should receive oxygen and if the rate is below 10 or above 29, assisted ventilation may be required. All trauma patients should receive high-concentration oxygen, irrespective of their respiratory rate.

> Normal respiratory rate in adults is 12–18 breaths per minute

It is important to recognize that hypoventilation may lead to carbon dioxide (CO_2) retention, which itself will alter the level of consciousness and result in brain injury.

During the primary survey life-threatening chest conditions should be identified; these include open chest wounds, flail chest and tension pneumothorax. The chest wall should be observed for symmetry and normal pattern of movement (there is "paradoxical movement" with a flail segment). A deviated trachea suggests a tension pneumothorax on the side *away* from the deviation and requires urgent medical intervention (see Chapter 33).

Mouth-to-mask ventilation, ventilation using a bag–valve–mask with reservoir or mechanical ventilation may be necessary to assist or replace ventilation if it is inadequate or absent. In all spontaneously breathing trauma cases oxygen at 15 litres per minute through a Hudson mask with an attached reservoir (giving an inspired concentration of about 90%) should be given.

A raised respiratory rate is an underrecognized sign of both hypoxia and hypovolaemia.

> Oxygen at high concentration saves lives

"C" – CIRCULATION AND CONTROL OF EXTERNAL HAEMORRHAGE

It is first essential to determine if the patient has a cardiac output and to start basic life support if this is absent.

External haemorrhage should be controlled where possible by direct pressure and elevation. Rarely, it is necessary to apply pressure over a pressure point or to use a tourniquet.

Circulatory status can be assessed by the pulse volume and pulse rate. Peripheral perfusion can be estimated by observing the capillary refill time: this is the time taken for the normal pink colour of the nail beds to return after 5 seconds of compression and is normally less than 2 seconds. This test is unreliable in the dark and in very cold conditions.

An early assessment of blood pressure is important. As a rough guide the presence of a:

- *carotid* pulse indicates a minimum blood pressure of 60 mmHg
- *femoral* pulse indicates a minimum blood pressure of 70 mmHg
- *radial* pulse indicates a minimum blood pressure of 80 mmHg.

Traumatic blood loss is corrected by placing at least one large-bore cannula (if possible, 14–16 gauge) and giving intravenous fluid (see Chapter 22). If the patient is not trapped and has critical injuries the infusion should be started en route to hospital, rather than delaying at the scene.

"D" – DISABILITY

The objective of assessing the neurological status is to provide a baseline for further observations. In the primary survey the AVPU scale is used.

A	>	Alert
V	>	responds to Verbal stimuli
P	>	responds to Painful stimuli
U	>	Unresponsive

In addition, pupillary size and reaction should be recorded.

"E" – EXPOSURE AND ENVIRONMENT

The patient needs to be exposed to allow clinical examination to exclude any obvious life-threatening conditions. In particular, exposure to inspect the chest is vital. It is important not to miss blood loss concealed by clothes or under the patient. Exposure should preserve the patient's dignity where possible and should protect from the extremes of temperature.

SUMMARY OF THE PRIMARY SURVEY

Life-threatening problems are identified and treated (wherever possible) during the primary survey. These problems may include maxillofacial trauma, for example (A), airway obstruction due to vomit in diabetic hypoglycaemia (A), severe pulmonary oedema following a heart attack (B), penetrating chest trauma (B) or blood loss due to trauma or bleeding duodenal ulcer (C). Whether the emergency is medical or traumatic, the approach remains the same. Sometimes a problem will be identified which the paramedic

cannot remedy on scene. The emphasis must then be on transferring the patient to hospital as rapidly as possible.

Assessment of the conscious level (using AVPU) and the pupils will give information about the primary problem (head injury or stroke) or about neurological complications that have ensued (e.g. deteriorating conscious level in untreated hypoglycaemia). Exposure (E) will prevent the missing of other significant injuries or useful clues (e.g. drug injection sites in a comatose patient or a purpuric rash in an unwell child indicating meningococcal septicaemia).

Prior to or during transport of all critical or seriously injured patients, communication either directly or through ambulance control should be made to the receiving hospital, giving a status report and requesting an appropriate response to meet the patient.

Resuscitation should be maintained en route to hospital. Monitoring should ideally include pulse, respiratory rate, blood pressure, level of consciousness, electrocardiogram (ECG) and pulse oximetry. It is still common practice in the UK to transport to the nearest hospital; it would be to the patient's advantage to transport directly to the *most appropriate* hospital.

A patient report form should be completed as soon as possible after arriving at hospital and should follow a clear handover of the patient. It is reasonable to allow the ambulance crew *45 seconds* to hand over the patient, during which *all* members of the receiving medical team listen, unless there is a problem with the airway or cardiopulmonary resuscitation is in progress. Only key information needs to be given at this stage – the mechanism of injury, the apparent and suspected injuries, the vital signs and the treatment given. This can be remembered by the acronym MIST.

M	>	Mechanism of injury
I	>	Injuries – apparent and suspected
S	>	Signs – abnormal vital signs
T	>	Treatment given

> **Remember in critical trauma:**
> A + B on scene
> C en route
> Do not allow the placing of intravenous lines to delay transfer

SECONDARY SURVEY

In trauma cases, a secondary survey may be performed in order to identify non-life-threatening injuries. In medical emergencies a similar approach to the patient may uncover vital clues to the patient's condition – injection marks, bruises, rashes, scars or informative tattoos.

If the patient's injuries are non-critical then a secondary survey may be undertaken. Depending on circumstances, this may best be done in the shelter and protection of the ambulance. The secondary survey should begin with reassessing the airway. In burns patients, for example, it is important to check for evidence of soot in the nose and on the lips or evidence of oedema of the upper airway.

> The secondary survey must never delay transfer to definitive care

HEAD

Pupil size and reaction are assessed. Evidence of bruising, lacerations, tenderness and other signs of fractures involving the skull or face should be identified. The nose and ears should be specifically inspected for blood and cerebrospinal fluid leakage (see Chapter 23).

NECK

The neck is assessed for signs of trauma, although in-line stabilization *must* be maintained. The larynx and trachea are palpated for evidence of injury and the latter for tracheal deviation. Assessment of the neck veins (distended in tension pneumothorax and cardiac tamponade) and carotid pulse should be made. The collar may need to be loosened while retaining stabilization to permit adequate examination.

CHEST

The chest is inspected for open wounds, contusion (bruising), seatbelt markings, a flail segment and respiratory rate and effort. Palpation may reveal local tenderness indicative of rib fractures, chest wall instability with a flail segment or surgical emphysema following a pneumothorax. The chest wall is auscultated for air entry and added sounds (e.g. wheeze) and percussion used to determine a haemothorax (dull, like a full barrel) or pneumothorax (resonant, like an empty barrel). Often this can only be adequately performed in the back of an ambulance because of the ambient noise at the scene.

ABDOMEN

The abdomen is inspected for open wounds, seatbelt markings and contusion. It is palpated for tenderness in all four quadrants. Swelling and tenderness can be seen in non-traumatic cases (e.g. bowel obstruction or ruptured abdominal aortic aneurysm).

PELVIS

In trauma cases the pelvis is usually "sprung" to determine tenderness and any instability; this involves pressing firmly on the front of each wing of the pelvis, but if a fracture is present this will be very painful and may exacerbate blood loss. This manoeuvre should not therefore be routinely performed outside hospital. Bleeding from the urethra (*per urethra*) may be noted, along with genital bruising which can be indicative of serious injury to the urethra, often following a pelvic fracture.

UPPER AND LOWER LIMBS

The limbs are inspected for swelling, deformity and wounds. They are palpated for fractures (a step in the cortex) or crepitus (broken ends grating together – very painful!).

The limb examination should include assessment of:

- motor response – test for active movements
- sensation – response to touch
- circulation – pulse and skin temperature.

Use the mnemonic MSC × 4.

M	>	Motor
S	>	Sensation
C	>	Circulation
×4	>	All four limbs

Limb injuries are treated as necessary, with dressings and splintage. Analgesia should be a high priority with suspected long-bone fractures (see Chapter 10). The choice may include:

- reassurance
- splintage (possibly with traction splint)
- nitrous oxide inhalation (Entonox, Nitronox)
- morphine.

Chapter 3

An introduction to clinical examination

CHAPTER CONTENTS

INTRODUCTION

Clinical examination remains the primary tool in the diagnosis of medical and traumatic problems in patients in pre-hospital care. In some respects, it is the oldest and most primitive tool we have for helping us to the right conclusion about a patient, but it remains the gold standard in the initial assessment of the patient. Unless clinical signs can be effectively and accurately elicited, their interpretation will be meaningless.

For the purposes of this chapter, examination will be described in the order used in the standard approach which is a common theme throughout this book – the ABCDE system.

> **A** irway with cervical spine control
> **B** reathing with oxygenation
> **C** irculation with haemorrhage control
> **D** isability
> **E** xposure

This systematic approach to the patient is described in detail in Chapter 2 and the individual components are discussed in the relevant chapters.

No examination is performed without clues from the history and attention should be paid to other information such as mechanism of injury, patterns of vehicle damage and damage to protective clothing or helmets. Often an assessment of A–D is made by a simple question: "Are you OK?". If this elicits a response such as "Yes, but my ankle hurts", this means the airway is clear, the patient is breathing enough to speak clearly, the brain is adequately perfused and the Glasgow Coma Score is either 14 or 15.

Recording the initial clinical findings is crucial, since many clinical diagnoses are made as a result of changes in clinical parameters over time, rather than a single "snapshot".

AIRWAY

The examination of the airway begins with a visual examination, to see if there is an obvious obstruction. It is equally important to listen carefully to hear if there is any evidence of obstruction. In many cases, when approaching the casualty, the first thing that is apparent is noisy breathing due to upper airways obstruction. This can give a gurgling, snoring or rasping sound and is indicative that there is obstruction of the airway that requires immediate attention. Assessment of the airway in victims of trauma should always include protection of the cervical spine by immobilization.

Possible abnormal noises originating in the upper airway include the following.

GURGLING

Gurgling suggests the presence of fluid in the airway, possibly blood, saliva or stomach contents that have been regurgitated. This will require suction if it is available.

SNORING

This is usually caused by the soft tissues of the nasopharynx and oropharynx flopping back against the posterior wall of the throat, partially obstructing the flow of air. It can be treated using simple airway opening manoeuvres, such as a head tilt or chin lift, or the use of simple airway adjuncts, or a combination of both.

STRIDOR

Stridor is caused by partial blockage of the upper airway by swelling (due to burns, infection, anaphylaxis) or a foreign body. An idea of the noise of stridor can be gained by making a forced maximal expiration.

HOARSENESS

Hoarseness has many causes, all relating to pathology around the larynx and vocal cords. This may be a result of simple laryngitis secondary to an upper respiratory tract infection but with a history of smoke inhalation or exposure to fire, it may represent a significant upper airway burn. In this case the patient requires urgent airway intervention by a specialist.

If there is no obvious noise, a more formal visual inspection is then carried out to assess for swelling, the presence of a foreign body, trauma or bleeding that may compromise the airway. An assessment of the airway goes hand in hand with an assessment of breathing and if there is no evidence of breathing, airway opening manoeuvres should be performed to ascertain if there is respiratory effort (see Chapter 6).

The airway reaches from the mouth or nose all the way to the lungs and can be divided into upper and lower parts. The airway can only be examined directly as far as the level of the vocal cords, but an examination of the airway is not complete without assessment of tracheal deviation. This is performed by placing the index finger into the suprasternal notch, palpating the trachea and feeling for any displacement to one side or the other. A conscious patient should be warned before this procedure is performed, as it may be uncomfortable. Tracheal deviation could be a sign that there is increased pressure in one side of the chest (e.g. with a tension pneumothorax) or reduced pressure in one side of the chest (e.g. due to total or lobar collapse or consolidation of a lung). The trachea will move towards the side of a collapse or consolidation and away from the side of a tension pneumothorax.

While examining the neck other findings should be sought. Swelling around the neck may be a result of trauma

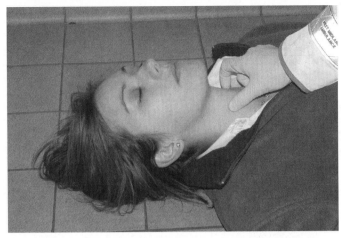

Figure 3.1 Assessment of the trachea

Box 3.1 Physical signs on neck examination

- Tracheal deviation
- Swelling and surgical emphysema
- Wounds
- Distended neck veins (see below)

and bruising, but may be due to other factors such as a generalized anaphylactic (allergic) reaction. The swelling should be palpated and if there is crepitus (a crackling feeling due to the presence of air within the tissues which is often compared to the popping of "bubble wrap" or palpating a bag of crisps) under the swelling, it may be that the patient has surgical emphysema. It is usually indicative of an underlying pneumothorax.

The neck contains several vital structures, some of which bleed if damaged, so particular attention should be paid to lacerations in this area and bleeding should be controlled at an early stage.

Features which should be sought when examining the neck are summarised in Box 3.1.

BREATHING

The assessment of breathing (and the respiratory system) should involve a four-stage process.

- Look
- Feel
- Percuss
- Auscultate (listen).

The first stage is to determine whether the patient is breathing. Whether or not breathing is present is determined by looking, listening and feeling for air movement from the mouth or nose. If the patient is not breathing, basic life support should be commenced (see Chapter 5).

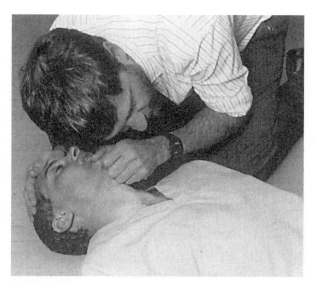

Figure 3.2 Look, listen and feel for breathing

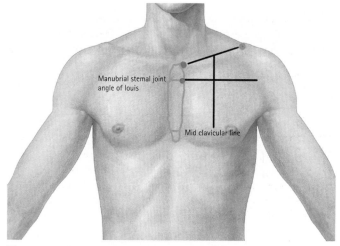

Figure 3.3 Surface anatomy of the chest: anterior view

If it is established that the patient is breathing, the four-stage assessment of the respiratory system should commence. Oxygen should be administered at this stage if appropriate.

DON'T FORGET THE OXYGEN

An assessment of breathing includes the following components.

LOOKING FOR VISUAL CLUES

The lungs are enclosed within the ribcage, which also protects some intra-abdominal structures, including the liver and spleen. The lungs are supported inferiorly by the dome-shaped diaphragm, which attaches to the lower margin of the ribcage at the front but extends further down at the back to the level of the lowest thoracic vertebra. Examination of the lung fields should therefore include the whole of the front of the chest and examination of the back down to this level. The sternum at the front of the chest provides bony protection for the heart which lies directly beneath, so injury to this area should raise suspicion of myocardial damage.

The first stage is to look at the patient to get a general impression of how hard he is working to breathe and for any external signs of injury such as pattern bruising or abrasions.

An assessment of the respiratory rate is next. The respiratory rate is one of the most important and sensitive indicators of severity of illness or injury. It should be measured over a given time period, for example 20 seconds, and multiplied by 3 to obtain a rate per minute. The normal respiratory rate for adults is 12–18 per minute.

Always count AND RECORD the respiratory rate

An assessment should now be made of whether there are signs of respiratory distress. The chest must be assessed for

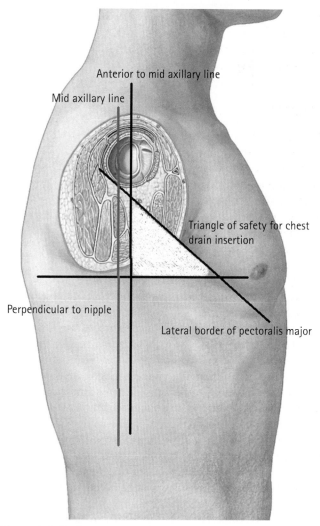

Figure 3.4 Surface anatomy of the chest: lateral view

symmetry of movement, body position, and signs of accessory muscle use (Figure 3.5). These are clues that may suggest that the patient is in respiratory distress. If there is increased work of breathing, accessory muscles of

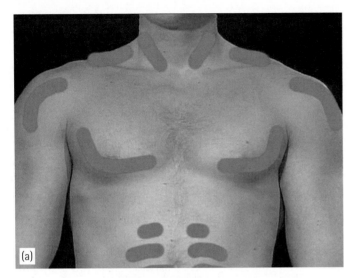

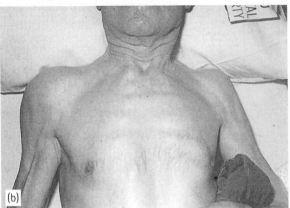

Figure 3.5 The accessory muscles of respiration. (a) Highlighted (b) clinical photograph

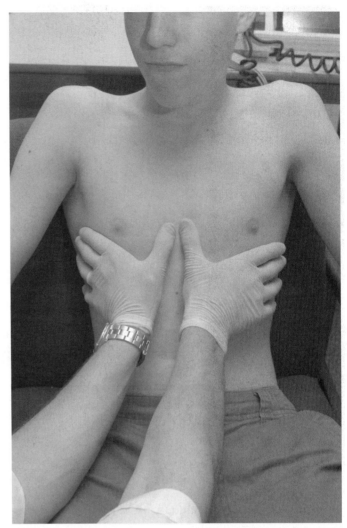

Figure 3.6 Assessing chest expansion. The hands are placed as shown and the thumbs drawn together until touching without removing the hands from the chest wall. The movement of the thumbs away from the midline is then assessed for equality and magnitude

respiration may be called into action. These may include intercostal muscles, strap muscles of the neck and abdominal muscles, which can often be detected clinically by watching the patient breathe. The presence of these findings suggests that the patient is having to work harder to get air into the lungs, due to either a respiratory problem or a circulatory problem. If a patient adopts a position such as sitting on the edge of the bed using the arms and shoulders to support the chest, this is also a sign of respiratory distress. If a patient is found in such a position, it is better to leave him in this position and not force him into a different position, such as lying flat.

If there is unequal movement of the chest, this suggests a problem on one side. There is reduced movement on the side of a pneumothorax, haemothorax or collapse of one lung. Asymmetry may represent an acute problem but may be a reflection of long-standing disease, such as previous surgery (e.g. a lobectomy for tuberculosis). If there is general hyperinflation of the chest, it may suggest chronic lung disease such as chronic obstructive pulmonary disease (COPD), but it may also occur in acute severe asthma.

PALPATION

Once visual inspection is complete, the chest should be palpated for equal expansion (Figure 3.6) and, in trauma, for any evidence of tenderness over the ribs or sternum. *Tactile fremitus* is a term given to transmission of vibration due to speech through the chest wall. It is increased in the presence of underlying solid lung (e.g. in consolidated lung secondary to pneumonia) but decreased in the presence of a collection of fluid outside the lung, such as a pleural effusion or haemothorax.

PERCUSSION

Percussion is a tool that helps determine the presence of fluid in the chest. It is a technique that was originally used by draughtsmen to determine how full their beer barrels were and can be used to distinguish between fluid, air-filled

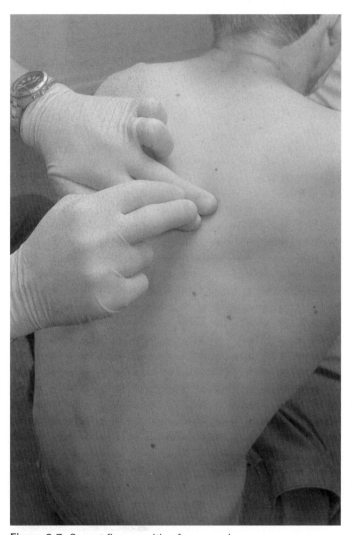

Figure 3.7 Correct finger position for percussion

cavity or solid organ (including consolidated lung). It is performed by tapping the end of the middle finger of one hand onto the middle phalanx of the same finger of the other hand, which should rest flat on the surface being examined (Figure 3.7).

It is imperative that the tip of the finger is used and not the pad of the finger, and only one finger should be used as the "hammer". Increased volume of percussion note is achieved by practice to improve technique, not by using two fingers, which produces a "double strike" and is unreliable.

A more hollow (resonant) sound than normal suggests an air-filled cavity beneath, a dull sound suggests a solid viscus and fluid is revealed by "stony" dullness. Only by practice can the user of this technique become proficient enough to learn reliable clinical information from its results. Percussion over the liver will give an indication of a dull percussion note compared with the more resonant note over normal lung.

> There is no substitute for endless practice of percussion

Table 3.1 Added sounds on auscultation

Added sound	Clinical meaning	Clinical example
Wheeze	Lower airway obstruction	Asthma
Stridor	Upper airway obstruction	Airway burn
Bronchial breathing	Solid lung	Pneumonia
Crepitations	Air spaces popping open	Pulmonary oedema

AUSCULTATION

Added sounds are the result of partial obstruction of air passages. If obstruction occurs high up in the respiratory tree in the larger airways, for example by inhalation of foreign body or swelling due to airway burn, the resultant effect produces *stridor*, a harsh noise produced on inspiration. If obstruction occurs lower down in the lungs in the smaller air passages, for example due to asthma, the resultant effect produces *wheeze*, a higher pitched noise on expiration.

Added sounds can sometimes be heard from the end of the bed but often a stethoscope is necessary to complete the examination. This can detect the presence or absence of air entry, added sounds and the presence of *bronchial breathing*. This is the noise that is transmitted from the larger airways through solid lung, the result of infection or collapse. *Crepitations* are crackling sounds that are typically heard in the lung bases in the presence of pulmonary oedema. They probably occur as a result of closed air passages popping open during inspiration, but are not specific to pulmonary oedema and may be present in a variety of clinical conditions.

During auscultation, the stethoscope should be placed on the front of the chest on both sides, in the axillae and at the bases, in order to gain a complete picture of both lung fields (Figure 3.8).

As a final note on respiratory examination, it is standard in most areas of prehospital care to have access to pulse oximetry and this should be considered routine in the examination of the sick or injured patient.

Special thought should be given to possible causes of a low oxygen saturation reading, such as cold and the use of metallic nail varnish ("conventional" nail varnish does not affect pulse oximetry), but it should be remembered that the most common cause of a low oxygen saturation reading is hypoxia.

CIRCULATION

Assessment of the circulation starts with establishing whether or not a pulse is present. If there is no pulse, basic life support should be commenced. The pulse can be palpated at several peripheral or central points, most commonly at the radial, carotid or femoral arteries.

The presence and nature of a pulse give the clinician an idea of the patient's haemodynamic status. If a pulse at the radial artery becomes impalpable but is still present at the carotid, this suggests the presence of a significant risk to vital organ perfusion.

After establishing the presence of a pulse, the next thing to do is establish its rate. This should be done by counting how many beats occur in a given time, for example 15 seconds, and multiplying by 4 to give a heart rate per minute. The normal heart rate for an adult is 60–100 beats per minute. A pulse faster than 100 beats per minute is by definition a tachycardia.

The character of the pulse is also important. A weak and thready pulse suggests a low blood pressure and a compromised cardiovascular state, whereas a strong and bounding pulse may indicate a hyperdynamic circulation and is found in conditions such as chronic lung disease and carbon monoxide poisoning.

Skin colour can also give a clue to the state of the patient. If the patient is very pale, he may have suffered significant blood loss.

Another method of assessing the patient's haemodynamic state is to measure the capillary refill time. This is performed by applying pressure to a nail bed for 5 seconds, then releasing the pressure and timing how long the nail bed takes to return to its normal colour. This is normal if it takes less than 2 seconds. Refill can be prolonged in the cold, so is often not as reliable as a pulse rate as a measure of circulation.

Non-invasive blood pressure measurement and a three-lead electrocardiogram trace (Figure 3.10) are also essential parts of the assessment of the circulation.

DISABILITY

Disability assessment should include examination of the conscious level, pupils and gross motor function. The conscious level can be assessed quickly using an AVPU score or more thoroughly using the Glasgow Coma Score.

THE AVPU SCORE

The AVPU score is a quick and easy assessment of conscious level. If a patient is alert and responsive, he scores "A". If he appears unresponsive, he should be asked the simple question: "Are you OK?". If this provokes an appropriate response, he scores "V", for verbal stimulus. If he still does not respond, more vigorous stimulation is necessary, by first gently shaking his shoulders and if he is still not responsive, by administering a painful stimulus, above the clavicles

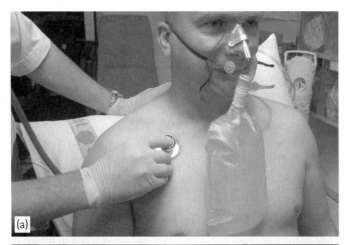
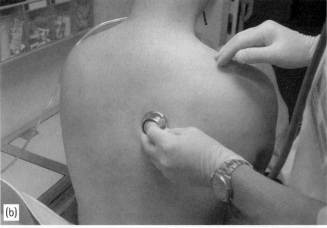
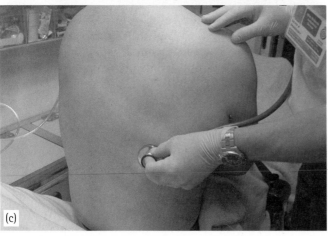

Figure 3.8 Positions of auscultation: front and back

Box 3.2 AVPU score		
Is the patient:		
● alert	SCORE	A
or does he:		
● respond to verbal stimulus	SCORE	V
● respond to painful stimulus	SCORE	P
or is he:		
● unresponsive	SCORE	U

Table 3.2 Clinical findings in lung pathology

Condition	Chest expansion	Trachea	Percussion	Breath sounds
Pneumothorax	Decreased – possibly hyperexpanded if tension	Deviation to opposite side	Increased resonance	Reduced
Haemothorax	Decreased	Deviated to opposite side or central	Dullness to percussion	Reduced
Collapse/consolidation	Decreased	Usually central*	Dullness to percussion	Reduced or bronchial breathing
Pleural effusion	Decreased	Central	Stony dullness to percussion	Reduced breath sounds

*may be deviated to ride of collapse.

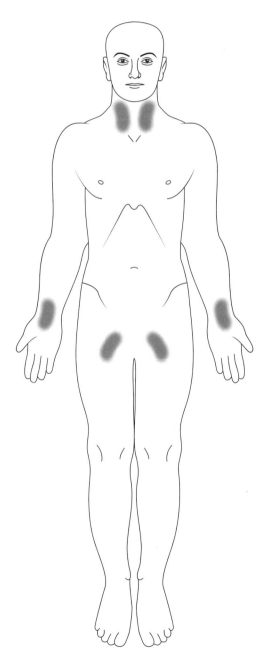

Figure 3.9 Position of radial (wrist), carotid (neck) and femoral (groin) pulses

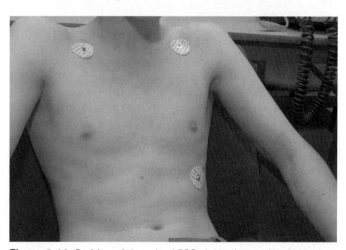

Figure 3.10 Position of three-lead ECG electrodes on the chest

such as applying pressure over a supraorbital nerve (Figure 3.11). Pressure on a finger nail bed should not be used as no response would be elicited in a patient with a spinal injury. If this provokes a response, the patient scores "P" for painful stimulus. If a response can still not be elicited, the patient scores "U" for unresponsive.

THE GLASGOW COMA SCORE

The Glasgow Coma Score (GCS) is used to make a more formal assessment of conscious level. It involves three components: the eye opening (E), verbal (V) and motor (M) responses, as outlined in Box 3.3. This assessment is made using the same approach as the AVPU score described above, assessing the stimulus needed for eye opening, the best verbal response to questioning, and the best motor response, if initially unresponsive, to a painful stimulus. If the verbal response is confused speech, this component score is V4, whereas if the patient only manages to groan and make incomprehensible sounds, it is V2. Similarly, when assessing motor response, localizing pain (M5) means reaching towards the site of the stimulus to remove it, whereas withdrawing from painful stimulus (M4) means simply pulling a limb away.

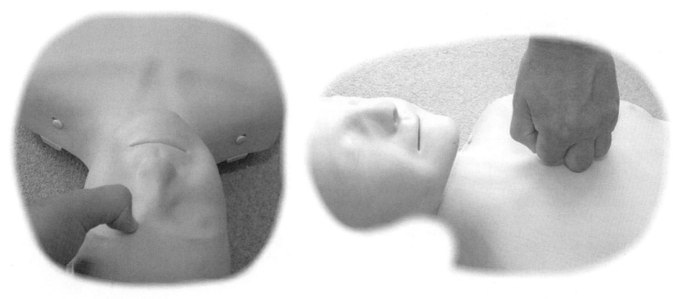

Supra orbital pressure   Sternal pressure

Figure 3.11 Administering a painful stimulus by applying pressure to the supraorbital nerve

---

Box 3.3 The Glasgow Coma Score

Eye opening response

Spontaneous	=	4
To verbal stimuli	=	3
To painful stimuli	=	2
No response	=	1

Best verbal response

Orientated	=	5
Confused	=	4
Inappropriate words	=	3
Incomprehensible sounds	=	2
No response	=	1

Best motor response

Obeys commands	=	6
Localizes pain	=	5
Withdraws from pain	=	4
Abnormal flexion	=	3
Abnormal extension	=	2
No movement	=	1

Abnormal flexion (M3) is flexion of all joints of the upper limbs and would suggest a decorticate posture, whereas abnormal extension (M2) is extension of the upper and lower limbs suggesting even more severe brain injury equating to a decerebrate posture (see Figure 3.12). These two forms of abnormal posturing are suggestive of raised intracranial pressure.

The GCS is scored from 3 (completely unresponsive) to 15 (fully alert and orientated). It was designed as an assessment of conscious level in victims of trauma, but its use is often extended to include medical patients. This is not without pitfalls, as can be demonstrated by a patient who has suffered a stroke and is fully conscious and alert, but is unable to speak, and therefore scores a GCS of only 11. It is thus often necessary to qualify a GCS with a more detailed description of the patient's problems. When handing over information about a GCS, it should always be broken down into its three components, (for example, "a GCS of 8 with E2 V3 M3"), since this conveys much more information about the patient's condition than the total alone.

After an assessment of conscious level, the pupils should be examined (Figure 3.13). The size, symmetry and reaction to light should be assessed so a bright light source is necessary. The pupils should constrict equally to a light stimulus. A unilateral dilated unreactive pupil (Figure 3.14) may be a sign of III cranial nerve damage due to intracranial swelling or haematoma on that side, although this is seldom seen until there is also depression of conscious level. It may also be due to other local factors such as direct trauma to the eye causing a traumatic mydriasis or to previous eye surgery. Bilateral pinpoint pupils may suggest administration of opiates and dilated pupils can be the result of drugs or activation of the sympathetic nervous system.

RAISED INTRACRANIAL PRESSURE (ICP)

When there is a rise in pressure within the closed space of the skull, due to bleeding or swelling, the brain and brainstem are squeezed, forcing the brainstem down towards the foramen magnum, the exit point at the base of the skull. This causes changes in cardiorespiratory parameters due to compression of the cardiac and respiratory centres in the brainstem, known as the Cushing response. This involves progressive bradycardia and hypertension, until eventually the blood pressure falls as a preterminal event. Since this is

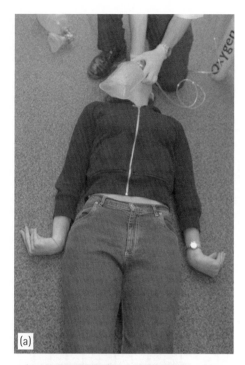

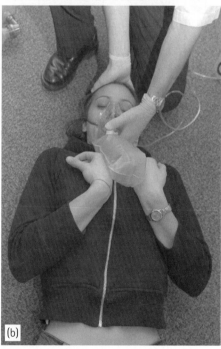

Figure 3.12 Decorticate (a) and decerebrate (b) posturing, suggesting severe brain injury

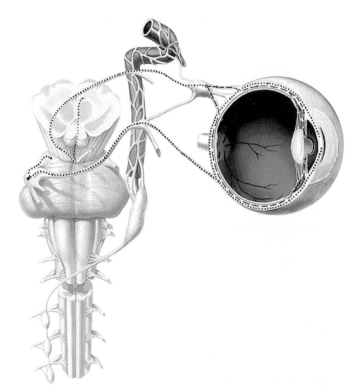

Figure 3.13 The pupillary responses: anatomical pathways

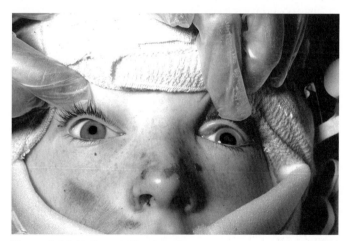

Figure 3.14 Unilateral dilated pupil

a progressive change, it is vitally important that the pulse and blood pressure are recorded regularly in patients with head injury, as this may give a clue to rising ICP (Figure 3.15). There may also be a reduction in conscious level, as the cortical activation systems in the brainstem are compressed, and cranial nerves may be affected, as outlined above with the III cranial nerve palsy causing pupillary dilation.

Finally, a gross assessment of peripheral motor and sensory function can be made by asking the patient to clench his fists and wiggle his toes and whether he can feel you touching his hands and feet. A more detailed examination of sensation is possible by assessing the response to light touch and pinprick sensation. It is important to touch the patient first where there is likely to be normal sensation, such as over the sternum or on the chin. Then the patient can be asked to close his eyes whilst sensation is checked down both sides of the body with either cotton wool or a pin, asking him to say "yes" whenever he feels the touch. In this way a map of normal sensation over the body can be made and should be documented. In the case of stroke, one side of the body may be paralysed, or in the case of spinal injury, there will be loss of sensory and motor function below the level of injury.

Table 3.3 Pupillary responses

Pupils	Common causes
Bilaterally constricted	Opiate overdose
Bilaterally dilated	Drugs, e.g. tricyclics
	Sympathetic response
	Dead
Unilaterally dilated	Raised ICP (see below)
	III cranial nerve palsy
	Traumatic mydriasis

EXPOSURE AND SECONDARY SURVEY

A brief assessment of head, torso and peripheral injuries is desirable at this stage. In cases of trauma, such an examination is the only way to ensure an important injury is not missed. This takes place under E of the primary survey and is confined to the identification of significant serious injuries.

The secondary survey is a detailed examination for *every* injury, however trivial. Usually, it is not appropriate even to begin this phase of the examination before arrival at hospital. The full secondary survey requires exposure of the patient and a detailed head-to-toe examination, including visualization of the tympanic membranes with an auroscope and a rectal examination. This will obviously not be necessary or appropriate in the majority of cases in the prehospital environment. A log roll will also be considered at this stage if appropriate.

EXAMINATION OF THE LIMBS

Each limb should be examined in turn, using the following method.

- Look
- Actively move
- Passively move
- Feel.

The first step is to look at the limb for signs of bruising or swelling. The most useful clue to an injury is an alert patient who can say where it hurts. The patient should then be asked to move the limb, ensuring that each joint is moved. For example, in the upper limb, the patient should be asked to move the arm at the shoulder, then to flex and extend the elbow and wrist, then finally to straighten out the fingers and make a fist. If possible, this should be followed by an examination of the joints being moved passively (in other words, by the examiner). After this, every part of each limb

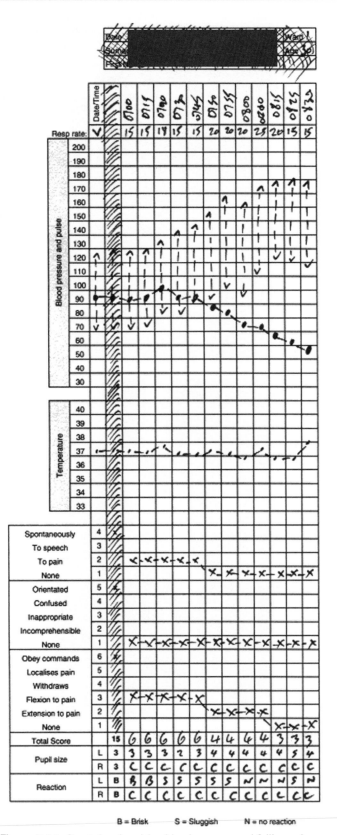

Figure 3.15 Chart showing rising blood pressure and falling pulse

should be palpated for swelling, crepitus, bruising and tenderness, which may indicate a significant injury.

CONCLUSION

Clinical examination remains the most important tool available for diagnosis in the prehospital environment. Like everything else, if a system is used then it is less likely that an important part of the examination will be missed. For ease of demonstration, a method of clinical examination has been described following the ABCDE system of prehospital care.

After this examination, findings should be documented and passed on to the place of definitive care, so any change in condition can be monitored.

Chapter **4**

Emergency services: structures and roles

INTRODUCTION

The emergency services in the United Kingdom consist primarily of the ambulance, police and fire services. In some circumstances other services will be involved in the management of emergencies involving injury and illness: Her Majesty's Coastguard; the voluntary aid societies (British Red Cross, St John and St Andrew Ambulance Associations); mountain and cave rescue teams; and volunteer doctors as part of the British Association for Immediate Care (BASICS). It is appropriate to consider these organizations collectively as the "emergency services".

Box 4.1 The emergency services

- Ambulance services
- Police
- Fire services
- HM Coastguard
- Air-sea rescue and mountain rescue
- Voluntary aid societies (St John and St Andrew Ambulance Associations, British Red Cross)
- Volunteer organizations (for example, British Association for Immediate Care, BASICS)

For the majority of health-related emergencies, the statutory ambulance service is the sole responder. However, it is common for the paramedic to work alongside colleagues from the police and fire services. Cooperation between all the emergency services is necessary to achieve the optimum outcome for patients. It is therefore vital to understand the roles and responsibilities of the members of the other services and organizations.

THE UK AMBULANCE SERVICE

Ambulance services in the United Kingdom were initially provided by local councils and it was only in 1974 that they belatedly became part of the National Health Service. More recently, ambulance services have become NHS trusts led by a board consisting of a chairman with executive directors (such as the chief executive and finance director) and non-executive directors who are appointed by the Department of Health, often from commercial or voluntary backgrounds. An increasing number of ambulance services employ a full- or part-time medical director.

Recent years have seen a rapid growth in the sophistication of the UK ambulance services. The modern ambulance service is divided into the accident and emergency (A&E)

service and a patient transport service. The ambulance service will have a central command and communications centre and may have involvement in other areas of healthcare such as NHS Direct.

PERSONNEL

Emergency ambulance staff are trained to standards produced by the Institute for Healthcare Development (IHCD) for paramedics and technicians. The paramedic syllabus for training has recently been revised, particularly to recognize the need for improvements in training for paediatric and obstetric emergencies. The professional status of paramedics has been recognized by *registration through the Health Professions Council* since September 2000. University education to degree level is increasingly available.

Each local training school for paramedics is required to have a paramedic steering group composed of local clinicians (from hospital and general practice), with additional representatives from pharmacy and nursing. This group oversees the training of paramedics at a local level and takes an advisory role in relation to guidelines for drug administration and treatment procedures.

The Joint Royal Colleges Ambulance Liaison Committee (JRCALC) provides medical advice and produces clinical guidelines at a national level.

DESPATCH

The A&E ambulance service predominantly responds to 999 calls from members of the public. However, a significant proportion of the workload is in response to either the requests of GPs to transport a patient urgently to hospital or requests for urgent interhospital transfer.

Traditionally the response to 999 calls has been in time order, according to the availability of resources. More recently, ambulance services have introduced systems to allow emergency calls to be prioritized on the basis of their urgency. The Advanced Medical Priority Despatch System (AMPDS) is the most commonly used system in the UK. It uses a structured process of interrogation of the caller by the despatcher to categorize patients as to whether their condition is potentially life-threatening, serious but not immediately life-threatening or not immediately life threatening or serious (Figure 4.1).

AMPDS also allows the despatcher to provide prearrival instructions to the caller, including how to provide basic life support for the patient in cardiac arrest prior to arrival of the ambulance. The despatcher therefore takes on a role in the initial assessment and management of a patient.

Most UK ambulance services continue to despatch a "lights and sirens" emergency ambulance to every 999 call irrespective of the priority assigned by the despatch system. With increased central pressure from the government to achieve performance standards, prioritization of calls and

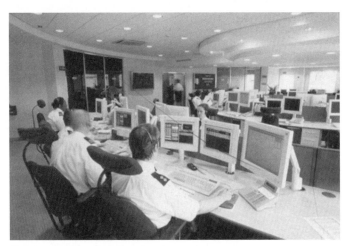

Figure 4.1 Ambulance service despatch centre

the use of alternative means of response to less urgent calls (such as diversion to NHS Direct) may become essential.

VEHICLES AND EQUIPMENT

Most of the UK population live within a relatively short distance of a fully staffed A&E department. Transport by UK ambulance services is therefore predominantly by road to the nearest A&E department. The number of air ambulance services has increased and these are provided predominantly by a combination of corporate sponsorship and charitable fund raising. The evidence of clinical benefit for the use of helicopters in prehospital care is somewhat conflicting, although it would appear to be a logical approach to the rapid transportation of a patient from a rural or remote area.

The equipment and drugs carried by frontline ambulances vary from region to region. All ambulances will carry a monitor-defibrillator and suction apparatus. Most will be equipped with a gas-powered ventilator and a pulse oximeter. The remainder of the equipment is currently poorly standardized.

PERFORMANCE STANDARDS

Historically UK ambulance services have been assessed on their ability to respond to emergency and urgent calls within time limits. New standards recognize that it is appropriate for the most urgent calls to receive the most urgent response. Therefore ambulance trusts are now required to respond to 75% of "category A" (most urgent) emergencies within 8 minutes.

The importance of the ambulance service in the management of coronary heart disease has been recognized in the National Service Framework (NSF), published in 2000. One target is to ensure a defibrillator is at a patient's side within 8 minutes if there are symptoms of a possible acute myocardial infarction. The NSF will also help to achieve the target

Box 4.2 Fire service assistance to the ambulance service

- Rescue of casualties from fire incidents
- Neutralization of hazardous materials – chemicals, radiation
- Release of entrapped casualty (transport and industrial accidents)
- Extrication of patients from inaccessible areas (for example, steep slope rescue)
- Assistance at major incidents (lighting, shelter, personnel for stretcher carry)

of 60 minutes from the time of the first call to the health service to thrombolysis being administered to eligible patients.

THE FIRE AND RESCUE SERVICE

Although the fire service has a primary duty to attend fires, it has developed the skills and knowledge to assist the health services in many functions (Box 4.2).

CLINICAL TRAINING AND EQUIPMENT IN THE FIRE SERVICE

The fire service is required to train its fire-fighters in first aid, including basic life support. Many services have provided further training to include use of medical devices such as a semi-automatic advisory defibrillator, cervical collar and spinal board.

Equipment carried by fire tenders mirrors the training provided to the crews. Oxygen, suction, cervical collars, first aid equipment and a folding stretcher with a winch capability are almost universally available.

COMMAND STRUCTURE

The fire service has a formal system of command. When attending an incident involving the fire service, it is important to identify and speak to the senior officer in order to ensure a coordinated response. The colour and markings on the fire-fighters' helmets identify seniority. Junior ranks wear yellow helmets whilst officers have white helmets. The helmets of anyone above the grade of fire-fighter will also be marked with black bands of varying number and thickness. The greater the number and width of the bands, the greater the seniority. The rank markings of the fire service are shown in Figure 4.2.

ENTRAPMENTS

Most entrapments occur as a result of road traffic accidents (Figure 4.3). However, other transport accidents, industrial and agricultural incidents and incidents involving collapse

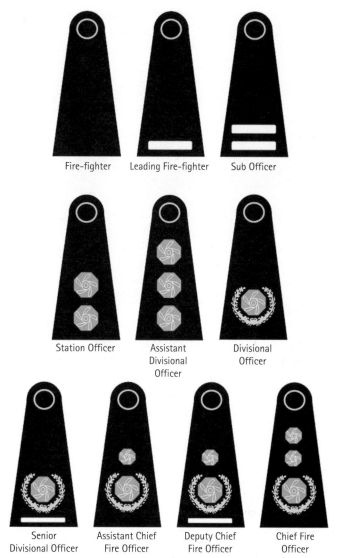

Figure 4.2 Fire service rank markings

of buildings may equally lead to entrapment of an injured patient. For the purposes of this chapter, the role of the fire service will be discussed in relation to entrapment following a road traffic accident.

The successful and orderly management of an entrapment can be divided into six phases commonly used by senior fire officers.

- Assessment and making the scene safe
- Stabilization and initial access
- Glass management
- Space creation
- Access
- Extrication.

An initial assessment of the scene is made on arrival to ensure safety for the patient and any personnel involved in the rescue. Hazards immediately related to the vehicle may include leaking fuel whilst the fire service will also take measures to control other hazards such as traffic passing

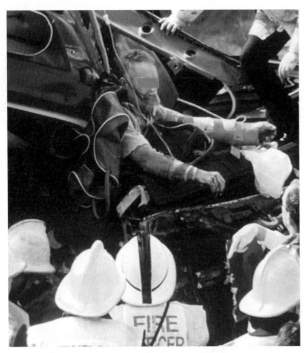

Figure 4.3 Entrapment following a road traffic accident

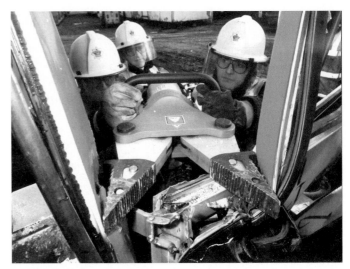

Figure 4.4 "Jaws of life"

close to the incident. On arriving at the scene of an accident, the paramedic should contact the Senior Fire Officer in order to determine whether it is safe to approach the patient.

Method of extrication

The method of extrication will be determined by the clinical urgency of the patient's condition. It is therefore vital for the paramedic to liaise closely with the Senior Fire Officer and to develop a plan for extrication once an initial assessment has been completed. On occasions, due to the urgency of the clinical situation or the risk to the patient from the environment, it may be necessary to remove the patient rapidly, omitting some of the stages that follow here.

The vehicle is stabilized with chocks to prevent further movement and ambulance service personnel will usually then enter the vehicle to assess the patient and initiate spinal immobilization. At an early stage glass is removed to improve access and remove a potential source of further injury to the patient and carers. The fire service may then start to create space around the patient to improve access for assessment and treatment prior to extrication. Fire tenders now carry a vast array of powerful hydraulic tools that can effectively dismantle a vehicle around a casualty in a matter of minutes (Figure 4.4). However, the speed of work may need to be slowed in order to protect the patient.

Finally the patient is extricated from the vehicle ensuring adequate spinal immobilization. Most fire-fighters are trained in the use of spinal boards and a coordinated effort managed by the paramedic but involving both fire and ambulance staff should ensure the spinal cord is not placed at risk.

INCIDENTS INVOLVING CHEMICAL OR RADIOACTIVE CONTAMINATION

The main principle governing the management of incidents involving hazardous material (chemical, radioactive material) is containment of the contamination to avoid exposure of the rescuers and the wider population.

The police will generally establish an outer cordon from which everyone except emergency service personnel is excluded. The contamination will be contained within the inner cordon, which is controlled by the fire service. Emergency services operating between the two cordons will not require the specialist personal protective equipment that is essential inside the inner cordon. Again, it is important for ambulance service staff to establish early liaison with the Senior Fire Officer to determine the nature of the hazard and the involvement of any casualties. It is a responsibility of the ambulance service to provide adequate decontamination facilities for patients. Reliance has previously been placed on improvised procedures by the fire service, but high-volume, high-pressure, cold and dirty water is inappropriate for decontaminating the injured.

MAJOR INCIDENTS

The role of any of the emergency services at a major incident will depend on the nature of the incident and all services must be prepared to act flexibly to deal with the challenges that a major incident presents. The primary objectives of the fire and rescue service at a major incident are shown in Box 4.3. In general the fire and rescue service will be able to supply a large volume of men and equipment early in the evolution of a major incident. The training of the fire-fighters in first aid may therefore come in useful when the number of casualties outnumbers the ambulance personnel present.

The emergency services will generally adopt a rigid command structure at a major incident. The Gold Commander is

Box 4.3 Objectives of the fire and rescue service at a major incident

- Saving life
- Prevention of escalation of the incident (control fires, contain chemicals)
- Protection of rescuers nd casualties
- Extrication of casualties, including first aid where necessary, and assistance with movement of injured to the casualty clearing station
- Control of access and egress from the inner cordon where hazards are existent
- Assistance in investigating the cause of the incident

Box 4.4 The generic police command hierarchy

- Chief Constable
- Assistant Chief Constable
- Superintendent
- Chief Inspector
- Inspector
- Sergeant
- Constable

usually located away from the incident and maintains a strategic oversight of the incident. The Silver Commander is on-site and delegates specific tasks to the Bronze (or sector) Commanders who are each responsible for a defined area of the incident.

THE POLICE

The primary duty of the police is to uphold the law and to bring justice to those who break it. The police will be involved jointly with the ambulance service in incidents where a crime has been committed such as an assault, a road traffic accident and a major incident (see below).

COMMAND STRUCTURE

A generic hierarchy of the police command structure is shown in Box 4.4 (this may differ slightly within the Metropolitan Police and within specialist police services including British Transport Police and Parks Police). Each police force covers a geographical area comprising several operational divisions. There are also specialized areas of policing such as traffic, firearms teams and air support.

Police service rank markings are shown in Figure 4.5.

AT A ROAD TRAFFIC ACCIDENT

The enforcement of road law is possibly the most effective intervention in preventing injury and death from road traffic

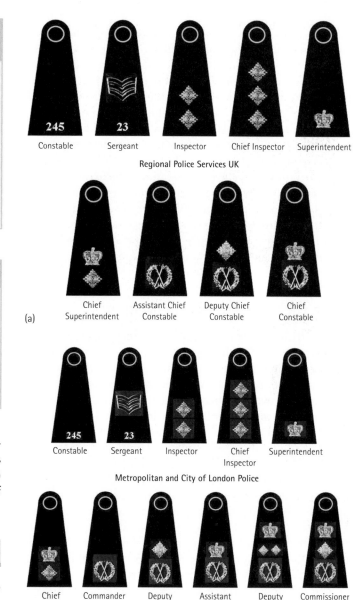

Regional Police Services UK

(a)

Metropolitan and City of London Police

(b)

Figure 4.5 Police service rank markings: (a) Regional police services UK; (b) Metropolitan and city of London police

accidents. The deterrent effect of the strict application of drink driving law and speed limits undoubtedly will save more lives than the most sophisti cated medical trauma system.

The primary duty of the police at the scene of a road accident is the preservation of life. Though seeking to preserve evidence at the accident site, they will not interfere with the process of treatment and evacuation of a patient. In the enforcement of drink driving law, the police will seek to measure the breath alcohol level of anyone they suspect of being a driver involved in an accident. It is an offence to refuse to provide a breath specimen.

In some areas of the UK police officers are being trained to respond to cardiac arrests as first responders tasked by the local ambulance service.

THE CRIME SCENE

At a crime scene, the police will be primarily concerned with the preservation of evidence where an offence may have been committed. The treatment and evacuation of patients from the scene of an incident will inevitably risk disturbing forensic evidence but the preservation of life is the first priority. It is also in the interests of all law-abiding members of the public to ensure that a crime scene is disturbed as little as possible. Ambulance service staff should therefore be aware of the police requirements to preserve evidence and avoid unnecessary contamination of a crime scene.

It is not uncommon for ambulance service staff subsequently to be asked to provide a witness statement as a professional witness. In this capacity a statement of the facts in relation to the incident is required. "Expert" interpretation of the facts is generally not required.

THE POLICE ROLE AT MAJOR INCIDENTS

The overriding duty of the police at a major incident is the preservation of life. Although they do not take a role in the treatment of injuries they play a major role in and are responsible for the effective coordination of the other emergency services. However, any major incident will require investigation and may subsequently result in criminal prosecution. The police will therefore also aim to protect evidence at the incident site to allow subsequent examination by scene of crime officers or by other specialized agencies such as the Air Accident Investigation Branch. In the United Kingdom the police have the role of coordinating the efforts of all the agencies involved (this is a fire service role in some other European countries). A group of senior officers is established that includes the Fire and Ambulance Incident Officers and representatives from the local authority and other agencies relevant to the specific incident.

The police will protect the scene of an incident by controlling access through an outer cordon. This prevents the access of unauthorized personnel who might not only place themselves in danger but also hinder the work of the other emergency services and destroy potentially valuable forensic evidence (it is not unknown for members of the public to visit the site of an incident to acquire "souvenirs" or even to steal personal effects from the deceased).

The police are responsible for the identification of the victims of the incident and for informing the relatives. Specifically the police are responsible for removing the bodies of fatalities to mortuary facilities and for collecting any evidence, which may subsequently aid in identification.

HM COASTGUARD

HM Coastguard is accessible through the 999 operator and should genuinely be regarded as the fourth emergency service. In incidents in coastal waters they will have primacy over other services and will take the traditional coordinator role that the police assume on land. Large multi-agency incidents will commonly be coordinated from the regional coastguard headquarters. Primacy is handed back to the police when on land.

VOLUNTARY AID SOCIETIES

The voluntary aid societies (VAS) (British Red Cross, St John and St Andrew Ambulance Associations) commonly provide medical care at mass gathering events (for example, football stadia and concerts). Their principal capability is to provide first aid but the societies will also deploy volunteer nurses, doctors and off-duty ambulance personnel to augment the emergency capability.

In the context of a major incident all voluntary aid society members will be responsible to the Ambulance Incident Officer from the statutory ambulance service, who will determine how VAS staff and VAS emergency ambulances are utilized.

BASICS

The British Association for Immediate Care (BASICS) consists of volunteer doctors (often but not exclusively general practitioners) functioning independently or in organized schemes to support their local ambulance service. There is no statutory role for this organization, although some ambulance services rely heavily on these volunteers to assist in the management of difficult cases at the roadside or in the home and in some circumstances (often in the more remote areas) to act as a first responder to a 999 call when ambulance resources are not immediately available.

BASICS doctors will invariably carry their own personal, medical and communication equipment. A raft of training and assessment programmes are now available to prepare them to practise in a hostile environment, culminating in the Diploma and Fellowship examinations in Immediate Medical Care of the Royal College of Surgeons of Edinburgh (RCSEd). The Faculty of Prehospital Care of the RCSEd is instrumental in setting national standards and promoting best medical practice in prehospital care for doctors and indeed for all professionals in this specialist field.

FURTHER READING

Greaves I, Porter K (eds) 1999 Pre-hospital medicine. Arnold, London

Hodgetts T, Mackway-Jones K (eds) 2002 Major incident medical management and support. BMJ Books, London

Section 2

RESUSCITATION SKILLS

Chapter 5

Basic life support

Cardiopulmonary resuscitation is not new. In the 16th century, Versalius reported how he had blown air into a patient via a reed, to try to revive the heart. In the 18th century, mouth-to-mouth breathing was described and by the 19th century descriptions of ventilation included chest compression and the arm lift method. It was not until the 1950s that expired air ventilation was proved to be both physiologically sound and superior to other mechanical methods.

Closed chest cardiac compression was first reported in 1878, but this was rapidly abandoned in favour of direct compression of the heart, usually via the abdominal route. By the 1950s, "open cardiac massage" was most commonly achieved via a thoracotomy, but this was abandoned following the rediscovery and development of "closed cardiac massage" by Kowenhoven and colleagues in 1960.

By 1961, expired air ventilation and closed chest cardiac compression were combined and Safar described the feasibility of teaching the public cardiopulmonary resuscitation (CPR), without the use of any equipment or surgical skills. The 1960s therefore can be regarded as the starting point of modern cardiopulmonary resuscitation.

WHAT IS BASIC LIFE SUPPORT?

Collapsed patients may require assistance to maintain their airway, breathing and circulation in order to prevent

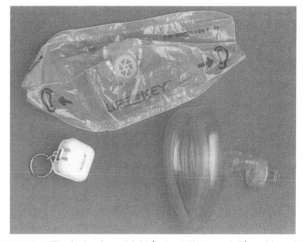

Figure 5.1 The Ambu face shield (top and bottom left) and Laerdal pocket mask (bottom right)

deterioration in their condition. When this is achieved without the use of equipment it is termed *basic life support* (BLS). When a simple protective shield is interposed between the mouth of the rescuer and patient, for example Ambu face shield, Laerdal pocket mask (Figure 5.1), the description "BLS with adjunct" is often used.

A patient's best chance of survival occurs when the collapse is witnessed and basic life support techniques are started immediately, as the brain is irreversibly damaged within 3–4 minutes of being deprived of oxygen. Therefore, BLS must be started in all patients who have collapsed suddenly, who are unresponsive and who are not breathing or have no major pulse palpable (or both).

During working hours paramedical staff will have access to a variety of equipment, in particular a defibrillator which they have been trained to use. The Resuscitation Council (UK) has therefore produced an "enhanced sequence of BLS" to be used under these circumstances to maximize the patient's chance of survival. However, it is important that the conventional sequence of BLS is understood in order that it can be taught to laypersons and for use on those occasions when you are confronted with a victim of cardiac arrest out-side the working environment!

THE SEQUENCE OF BLS FOR LAYPERSONS

In order that the rescuer suffers no harm and BLS is carried out effectively and in the most efficient manner, the following sequence of actions should be performed.

- *Safety check*: to avoid danger to the rescuer and patient
- *Evaluation*: to identify whether the patient has any spontaneous ventilation or a palpable pulse
- *Airway control*: to obtain and maintain a patent airway
- *Ventilatory support*: to establish artificial ventilation using expired air
- *Circulatory support*: to establish an artificial circulation by external cardiac compression.

THE SAFE APPROACH

On discovering or being asked to attend to a collapsed patient, the first response must be to *shout* for help. Basic life support techniques are physically demanding and are more effective if performed by two rescuers. Furthermore, the arrival of help will allow the performance of other simple tasks.

People collapse anywhere, at any time and from many different causes. Rescuers should therefore *approach* a collapsed person with care, never putting themselves (or others) at risk. This is clearly important when the collapse occurs outside a hospital environment, where there may be gas, toxic fumes, traffic, electricity or fire endangering the rescuer.

If it is perceived that there are risks either to the victim or rescuer, then the patient must be moved to a place of greater safety which is *free from danger* before starting resuscitation.

Finally, the rescuer must *evaluate* the patient's ABC (airway, breathing and circulation). Not all collapsed patients will need artificial ventilation and external cardiac compressions.

In summary:

S	>	Shout for help
A	>	Approach with care
F	>	Free from danger
E	>	Evaluate the ABC

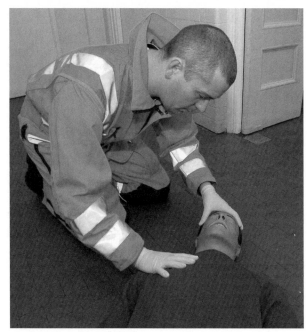

Figure 5.2 "Are you all right?"

PATIENT EVALUATION

The first step is to see if the patient is responsive. This is achieved by placing one hand on the patient's forehead and shaking the shoulder gently with the other hand. At the same time the rescuer asks loudly, "Are you all right?" (Figure 5.2). One of two things may now happen and will determine further action.

The patient responds by either talking or moving

If it is safe to do so, leave the patient in the position in which he or she was found and summon medical assistance or prepare for transfer. However, remember that the patient may deteriorate before help arrives, so regular reassessment is mandatory.

- The head is held stable during the assessment to guard against the possibility of aggravating an injury to the cervical spine
- Always remember that the patient may be deaf, therefore ensure he or she can see your lips moving when assessing responsiveness
- In the responsive patient, where there is obvious trauma, immobilize the cervical spine by manual in–line stabilization (Figure 5.3)

There is no response to voice or touch

If no assistance has arrived, shout for help again. Then evaluate the state of the patient's airway, breathing and circulation.

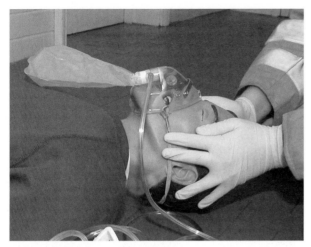

Figure 5.3 In-line cervical stabilization

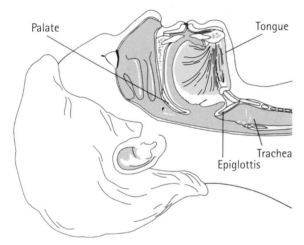

Figure 5.4 Vertical section through the airway

Palate

Tongue

Trachea

Epiglottis

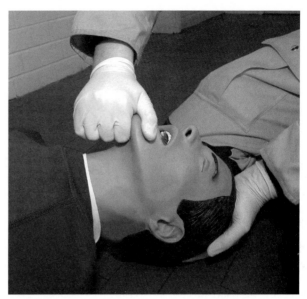

Figure 5.5 Head tilt, chin lift

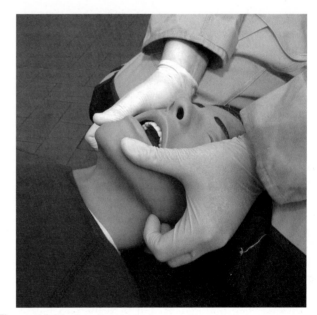

Figure 5.6 The jaw thrust

AIRWAY CONTROL

In most unconscious patients the airway will become obstructed at the level of the hypopharynx. The reduced tone in the muscles of the tongue, jaw and neck allow the tongue to fall against the posterior pharyngeal wall (Figure 5.4). The following manoeuvres are designed to achieve a clear airway.

Head tilt plus chin lift

The rescuer's hand nearest the head is placed on the forehead, gently tilting (extending) the head backwards. The chin is then lifted using the index and middle finger of the rescuer's other hand (Figure 5.5). If this causes the mouth to close, the lower lip should be retracted downwards by the thumb. This is the "triple airway manoeuvre" – head tilt, chin lift, mouth open.

Jaw thrust

If the above technique fails to open the airway or there is a suspicion that the cervical spine may have been injured,

then the jaw thrust alone is used. The patient's jaw is thrust upwards (forwards) by applying pressure behind the angles of the mandible. The rescuer uses the fingertips, with the base of the thumbs resting on the patient's cheeks (Figure 5.6).

Finger sweep

If there is any evidence that foreign material may be contributing to airway obstruction, the mouth must be opened and inspected. Obvious material may be removed by placing a finger in the mouth and gently sweeping from side to side, hooking out loose material (Figure 5.7). At the same time, broken, loose or partial dentures should be removed, but

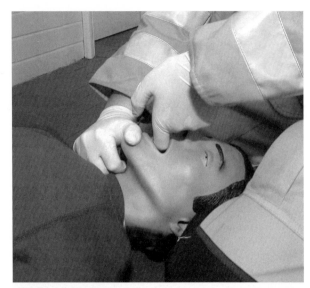

Figure 5.7 The finger sweep

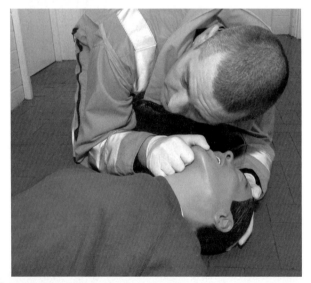

Figure 5.8 Look, listen, feel

well-fitting dentures may be left in place (see below). A blind finger sweep is not recommended, as this may further impact a foreign body.

BREATHING

Whilst keeping the airway patent using one of the above techniques, the patient's breathing must now be rapidly evaluated in the following manner.

- *Look* down the line of the chest to see if it is rising and falling.
- *Listen* at the mouth and nose for breath sounds, gurgling or snoring sounds.
- *Feel* for expired air at the patient's mouth and nose with the side of your cheek.

Look, listen and feel for no longer than 10 seconds before deciding whether breathing is absent (Figure 5.8).

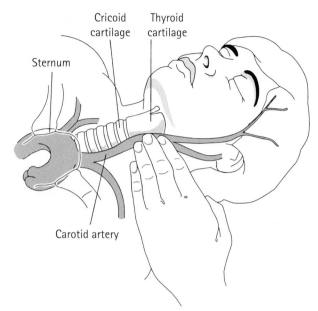

Figure 5.9 Feeling for the carotid pulse

The patient is breathing

Place the patient in the recovery position (see later) unless it is unsafe to do so because of other injuries (e.g. to the cervical spine). Check regularly for breathing. The majority of these patients will require urgent hospital transfer. It is essential at this point that either someone is sent to summon such help or, if you are alone, you must leave the patient and go for help.

The patient is not breathing

Help must be sought immediately, either by sending someone else or going yourself, even if this means temporarily leaving the patient. On return, give two breaths of expired air (see below). If difficulty is encountered achieving this, make up to five attempts to achieve two effective breaths. Once this has been achieved, assess the circulation.

CIRCULATION

A check must now be made for evidence of the patient's circulation by looking for any movement, including breathing (more than just an occasional gasp) or swallowing. This should take no more than 10 seconds.

At this point it is appropriate for a healthcare professional to utilize their knowledge and skills and perform a pulse check. In an emergency, central arteries are more reliable and the carotid artery is usually the most accessible and acceptable. The carotid arteries are found on either side of the neck in the "gutter" between the larynx and sternomastoid muscles (Figure 5.9). An alternative, but less socially acceptable, is the femoral artery in the groin. Again, take no more than 10 seconds to make the assessment.

The patient is not breathing but does have a pulse

If a pulse is present, continue with ventilation, 10–12 per minute, reassessing the circulation approximately every minute. If the signs of a circulation or the pulse disappear, chest compressions must be started (see below).

The patient is not breathing and has no signs of a circulation

This is often referred to as a "cardiac arrest" and requires CPR to be commenced immediately. CPR consists of expired air ventilation plus external cardiac compressions – see below.

The only exceptions to this sequence of events are cases of trauma, drowning or infants and children, when a single rescuer should perform resuscitation for one minute before going for help.

TECHNIQUES OF EXPIRED AIR VENTILATION

To successfully ventilate a patient with expired air there must be a clear path, with no leaks, between the rescuer's lungs and the patient's lungs.

MOUTH-TO-MOUTH VENTILATION

1. The patient's airway is kept patent by the rescuer using the palm of the uppermost hand to perform a head tilt, leaving the index finger and thumb free to pinch the patient's nose to prevent leaks. The fingers of the lower hand are then used to perform a chin lift and if necessary, the thumb is used to open the mouth.
2. The rescuer takes a deep breath in and makes a seal with his or her lips around the patient's mouth. Well-fitting dentures should be left in the patient's mouth as they help maintain the contour of the mouth and make it easier to create a good seal. Poorly fitting false teeth or dental plates should be removed, as they may obstruct the airway.
3. The rescuer blows gently into the patient's mouth for 2 seconds, at the same time listening for leaks and looking down the patient's chest to ensure that it rises (Figure 5.10a).
4. While maintaining the head tilt and chin lift, the rescuer moves away from the patient's mouth to allow passive exhalation for 2 seconds, watching to make sure the chest falls (Figure 5.10b).

MOUTH-TO-NOSE VENTILATION

Mouth-to-nose ventilation is used where mouth-to-mouth ventilation is unsuccessful, for example if an obstruction in the mouth cannot be relieved or when the rescuer is a child (child's mouth would not completely cover adult's mouth). The airway is maintained as already described but the mouth is closed with the fingers of the lower hand. The seal is made with the rescuer's lips around the base of the patient's nose. Inflation is as above, checking to ensure that the chest rises. The mouth is opened to assist expiration, with the rescuer watching to ensure that the chest falls.

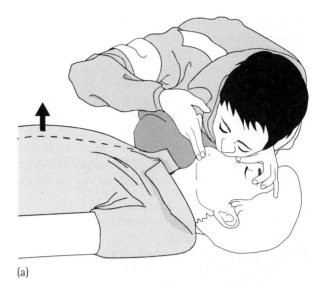

(a)

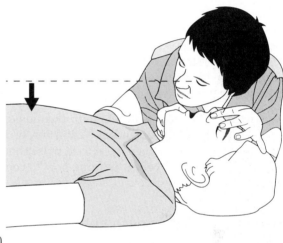

(b)

Figure 5.10 (a, b) Mouth-to-mouth (expired air) ventilation

Box 5.1 Common causes of inadequate ventilation

- *Obstruction* – failing to maintain head tilt or chin lift
- *Leaks* – inadequate seal around the mouth or failure to occlude the patient's nose
- *Inflating too hard* – trying to overcome an obstructed airway, resulting in gastric distension and regurgitation
- *Foreign body* – unrecognized in the patient's airway

Each complete cycle of expired air ventilation should take approximately 4 seconds, thereby allowing 15 breaths per minute.

TECHNIQUE OF CARDIOPULMONARY RESUSCITATION

A patient who is not breathing and has no pulse should be placed in the supine position on a firm surface and CPR commenced. As described above, two expired air ventilations are given and these are followed immediately by 15 external cardiac compressions (see below). This cycle (15 compressions : 2 breaths) is performed continuously, each time remembering to tilt the head and lift the chin to create a patent airway and checking the correct position of the hands before commencing chest compressions.

If two or more laypersons are present, then they should take turns to perform single-person CPR using the 15:2 ratio. However, if two or more healthcare professionals are present, two-person CPR is preferred using the following technique.

- A ratio of 15 compressions : 2 breaths is used.
- Rescuers should work from opposite sides of the victim to facilitate change of tasks.
- Two rescue breaths must be performed immediately after the 15th compression, with compressions recommencing immediately after the second inflation without waiting for passive expiration.
- A patent airway must be maintained at all times.
- The person performing external cardiac compressions can leave the hands on the sternum between each series of compressions, but in doing so the pressure must be *totally* released so as not to interfere with the efficacy of ventilation.

Once started, CPR must not be interrupted unless the patient shows signs of spontaneous ventilation or movement. If this does happen, then the carotid pulse should be reassessed for 5 seconds before deciding how to continue. However, such an occurrence is *extremely rare*.

EXTERNAL CARDIAC (CLOSED CHEST) COMPRESSION

The exact mechanism by which external cardiac compression results in blood flow is unclear. It is probably a combination of direct compression of the heart between the sternum and the spine, along with a sudden rise in the intrathoracic pressure during compression generating forward flow in the arteries. Whatever the mechanisms, at its best it can achieve a maximum flow 30% of normal. The position of the hands is critical for maximal effect.

1. The rescuer takes up a position on one side of the patient.
2. The patient's chest is exposed and the xiphisternum identified (this is the bony prominence in the midline at the junction of the lower borders of the ribs).
3. The index and middle fingers of the rescuer's lower hand are placed on the xiphisternum and without removing them, the heel of the other hand is placed adjacent to the index finger on the sternum (Figure 5.11).
4. The lower hand is removed and placed on the back of the hand resting on the sternum, interlocking the fingers.
5. The sternum is alternately depressed 4–5 cm and released. This is repeated at a rate of 100 per minute, with compression and relaxation each taking the same length of time.
6. External cardiac compressions are best performed with the rescuer leaning well forward over the patient, with straight

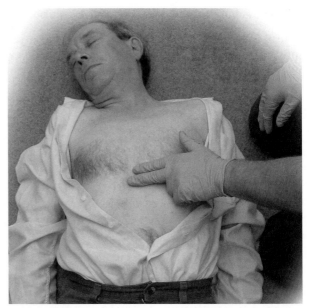

Figure 5.11 Correct hand position for external cardiac compression (above the two fingers)

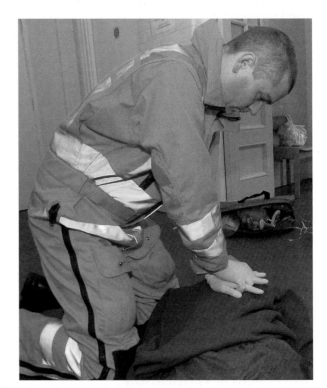

Figure 5.12 External cardiac compression

arms. This allows the rescuer to use upper body weight to achieve compression rather than using the arm muscles, which will tire rapidly and reduce efficiency (Figure 5.12).

TRANSMISSION OF DISEASE DURING RESUSCITATION

Recently there has been increasing concern over the possible transmission of infection, particularly HIV, during mouth-to-mouth ventilation. Although there have been instances of transmission of infection, most have been bacterial rather than viral. The greatest risk of transmission of HIV or hepatitis B and C viruses is via blood contamination, as a result of accidental injury with a needle. Following a documented case of transmission of tuberculosis during resuscitation, when mouth-to-mouth ventilation is performed on a victim known to be or suspected of suffering from tuberculosis, the rescuer should subsequently undergo appropriate screening for the disease.

As a result of concerns about the above or if for any reason there is a reluctance to perform expired air ventilation in a patient who has collapsed and is apnoeic and pulseless, then chest compressions alone should be performed, preferably while a second person maintains a patent airway. Chest compressions alone are superior to no BLS at all.

Basic life support procedures are summarized in Figure 5.13.

PARAMEDIC BLS

A paramedic crew responding to a collapsed person will have additional training, skills and equipment immediately available, which should be used to maximize the patient's chances of being successfully resuscitated. In recognition of this situation, modifications should be made to the above sequence of BLS. The following are based on the recommendations of the Resuscitation Council (UK) for in-hospital BLS.

Box 5.2 Common causes of ineffective external chest compressions

- Wrong hand position
  - Too high – the heart is not compressed
  - Too low – the stomach is compressed and the risk of aspiration increased
  - Too far laterally – will injure underlying organs
- Overenthusiastic effort
  - Causes cardiac damage
  - Fractures ribs, causing damage to underlying organs, particularly lungs and liver
- Inadequate effort
  - The rescuer is not high enough above the patient to use his or her body weight
  - Fatigue during prolonged resuscitation or poor technique
- Failure to release between compressions
  - Prevents venous return and filling of the heart
- Inadequate or excessive rate

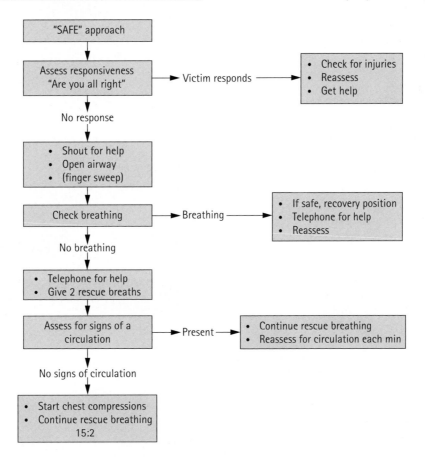

Note:
- Get help immediately if more than one rescuer
- Perform CPR for 1 min before getting help if arrest due to trauma, drowning, drugs or victim is an infant or child.

Figure 5.13 Summary of layperson basic life support procedures

As there will generally be more than one trained person present, it will be possible for a paramedic crew to undertake actions simultaneously.

- Having established that the victim is unresponsive, one person should check for breathing, at the same time assessing for signs of a circulation and feeling for a carotid pulse.
- The second person should rapidly collect the appropriate resuscitation equipment, including a defibrillator.
- Having confirmed the diagnosis of cardiac arrest, the defibrillator electrodes should be applied as quickly as possible.

- At the same time ventilation should commence using a bag–valve–mask with supplemental oxygen rather than expired air ventilation.
- If indicated, a shock must be administered, either manually or via an automated external defibrillator (AED).
- If there is any delay or a shock is not indicated, chest compressions and ventilations in a ratio of 15:2 should commence.

> Attempts at defibrillation must not be delayed while BLS is performed

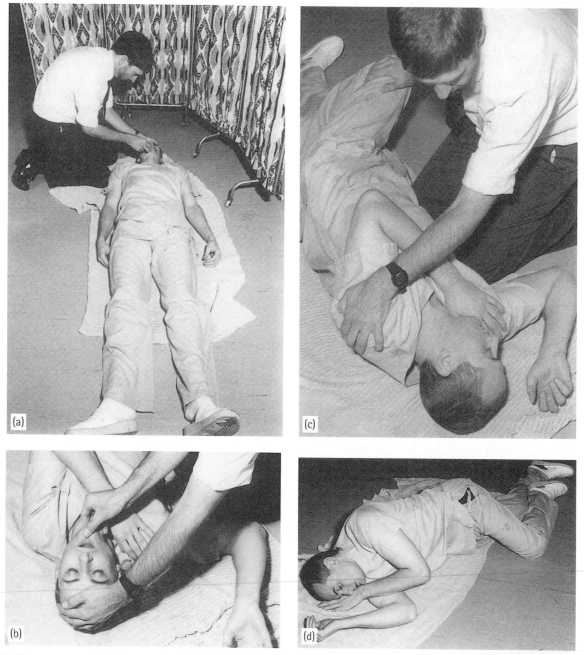

Figure 5.14 The recovery position

THE RECOVERY POSITION

In the unconscious patient who is breathing and has a pulse, the airway is best maintained and the risk of aspiration of gastric contents minimized by placing the patient in the *recovery position*. There is more than one method that a single rescuer can use. The following is an adaptation of the method supported by the European Resuscitation Council.

1. Place the patient supine, with legs extended, and ensure the airway is open (head tilt, chin lift) (Figure 5.14a).
2. Kneeling against the patient's chest, move the patient's closest arm away from the body so that it lies at 90°, then flex the elbow to 90° so that the palm lies facing upwards.
3. Bring the patient's far arm to lie across the chest, so that the back of the hand lies against the cheek (Figure 5.14b).
4. Flex the far leg at the hip and knee, keeping the foot on the ground. Grasp the far shoulder.
5. Roll the patient by pulling the shoulders towards you, while using the bent leg as a lever – this is achieved by gently pulling the flexed knee towards you and pressing down (Figure 5.14c).
6. Adjust the upper leg so that both the hip and the knee are flexed to 90°. Adjust the hand under the cheek to help maintain the head tilt (Figure 5.14d).
7. Finally, the airway, breathing and pulse are checked regularly.

In the recovery position, gravity helps keep the tongue away from the posterior pharyngeal wall, thereby preventing airway obstruction while at the same time allowing any vomit or secretions to drain out of the patient's mouth.

If there is *any* suspicion of a spinal injury, then the log roll is the preferred method of positioning the patient on their side. However, if there is insufficient manpower to do this, these patients may have to be turned into the recovery position. The airway takes precedence over C-spine.

THE CHOKING PATIENT

Although almost any foreign body can cause airway obstruction, in adults it is usually food, as a result of trying to eat, talk and breathe simultaneously. This has been misleadingly termed the "*café coronary*". In these circumstances adults show signs of acute airway obstruction, with extreme distress and activity to try to dislodge an obstruction. If the obstruction is incomplete, there may be severe coughing and inspiratory stridor.

If the patient is still conscious and unable to cough, then back blows should be used initially. Standing to one side of the patient, the rescuer should encourage the patient to lean forwards. While supporting the chest with one hand, five firm blows are delivered between the scapulae. If the obstruction is relieved quickly, all five blows need not be delivered.

> If this fails then proceed rapidly to the abdominal thrusts

ABDOMINAL THRUSTS

These can be performed with the patient standing, sitting or kneeling down. The aim is to produce a rapid rise in the intrathoracic pressure (by forcing the diaphragm into the chest) which will expel the foreign body.

If the patient is standing, the rescuer should move behind the patient and pass both arms around the body at the level of the upper abdomen. The rescuer makes one hand into a fist and places it firmly in the patient's epigastrium. The rescuer's other hand is then placed over the fist and both together forced vigorously upwards and backwards into the epigastrium (Figure 5.15); this should be repeated up to five times. With luck this will force the object into a position where the patient can remove it by coughing or it can be hooked out with a finger. If this fails to dislodge the foreign body, the sequence of five back blows and five abdominal thrusts should be repeated until the patient recovers or becomes unconscious. When the patient is unconscious, he or she should be placed supine. Tilt the head back and remove any visible obstruction. Perform a chin lift and check for breathing: if absent try to deliver two effective rescue breaths in up to five attempts. If breaths cannot be delivered,

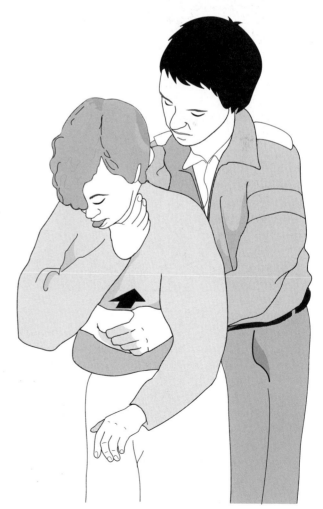

Figure 5.15 Abdominal thrusts

give 15 chest compressions (regardless of circulatory status). Next check the mouth for visible obstructions and check for breathing. If absent, repeat this cycle.

If this fails to remove the obstruction as soon as ALS equipment is available perform a laryngoscopy and visualise the object. If it is possible to do so without risk of worsening the obstruction, remove the object using Magill's forceps. If this proves impossible a cricothyroidotomy should be performed without further delay and the patient transferred urgently to hospital.

FURTHER READING

Baskett PJF, Bossaert L, Carli P, et al 1996 Guidelines for the basic management of the airway and ventilation during resuscitation. A statement by the Airway and Ventilation Management Working Group of the European Resuscitation Council. Resuscitation 31: 187–200

Driscoll PA, Gwinnutt CL, Mackway-Jones K eds 2000 Advanced cardiac life support – the practical approach, 3rd edn. Arnold, London

Handley AJ, Becker LB, Allen M, van Drenth A, Montgomery WH 1997 Single rescuer adult basic life support. An advisory statement by the Basic Life Support Working Group of the International Liaison Committee on Resuscitation. Resuscitation 34: 101–107

Chapter 6

Basic management of the airway and ventilation

INTRODUCTION

The airway is the first priority during resuscitation and airway management skills are essential for those involved in emergency care. In the presence of airway obstruction, hypoxia leading to circulatory arrest and irreversible central nervous system damage can be expected to occur within 3–4 minutes. Basic airway management requires relatively simple skills, but emergency conditions are often difficult and add to the stress of the situation. Advanced airway management demands much more skill and experience. To be effective, airway management requires an understanding of functional airway anatomy and physiology and the possession of skills which allow one to assess and intervene rapidly.

The basic skills of maintaining an open airway are vitally important and should be mastered before embarking upon advanced airway management techniques.

ANATOMY OF THE RESPIRATORY SYSTEM

The anatomy of the respiratory tract is illustrated in Figures 6.1–6.3.

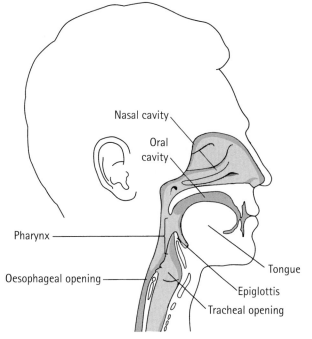

Figure 6.1 The upper airway

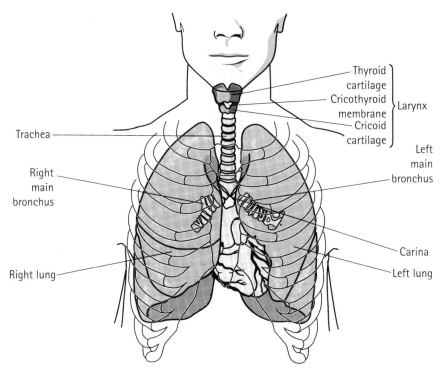

Figure 6.2 The lower airway

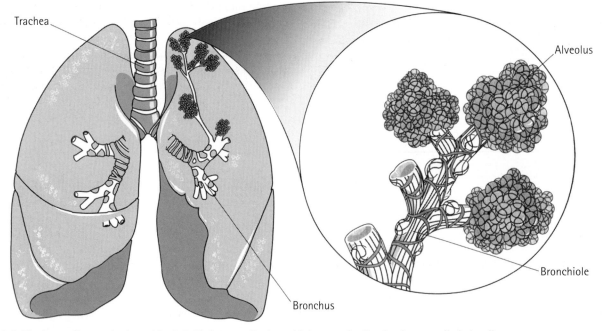

Figure 6.3 The lower airway: the bronchi subdivide into smaller bronchioles, terminating in air sacs called alveoli

THE UPPER AIRWAY

The upper airway extends from the mouth and nose to just below the larynx (Figure 6.1).

The nose

The nasal cavity extends from the nostrils to the nasopharynx. The roof of the nasal cavity contains the receptors for the sense of smell and lies below the anterior aspect of the base of the skull, which is quite thin. Thus, nasal tubes inserted when the base of the skull is fractured may enter the cranial cavity.

The floor of the nasal cavity is formed from the hard and soft palates. Inside, the nose is lined with a thick, vascular mucous membrane. The conchae (or turbinates) project into the nasal cavity from the side and may be damaged during nasal intubation, causing haemorrhage. The paranasal sinuses open into the nasal cavity below the conchae. The naso-lacrimal duct and the eustachian tube also drain into the nasal cavity.

The nasal cavity is divided by the nasal septum, which in older children and adults is often deviated to one side, making one nostril narrower than the other. The main nasal air passage lies in the floor of the nasal cavity; correctly placed nasal tubes will be directed backwards along the upper aspect of the palate. The nasal cavity continues as the nasopharynx, starting above and behind the soft palate. Above the nasopharynx lies the base of the skull and behind it the first cervical vertebra. The lateral walls are made up of the superior constrictor muscle and the pharyngobasilar membrane.

The nasal blood supply is from the ophthalmic, maxillary and facial arteries. Most nose bleeds arise from the front lower part of the nasal septum which receives a blood supply from branches of the maxillary and facial arteries. The nerve supply of the nasal cavity originates from the olfactory nerve which supplies the smell receptors and from branches of the trigeminal nerve which supply sensation.

At the back of the nasopharynx there is a collection of lymphoid tissue, the adenoid or nasopharyngeal tonsil. In children, adenoids may enlarge and obstruct the airway and the eustachian tube. Enlarged adenoids are likely to bleed if damaged by a nasal tube.

The functions of the nasal cavity include providing the respiratory airway, the sense of smell, humidification, heat exchange, filtering of particulate matter and speech enunciation.

The mouth

The oral cavity is bound by the lips, cheeks and teeth in the front and at the side, the hard and soft palates above, the tongue below and the oropharyngeal isthmus behind.

The soft palate contains muscles which act in a coordinated manner to close off the mouth from the nasopharynx during speech and swallowing.

The oropharynx

The oropharynx communicates with the oral cavity and the nasopharynx and extends from the soft palate to the tip of the epiglottis. The tonsils are situated at the sides. In children, tonsillar enlargement and infection (tonsillitis or tonsillar abscess – quinsy) may cause airway obstruction.

The laryngopharynx

The laryngopharynx is the continuation of the oropharynx and extends from the tip of the epiglottis to the lower border of the cricoid cartilage at the level of the sixth vertebral body. The laryngeal inlet is normally protected from aspiration during swallowing. When swallowing occurs, breathing is temporarily interrupted, contraction of the pharyngeal constrictor muscles forces the bolus into the oesophagus and elevation of the larynx assists in closing the laryngeal inlet. The inlet is also protected by tilting of the epiglottis backwards and downwards. Nerve damage, head injury or intoxication with alcohol or drugs, causing a depressed level of consciousness, impairs these mechanisms and depresses these protective reflexes. In these situations there is a great risk that vomiting or regurgitation will result in aspiration of foreign material into the lower airway and lungs.

The larynx

The larynx lies between the laryngopharynx and the trachea and is made up of cartilages, membranes and ligaments. The principal cartilages are the thyroid, cricoid and arytenoids. The cricothyroid membrane joins the cricoid cartilage to the thyroid cartilage. The free upper border forms the vocal cords at the level of the thyroid cartilage notch behind the laryngeal prominence (Adam's apple). When separated, the vocal cords form the narrowest part of the adult airway. The larynx is supplied from the vagus nerve via its superior and recurrent laryngeal branches.

THE LOWER AIRWAY

The lower airway continues as the trachea and bronchi (Figures 6.2, 6.3). The adult trachea is 10–12 cm long, 2.5 cm in diameter and has 16–20 C-shaped cartilages. It divides at the carina, at the level of the sternal angle and the fourth or fifth thoracic vertebra. The right main bronchus continues more vertically than the left, accounting for the tendency for aspirated material or intubation with a long tracheal tube to enter the right rather than the left side. The left main bronchus is usually about 5 cm long. The nerve supply is via the recurrent laryngeal nerve.

ANATOMY AND PHYSIOLOGY OF THE PAEDIATRIC AIRWAY

Neonates breathe principally through their noses, so nasal obstruction may be immediately life-threatening. The infant head is relatively large compared with adults so in the supine position the neck tends to be flexed; placing a pillow under the head may actually obscure the view of the larynx and increase obstruction. The tongue, tonsils and adenoids are relatively large in children, increasing the risk of upper airway obstruction, and may interfere with laryngoscopy. At laryngoscopy, the larynx is more anterior. The epiglottis tends to be a large, floppy structure which may need to be lifted directly with the laryngoscope blade to obtain a view of the larynx.

The neonatal trachea is narrow (3–4 mm) and short (4–5 cm), increasing the risks of bronchial intubation. Up to the age of approximately 10 years, the cricoid cartilage represents the narrowest part of the upper airway. Damage at this level is associated with scarring and narrowing; the risk is reduced by using uncuffed tracheal tubes. In adults, the narrowest part of the airway is at the level of the vocal cords.

Reflexes are sensitive in children and instrumentation of the airway in those not profoundly unconscious can result in laryngospasm, bronchospasm, bradycardia and even cardiac arrest.

Oxygen consumption is relatively much higher in the child because of the raised metabolic rate. This results in a high respiratory rate. The increased oxygen consumption results in rapid cyanosis if upper airway obstruction or apnoea occurs.

AIRWAY ANATOMY AND PHYSIOLOGY DURING PREGNANCY

In pregnancy (see Chapters 50 and 51) capillary engorgement may cause significant mucosal swelling in the upper airway and this may be exacerbated by the oedema of preeclamptic toxaemia (PET) and upper respiratory tract infections. This swelling, together with the weight gain and breast enlargement associated with pregnancy, can make intubation more difficult. The increased oxygen consumption, coupled with a reduced oxygen reserve, results in rapid cyanosis in the presence of upper airway obstruction or apnoea.

RESPIRATORY CONTROL

CENTRAL CONTROL

Central nervous system control of respiration is mediated through respiratory centres in the brainstem. These centres receive input from other areas of the brain and from the contents of the blood perfusing them. Sleep, sedatives, alcohol, many analgesic drugs and injury to the respiratory centres result in a reduction in ventilation (hypoventilation) (Table 6.1). This reduction in ventilation may result from a fall in respiratory rate or tidal volume (the volume of air inhaled with each breath) or from a fall in both.

Ventilation is stimulated by a rise in arterial carbon dioxide or a fall in arterial oxygen. However, very high levels of carbon dioxide and very low levels of oxygen *depress* ventilation.

Ventilation is also stimulated by a fall in blood pH (rise in level of blood acidity) which may occur, for example, in a hyperglycaemic diabetic coma.

Breathing is normally controlled by the partial pressure of carbon dioxide in arterial blood ($Pa\text{CO}_2$). In some patients with chronic obstructive pulmonary disease (COPD), previously termed chronic bronchitis, who have grown accustomed to a high $Pa\text{CO}_2$, this drive has been replaced by a hypoxic drive dependent on low partial pressures of oxygen in arterial blood ($Pa\text{O}_2$).

> In other words, low levels of blood oxygen rather than high levels of blood carbon dioxide act as a stimulus to breathing

If high inspired concentrations of oxygen are given to these patients, this drive is lost and a reduction of ventilation with further carbon dioxide retention and decreasing consciousness may occur. However, it is important to remember

Table 6.1 Causes of hypoventilation

Mechanism	Cause
Thoracic cavity disruption	Penetrating trauma Flail chest
Respiratory muscle failure	Drugs and poisons Muscular dystrophy Myasthenia gravis Muscle relaxant drugs
Respiratory nerve failure	Spinal cord injury Neurological disease
Respiratory centre depression	Hypercarbia Hypotension Head injury Electrocution Poisoning Brain haemorrhage Brain infarction Brain thrombosis Brain infection Opiate drugs
Lung failure	Lung contusion Lung disease Pneumothorax Haemothorax Obesity Pregnancy

that a high carbon dioxide content kills slowly, but a low oxygen content kills quickly.

> The need to provide immediate adequate oxygenation takes precedence

Cyanotic patients should always be treated with high oxygen concentrations.

PERIPHERAL CONTROL

Adequate ventilation also requires an intact chest wall and intrapulmonary mechanics. Peripheral causes of impaired ventilation (see Table 6.1) include obstruction of the upper airway, most commonly due to the tongue. Peripheral nerve damage or blockade involving the phrenic and intercostal nerves may be seen with spinal cord damage. The phrenic nerves originate from cervical spinal roots C3–5; therefore diaphragmatic function will be maintained with cord lesions below this level.

AIRWAY AND VENTILATION ASSESSMENT

Airway obstruction may arise from a number of causes at a variety of levels in the respiratory tract. These are listed in Table 6.2.

Table 6.2 Causes of airway obstruction

Cause	Leads to
Coma / Mandible trauma	Tongue displacement
Anaphylaxis	Tongue oedema
Foreign body / Maxillary trauma	Oropharynx obstruction
Irritants	Laryngeal spasm
Foreign body	Laryngeal obstruction
Laryngeal trauma	Laryngeal oedema/obstruction
Infection / Anaphylaxis	Laryngeal oedema
Foreign body	Tracheal or bronchial obstruction
Irritants / Anaphylaxis / Infection / Near-drowning / Neurogenic shock / Cardiac failure	Pulmonary oedema

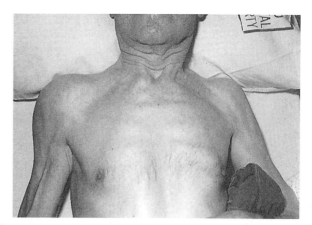

Figure 6.4 The accessory muscles of respiration

The history should include the circumstances of the immediate event and any pre-existing conditions of relevance such as asthma, congenital anatomical deformity and previous injury or disease of the spine or craniofacial region.

Airway and ventilation problems may be delayed in onset. The effects of smoke or chemical inhalation may not develop until hours after the event.

Physical assessment of the airway and ventilation involves looking, listening and feeling for chest movement and air flow. During the examination, attention should be directed to the respiratory rate, the presence of cyanosis (a blue discolouration due to lack of oxygen in the blood) and/or agitation and the use of the accessory muscles of respiration (Figure 6.4) and abnormal movement of the abdominal muscles.

Noisy breathing during inspiration generally indicates obstruction *above* the level of the larynx, whereas an expiratory wheeze usually indicates that the problem lies *at or below* the larynx. Characteristically, the patients who are choking indicate their predicament by clasping their neck or pointing to their larynx.

The examination steps to assess airway and ventilation are set out in Table 6.3.

SIMPLE AIRWAY MANAGEMENT

Upper airway patency can generally be reestablished by simple manual and positional manoeuvres involving correct alignment of the head, neck and mandible. Simple adjuncts may further improve the situation.

Table 6.3 Assessment of the airway and ventilation

	Airway	Ventilation
Check for	Unconsciousness	Unconsciousness
Look for	Cyanosis Pallor Blood Excessive salivation Stomach contents Foreign body Maxillofacial injury Neck trauma Broken dentures	Penetrating injury Cyanosis Pallor Respiratory rate Chest movements (adequate; flail; equal) Use of accessory muscles Use of abdominal muscles Chest wall bruising
Listen for	Voice quality Air entry Wheeze – inspiratory/ expiratory Abnormal sounds (stridor)	Voice quality Air entry Wheeze – inspiratory/ expiratory Added sounds (crackles)
Feel for	Air flow on your cheek	Chest movement Subcutaneous emphysema

HEAD TILT

Backward tilt of the head overcomes obstruction from the relaxed tongue in the majority of cases. The manoeuvre stretches the muscles in the front of the neck and lifts the base of the tongue away from the posterior pharyngeal wall (Figure 6.5). Ideally, the patient's head should be placed on a small pillow.

CHIN LIFT

The tongue is a muscle which is attached to the mandible and relief of the obstruction may be provided by lifting the chin (Figure 6.6). Both head tilt and chin lift are contraindicated if there is a risk of cervical spine injury.

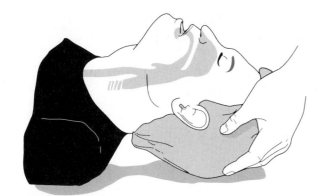

Figure 6.5 Head tilt

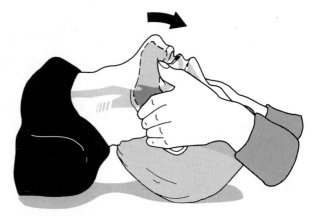

Figure 6.7 Jaw thrust

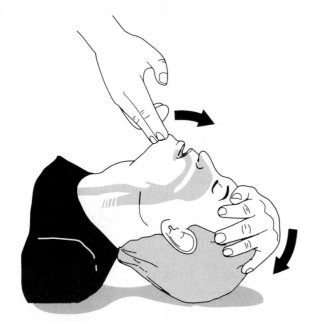

Figure 6.6 Chin lift

JAW THRUST

Jaw thrust provides an amplified effect of chin lift. The technique involves lifting the mandible upwards and forward with the index, middle and ring fingers and using the thumbs to open the mouth to allow air entry (Figure 6.7).

POSITIONAL METHODS OF AIRWAY ALIGNMENT IN PATIENTS WITH SUSPECTED CERVICAL SPINE INJURY

Great care should be taken with airway alignment in patients with suspected cervical spine injury. Flexion and rotation of the neck are the most dangerous movements. At all times manual in-line stabilization should be applied by an assistant.

> The safest way to achieve airway patency in patients with suspected cervical spine injury is by jaw thrust

Extension of the head on the neck should be minimized to that just necessary to establish an airway. It is important to remember, however, that airway obstruction is immediately lethal and airway management takes precedence.

RECOVERY POSITION

Once airway patency and adequate spontaneous ventilation are assured, the patient should be turned into the recovery position (Figure 6.8). In the majority of cases, patients with suspected spinal injuries are best managed on their back with full immobilization and appropriate airway care. Rarely, it will be necessary to log roll a patient with a potential spinal injury if their airway is at risk from profuse vomiting which cannot be cleared using suction. In such cases, this manoeuvre should be accomplished by a team consisting of a minimum of four people with the patient's head and neck supported in neutral alignment at all times (Figure 6.9). The attendant supporting the head and neck should give the commands. If manpower is insufficient, it may be necessary for a single rescuer to turn a patient with a possible spinal injury into the recovery position if there is no other way of maintaining a patent airway.

CLEARANCE OF THE AIRWAY OBSTRUCTED BY FOREIGN MATERIAL

In conscious patients, airway obstruction from a foreign body which is not relieved by spontaneous coughing must be cleared by back blows (Figure 6.10). In adults, the usual obstruction is a bolus of unchewed food; in children and patient's with learning difficulties or confusion it can be a variety of objects.

The manoeuvre can be carried out with patients lying on their side or in the sitting or standing position leaning

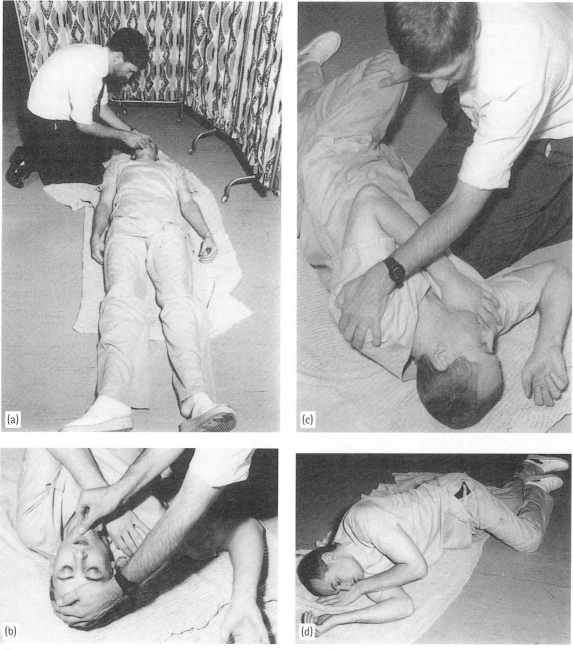

Figure 6.8 The recovery position

forward. Children can be placed head down lying along the rescuer's thigh or arm (Figure 6.11).

Abdominal thrusts (the Heimlich manoeuvre) may expel an impacted foreign body from the upper airway in a conscious patient when back blows have failed. The rescuer stands behind the patient with hands clasped together in a fist just below the patient's ribcage margin. A series of sharp upward thrusts raise the intrathoracic pressure and the object may be forcibly dislodged (Figure 6.12). This manoeuvre is not without danger of causing visceral injury to the stomach, spleen and liver and it is *not* recommended for infants

and small children. While the patient remains conscious, cycles of five back blows and five abdominal thrusts can be repeated.

In patients who are (or become) unconscious due to airway destruction, tilt the head back and remove any visible foreign object. Perform a chin lift and check for breathing: if this is absent try to deliver two rescue breaths in up to 5 attempts. If breaths cannot be delivered, give 15 chest compressions (regardless of circulatory status). Next check the mouth for visible obstructions and check for breathing. If this is absent, repeat this cycle until ALS equipment

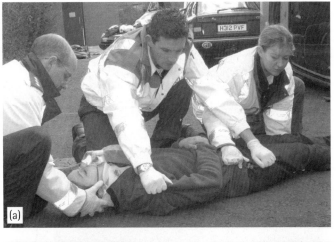

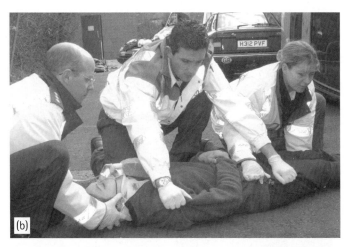

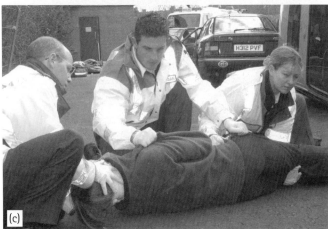

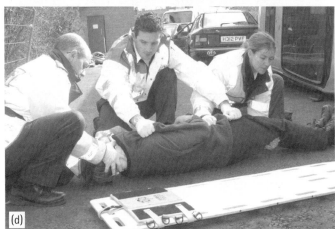

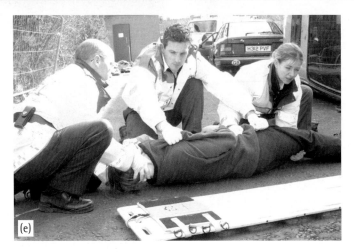

Figure 6.9 The "log roll"

(laryngoscope, Magill's forceps, and cricothyretomy kit) is available.

The best way of removing liquid material from the oropharynx is by direct suction using a wide-bore or Yankauer suction catheter, which is a stiff, angled catheter (Figure 6.14). Ideally the suction end should be manipulated under direct vision using a laryngoscope. A flexible catheter can be used to clear the lumen of an airway adjunct, such as a nasopharyngeal airway, tracheal tube or laryngeal mask.

Portable suction apparatus

Several manufacturers produce portable suction apparatus which may be powered electrically, by hand or by foot. The following points should be considered when choosing a particular model.

- Performance – generation of sufficient vacuum (600 mmHg) and flow rate (35 l/min) of free air
- Suitable fitments for Yankauer, flexible and wide-bore catheters.

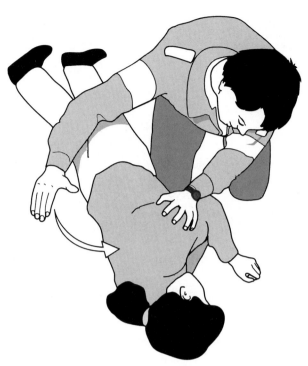

Figure 6.10 Back blows

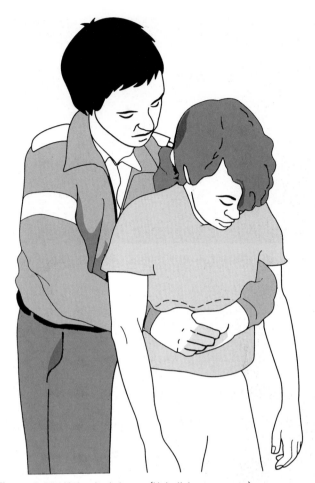

Figure 6.12 Abdominal thrusts (Heimlich manoeuvre)

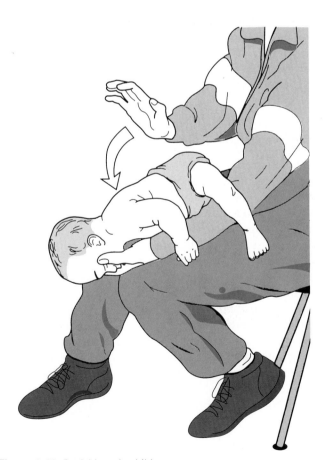

Figure 6.11 Back blows in children

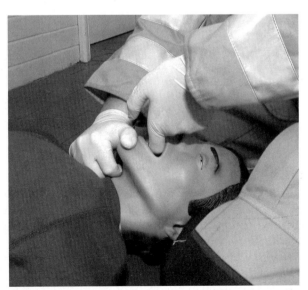

Figure 6.13 The use of the finger sweep to remove a foreign body

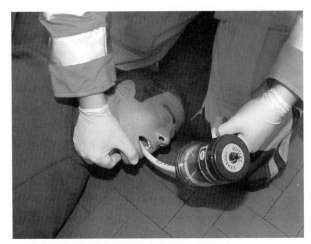

Figure 6.14 Clearance of the airway using suction

- Suitable power options of mains, rechargeable battery or 12-volt supply or hand or foot power where appropriate
- Compact size and height for portability
- Adequate-sized container for aspirated material
- Ease of disassembly, cleaning and reassembly without error
- Reliability and robust manufacture.

The neonatal aspirator is used to clear mucus from the mouth and nose of the newborn. It consists of a soft, flexible catheter attached to a small collecting chamber. A suction tube is attached to a second chamber which is placed in the mouth of the operator. Suction is generated in the operator's mouth and mucus is aspirated from the baby via the catheter into the collecting chamber. Only double-chambered mucous aspirators should be used to minimise the risk of cross infection.

SIMPLE AIRWAY ADJUNCTS

In some patients it is difficult to establish and maintain a clear airway using manual methods alone. Simple airway adjuncts may improve the position considerably. Three airway adjuncts, the oropharyngeal airway, cuffed oropharyngeal airway (COPA) and nasopharyngeal airway, are considered here. More advanced airways are considered in Chapter 6.

Oropharyngeal airway

The oropharyngeal airway controls backward displacement of the tongue and provides a free air passage from the mouth to the hypopharynx. It reduces the need for prolonged application of jaw thrust.

The airway is introduced through the mouth in an inverted position and rotated through 180° as it passes the edge of the palate. The distal end locates in the oropharynx (Figure 6.15). The airway may also be introduced directly using a tongue spatula or laryngoscope. This method is recommended in infants and small children. The oropharyngeal airway comes

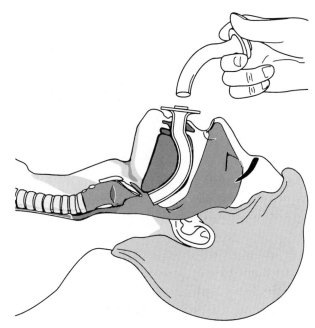

Figure 6.15 Inserting the oropharyngeal airway

in a range of six sizes suitable for an infant (size 000) to a large adult (size 4). The correct size for any individual equates to the distance from the corner of the mouth to the tragus of the ear or from the incisors to the angle of the mandible.

In patients with active protective reflexes insertion of the airway may provoke vomiting, retching or laryngeal spasm. The airway should be removed at the first sign of such intolerance.

Cuffed oropharyngeal airway

The cuffed oropharyngeal airway (COPA) is a device which has been recently introduced. It is similar in basic design to the conventional oropharyngeal airway but has two valuable additional features: a large-volume oropharyngeal cuff which is designed to produce a seal at this level and a standard 22 mm fitting at the oral end which connects to a self-inflating bag or automatic resuscitator (Figure 6.16). Experience has shown that artificial ventilation is made easier by using the COPA compared with the conventional airway because there is no need to apply a face mask with an airtight seal. Nevertheless, most patients will require a degree of chin lift or jaw thrust to maintain clear airway alignment during both spontaneous and positive pressure ventilation.

The oropharyngeal cuff also offers some protection against aspiration from blood emanating from the nasal and oral cavities but does not prevent aspiration of regurgitated gastric contents.

The insertion technique is similar to that used for the conventional oropharyngeal airway but care must be taken to avoid damaging the thin-walled cuff on the teeth. The cuff volume is of the order of 100 ml and a suitable syringe must be available.

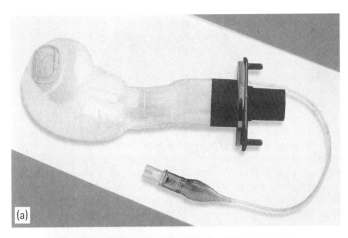

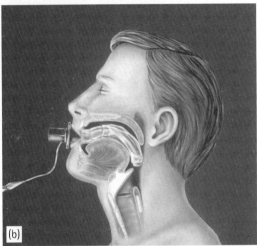

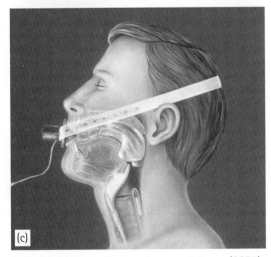

Figure 6.16 (a)–(c) The cuffed oropharyngeal airway (COPA)

Nasopharyngeal airway

The nasopharyngeal airway consists of a bevelled tube with a flange at the proximal end. It should be made of soft material to minimize intranasal damage.

The airway is introduced, well lubricated, into either nostril (generally the right is attempted first because of the direction of the distal bevel). It should be directed backwards

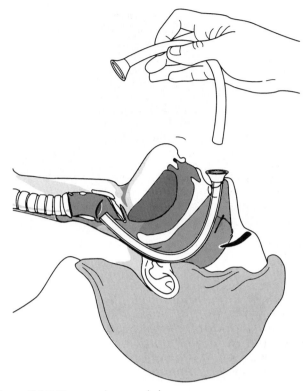

Figure 6.17 The nasopharyngeal airway

(*not* upwards) along the roof of the palate so that the tip lies in the hypopharynx, just above the larynx (Figure 6.17). If resistance to the passage of the airway is encountered it should be withdrawn and an attempt made through the other nostril. Suction should be on hand to control any bleeding.

The correct size of airway equates approximately with the diameter of the patient's nostril – an airway of 6.0 or 6.5 mm internal diameter will be suitable for the majority of adults.

The nasopharyngeal airway is particularly valuable in patients with maxillofacial injuries or a clenched jaw. Once in place, it is better tolerated than an oropharyngeal airway.

SIMPLE VENTILATION TECHNIQUES

Techniques of expired air ventilation without adjuncts were discussed in Chapter 4. This chapter deals with simple adjuncts for artificial ventilation. More advanced equipment is discussed in Chapter 6. The following devices are described in this chapter:

- the simple foil type
- the tube flange type
- the mask type
- the self-inflating bag–valve device.

THE SIMPLE FOIL

Foil devices were introduced for use by members of the public in an effort to minimize direct contact with the patient during expired air ventilation. These foils consist of

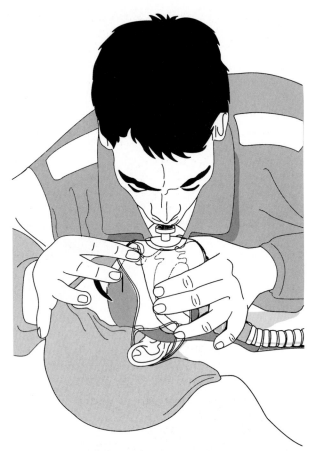

Figure 6.18 The foil device used for expired air ventilation. From Baskett PJF 1993 Resuscitation handbook, 2nd edn, with permission from Gower Medical Publishing

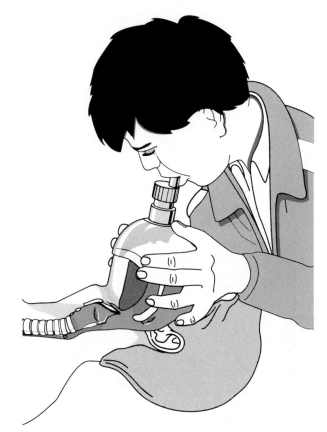

Figure 6.19 Mouth-to-mask ventilation

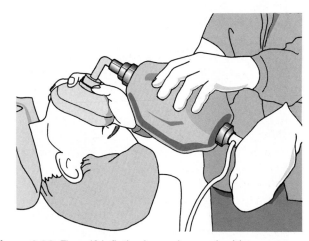

Figure 6.20 The self-inflating bag–valve–mask with oxygen reservoir

a plastic film which is applied to the oronasal region. There is a central orifice with a textile filter or one-way valve which is aligned with the patient's mouth. Expired air ventilation is applied in the usual way (see Chapter 4) with the patient's nostrils occluded with the fingers of one hand, while the other hand applies chin lift and seals the foil to the face (Figure 6.18). On occasion the foil may tear when in contact with the patient's or rescuer's teeth.

THE MASK DEVICE

A moulded face mask, made from transparent material, is fitted with an inflation port incorporating a one-way valve which directs the patient's exhaled air away from the rescuer and traps macroscopic particles. Some models incorporate an additional port for supplemental oxygen. The oxygen flow rate should be set at the maximum available.

The mask is applied over the mouth and nose with both hands, applying jaw thrust and head tilt to draw the face into the mask. The mask is sealed to the face with the index fingers and thumb of each hand (Figure 6.19).

THE SELF-INFLATING BAG–VALVE DEVICE

The self-inflating bag–valve device is designed to inflate the patient's lungs with air or an air and oxygen mixture.

Inflation of the lungs is provided through a valve which directs the air/oxygen to the patient and vents exhaled air to the atmosphere. Oxygen enrichment (only achieving an inspired concentration of up to 50% – FiO_2 0.5) can be provided through a port adjacent to the unidirectional air inlet valve. Much better inspired concentrations can be achieved (FiO_2 0.9, an inspired oxygen concentration of 90%) when an oxygen reservoir bag is attached to the air inlet valve and the flow rate adjusted to 10–15 l/min (Figure 6.20). The aim is to adjust the flow rate to ensure that the reservoir bag remains at least partially inflated at all times. If this is achievable with a flow rate of 10 l/min then a valuable resource can be conserved.

The self-inflating bag may be used with a face mask or may be attached to a tracheal tube or laryngeal mask airway (see Chapter 6). Use of the bag and face mask by one operator requires significant skill – the mask must be applied to the face with an airtight seal and the airway maintained in correct alignment, all with one hand. Expertise only comes with considerable practice. Importantly, operators may not be aware of their ineptitude and incorrect technique may result in hypoventilation, due to a leak between the face and mask, or inflation of the oesophagus due to imperfect airway alignment. For these reasons the two-person technique is advocated, one person using two hands to hold the mask with the airway aligned and the other inflating the patient's lungs by squeezing the bag.

A modified patient valve can permit positive end-expiratory pressure (PEEP) to be applied when the bag is used with a tracheal tube. The use of PEEP may be particularly valuable in patients with pulmonary oedema following exposure to irritants, smoke inhalation, near-drowning, aspiration and cardiac failure. The effect of PEEP is to maintain some pressure in the airways, even at the end of expiration, which reduces and even reverses the leakage of fluid into the alveoli (as occurs in pulmonary oedema). The "downside" is that the positive intrathoracic pressure reduces cardiac filling and may lead to a reduction in blood pressure, especially in hypovolaemic patients.

Some bag–valve devices can also be fitted with a filter on the intake valve to permit operation in contaminated atmospheres.

VENTILATION VOLUMES

For many years the American Heart Association has advocated a tidal volume of 800–1200 ml in adult patients with cardiac arrest. It is likely that such volumes are excessive, particularly in patients with cardiac arrest who produce relatively little carbon dioxide. Inflation with such high volumes in the patient with an unprotected and unsecured airway is likely to produce high inflation pressures with oesophageal and gastric inflation and hypoventilation of the lungs owing to leakage between the face and mask. Inflation pressures in these circumstances can only be minimized by a prolonged inspiratory period, which encroaches on the time for chest compressions.

Current resuscitation guidelines suggest using inflation volumes of 10 ml/kg (600–900 mls in an adult) if non-enriched atmospheric air is used. If supplemental oxygen is available, the volume of each inflation should be limited to 400–600 mls (7 ml/kg).

CRICOID PRESSURE

The unconscious patient with an insecure airway is continually at risk of regurgitation of gastric contents and pulmonary aspiration. True security of the airway can only be provided by tracheal intubation or use of other advanced airway adjuncts, including the surgical airway.

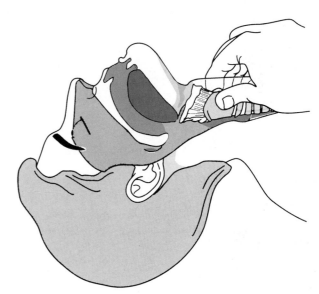

Figure 6.21 Cricoid pressure

Cricoid pressure (Sellick's manoeuvre) during artificial ventilation in the patient with the unsecured airway substantially reduces the risk of gastric regurgitation. The technique should always be used in this situation when sufficient personnel are available. Cricoid pressure is applied to either side of the cricoid cartilage using the thumb and forefinger of one hand. The other hand may provide counterpressure at the back of the neck (Figure 6.21) and this technique should always be used in cases of suspected cervical spine injury.

OXYGEN THERAPY IN THE SPONTANEOUSLY BREATHING PATIENT

All patients with airway or ventilatory compromise, major trauma or cardiac disease should be given oxygen. High inspired concentrations can only be achieved with an oxygen mask that incorporates reservoir bag. This is recommended in all of the above examples and the oxygen flow

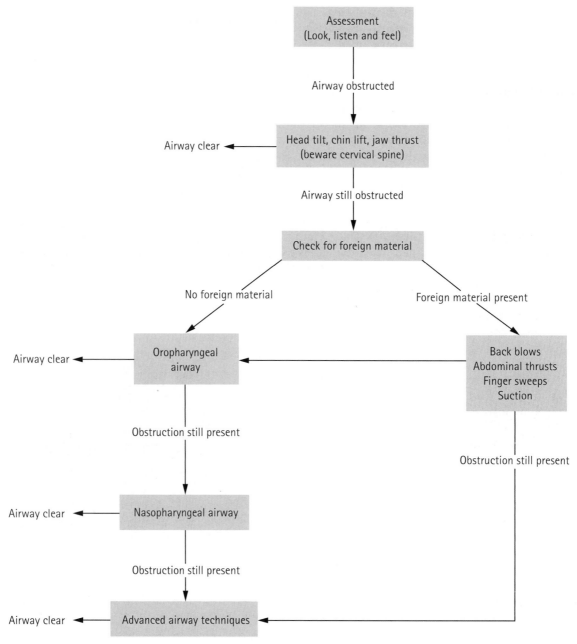

Figure 6.22 A protocol for simple management of the airway

rate should be set at 10–15 l/min, to ensure the reservoir bag remains inflated.

Patients with severe chronic obstructive pulmonary disease (COPD) depend, to some extent, on a hypoxic drive to stimulate their respiratory centre (see above). In these patients, when they are breathing spontaneously, a high inspired oxygen concentration may *reduce* the respiratory drive and lead to hypoventilation and an accumulation of carbon dioxide which has deleterious effects on the circulation and intracranial pressure. In such patients oxygen should be administered at a concentration of 24–28% using a Venturi mask. However, if cyanosis develops or oxygen saturation falls the attendant should not hesitate to assist ventilation using a high inspired oxygen concentration (see Chapter 6).

MANAGEMENT PROTOCOLS

Management protocols are useful in prehospital care. "Decision tree" algorithms for management of the airway and ventilation are given in Figures 6.22 and 6.23.

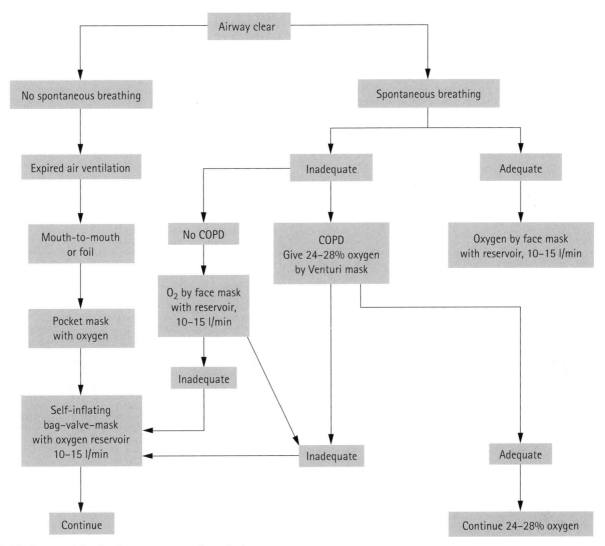

Figure 6.23 A protocol for simple management of ventilation

FURTHER READING

American Heart Association 1992 National Consensus Conference Standards and Guidelines for Cardiopulmonary Resuscitation (CPR) and Emergency Cardiac Care (ECC). Journal of the American Medical Association 268: 2171–2307

Baskett PJF 1993 Resuscitation Handbook, 2nd edn. Mosby, London

Baskett PJF, Dow AAC, Nolan JP 1994 Practical procedures in anaesthesia and critical care. Gower Medical Publishing, London

Committee on Trauma of the American College of Surgeons 1993 Advanced trauma life support instructor manual. American College of Surgeons, Chicago

European Resuscitation Council (Ed Bossaert L) 1998 Guidelines for resuscitation. Elsevier Science, Amsterdam

Chapter 7

Advanced management of the airway and ventilation

Management of the airway and ventilation using advanced techniques complements the basic methods but does not in any way replace them.

Advanced airway techniques are designed to secure the airway against aspiration of foreign material and to allow positive pressure ventilation without danger of inflating the stomach or leak at the mouth/mask interface.

The "gold standard" for airway control in prehospital care is tracheal intubation using a cuffed tracheal tube. However, the technique of tube placement under direct vision using a laryngoscope requires extensive and prolonged training and regular practice to maintain the skill. Excessive movement of the head and neck during laryngoscopy and intubation may aggravate a cervical spine injury.

For these reasons other techniques have been introduced to aid tracheal intubation and alternative devices have been developed which may be introduced blindly without the need for direct laryngoscopy.

CONVENTIONAL TRACHEAL INTUBATION

Conventionally the tracheal tube is passed through the mouth using a laryngoscope to visualize the vocal cords which form the gateway to the trachea. The tube may also be passed through the nose and directed into the trachea blindly or with the aid of a laryngoscope.

Tracheal intubation can be used for any age group and a range of tube sizes is available to accommodate neonates to large adults. Tubes of internal diameter greater than 6.5 mm are available with a cuff to seal the airway, permitting leak-proof positive pressure ventilation and preventing aspiration of foreign material into the lungs. In children and babies a good seal usually occurs without a cuff as the larynx and cricoid ring grip the tube sufficiently. The absence of a cuff in children reduces mucosal damage and the risk of subsequent stenosis.

SIZE OF TUBE

Tubes of size 7–9 mm will fit most adults. An 8 mm tube is a useful size to carry for all-purpose emergency use. Tubes are made longer than is generally needed and should be cut to a length of 21–25 cm. The length required in any individual will be twice the distance from the corner of the mouth to the angle of the jaw.

For children the correct size can be calculated using the following formulae:

$$\text{correct internal diameter (mm)} = \frac{\text{(age of child in years)}}{4} + 4$$

$$\text{correct length (cm)} = \frac{\text{(age of child in years)}}{2} + 12$$

Once the correct diameter has been calculated it is important to have the next biggest and the next smallest tube available to ensure a good fit.

The length should be increased by up to 2 cm if the nasal route is to be used.

In children, to ensure a good seal, it is important that the full range of ET tube sizes (including half sizes) are available.

EQUIPMENT FOR CONVENTIONAL TRACHEAL INTUBATION

The following equipment is required (Figure 7.1).

- Appropriate sized laryngoscope in working order
- Appropriate range of tubes cut to correct length with connections (15 mm) to fit the ventilating apparatus
- Scissors
- Suction apparatus
- Lubricant on a gauze swab (only occasionally required in the prehospital setting)
- 20 ml syringe for cuff inflation
- Clamp to secure the cuff inflation port (unless a one-way valve is fitted)
- Flexible bougie and stylet
- Magill's forceps

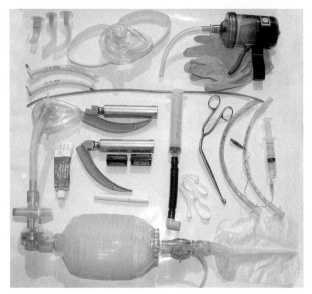

Figure 7.1 Intubation equipment. With kind permission of *First Person on Scene Intermediate Manual IHCD* at Excel (2004)

- Tape or tie to secure tube in place
- Apparatus to inflate the lungs (bag–valve or automatic resuscitator)
- Pulse oximeter to monitor patient during and after intubation attempt (optional)
- End-tidal CO_2 apparatus to detect correct tube placement (preferred device, described later in this chapter) or
- Syringe or bulb oesophageal intubation detector.

INDICATIONS

The indications for conventional tracheal intubation in the prehospital setting are set out below.

- Airway obstruction or potential airway obstruction in the profoundly unconscious patient with no gag reflex
- Patient at risk of aspiration of foreign material (e.g. gastric contents, blood from maxillofacial trauma)
- Patient requiring positive pressure ventilation, for example, in cardiorespiratory arrest
- To gain access to the lower respiratory tract to aspirate secretions or foreign material.

CONTRAINDICATIONS

Tracheal intubation is contraindicated in the absence of a skilled operator and the necessary equipment. It is also contraindicated in patients who are not profoundly unconscious and have an intact gag reflex. Forced intubation in, for instance, the lightly unconscious patient with a head injury will do more harm than good by raising the intracranial pressure and reducing the perfusion of the brain. In such circumstances simpler methods of airway management, such as insertion of a nasopharyngeal or oropharyngeal airway, will have to be used.

Relative contraindications include immobility of the head and neck, or distorted anatomy due to tumour, infection or oedema – all of which impair the view of the larynx and the glottis opening.

On no account should attempts be made to intubate children with croup or infections such as acute epiglottitis, unless respiratory arrest has occurred. Intervention with a laryngoscope in such patients may provoke bleeding or further oedema and convert a partial airway obstruction to a complete airway obstruction. However, once complete obstruction has occurred a cautious intubation attempt may prove life-saving. If this is not immediately successful, it will be necessary to proceed urgently to needle cricothyroidotomy.

TECHNIQUE FOR OROTRACHEAL INTUBATION USING LARYNGOSCOPY (Figure 7.2)

1. Ensure that all equipment functions correctly and that tubes and bougies are well lubricated if necessary.
2. If possible, the patient, should be supine with the head and neck aligned in the clear airway position (preferably with the head on a small pillow or rolled-up blanket).
3. Holding the laryngoscope in your left hand, insert the curved blade into the right-hand corner of the patient's mouth, ensuring that the lip is not caught between the blade and lower teeth (Figure 7.2a).
4. Advance the blade, aiming for the larynx in the midline, and displacing the tongue towards the left-hand side of the mouth to leave a clear view.
5. When the tip of the blade reaches laryngeal level, lift the handle forwards and upwards. Slide the tip of the blade into the recess between the epiglottis and the base of the tongue.
6. Maintain the backwards tilt of the head by pressing on the occiput with your other hand and against the tip of the blade to get the best view of the glottic opening. Cricoid pressure will generally improve the view and should be used in all patients in the field.
7. Pass the tracheal tube from the right-hand side of the mouth through the glottic opening, rotating it 90° counterclockwise if necessary to ease entry between the vocal cords.
8. If a full view of the glottis is not possible a bougie may be passed under direct vision through the cords and the tube introduced over the bougie into the trachea. The bougie is then withdrawn. Alternatively, a malleable stylet may be placed inside the lumen of the tube and bent to a curve suitable for introduction of the tube through the glottis.
9. Once the tube has passed between the vocal cords it should be advanced so that the cuff lies below the larynx.
10. The cuff should be inflated with air (or sterile water if the patient is to be transported at altitude or in a decompression chamber). Sufficient air should be introduced to eliminate any leak at the peak of positive pressure ventilation. Cuff inflation volumes requiring more than 15 ml should lead to a suspicion that the tube is misplaced in the oesophagus or that the cuff itself has developed a leak.
11. Check that the tube is in the trachea by observing bilateral chest movement and listening for air entry over both upper lobes. Unilateral chest movement (generally on the right) may indicate that the tube has gone down too far and has entered the main bronchus. A check should also be made that air entry is not heard in the epigastric area. Other methods of checking correct tube placement are described later in this chapter.
12. Secure the tube in place with a tie or tape.

The entire process of intubation should be accomplished in 30 seconds or less. If the attempt is taking longer then it should be temporarily abandoned and the patient ventilated with oxygen via a face mask for 1–2 minutes before trying again. Note, however, that ventilation via a mask between intubation attempts is pointless if the airway remains obstructed. No more than two attempts should be made before moving to other measures.

PROBLEMS AND HAZARDS ASSOCIATED WITH OROTRACHEAL INTUBATION

Tracheal intubation attempts using direct laryngoscopy are not without hazards.

- Trauma to lips, teeth, tongue and structures in the pharynx and larynx (a common problem is using the teeth as a fulcrum, causing damage to crowns particularly).
- Oesophageal intubation (this in itself is not a major problem unless it is undetected; however, undetected oesophageal intubation generally leads to serious hypoxic brain damage or death and represents probably the most serious technical error a paramedic can make).
- Intubation of a single bronchus will lead to hypoxia and collapse of the opposite lung.
- Aspiration of foreign material such as stomach contents or blood during the intubation attempt.
- Kinking of the tracheal tube.
- Overinflation of the cuff leading to pressure damage of the tracheal mucous membrane or ballooning of the cuff over the lumen of the tube.
- Exacerbation of cervical spine injury (see Chapter 29).
- Trauma from the tip of a stylet protruding from the end of the tube (stylet used to stiffen or shape the tube during a difficult intubation).

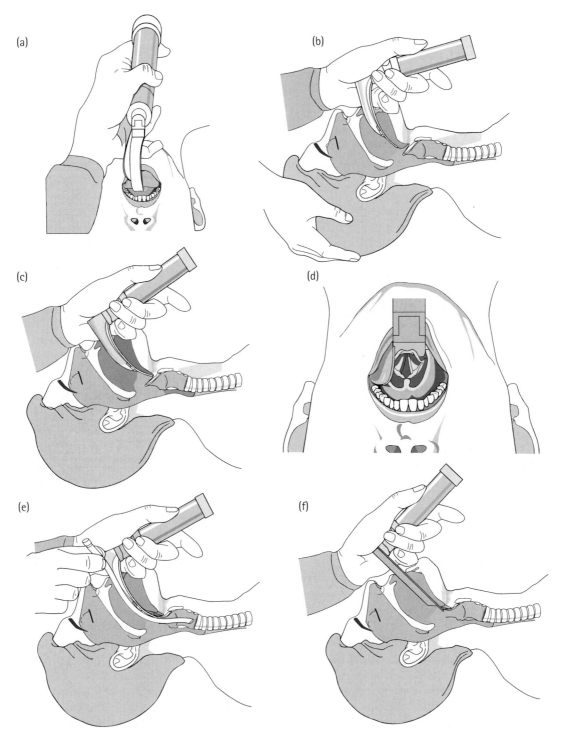

Figure 7.2 Orotracheal intubation. (a–e) Adult intubation; (f) use of straight-bladed laryngoscope in infants. From Baskett PJF 1993 *Resuscitation handbook*, 2nd edn, with permission from Gower Medical Publishing

NASOTRACHEAL INTUBATION

Nasotracheal intubation is sometimes used when the patient has trismus and is preferred by some authorities in patients with suspected cervical spine injury because it may be accomplished with the head and neck in the neutral position. However, it is generally agreed that the nasal route requires more technical skill and may take longer. There is also a risk of bleeding from the nose. *It is not recommended for use by paramedics untrained in this technique.*

Some ET tubes are available with a flexible tip which allow the curve to be varied by traction on a ring pull to negotiate the curve from the nasopharynx towards the glottic opening (Figure 7.3).

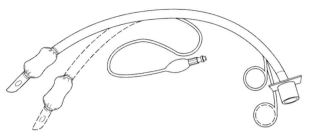

Figure 7.3 A nasotracheal tube. From Baskett PJF 1993 Resuscitation handbook, 2nd edn, with permission from Gower Medical Publishing

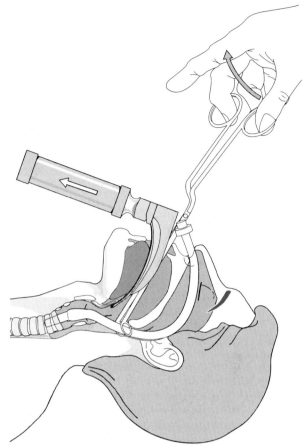

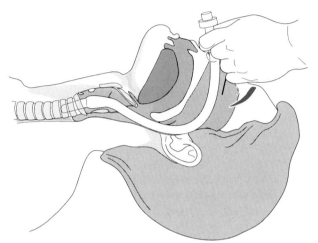

Figure 7.4 Blind nasal intubation. Adapted from Baskett PJF 1993 Resuscitation handbook, 2nd edn, with permission from Gower Medical Publishing

Figure 7.5 Nasal intubation by direct laryngoscopy. Adapted from Baskett PJF 1993 Resuscitation handbook, 2nd edn, with permission from Gower Medical Publishing

Two methods of nasal intubation may be used in prehospital care.

- Blind nasal intubation (Figure 7.4)
- Nasal intubation assisted by direct laryngoscopy and Magill's forceps (Figure 7.5).

TECHNIQUE OF BLIND NASOTRACHEAL INTUBATION

1. The patient is positioned as for orotracheal intubation. The head and neck may be placed in the neutral position, avoiding hyperextension.
2. The tube should be sized for the patient and well lubricated. A suitable tube will have a similar diameter to the patient's own nostril (7–8 mm for an adult).
3. The tube is introduced through the most patent nostril (generally the right side is attempted first) and passed directly backwards (*not* upwards) through the nasal cavity along the floor of the nose to enter thenasopharynx.
4. In patients who are breathing spontaneously the mouth and opposite nostril should be occluded manually and breath sounds should be listened for as the tube is steered towards the larynx and onwards through the glottis into the trachea. Generally a cough heralds successful passage through the cords.

5. The technique may also be used in the apnoeic patient, although it is more difficult. Considerable skill and practice, and optimal head and neck positioning, are required to steer the tube through the glottic opening.
6. Secure the tube and check for correct positioning as in orotracheal intubation.

TECHNIQUE OF NASOTRACHEAL INTUBATION USING DIRECT LARYNGOSCOPY AND MAGILL'S FORCEPS

1. Proceed as with blind nasal intubation until the tip of the tube lies just above the glottis.
2. Introduce the laryngoscope as for orotracheal intubation and view the glottis.
3. Grasp the tube with Magill's forceps 1–2 cm from its tip and steer it through the glottic opening.
4. Secure the tube and check for correct positioning as in orotracheal intubation.

HAZARDS OF NASOTRACHEAL INTUBATION

Nasal intubation is associated with the same hazards as orotracheal intubation. Additionally, the nasal passage and adenoids may be damaged with associated bleeding, which may obscure the view at direct laryngoscopy. The tube may enter a false passage beneath the mucous membrane of the nasopharynx. In patients with a fracture of the base of the skull, a tube directed upwards instead of backwards may penetrate the cribriform plate and enter the cranial cavity.

> Nasal intubation is not generally recommended in the prehospital environment

AIDS TO OROTRACHEAL INTUBATION AVOIDING DIRECT LARYNGOSCOPY

Two techniques have been introduced in an effort to avoid the difficulties and hazards associated with direct laryngoscopy at intubation and to enable the tracheal tube to be introduced blindly via the mouth.

- The intubating laryngeal mask
- The lighted stylet.

THE INTUBATING LARYNGEAL MASK

The intubating laryngeal mask was introduced in 1997. It is a variant of the conventional laryngeal mask airway (see Fig. 7.8) which is specifically designed to facilitate blind tracheal intubation using a flexible reinforced Brain tracheal tube (Intavent, UK). The midline position of the bevel of this tube is designed to increase the chances of successful blind intubation.

The intubating laryngeal mask (ILM) is shown in Figure 7.6. The mask element is similar to the conventional laryngeal mask airway (LMA) but it is fitted to a rigid, silicone-covered, pre-curved metal tube which has a standard fitting for connection to a self-inflating bag or automatic resuscitator. A handle is fitted at the proximal end to introduce the device and manipulate it to the correct position. The device is currently available in sizes 3 (child age 10–14), 4 (adult female or small male), 5 (normal to large adult male). It is a reasonable device and after use should be cleaned and autoclaved according to the manufacturer's instructions.

The device is introduced in the head and neck neutral position, which is of special value in patients with suspected cervical spine injury. On its own, the ILM provides a clear airway in a large majority of cases (98%) and is probably easier to position than the conventional LMA. Mouth opening of more than 2 cm is needed. Tracheal intubation using the ILM naturally requires training but proficiency is probably acquired more rapidly than with conventional intubation using a laryngoscope. The device can usually be easily inserted in cases of known difficult conventional intubation. The ILM can be inserted with the operator placed at the patient's side if access to above the head is difficult.

Indications

The device should be used, by trained personnel, in unconscious patients with suspected cervical spine injury when an airway is required. It may also be used in patients with known or anticipated difficult intubation or if access to above the patient's head is difficult or impossible. According to the training received, it may be preferable to conventional tracheal intubation using a laryngoscope in other patients.

Technique

1. Test the cuff for leaks and lubricate the back and sides, but not the aperture, of the LMA at the distal end.
2. Test the tracheal tube cuff for leaks.
3. Lubricate the tracheal tube and slide it in and out of the ILM until it moves easily.
4. Deflate the cuff of the ILM completely.
5. With the head and neck in the neutral position, grasp the handle of the ILM and position it over the patient's lower neck and upper chest.
6. Introduce the top of the mask behind the upper incisors and, using a rotating movement, roll the mask along the surface of the palate and down into the hypopharynx.
7. Inflate the cuff of the ILM (20 ml for size 3, 30 ml for size 4 and 35–40 ml for size 5).
8. Connect a ventilating device to the ILM and check for chest movement and leaks around the cuffs (Figure 7.6d).
9. Make final adjustments to the position with the handle to achieve inflation with least resistance. Usually a slight elevation of the mask will achieve the best position.
10. Holding the handle firmly in this position, introduce the tracheal tube into the ILM and attempt to pass it through into the trachea. Passage without resistance will occur in the majority of cases.
11. If resistance occurs, partially remove the ILM by rotation of the handle and then reintroduce it. This may dislodge a downfolded epiglottis.
12. When it is thought that the tracheal tube is in position, inflate the cuff and check for bilateral lung inflation and the absence of gastric inflation.
13. The ILM can now be removed. Deflate the cuff of the ILM.

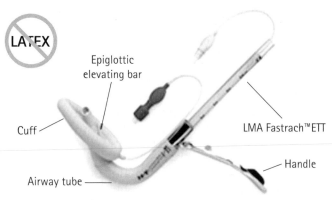

LATEX

Epiglottic elevating bar

Cuff

LMA Fastrach™ETT

Airway tube

Handle

Figure 7.6 The intubating laryngeal mask

14. Remove the connector from the tracheal tube and, using a pusher, hold the tracheal tube in place while removing the ILM with a rotation action.
15. Once removal of the ILM is nearly complete, grasp the tracheal tube in the mouth to prevent its dislocation and complete removal of the ILM, ensuring the tracheal tube pilot balloon passes easily through the ILM.
16. Replace the tracheal tube connector and check again for correct tracheal tube placement.

The ILM is finding a place in hospital anaesthetic and emergency department practice. Initial experience has proved very promising (96% success in blind tracheal intubation). It is likely, after trials have been completed, to find a place in prehospital paramedic practice.

THE LIGHTED STYLET

Another intubation method uses a malleable lighted stylet (Laerdal Medical) passed through the lumen of the tracheal tube so that the light at the end does not quite emerge from the distal end of the tube (Figure 7.7). Bent to a "J" shape, the tube is introduced directly through the glottis into the

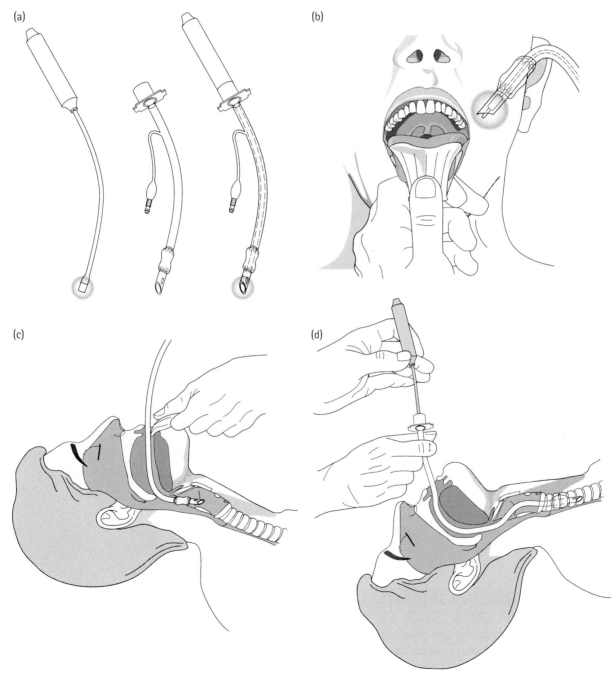

Figure 7.7 The lighted stylet. From Baskett PJF 1993 Resuscitation handbook, 2nd edn, with permission from Gower Medical Publishing

trachea. Correct positioning just above the glottic opening is confirmed by maximal transillumination in the midline.

Technique

1. The tracheal tube and lighted stylet are lubricated and confirmed to be in working order.
2. The lighted stylet is introduced into the tube so that the lighted end does not quite emerge from the distal end of the tube.
3. The tube and wand are bent into a "J" shape so that the base of the "J" is equal in length to the distance from the tip of the chin to the thyroid cartilage (Adam's apple). The proximal end of the tube is clipped to the wand handle.
4. With the patient's head and neck in the neutral position and the tongue pulled forward wrapped in a gauze swab, the tube is introduced into the mouth and passed backwards over the tongue, aiming for the larynx in the midline.
5. As the tube enters the hypopharynx transillumination will be observed. The position of the tube should be adjusted so that the transillumination is in the midline.
6. Advance the tube. If it passes easily and transillumination intensifies, it has passed into the trachea. If the light intensity dims the tube is lying in the oesophagus. Cricoid pressure may be of assistance.
7. Transillumination on either side of the midline with difficulty in tube advancement means that the tip is in the piriform fossa to the side of the larynx. The tip of the tube should be repositioned in the midline.
8. Once the tube is correctly placed, the lighted stylet should be unclipped from the proximal end and withdrawn from the tube.
9. Correct placement in the trachea should be confirmed using the usual methods and the tube should be secured in place with a tie or tape.

Problems and hazards

- Inability to introduce and locate the tube correctly, resulting in persistent lodging in the piriform fossa or in front of the epiglottis.
- Local trauma to the pharyngeal and laryngeal structures.
- Oesophageal intubation.
- Difficulty in detecting maximal transillumination in ambient bright light.

Although used in hospital practice, the lighted stylet and its variants have not yet undergone extensive trials in the prehospital arena and therefore are not recommended at present for paramedic use.

ALTERNATIVES TO TRACHEAL INTUBATION

Alternatives to tracheal intubation have been introduced to circumvent some of the problems associated with direct laryngoscopy and intubation. These problems include the considerable technical skill required, the need for extensive

training on human patients, the need for regular practice, the potential for patient injury during the procedure and the risk of unrecognized oesophageal intubation.

Two devices have potential for use in prehospital care:

- the laryngeal mask airway
- the Combitube.

THE LARYNGEAL MASK AIRWAY

The laryngeal mask airway (LMA or Brain airway) has found a niche in airway management during anaesthesia since its introduction into clinical practice in the mid-1980s (Figure 7.8).

The advantage of the LMA is that it can provide an airway without the training and skill required for laryngoscopy

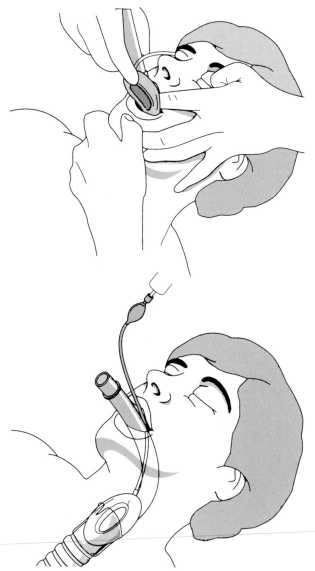

Figure 7.8 The laryngeal mask airway. Adapted from Baskett PJF 1993 Resuscitation handbook, 2nd edn, with permission from Gower Medical Publishing

and tracheal intubation. The incidence of trauma, sore throat and laryngeal spasm is considerably less than with tracheal intubation. The technique is easily learnt by nurses and paramedics.

While not guaranteeing absolute protection of the airway in every case, the LMA does offer considerably greater security than most other airways except the tracheal tube.

The LMA has been reported to have been successful in the management of the airway by nurses during cardiopulmonary resuscitation and a similar study is in progress to assess the performance of paramedics and emergency medical technicians with the device in prehospital care.

The LMA consists of a wide-bore tube with a standard 15 mm connector at the proximal end. At the distal end is an elliptical cuff designed to seal the hypopharynx around the laryngeal opening. The airway comes in a range of sizes suitable for an infant to a large adult (Table 7.1) and may be reused up to 40 times. Disposable versions are also available. After use it should be cleaned and autoclaved according to the manufacturer's instructions. If necessary, a 6.0–6.5 mm tracheal tube may be passed through the lumen of the size 4 and size 5 masks into the trachea but this is unreliable and the intubating laryngeal mask is much better suited for this purpose (see p 66).

Indications

The LMA is indicated when an airway is required in an unconscious patient and tracheal intubation is precluded by lack of available expertise or equipment or has proved difficult or impossible.

Technique (Figure 7.8)

1. Test cuff inflation for leaks and then lubricate the back and sides, but not the aperture, of the cuff and the distal part of the tube.
2. Deflate the cuff completely.
3. The patient should be supine with the head and neck in the clear airway position.

4. The mouth should be opened by an assistant depressing the chin.
5. The tube is held like a pen in the gloved hand and introduced into the mouth with the aperture facing the tongue. *As the LMA is advanced it should be applied to the roof of the palate.*
6. Once the hand cannot go further inside the mouth, it should be moved to the proximal end of the tube and the mask pressed into position until resistance is felt as it locates in the hypopharynx. The coloured line on the tube should be aligned with the nasal septum.
7. The cuff is inflated with the correct amount of air for the size (see Table 7.1). As the cuff is inflated the tube rises out of the mouth by approximately 1 cm.
8. Confirm that a clear airway exists by listening for spontaneous breathing or check for chest movement and breath sounds during inflation with a bag attached to the tube.
9. Insert the bite block or oropharyngeal airway alongside the tube and secure it in place with a tie or tape.

Note: normally the operator will be positioned at the head of the patient to introduce the tube, but if access to this position is impossible the operator may stand or kneel in front of the patient and introduce the tube from below.

Problems and hazards

Laryngeal mask airways leak around the cuff if inflation pressures greater than 20 cmH$_2$O are generated. This can generally be overcome by careful attention to the ventilation pattern using slow flow rate inflation, but this may present difficulties in those with bronchospasm or chronic obstructive pulmonary disease.

Rejection of the LMA, straining, coughing and laryngeal spasm may occur in patients who are not profoundly unconscious and who retain active reflexes. Such limitations may confine LMA use in prehospital care to cardiorespiratory arrest, near-drowning, drug overdose to the point of respiratory arrest and in trauma, except for the profoundly unconscious. Oropharyngeal trauma may be aggravated by the LMA.

Incorrect placement may occur if the tip of the cuff folds back on itself, catches in the epiglottis or rotates during insertion. If this occurs withdraw the LMA, deflate the cuff completely and try again, adhering precisely to the manufacturer's recommended technique for insertion.

The LMA offers a method of establishing a clear airway in the unconscious patient before tracheal intubation skills and equipment are available or if tracheal intubation proves difficult. It is not intended as a long-term airway and does not offer absolute protection against pulmonary aspiration, although the incidence is very small indeed.

A new variant of the LMA, the Proseal, is currently undergoing trials. This version incorporates a separate drainage tube to divert any regurgitated gastric contents to the exterior. The Proseal also incorporates a modified cuff design which permits much higher seal pressures. If trials

Table 7.1 Laryngeal mask sizes			
Patient	Weight (kg)	Size	Cuff volume (ml)
Neonate/infant	Up to 6.5	1	2–4
Infant/child	6.5–15	2	10
Child	15–30	2.5	15
Small adult/child	30–50	3	20
Adult	50–75	4	30
Large adult	>75	5	40

are encouraging the Proseal may well displace the conventional LMA in prehospital practice.

THE COMBITUBE

The Combitube (Figure 7.9) is a single-use disposable device which has been introduced as an alternative to tracheal intubation. It is a preformed double-lumen tube which is passed blindly through the mouth, avoiding the need for laryngoscopy. Ventilation of the lungs is possible whether the tube enters the trachea or the oesophagus.

The channels of the tube are designated "tracheal" or "oesophageal". The tracheal tube has an open distal end and the oesophageal tube has a blind end with openings

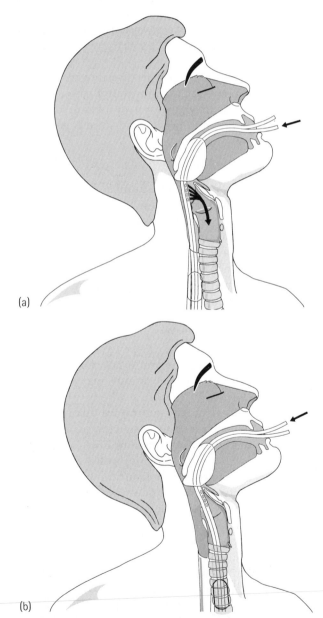

Figure 7.9 The Combitube (a) oesophageal placement; (b) tracheal placement. From Baskett PJF 1993 Resuscitation handbook, 2nd edn, with permission from Gower Medical Publishing

situated at the level just above the larynx. There is a small-volume (10–20 ml) cuff situated at the distal end of the oesophageal tube and a large-volume (100 ml) cuff designed to occupy the hypopharynx. If the tube passes directly into the trachea the distal cuff is inflated and the ventilating apparatus is attached to the tracheal tube. The hypopharyngeal cuff is redundant. If the tube passes into the oesophagus (more usual), both distal and hypopharyngeal cuffs are inflated and the ventilating apparatus is connected to the oesophageal tube. Inflation of the lungs occurs through the openings at the laryngeal level, the inflating gas being prevented from passing into the oesophagus by the distal cuff and from leaking into the mouth and nose by the hypopharyngeal cuff.

The Combitube is not currently available in sizes suitable for children.

Technique

1. Lubricate the Combitube.
2. With the patient supine and the head and neck aligned in the clear airway position, introduce the tube through the mouth to a distance of approximately 24 cm.
3. Inflate the distal cuff and ventilate the patient through the tracheal tube port. If it is confirmed that the tube is located in the trachea (see below), continue ventilation by this route.
4. If the tube has passed into the oesophagus, as is more usual, then both cuffs should be inflated and the patient ventilated through the oesophageal tube port.
5. Confirm that the lungs are being ventilated (see below) and that gas is not entering the stomach.

Problems and hazards

- The device is bulky and may be difficult to introduce into a small mouth. The cuffs may be damaged by sharp teeth.
- Hypopharyngeal injuries may be aggravated.
- There is a potential for ventilating the oesophagus and stomach if the tube position is incorrectly identified.
- The tube may be rejected and coughing and straining may occur if the patient is not profoundly unconscious.
- If the tube has passed into the oesophagus direct suction cannot be applied to the trachea for the suction catheter will not pass through the side holes.
- Ventilation may be difficult if the tube is pushed too far down the oesophagus, thereby obliterating some of the side holes.

The Combitube also offers a potential alternative to tracheal intubation in instances where expertise and equipment are not immediately available. There have as yet been no reports of large-scale trials of its use by ambulance personnel in prehospital care and positive recommendations for use must await such clinical experience.

THE PHARYNGOTRACHEAL LUMEN AIRWAY

This device is no longer in use and not recommended.

DETECTION OF CORRECT TUBE PLACEMENT

An undetected misplaced tracheal tube is the most serious complication of airway management. A protocol to check correct placement should follow each intubation attempt. If there is the slightest doubt that the tube is not in the trachea the rule is that it should be removed and the patient oxygenated by alternative methods.

> If there is any doubt about the correct placement of a tracheal tube – remove it!

Four methods are available in the emergency setting for detecting that the tube is correctly placed in the trachea.

CLINICAL METHODS

Clinical methods include:

- visualizing the tube passing between the vocal cords during the intubation attempt
- palpation of the tube as it passes through the larynx
- during positive pressure inflation applied to the tube, note:
  - absence of leak around the inflated cuff
  - bilateral chest expansion
  - breath sounds in both axillae
  - absence of sounds in the epigastric area.

These methods are generally effective in the majority of cases but are not totally reliable. Fortunately, there are simple, inexpensive methods to supplement the clinical methods.

TRANSILLUMINATION

A lighted stylet passed down the lumen of the tube (see Figure 7.7) shows bright transillumination when the tube is in the trachea. A dull glow suggests that the tube is in the oesophagus. The method is subject to observer variation and is not reliable in bright light.

DETECTION OF CARBON DIOXIDE

Detection of carbon dioxide emerging from the tube generally indicates that it is in the trachea. A simple, inexpensive colorimetric device is available and is a reliable carbon dioxide detector. Miniaturized electronic devices are also available which provide a capnograph trace and digital readings. However, carbon dioxide can also emerge from the oesophagus if the patient has recently had a carbonated drink.

During cardiac arrest carbon dioxide is not produced and therefore will not be detected even in a correctly placed tube. However, effective cardiopulmonary resuscitation results in some carbon dioxide production and indeed, the amount of carbon dioxide detected provides a prediction of outcome.

End-tidal CO_2 monitoring represents the gold standard for confirming ET tube placement.

THE OESOPHAGEAL DETECTOR

The oesophageal detector consists of a 50 ml syringe or self-inflating bulb joined by an airtight connection to the tracheal tube (Figure 7.10). If the tube is correctly placed, free aspiration of air into the syringe occurs. If the tube is located in the oesophagus aspiration attempts meet with resistance as the oesophagus collapses.

AIRWAY MANAGEMENT IN SUSPECTED CERVICAL SPINE INJURY

Special care must be taken during management of the airway in patients with suspected cervical spine injury. Aggravation of the injury must be avoided by the application of manual in-line stabilization of the head and neck in the neutral position during the attempt to secure the airway (Figure 7.11). However, the importance of a clear airway is paramount, as a continuously obstructed airway is fatal.

Certain important principles should be borne in mind during management of such patients.

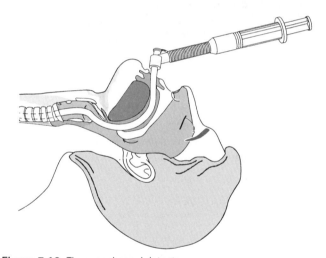

Figure 7.10 The oesophageal detector

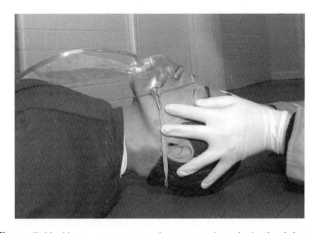

Figure 7.11 Airway management in suspected cervical spine injury

- Flexion and rotation of the head and neck are the most dangerous movements.
- Oral intubation using direct laryngoscopy can be safely accomplished by a skilled operator in the vast majority of cases.
- In cases of real or anticipated difficulty with intubation using direct laryngoscopy, the intubating laryngeal mask may be used. The laryngeal mask airway or the Combitube may be used if tracheal intubation is not possible.
- Patients with severe maxillofacial injury in whom the airway cannot be secured should be managed by needle cricothyroidotomy and jet ventilation or surgical cricothyroidotomy and tracheal intubation.

AIRWAY MANAGEMENT IN PATIENTS WITH PHARYNGEAL OR LARYNGEAL OEDEMA

Oedema in the pharyngeal or laryngeal region can be related to thermal injury, anaphylaxis or acute infection such as epiglottitis. Blind techniques such as use of the lighted stylet, ILM or alternatives to tracheal intubation (LMA, Combitube) are contraindicated.

> *Oral intubation should only be attempted by a skilled anaesthetist using deep inhalational anaesthesia*

In the prehospital setting the airway should be managed by basic positional methods and a high inspired oxygen concentration, with rapid transfer to a hospital. Life-threatening airway obstruction should be treated by needle cricothyroidotomy and jet ventilation or surgical cricothyroidotomy (see below). Patients with inhalational thermal injury should be intubated early before serious oedema develops.

THE SURGICAL AIRWAY

The surgical airway is indicated in patients with life-threatening airway obstruction where basic positional methods and endotracheal intubation (or alternatives) have failed.

In prehospital care access to the trachea should be made through the cricothyroid membrane unless there is severe trauma in this region. Tracheostomy in the emergency situation is very difficult and is usually hampered by severe bleeding from the thyroid vessels.

A number of methods of gaining access to the airway through the cricothyroid membrane have been developed. These include:

- needle cricothyroidotomy
- surgical cricothyroidotomy
- blind stab techniques using specially designed equipment
- percutaneous dilation methods.

All these methods are difficult and hazardous in the prehospital situation with a gasping patient. They should only be undertaken in extreme circumstances. In the first instance the recommended method is needle cricothyroidotomy.

NEEDLE CRICOTHYROIDOTOMY

The procedure is shown in Figure 7.12.

1. A 14 gauge intravenous cannula directed slightly towards the feet (caudally) is introduced through the cricothyroid membrane, while aspirating continually through an attached 20 ml syringe until a free flow of air is obtained.
2. The needle is withdrawn, leaving the cannula in situ.
3. Correct placement of the cannula is reconfirmed by free aspiration of air.
4. A 14 gauge cannula is of insufficient diameter to allow any significant spontaneous ventilation to occur. Positive pressure ventilation can be provided using a self-inflating bag attached to a 3 mm tracheal tube connector which will fit a Luer intravenous connection. *Ventilation provided by this method is marginal and sufficient only to buy a few minutes' time until an alternative is available.*
5. Adequate ventilation *can* be provided using a high-pressure jet injector system. The cannula is connected by non-compliant tubing to an oxygen cylinder fitted with a regulator, which will produce a pressure in the region of 400 kPa. This is the pressure produced by an oxygen cylinder before a flow meter is attached and requires a special fitting.
6. Inflation is produced by a finger intermittently occluding a hole in the tubing or by a specially designed system with a manually operated trigger which produces inflation when depressed. Alternatively, a "Y" connector may be used to connect the tubing to the cannula, with the stem of the "Y" towards the patient and one of the top ends attached via the tubing to the oxygen supply. The open branch can be intermittently occluded to produce insufflation. Each inflation must be very carefully observed and the trigger immediately released when normal chest expansion occurs, in order to avoid lung barotrauma.
7. Time must be left for lung deflation (1 second inflation: 4 seconds deflation). For the technique to be safe there must be a clear route through the larynx and mouth for the expired gases, otherwise lung barotrauma will occur with gross, life-threatening subcutaneous and mediastinal emphysema.

SURGICAL CRICOTHYROIDOTOMY

Surgical cricothyroidotomy (Figure 7.13) may occasionally be performed by a medical practitioner before the patient reaches hospital.

1. A 2–3 cm transverse stab incision is made through the cricothyroid membrane.
2. The scalpel handle is then placed in the incision and rotated 90° to the vertical.
3. A pair of forceps may be inserted into the wound to maintain the track.
4. A 6–7 mm lubricated tracheal tube (tracheal/tracheotomy) is inserted through the incision and directed towards the lower trachea.

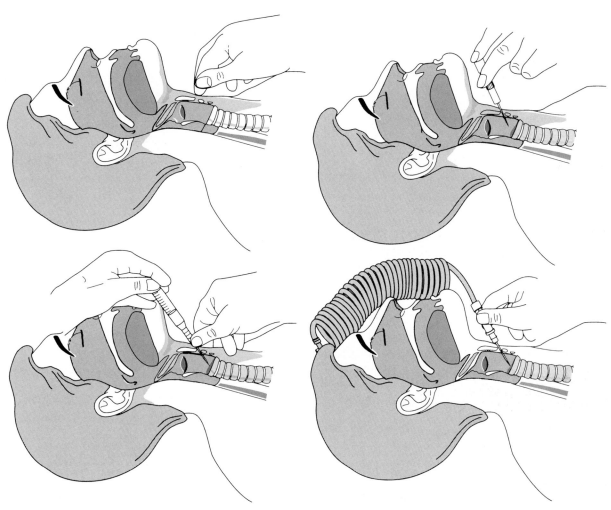

Figure 7.12 Needle cricothyroidotomy

5. The cuff is inflated and the tube is secured with a tape and connected to the ventilating apparatus.

This method provides the optimum emergency surgical airway.

BLIND STAB TECHNIQUES

Access to the trachea can be achieved with methods that use a blind stab through the skin, subcutaneous tissues and cricothyroid membrane. A bougie (Portex Mini-Trach II) (Figure 7.14) or expandable trocar system (Nu-Trach) is passed through the incision and directed into the trachea and a tube inserted over the bougie or through the trocar. With the Mini-Trach system a 4 mm uncuffed tube is provided which is adequate for only about 1 hour. Using serial dilations, however, a tube of 6.5 mm can be inserted. With the Nu-Trach, tubes of 6–6.5 mm can be placed directly.

Blind stab techniques present considerable problems in the gasping patient in the emergency setting and it can be very difficult to find the passage through the skin incision and into the trachea. This is because the larynx moves under the skin, with the result that the incision in the cricoid membrane is no longer directly beneath the skin incision.

PERCUTANEOUS DILATIONAL CRICOTHYROIDOTOMY

The Melker percutaneous dilational cricothyroidotomy kit is shown in Figure 7.15. The technique should only be performed by a medical practitioner.

1. A needle is inserted through the cricothyroid membrane into the trachea and correct placement is confirmed by aspiration of air. A guidewire is passed through the needle and the needle removed.
2. An incision is made in the skin alongside the guidewire and extended to pierce the cricothyroid membrane beneath.
3. A dilator is passed over the guidewire into the trachea and moved up and down to ensure a hole of sufficient size in the membrane.

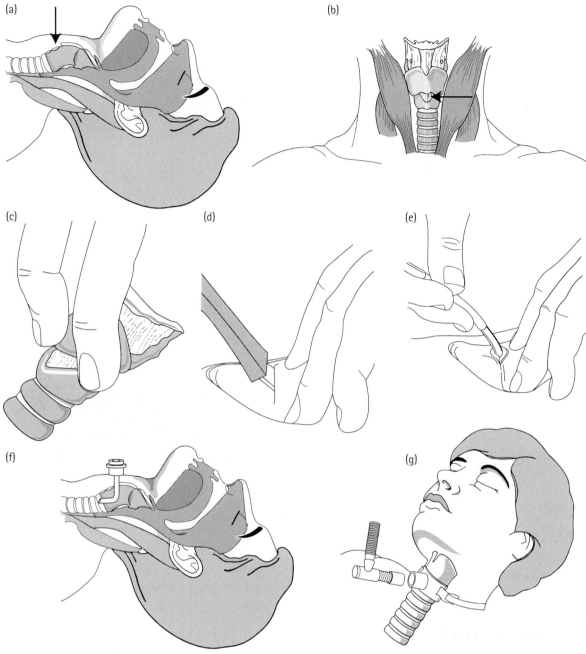

Figure 7.13 Surgical cricothyroidotomy

4. A 6–6.5 mm lubricated tube is passed over the dilator into the trachea.
5. The dilator is removed and the tube is secured with a tie; the tube cuff is inflated and the tube connected to the ventilation apparatus.

For prehospital use the best methods of achieving a surgical airway are needle cricothyroidotomy or direct surgical cricothyroidotomy.

The percutaneous dilation method is not appropriate for routine prehospital use.

ADVANCED VENTILATION TECHNIQUES

Oxygen-powered resuscitators have been designed to take over from the self-inflating bag. They are driven from a high-pressure (400 kPa) oxygen source, so are valuable in contaminated atmospheres. The devices may be connected to a face mask, tracheal tube, laryngeal mask, Combitube or intubating laryngeal mask. The equipment should be designed to restrict the inspiratory flow rates to a maximum of 40 litres per minute and should incorporate a blow-off valve with automatic warning if the inflation pressure exceeds 60 cmH$_2$O in adults.

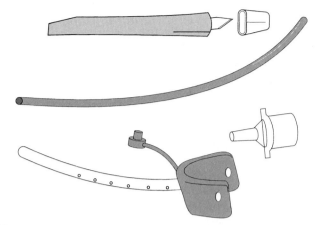

Figure 7.14 The Portex Mini-Trach system

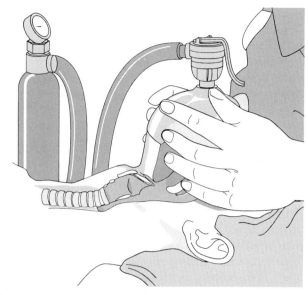

Figure 7.16 A manually triggered resuscitator

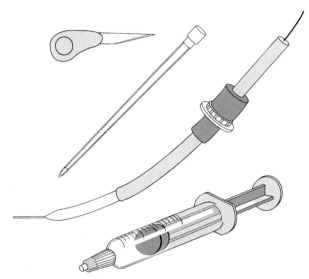

Figure 7.15 Percutaneous dilational cricothyroidotomy equipment

Two types are available:

- manually triggered resuscitators
- automatically triggered resuscitators.

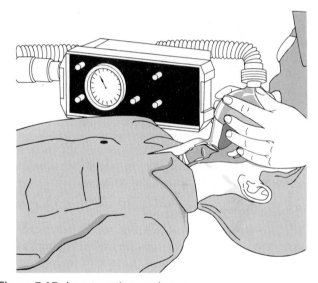

Figure 7.17 An automatic resuscitator

MANUALLY TRIGGERED RESUSCITATORS

Manually triggered resuscitators (Figure 7.16) are triggered by pressing a lever or button at the patient valve. Both hands are used to ensure an airtight fit and to maintain airway alignment if a face mask is used but there is a lack of direct "feel", compared with a self-inflating bag, during the inspiratory phase. This may increase the risk of gastric inflation, and consequently these devices are not recommended for use in the prehospital setting.

Unlike the automatic resuscitator, one operator is committed to providing continuing ventilation, even when a tracheal tube is in place. Some models have a triggered demand valve to provide assisted ventilation in time with the patient's own inspiratory efforts.

AUTOMATIC RESUSCITATORS

Automatic resuscitators (Figure 7.17) cycle between inspiration and expiration using a fluid logic system or by electronic control. For prehospital work, cycling should be related to volume and time, not to pressure.

The automatic resuscitator provides consistent automatic ventilation at the preset tidal volume, rate and respiratory pattern. If a tracheal tube, Combitube, laryngeal mask or intubating laryngeal mask is in place the rescuer is free to attend to other tasks, such as venous cannulation, splinting or defibrillation.

Automatic resuscitators vary in versatility in terms of variation of the inspiratory and expiratory pattern. Some models have the option of ventilation with air/oxygen mixtures to conserve oxygen supplies and some incorporate a demand valve to synchronize with the patient's own inspiratory efforts.

Models with a low inspiratory flow rate and a blow-off valve with an audible warning signal (e.g. Pneupac) are most satisfactory. They are said to carry less danger of gastric inflation than a self-inflating bag when used with a face mask.

VENTILATION PATTERNS

INSPIRATORY FLOW RATES

High inspiratory flow rates are associated with a higher incidence of gastric inflation in the unprotected airway owing to a raised inflation pressure. There is also reduced alveolar ventilation with a tendency to lung collapse.

In normal adult patients the inspiratory phase should occupy 1.5–2 seconds and longer if there is an increased resistance to inspiration. Resuscitators should not generate inspiratory flow rates in excess of 40 litres per minute.

EXPIRATORY FLOW RATES

Generally the expiratory time should be about twice as long as the inspiratory time. It may need to be even longer in patients with increased expiratory resistance, for example, bronchospasm due to asthma or chronic pulmonary disease.

POSITIVE END-EXPIRATORY PRESSURE

Valves can be fitted to resuscitators or self-inflating bags which provide an obstruction to expiratory pressure above zero. Such valves can usually operate with a range of 0–10 cmH$_2$O positive end-expiratory pressure (PEEP). Usually 5 cmH$_2$O PEEP is sufficient.

PEEP allows recruitment of collapsed or oedematous alveoli and so increases the oxygen saturation in the systemic circulation. The technique is valuable in near-drowning, smoke inhalation and some cases of primary cardiac arrest due to cardiac origin. However, it may be associated with a fall in cardiac output and blood pressure, particularly in hypovolaemic patients. It is not a technique generally available in prehospital care.

NEBULIZERS

Nebulizers are increasingly used for the prehospital management of bronchospasm. Salbutamol is commonly available for paramedic and technician use and when given by nebulizer, it is rapidly effective.

The most appropriate nebulizer for prehospital care is the gas-driven type. Oxygen, the carrier gas, is passed through a nozzle and generates an area of low pressure around it. The liquid drug placed beneath this area of low pressure is drawn up into the gas stream as droplets and carried forward to the face mask for inhalation. Although simple gas-driven nebulizers may not produce droplets of sufficiently small size to reach the extremes of the bronchial tree, in the main the droplets are small enough to be effective in the proximal areas, provided the flow rate is set at the level recommended by the manufacturer of the nebulizer.

The nebulizer (normally containing 2.5 ml) can be refilled and used several times in refractory cases.

FURTHER READING

American Heart Association 1992 National Consensus Conference Standards and Guidelines for Cardiopulmonary Resuscitation (CPR) and Emergency Cardiac Care (ECC). Journal of the American Medical Association 268: 2171–2307

Baskett PJF 1993 Resuscitation Handbook, 2nd edn. Mosby, London

Baskett PJF, Daw ACC, Nolan JP 1994 Practical procedures in anaesthesia and critical care. Gower Medical Publishing, London

Colquhoun M, Handley AJ, Evans TR (eds) 1999 The ABC of resuscitation, 4th edn. BMJ Books, London

Committee on Trauma of the American College of Surgeons 1993 Advanced trauma life support instructor manual. American College of Surgeons, Chicago

Driscoll P, Skinner D, Earlam R (eds) 2000 The ABC of major trauma, 3rd edn. BMJ Books, London

Eaton CJ 1999 Essentials of immediate care, 2nd edn. Churchill Livingstone, London

European Resuscitation Council (Ed. Bossaert L) 1998 Guidelines for resuscitation. Elsevier Science, Amsterdam

Finucane BT, Santora A 1996 Principles of airway management, 2nd edn. Mosby Year Book, St Louis, Missouri

Hagberg CA 2000 Handbook of difficult airway management. Churchill Livingstone, Philadelphia

Chapter 8

Intravenous access

The ability to gain access to the circulation is an essential skill which all those involved in the care of critically ill or injured patients must acquire. Intravenous access allows a number of therapeutic options:

- Fluid can be given to restore or maintain a patient's circulation.
- Drugs can be administered – for example, adrenaline during a cardiac arrest: this eliminates the delays and uncertainty following intramuscular or subcutaneous administration.
- A blood sample can be taken: this can be sent ahead to the receiving hospital so that crossmatched blood is available when the patient arrives.

The most common technique used to achieve venous access is by percutaneous puncture of a peripheral vein using a metal needle and subsequent introduction of a small-bore plastic tube or cannula into the vein. In small children this technique is relatively difficult as their veins are smaller and not easily identifiable and the intraosseous route is being used with increasing frequency. However, in some patients it may be necessary to surgically expose a vein and insert a cannula under direct vision, the "cut-down" technique, which may rarely be performed by a medical team at the scene of an entrapment.

Venous cannulation is an invasive procedure and must not be treated with complacency; nor should intravenous cannulation be attempted simply because it appears feasible.

Studies in both the UK and USA have found that up to two-thirds of the cannulae inserted prehospital are never used therapeutically. Furthermore, insertion before reaching hospital does not shorten the time to the subsequent intravenous administration of any treatment in the emergency department. In an increasingly cost-conscious health service, an intravenous cannula should only be inserted when clinically indicated. In general, in trauma, intravenous access should only be gained at the scene if the patient is trapped or for the provision of analgesia if appropriate. Otherwise, cannulation should be performed en route to hospital. In medical emergencies, early cannulation may be necessary for therapeutic interventions such as the administration of a thrombolytic.

When a patient does require an intravenous cannula, insertion is most likely to be successful and potential problems minimized if the person performing cannulation:

- Has knowledge of the anatomy of the site chosen
- Is familiar with the equipment to be used
- Understands the technique to be used
- Is aware of the potential complications.

Obtaining intravenous access is a skill which is best learnt and maintained by practice and once acquired, if used appropriately will enhance patient care and help save lives. The following description is only intended as a guide and is not a substitute for practice under the guidance of an expert.

ANATOMY

VEINS USED FOR INTRAVENOUS ACCESS

The veins most commonly used are the superficial peripheral veins in the upper limbs. If for any reason these are not accessible then the saphenous vein at the ankle can be used. In cases where turning the head to one side (for ease of access) is not contraindicated (as it is in trauma), cannulation of the external jugular vein may be considered.

The dorsum of the hand and forearm

The veins in the upper limb appear at first to be very variable in their layout, but certain common arrangements are found.

The veins draining the fingers unite to form three *dorsal metacarpal veins*. Laterally these are joined by veins from the thumb and continue up the radial border of the forearm as the *cephalic vein* (Figure 8.1).

Medially the metacarpal veins unite with the veins from the little finger and pass up the ulnar border or forearm as the *basilic vein*. There is often a large vein in the middle of the ventral (anterior) aspect of the forearm, the *median vein of the forearm* (Figure 8.2).

The antecubital fossa

Although the veins in this area are prominent and easily cannulated, there are many adjacent important structures which can be easily damaged. The cephalic vein passes through the antecubital fossa on the lateral side and the basilic vein enters the antecubital fossa medially, just in front of the medial epicondyle of the elbow. These two large veins are joined by the *median cubital* or *antecubital vein*. The median vein of the forearm also drains into the basilic vein (Figure 8.2).

Other structures of importance

- The brachial artery lies beneath the median cubital vein, deep to the biceps tendon, and can be felt pulsating beneath this vein.
- Medial to the brachial artery is the median nerve.
- Branches of the medial cutaneous nerve of the forearm lie adjacent to the basilic vein and the lateral cutaneous nerve of forearm lies adjacent to the cephalic vein.

The ankle

The most accessible vein in the ankle region is the long saphenous vein. It is consistent in its location, found 2 cm in front

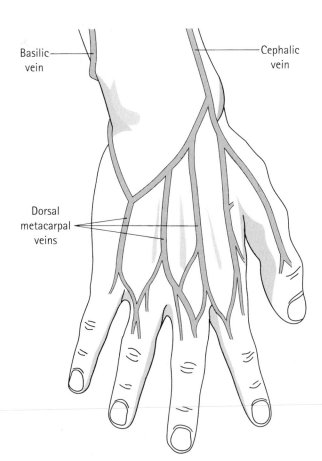

Figure 8.1 Veins of the hand and forearm

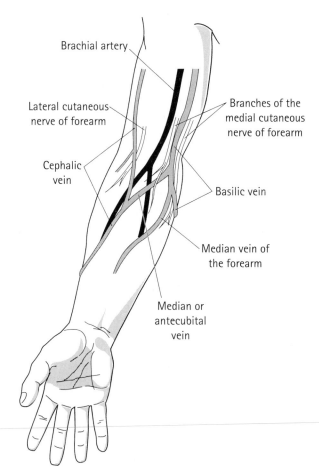

Figure 8.2 Veins and other structures of the forearm and antecubital fossa

and 2 cm above the medial malleolus in adults (Figure 8.3). It is associated closely with the saphenous nerve.

The neck

Although there are many large veins in the neck, the most easily identified and accessible is the external jugular vein. This begins at the angle of the mandible and runs downwards and forwards to pass behind the middle of the clavicle (Figure 8.4). The vein is relatively superficial, covered only by a thin sheet of muscle (platysma), fascia and skin. Its use is precluded by the application of a semi-rigid collar or in any case where there is a possibility of spinal injury.

EQUIPMENT

A variety of devices of different lengths and diameters are used to secure venous access. The term "cannula" is here used for those of 7 cm or less in length, and "catheter" for those longer than 7 cm. The outside diameter of the device is quoted either in millimetres or in terms of its "gauge". Diameter increases with decreasing gauge (see Table 8.1).

CANNULAE

The most popular device used in the UK to achieve venous access is the cannula over needle (for example, Venflon). These devices are available in a variety of sizes, from 12 to 27 gauge. They consist of a plastic (PTFE or similar material) cannula which is mounted on a smaller diameter metal needle, the bevel of which protrudes from the cannula. The other end of the needle is attached to a transparent "flashback" chamber, which fills with blood indicating that the needle bevel lies within the vein (Figure 8.5a). Some devices have flanges or wings to facilitate attachment to the skin (Figure 8.5b). All cannulae have a standard Luer connector for attaching a giving set and some have a valved injection port through which drugs can be administered (Figure 8.5c).

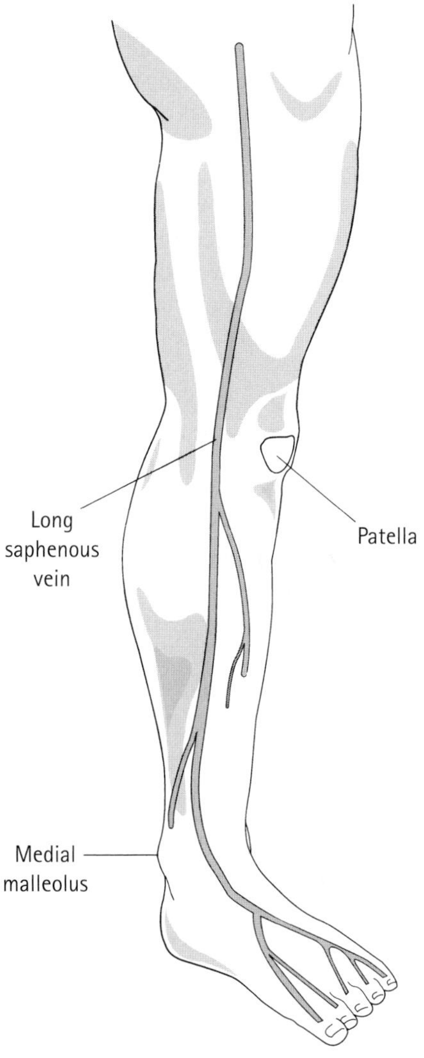

Figure 8.3 The long saphenous vein

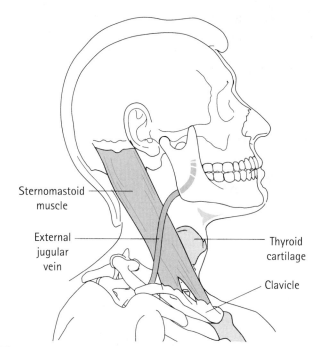

Figure 8.4 The right external jugular vein

Table 8.1 Rate of water flow through different sizes of Venflon cannulae

Colour	Diameter (mm)	Gauge	Length (mm)	Flow (ml/min)
Pink	1.0	20	32	54
Green	1.2	18	45	80
Grey	1.7	16	45	180
Brown	2.0	14	45	270

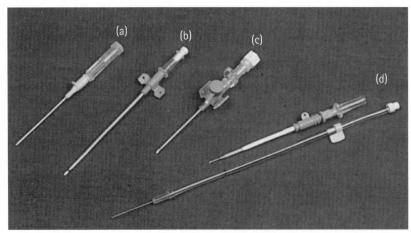

Figure 8.5 Intravenous cannulae: (a) Cannula over needle; (b) cannula over needle with wings; (c) cannula with injection port; (d) Seldinger needle

An alternative method is the Seldinger technique. The vein is initially punctured percutaneously with a small needle, through which a blunt, flexible wire is inserted into the vein. The needle is then withdrawn, leaving the wire in the vein and finally, a relatively large cannula is inserted (sometimes over a dilator) into the vein. The technique can therefore be used to allow the insertion of a large-diameter catheter without having to use a large-diameter needle (Figure 8.5d).

The Seldinger technique is useful when cannulating the external jugular vein. Although it is commonly used in the emergency department, it is not currently widely used in the prehospital environment.

TECHNIQUE OF INTRAVENOUS CANNULATION

The superficial veins are situated immediately under the skin in the superficial fascia along with a variable amount of subcutaneous fat. The veins are relatively mobile within this layer and are also capable of considerable variation in their diameter. These details are of particular importance when it comes to inserting an intravenous cannula. The size of cannula used will depend upon its purpose: large ones are required for rapid fluid administration, smaller ones for drug administration.

Although in principle the largest cannula possible should be inserted, there is no point attempting to insert a large cannula into a very small vein and failing. The largest cannula which can *successfully* be inserted into the vein should always be chosen.

> As with any procedure where there is a risk of contact with body fluids, gloves should be worn by the operator

CANNULA OVER NEEDLE

1. Choose a vein capable of accommodating the size of cannula needed, preferably one that is both visible and palpable (Figure 8.6). The junction of two veins is often a good site as the "target" is larger and the veins tend to be less mobile.

2. The vein should be allowed to dilate as this increases the success rate of cannulation. In the limb veins this is usually achieved by using a proximal tourniquet which stops venous return from the limb but permits arterial flow into the limb. Further dilation can be encouraged by gently tapping the skin over the vein. When cannulating the external jugular vein, if it is safe to do so, the patient can be tipped slightly head down to encourage the vein to dilate. Turning the patient's head to the opposite side will also facilitate cannula insertion.

3. The skin over the vein should be cleaned. If alcohol-based agents are used, they must be given time to work (2–3 minutes), ensuring that the skin is dry before proceeding further. This is not appropriate when rapid access is needed, such as during a cardiac arrest.

4. The vein should now be immobilized in order to prevent it being displaced by the advancing cannula. This is achieved by pulling the skin over the vein tight, with the operator's free hand (Figure 8.7).

5. Holding the cannula firmly, at an angle of 10–15° to the skin, it should be advanced through the skin and into the vein. Often a slight loss of resistance is felt as the vein is entered. This should be accompanied by the appearance of blood in the flashback chamber of the cannula (Figure 8.8). However, the appearance of blood indicates only that the tip of the needle is within the vein, not necessarily any of the plastic cannula.

6. While keeping the skin taut, the next step is to reduce the angle of the cannula slightly and advance it a further 2–3 mm into the vein. This is to ensure that the first part of the plastic cannula lies within the vein. Care must be taken at this point not to push the needle out of the back of the vein.

7. The needle is now withdrawn 5–10 mm into the cannula so that the point no longer protrudes from the end. As this is done, blood will often be seen to flow between the needle body and the cannula, confirming that the tip of the cannula is within the vein (Figure 8.9).

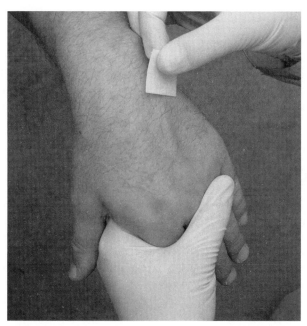

Figure 8.6 Vein ready for cannulation

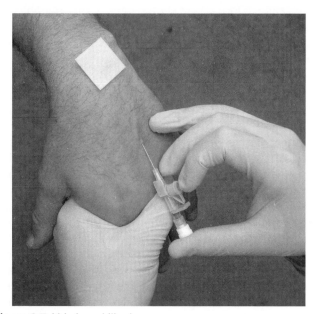

Figure 8.7 Vein immobilized

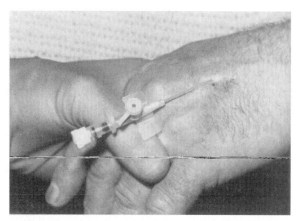

Figure 8.8 Inserting an intravenous cannula: the "flashback"

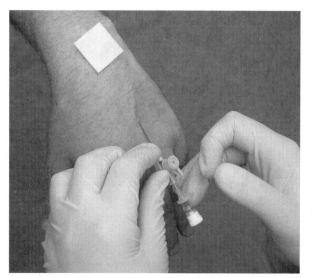

Figure 8.9 Inserting an intravenous cannula: withdrawing the needle

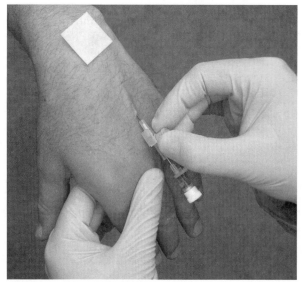

Figure 8.10 Inserting an intravenous cannula: the cannula inserted

8. The cannula and needle are advanced along the vein together. The needle is retained within the cannula to provide support and prevent kinking at the point of skin puncture (Figure 8.10).
9. Once the cannula is inserted as far as the hub, the tourniquet should be released and the needle completely removed and disposed of safely.
10. Confirmation that the cannula lies within the vein should be made by injection of a saline flush. The tissues around the site must be observed for any signs of swelling that may indicate that the cannula is incorrectly positioned. Finally, the cannula should be secured using adhesive tape (e.g. Elastoplast) or a specific cannula dressing (e.g. Vecafix).

COMPLICATIONS

There are a number of complications associated with venous cannulation. Most of them are minor; however, this must not be used as an excuse for carelessness and poor technique. The complications are conveniently divided into "early" and "late".

EARLY COMPLICATIONS

Failure of cannulation

This is the most common complication, usually as a result of pushing the needle completely through the vein, and is due to inexperience or poor technique, usually when the angle between the cannula and the skin is too large at the time of insertion. If possible, it is always best to start distally in a limb and work proximally. In this way, if further attempts are required, fluid or drugs will not leak from previous puncture sites.

Haematoma

These are usually secondary to failed cannulation when inadequate pressure has been applied to prevent blood leaking from the vein. They are made worse by forgetting to remove the tourniquet. Simply bending the arm is not adequate to prevent bleeding from a puncture site – direct local pressure is required.

Extravasation

Leakage of fluid or drugs into the tissues is commonly a result of failing to recognize that the cannula is not within the vein before beginning the infusion. Pressurized infusions are more likely to extravasate, but the commonest cause of this problem is failure to establish whether the cannula is correctly sited before beginning the infusion. Once the problem is identified, the cannula must no longer be used. Damage to the adjacent tissues will depend primarily upon the nature of the extravasated fluid.

Damage to local structures

This is secondary to poor technique and lack of knowledge of the local anatomy. The greatest risks are when attempting to cannulate the external jugular vein.

Air embolus

Air embolus occurs when the pressure in the veins is lower than in the right side of the heart and air is entrained. It is usually prevented from occurring via the peripheral veins as they collapse when empty, but a cannula will splint the vein open. It is most likely to happen in the external jugular vein, particularly if the patient is in a head-up position.

Breakage of the cannula

The plastic cannula can be sheared, allowing fragments to enter the circulation. This is usually a result of trying to reintroduce the needle into the cannula after it has been withdrawn. The safest action is to withdraw the whole cannula and attempt cannulation at another site with a new cannula.

LATE COMPLICATIONS

Infection and inflammation

Localized infection at the site of the skin puncture is more common in cannulae inserted in the prehospital environment. At its worst, it can lead to local abscess formation or systemic infection. The risk of infection occurring can be minimized by cleaning the skin and not palpating the vein after the skin has been cleaned.

Inflammation of the vein, thrombophlebitis, is related to the length of time the vein is in use and irritation caused by the substances flowing through it. Drugs in high concentration and fluids with extremes of pH or high osmolality are the main causes. Once a vein shows signs of thrombophlebitis (tenderness, redness and deteriorating flow), the cannula must be removed to prevent subsequent infection or thrombosis which may spread proximally.

INTRAOSSEOUS ACCESS

Percutaneous venous cannulation is often more difficult in children, particularly when they are critically ill. The intraosseous route has been demonstrated to provide rapid and effective access to the circulation. It allows the administration of fluids and drugs, with circulating levels of drugs being comparable to those achieved when given via a central vein. Furthermore, aspirated marrow can be used to test blood glucose level and to crossmatch blood in the absence of a blood sample. It is a technique most suited to children less than 6 years old, since beyond this age the vascular red marrow is gradually replaced by fatty yellow marrow.

ANATOMY

The proximal tibia is the most commonly used site for intraosseous access, alternatives being the distal tibia and distal femur.

Three sites can be used for intraosseous access (Figure 8.11).

● The anteromedial surface of the tibia, 2–3 cm below the tibial tuberosity
● The distal tibia, just proximal to the medial malleolus
● The anterior surface of the femur, 3 cm above the lateral condyle.

These sites are relatively free of other local important structures. The most relevant feature to be borne in mind is the

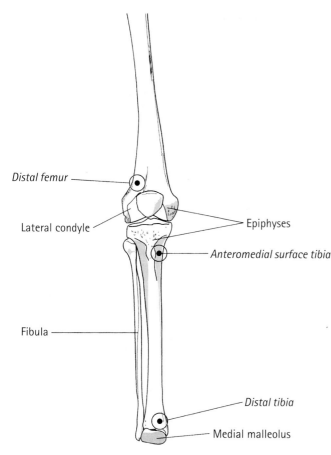

Figure 8.11 Distal femur, Lateral condyle, Epiphyses, Anteromedial surface tibia, Fibula, Distal tibia, Medial malleolus

Figure 8.11 Sites for intraosseous access in the lower limb

proximity of the epiphyses (growth plates). Damage to these could interfere with subsequent bone growth and development.

EQUIPMENT

A needle specifically designed for intraosseous access must be used. As they have to pierce the bone cortex, such needles are made entirely of metal. They come in a variety of designs but they all have certain features in common. The needles have a short shaft, with a central solid trocar, which has a large handle. The trocar must be unscrewed before it can be removed from the needle. The external end of the needle has a standard Luer fitting. Some needles have a screw thread to improve their security in the bone (Figure 8.12). If possible, a threaded needle should be used.

Intraosseous needles come in a range of sizes:

- 16–20 gauge for children younger than 18 months
- 12–16 gauge for children older than 18 months.

TECHNIQUE

1. An appropriate site is chosen, taking care to avoid placing the needle in a fractured bone. Placement of a needle in a distal bone (e.g., the tibia) in the presence of a proximal fracture (for

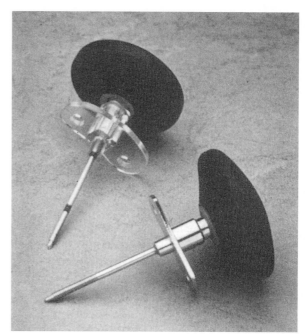

Figure 8.12 Intraosseous needles

example, of the femur) is acceptable. If the proximal tibia is used, it may help to place a firm support behind the knee.
2. If time permits, the skin over the site should be thoroughly cleaned. If the patient is conscious and time permits, local anaesthetic solution should be infiltrated into the skin and underlying periosteum.
3. The needle is then introduced at 90° through the skin to make contact with the bone and then advanced using a screwing action with threaded needles or a "bradawl"-type action with unthreaded needles, at the same time applying firm pressure.
4. A loss of resistance is felt as the cortex is penetrated by an unthreaded needle and the marrow cavity entered. The needle should feel as if it is "gripped" by the bone and should hold its position once released (Figure 8.13).
5. The trocar is unscrewed and removed and correct placement confirmed by the ability to aspirate bone marrow. This should always be used to check blood glucose level. Further confirmation is provided by being able to flush 5 ml of saline through the needle without resistance or signs of extravasation.

COMPLICATIONS

Complications are very rare and are mainly theoretical.

- Failure to enter the bone marrow cavity is the most common problem.
- If the needle is incorrectly placed, fluid may extravasate and prolonged infusion could cause a compartment syndrome. A second attempt at placement in the same bone will result, if successful, in leakage from the hole left by the previous attempt.
- Infection in the skin, abscess formation and ultimately osteomyelitis may occur, but these complications appear to be related to prolonged use of a needle.

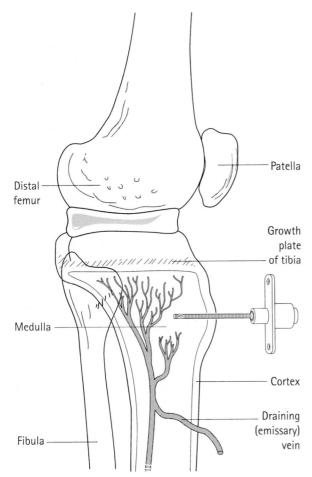

Distal femur

Patella

Growth plate of tibia

Medulla

Cortex

Draining (emissary) vein

Fibula

Figure 8.13 An intraosseous needle in place in the proximal tibia

- Damage to the growth plate of the bone could occur as a result of careless placement and in very young children, a fracture might occur if excessive force is used.

FLUID FLOW THROUGH CANNULAE AND CATHETERS

There are four factors that affect the rate at which fluid will flow through a cannula or catheter (Table 8.1).

- *The diameter*: this is the most important factor, with flow being proportional to the fourth power of the radius. This means that

doubling the diameter should result in flow increasing 16-fold (2^4). This is rarely achieved in practice but an increase of 4–5-fold can be expected.
- *The length*: flow is inversely proportional to the length of the cannula, therefore doubling the length will halve the flow.
- *The viscosity of the fluid*: flow is inversely proportional to the viscosity, therefore increasing viscosity reduces flow. Hence colloids and blood flow much more slowly than crystalloids particularly when they are cold.
- *The pressure applied*: increasing the pressure across the cannula will increase the flow. This is usually achieved by increasing the pressure of the fluid being administered, either by raising the height of the drip above the patient or by using external pressure.

FLOW THROUGH INTRAOSSEOUS NEEDLES

Fluid administration via an intraosseous line in children is most safely and effectively achieved by the administration of boluses by injection using a syringe and a three-way tap.

FURTHER READING

Advanced Life Support Course SubCommittee (eds) 1998 Advanced life support course provider manual, 3rd edn. Resuscitation Council (UK), London

Driscoll PA, Gwinnutt CL, Mackway-Jones K (eds) 2000 Advanced cardiac life support: the practical approach, 3rd edn. Arnold, London

Evans RJ, McCabe M, Thomas R 1994 Intraosseous infusion. British Journal of Hospital Medicine 51: 161–164

Halter M, Lees-Mlanga S, Snooks H, Koenig KL, Miller K 2000 Out-of-hospital intravenous cannulation: the perspective of patients treated by the London Ambulance Service paramedics. Academic Emergency Medicine 7: 127–133

Henderson RA, Thomas DP, Bahrs BA, Norman MP 1998 Unnecessary intravenous access in the emergency setting. Prehospital Emergency Care 2: 312–316

Tonks A 1992 How to put up a drip. Student British Medical Journal 1: 57–59

Section 3

MEDICINE

Chapter 9

Taking a medical history

INTRODUCTION

Obtaining a medical history is a core skill for any healthcare professional. It takes practice, discipline and empathy for the patient and it requires a structure. This structure serves two purposes. First, it acts as an *aide-mémoire*, so that the practitioner does not omit any vital questions or observations, and second, it facilitates the recording of the information in a way that will be accessible to other practitioners. Obtaining the medical history must not interfere with the initial management priorities of airway, breathing and circulation. Assessment and immediate appropriate action for any compromise of airway, breathing or circulation must take place first. Some elements of the history can be obtained during this action but the priorities of opening an airway, ensuring adequate ventilation and establishing adequate circulation to allow organ perfusion take precedence at all times.

This chapter describes a structure which is widely used in medicine and the allied professions. The skills of observation and retention of information until it can be written down must be practised over and over again until they become second nature.

In medical illness the history affords 70% of the information on which most diagnoses are made. If at the end of history taking a list of differential diagnoses is not apparent, then it is likely that a range of investigations in hospital will be necessary before the diagnosis becomes clear. The history is much more important than the physical examination in establishing a diagnosis.

The purposes of history taking are to:

- establish what has happened (*the history*)
- establish what the patient feels to be wrong (*the symptoms*)
- establish the background to the current events (*the past medical history*)
- establish what medication the patient is taking
- help establish a list of possible diagnoses (*the differential diagnosis*)
- help establish priorities for treatment
- obtain information that will not be available later (e.g. from the scene)
- establish a baseline from which subsequent monitoring can start (e.g. of the conscious level).

STRUCTURE OF THE HISTORY

However detailed or simple a medical history is being taken, a structured approach is essential. While at the scene a detailed history is not usually appropriate. A brief outline history is ample – and "AMPLE" is a useful mnemonic to remember what constitutes an adequate history from the scene.

A > ALLERGIES

In all emergencies other than cardiac arrest, it is important to try to establish any known allergies before drugs are administered.

M > MEDICINES

The presence of medications in the bloodstream may influence the response to injury or illness or to any other drugs which may be given. A knowledge of what medication the patient has been taking may indicate the severity and duration of any preexisting illness. A knowledge of the patient's medication may give vital clues, for example, in the management of a patient with breathlessness.

P > PAST MEDICAL HISTORY

The past medical history has a major bearing on responses to treatment and possible outcomes from illness or injury. It also offers vital clues as to what the current problem may be. Particular note should be made of any known cardiac disease, respiratory disease or such chronic conditions as diabetes or epilepsy.

L > LAST FOOD AND DRINK

A full stomach is a major risk factor for regurgitation and consequent airway compromise. It is also helpful to obtain information about the patient's nutritional status and general level of self-care.

E > EVENTS LEADING UP TO THE CURRENT PROBLEM

This is the core of the history. The other elements are important but this is the key to understanding what is happening to the patient now.

It is not necessary to go through the questions in the order in which they appear above. The events leading up to the current problem and the past medical history are usually the first two to be addressed. Not all of the information needs to be acquired at the scene; some can be acquired en route. In extremely urgent situations, rather than attempting to laboriously establish the drug history in detail, all medications should be gathered together and taken to hospital with the patient.

Nevertheless, the mnemonic "AMPLE" is a way of ensuring that all the relevant information is gathered and that nothing significant is forgotten.

> AMPLE is a series of "pegs" to hang the history on

SOURCES OF INFORMATION

THE SCENE

Gleaning information from the scene requires the practitioner to be a trained observer. If an important detail is not specifically looked for, it is unlikely to be found. Two pairs of eyes are better than one. Wherever possible, observations should be collated with those of a colleague before they are recorded. There may be vital clues at the scene and in the vast majority of cases only ambulance service personnel will have the chance of interpreting them and carrying the information to those who will subsequently be caring for the patient. Figure 9.1 is an example of a scenario and Box 9.1 suggests the information that may be gleaned from it.

THE PATIENT

When dealing with a conscious patient, the opening questions must be directed to the patient, even if he appears confused or aggressive. The response to initial questioning may or may not be meaningful but will give information as to the degree of cooperation with subsequent questions that can

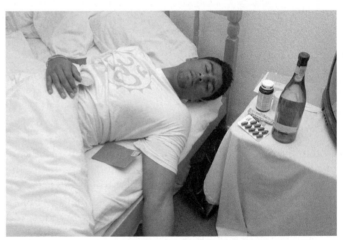

Figure 9.1 Information gathering at the scene: the call to a patient's home. See the questions in Box 9.1

Box 9.1 Information to be gleaned at the scene

You are called to the patient lying ill in bed (Figure 9.1).

- Are the patient and the surroundings clean and tidy?
- Are there carers present?
- Is it an environment to which the patient could return?
- Are there bottles of medication which could be taken to the hospital?
- Are there empty pill bottles indicating a possible overdose?
- Is there evidence of alcohol or drug abuse?
- If the patient is unconscious are there any clues at the scene that might help establish the duration or cause of the unconsciousness?

be expected. If there is no meaningful response, further information can then be sought from bystanders or witnesses.

THE WITNESSES

Even if the patient is conscious and cooperative, witnesses may help with information about the mechanism of injury not necessarily known to the patient. If the patient is unconscious, witnesses should be asked about the duration of the unconsciousness and specifically asked if the patient is getting worse, getting better or staying the same. Some witnesses or

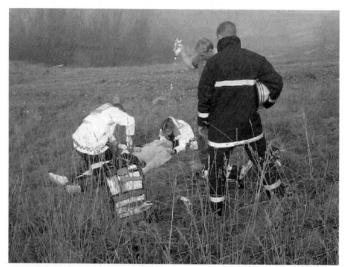

Figure 9.2 Information gathering from the scene. An unkempt young man is found collapsed and unconscious on waste ground where young people are known to congregate. What specific details should be sought by the practitioner?

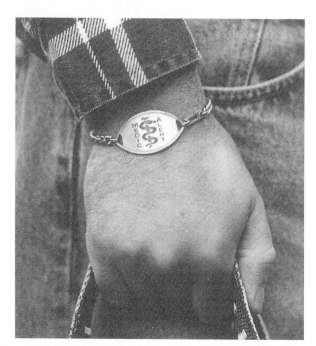

Figure 9.3 A Medic-Alert bracelet

bystanders may know the patient and be able to give background information.

MEDICAL INFORMATION DEVICES

Only a few patients in this country wear Medic-Alert bracelets or necklaces (Figure 9.3) but they are always worth looking for. Horse riders may carry medical information in a recess inside their crash helmet.

Many patients have lists of medication on their person and the elderly often carry containers with compartments for timed administration of tablets.

THE ART OF QUESTIONING

Obtaining information from frightened, ill or injured patients is made easier by a positive, confident and friendly approach. It is much less disorientating for patients if they can see who is talking to them. Patients who are confused or deaf may be reassured more by a smile than by the words that are spoken.

All patient contacts should begin with an introduction. The degree of familiarity will obviously depend on the age of the patient and the circumstances. Older patients appreciate the correct use of their surname and title, at the very least on first introductions. First names and terms such as "love", "mate" and "darling" are best avoided. The introduction should include your name and role and the fact that help has now arrived.

Maintain conversation with the patient

The patient's name and age should be established and his name used during the subsequent conversation. Whenever possible, practitioners should position themselves at the same level as the patient; for example, kneeling beside a patient who is lying on the floor. Eye contact should be maintained if possible. These manoeuvres take seconds but help establish empathy with the patient and make it likely that subsequent questions will be answered helpfully.

The questions which are asked will be dictated by the circumstances. Assessment and correction of any problems in airway, breathing and circulation will take priority. The circumstances and the urgency of the situation will dictate how many questions are asked at the scene, how many can be asked en route and how many will need to be left to the hospital staff.

In general terms questioning should begin with broad, open questions; for example: *"Tell me what's the matter"*. Questions such as this allow patients to express what they perceive to be wrong. An open question can be followed by a more focused question. For instance, if the answer to the question above is *"I've got a pain in my chest"*, then the next question might be along the lines of *"Tell me about the pain"*. If, after the patient has volunteered more information, still more detail is needed, questions can become more focused, for example:

"What's the pain like?"
"How long have you had it?"
"Have you ever had a pain like this before?"
"What makes the pain worse?"

The transition from open questions to more focused questions is dictated by a knowledge of what information is needed to help with decision making in any given clinical situation. Knowing the right questions to ask requires a thorough knowledge of the conditions in the differential diagnosis. It is a useful exercise to compile and learn lists of relevant questions for a specific clinical symptom. Examples might include chest pain and shortness of breath. Having, for example, a set of "chest pain questions" which can be modified as more information becomes available reduces the chance of important questions being forgotten and allows the focusing of the questioning.

It requires discipline to remember all the answers so that they can be formulated into a chronological statement of what the patient has said. It is important not to change the history when writing it down and whenever possible, the patient's own expressions should be used in inverted commas to describe the symptoms.

(Chest pain) *"like an iron band round my chest"* is virtually specific to myocardial ischaemia.

(Sudden pain) *"like a severe blow in the back of the neck"* suggests subarachnoid haemorrhage.

PASSING ON THE INFORMATION

The key points of the history should be recorded with brevity and clarity. In many situations a printed form assists recording of the history and findings at the scene. Such documentation makes it easier for subsequent carers to refer back to information that might be lost if it is not recorded and kept with the patient.

Another way to transmit information is by telling the receiving doctor, or other professional, what has been found. This can be done succinctly and quickly, but requires practice and discipline. The summary should include the patient's name (if known), the patient's age (if known), the events surrounding the involvement of the emergency medical services and any past history that has been gleaned. Most people cannot receive more information than that at the early part of the handover. Many receiving rooms have a chalkboard or flipchart on which prehospital personnel can record information that may be useful later. The receiving doctor or other professionals will need a brief handover initially but will generally have more time to receive information after they have completed the primary survey, which may only take a very few minutes. Nevertheless, it is essential that prehospital personnel are actively involved in the handover and do not leave until they have imparted all the information that they think is relevant to the case. Good emergency departments will ensure a brief period of undivided attention to the incoming crew for the initial brief handover. A copy of the prehospital record must accompany the inpatient notes to allow a complete picture of the injury or illness to be recorded.

CONCLUSION

History taking is a core skill which requires practice. The key is knowing which questions to ask and asking them in a thorough, logical manner without significant omissions. The relevant questions will vary according to the clinical scenario or presenting complaint. Experience and a knowledge of individual systems and the symptoms associated with their pathology will assist in effective, focused information gathering.

FURTHER READING

Munro 1996 Macleod's clinical examination. Churchill Livingstone, Edinburgh

Marsh 1998 History and physical examination. Elsevier, London

Chapter 10

Therapeutics

Clinical pharmacology concerns how drugs are used in the treatment of illness and disease. It involves the four specialist disciplines of pharmaceutics, pharmacokinetics, pharmacodynamics and therapeutics. *Pharmaceutics* concerns the chemical process of creating and formulating drugs and medicines to allow them to be administered in different ways and by different routes. *Pharmacokinetics* concerns how the body handles drugs and medicines once they have been given while *pharmacodynamics* concerns the biochemical and physiological actions of drugs once they reach their site of action (how drugs act on the body). *Therapeutics* is the practical application of clinical pharmacology and concerns the beneficial and toxic effects of drugs in clinical conditions.

This chapter discusses the general principles of therapeutics in the prehospital environment and describes in detail those drugs that are most commonly used.

WHAT IS A DRUG?

The World Health Organization defines a drug as *"any substance or product that is used or intended to be used to modify or explore physiological systems or pathological states for the benefit of the recipient"*. Put simply, a drug is a chemical that has an effect on the function of the body. Individual drugs are the active ingredients of medicines that also contain other substances to help maintain the stability of the drug or allow it to be delivered in a particular way.

HOW ARE DRUGS REGULATED?

The Medicines and Healthcare Products Regulatory Agency (MHRA) is responsible for licensing drugs in the UK. Before a drug is allowed onto the commercial market it must undergo a period of intense research. The safety profile of a drug is established using both animal and human studies. Eventually a drug may be granted a product licence which allows the drug to be legally sold. Such licences are granted country by country, so a drug that is used on a day-to-day basis in the UK may not be legally allowed in another country.

Depending on the drug's safety record and potency, it may be given one of several legal categories. When a medicine is licensed it is classified as either a prescription-only medicine (PoM), such as adrenaline, a pharmacy medicine (P), such as loperamide (a treatment for diarrhoea), which can be sold only from registered pharmacies under the supervision of a pharmacist, or a general sales list medicine such as aspirin. Some drugs may also come under the Misuse of Drugs Regulations 1985 and are described as "controlled drugs". Special arrangements must be made to safeguard these drugs and document their use.

The use of drugs and medicines is controlled under the Medicines Act of 1968 and its amendments. Most emergency drugs are PoMs. Only a registered medical practitioner and some nurses can prescribe PoMs. However, a mechanism for exemption exists within the Medicines Act which allows ambulance paramedics who hold a certificate of proficiency in paramedic skills issued by, or with the approval of the Secretary of State, to supply and administer PoMs in circumstances specified by local paramedic steering committees or their equivalent. The Joint Royal Colleges Ambulance Liaison Committee (JRCALC) is the body that makes applications for exemption for the drugs listed in the formulary below. The JRCALC National Clinical Guidelines for use by UK ambulance services provide the most up-to-date list of relevant drugs (see www.asancep.org.uk/JRCALC/guidelines).

WHY SO MANY NAMES?

Each drug has several "names". The first of these, the *chemical name*, describes the drug's chemical structure. It is often too long and unwieldy to use on a day-to-day basis and hence each drug is given a simplified version known as its *generic* or *non-proprietary name*. As different drug companies will sell the same drug in a competitive market, each company will give the drug a third *trade* or *proprietary name* that identifies it to their company. Hence for metoclopramide, a drug commonly used with morphine to prevent nausea, the following names exist.

- Chemical name: 4-amino-5-chloro-*N*-[2-(diethylamino)ethyl] 1-2-methoxybenzamide
- Generic name: metoclopramide
- Trade name: Maxolon.

Other trade names for common emergency drugs are Crystapen for benzylpenicillin, Diazemuls for diazepam emulsion, GlucaGen for glucagon, Nubain for nalbuphine and Syntometrine for ergotamine with oxytocin.

A recent European Directive required the use of the international non-proprietary name for all medicinal substances. In most cases the names used in the UK and elsewhere were identical but there are three emergency drugs which have different names in the UK. These are adrenaline (epinephrine), lignocaine (lidocaine) and frusemide (furosemide). To prevent confusion, these drugs are likely to have both names written on the packs and ampoules for several years.

HOW ARE DRUGS GIVEN?

In order for a drug to produce an effect, it must be able to reach the site of action and then interact with the body on a cellular or biochemical level. These effects are governed by the properties of the drug:

- the chemical structure and formulation of the drug (pharmaceutics)
- the absorption, distribution, metabolism and excretion of the drug (pharmacokinetics)
- the biochemical and physiological effects of drugs (pharmacodynamics).

The basic actions of drugs used in prehospital care are provided in the formulary below. Further details of pharmaceutics, pharmacokinetics and pharmacodynamics can be obtained from standard pharmacology texts. It is useful, however, to have a clear understanding of some basic principles. For a drug to have a desired effect it should:

- reach its target organ at the right time
- reach its target organ in an appropriate dose
- reach its target organ in active form
- stay at the target organ for an appropriate period of time.

To reach the target organ, drugs can be administered in a variety of different ways. These are divided into *enteral* routes, via the alimentary canal (including oral, rectal, sublingual or buccal), and *parenteral* routes, which includes all routes not via the alimentary canal (intravenous, intramuscular, subcutaneous, inhalational and transdermal).

ENTERAL ROUTES

Oral

The oral route is the most common and convenient method of administration of drugs in medical practice. It is also usually the cheapest and simplest. Drugs are rarely given orally in prehospital care because the onset of action is generally slow (typically 30 minutes) and it is normal practice to keep patients nil-by-mouth prior to arrival at hospital. Many emergency drugs are inactivated by the liver if taken by mouth (e.g. atropine and lidocaine). There are, however, some situations where oral administration is appropriate. The most obvious example is the administration of glucose in hypoglycaemia (either in liquid form or as granulated sugar or sugar lumps – two teaspoons of sugar or three sugar lumps contain approximately 10 g of glucose). Oral analgesic agents such as paracetamol and ibuprofen may be useful when there is delay to treatment or the patient's injuries are such that it is not necessary for the patient to remain nil-by-mouth.

Rectal

Drugs may be given rectally in the form of suppositories or via a tube and are absorbed via the wall of the rectal passage. This method is suitable for patients who are nauseated, unconscious or unable to swallow or who have no intravenous access (for example, rectal diazepam in patients with seizures). Effects are seen 5–15 minutes after administration.

Sublingual

Tablets may be placed or an aerosol may be sprayed under the tongue (e.g. glyceryl trinitrate tablets and spray). The effect is very rapid (within 2–3 minutes). This route is ideal where rapid administration is required (for example, patients with angina), where patients are unable to swallow or where nausea and vomiting are present.

Buccal

Tablets absorbed via the mucous membrane of the gum (for example, modified-release glyceryl trinitrate). Effects can be seen within 2–3 minutes but can last much longer with modified-release preparations that slowly dissolve against the gum.

PARENTERAL ROUTES

Dermal patches

Patches impregnated with drug are placed on the skin and the drug is absorbed through the layers of the skin. This route is ideal for drugs that can be given slowly and that are rapidly inactivated (metabolized) when they enter the body, such as glyceryl trinitrate. Dermal patches are not used in prehospital care.

Intradermal

The intradermal route involves injection directly into the layers of the skin. Absorption is slow. This method is most commonly used for allergy testing. It is not used in prehospital care.

Intramuscular

The intramuscular (IM) route involves injection into muscle tissue where the blood supply absorbs the drug. This is a simple technique requiring less training than the administration of an intravenous injection and it may be life saving in patients where venous access is difficult (e.g. IM benzylpenicillin for suspected meningitis or meningococcal septicaemia). Absorption is slower than intravenous administration but faster than subcutaneous.

Subcutaneous

Injection of drug into the fatty tissue beneath the skin leads to slower absorption than that of intravenous or IM injection. It has been advocated for drugs that can have harmful consequences if absorbed too quickly.

Intravenous

Either as a slow intravenous (IV) injection or as an infusion where a drug is diluted in a bag of fluid. Direct introduction of a drug into the cardiovascular system provides a direct route to the target organs. This method has the highest risk of side-effects. It is the route by which most emergency drugs are given.

Endotracheal

The endotracheal route permits rapid absorption; it is useful when rapid administration is required and IV access is difficult or unobtainable. Drugs are injected at double the usual dose in a volume of 20 ml via a catheter placed in the endotracheal tube. Epinephrine and atropine can be given via an endotracheal tube in the early stages of cardiac arrest.

Inhaled or nebulized

Administration of liquid drugs as fine droplets in oxygen or air gives rapid effects, occurring in minutes (for example, salbutamol in acute asthma).

Intraosseous

A rigid needle is inserted directly into the bone marrow of a long bone. This is most often used in children and this route can be used to administer most drugs and fluids (the upper tibia is the preferred site).

PHARMACOKINETICS AND PHARMACODYNAMICS

Once a drug has been administered, the body acts on the drug in a number of ways. The absorption, distribution, metabolism and excretion of different drugs can be very complex. When the drug reaches the target organ it brings about biochemical and physiological effects through a variety of mechanisms: it may stimulate or block receptors, it may prevent chemicals moving across cell walls, it may inhibit or alter enzyme function or it may simply change the characteristics of other body chemicals. In emergency care, most drugs are manufactured in the most appropriate form for rapid administration and action. It is rarely necessary for prehospital practitioners to have to weigh up the advantages and disadvantages of different formulations of the same drug.

Pharmacokinetics uses complex mathematics to describe the processes of absorption, distribution, metabolism and excretion. One useful term that describes part of this process is the *half-life* (tfi). This is the time it takes for the plasma concentration of a drug in the body to halve. In most cases it is constant regardless of how much drug is initially given. After one half-life only 50% remains, after two half-lives only 25% remains and so on. It therefore takes between four and five half-lives for most of the drug to be eliminated. This is important because drugs with a long half-life take a long time to be eliminated compared to those with a short half-life. Naloxone, the antidote to morphine, has a much shorter half-life than morphine itself.

PREHOSPITAL FORMULARY

There are a wide range of emergency conditions which can be quickly and effectively treated by the administration of the appropriate drug. In many cases, giving the drug as soon as possible maximizes its effectiveness and prevents the patient from deteriorating further. There is little point in restricting the use of key emergency drugs to hospitals, medical centres or medical practitioners when they can be safely and effectively given in the prehospital environment by appropriately trained personnel. A simple glance at the drugs listed in the formulary will confirm that effective prehospital care cannot be provided without the use of these key drugs. Consider, for example, how the use of drugs at an early stage may influence the management of the following emergencies.

- Cardiac arrest
- Cardiac arrhythmias (bradycardia, VT)
- Acute asthma
- Anaphylaxis
- Hypoglycaemic coma
- Status epilepticus
- Myocardial infarction
- Left ventricular failure
- Meningococcal disease
- Acute angina
- Severe pain
- Opioid overdose
- Postpartum haemorrhage.

The following list of drugs includes those available for administration by paramedics for "the immediately necessary treatment of the sick or injured". Each drug is described in terms of main prehospital use, other uses for the drug, principal pharmacological actions, preparations generally available, indications for when it should be used, conditions requiring caution, contraindications (when it must not be used), side-effects which may be seen, method of administration and dose. Local protocols define the indications, dosage and administration of individual drugs and these should always be followed. Doses should always be checked with the British National Formulary (www.bnf.org) or local formulary when preparing protocols. Prior to administration, the packaging should be checked for damage and the drug itself checked for clarity. Only drugs that are within their expiry date should be used. Dose calculations should always be checked.

The drugs are listed alphabetically according to their recommended international non-proprietary name. Where the British Approved Name differs, this is given in brackets.

AMIODARONE

Main prehospital use

VF or pulseless VT refractors to 3 countershocks
VT with chest pain, heart failure, or heart rate >150 bpm

Action

An antiarrythmic drug which lengthens cardiac action potential and effective refractory period

Preparations

30 mg/ml 10 ml ampoule for intravenous injection

Indications

Replaces lidocaine for:

VF or pulseless VT
VT with either chest pain, heart failure, or heart rate >150 bpm provided SBP >90 mmHg

Cautions

None in cardiac arrest situations

Contraindications

None in cardiac arrest situations
For **VT: hypotension** (BP <90 mmHg), bradycardia, heart block, thyroid dysfunction, iodine allergy, respiratory failure, congestive heart failure, decompensated cardiomyopathy, pregnancy, breast feeding.

Side-effects

Not relevant in cardiac arrest situations
Following treatment for VT: severe bradycardia, vasodilation and hypotension, bronchospasm, arrhythmias (*torsade de pointes*)

Dose

Cardiac arrest 300 mg by slow intravenous injection over at least 3 mins (single dose)

   VT 150 mg over 10 mins (3 mins if life-threatening). May be repeated once after 10 mins

ASPIRIN

Aspirin (acetylsalicylic acid) decreases platelet aggregation and inhibits clot formation on the arterial side of the circulation. Its use can reduce mortality associated with myocardial infarction and unstable angina. When indicated, a 300 mg tablet should be given regardless of any previous aspirin taken that day. In children under 12 years old, aspirin is associated with Reye's syndrome (acute encephalopathy and liver damage) and is contraindicated.

Main prehospital use

Acute coronary syndromes

Other uses

Prevention of thrombotic cardiovascular or cerebrovascular disease
Simple oral analgesic and mild antiinflammatory

Action

Antiplatelet activity prevents or limits formation of clots
Decreased perception of pain
Antipyretic (lowers temperature)

Preparations

Dispersible tablet 300 mg

Indications

Adults with ischaemic chest pain

Cautions

Asthma
Pregnancy
Kidney or liver failure
Gastric or duodenal ulcer

Contraindications

Known hypersensitivity
Children under 16 years
Patients with known clotting disorders (e.g. haemophilia)

Side-effects

Gastric irritation and bleeding
Bronchospasm in some asthmatics

Administration

Place on the tongue and chew or dissolved in water and drink

Dose

300 mg single dose

ATROPINE

Main prehospital use

Management of asystolic cardiac arrest and symptomatic bradycardia (heart rate <60)

Other uses

Organophosphate poisoning

Action

Blocks vagal (parasympathetic) tone – blocks effect of vagus nerve at sinoatrial and atrioventricular nodes, thus increasing sinus automaticity and facilitating AV node conduction
Reduces likelihood of VF triggered by hypoperfusion associated with extreme bradycardia

Preparations

10 ml disposable syringe with 1 mg (100 µg/ml)
10 ml disposable syringe with 3 mg (300 µg/ml)
1 ml ampoule with 600 µg/ml

Indications

1. Management of asystolic cardiac arrest or PEA with heart rate <60
2. Symptomatic bradycardia associated with any of:
   - pulse <40 bpm
   - systolic BP <90 mmHg
   - ventricular arrhythmias requiring supression
   - inadequate perfusion (e.g. confusion)
3. Heart rate <60 and any indication of high risk of asystole:
   - recent asystole
   - mobity II AV block
   - complete heart block with wide QRS
   - ventricular pauses 73 secs
4. Organophosphate poisoning.

Cautions

Give cautiously to avoid tachycardia post myocardial infarction (increases myocardial oxygen demand and worsens ischaemia)

Contraindications

Bradycardia associated with hypothermia

Side-effects

Dilation of pupils and blurred vision
Dry mouth
Urine retention
Confusion
Tachycardia

Administration

IV or endotracheal (requires double dose and dilution to 20 ml)

Dose

0.5–3 mg IV for symptomatic bradycardia or high risk of asystole

3 mg IV in asystole or PEA with heart rate <60

Children, 20 µg/kg (maximum cumulative dose 0.1 mg, minimum 100 µg)

Organophosphate poisoning, 2 mg IV repeated as required until skin becomes flushed and dry, pupils dilate and tachycardia develops

BENZYLPENICILLIN

Benzylpenicillin is one of the penicillin group of drugs. It interferes with bacterial cell wall production and kills a range of bacteria which include those commonly responsible for meningococcal septicaemia and meningitis. Although the most important side-effect of benzylpenicillin is an allergic reaction, very few patients are at risk of anaphylaxis. Many patients think that they may be allergic to penicillin because of transient rashes or an episode of diarrhoea. If a patient is suspected of having meningococcal septicaemia, only a genuine (proven) history of penicillin allergy should stop benzylpenicillin being given.

Main prehospital use

The treatment of meningococcal septicaemia

Other uses

None prehospital

Action

Bactericidal by interfering with bacterial cell wall synthesis

Preparations

Ampoule containing 600 mg of penicillin G (benzylpenicillin) in powder form

Indications

Meningococcal septicaemia
Meningitis

Cautions

Previous side-effects after penicillin
Renal impairment

Contraindications

Genuine penicillin allergy

Side-effects

Rare in context of severe infection
Hypersensitivity reactions (e.g. urticaria)
Anaphylaxis (rare)
Convulsions in high doses
Hypotension (due to action of drug in releasing toxins. Manage with IV fluid challenges)

Administration

IV or IM

Dose

Dissolve each 600 mg in 10 ml sterile water for IV use, and 2 ml sterile water for IM use. Give:

- adult and child older than nine – 1200 mg (20 ml IV, 4 ml IM)
- child 1–9 years – 600 mg (10 ml IV, 2 ml IM)
- infant – 300 mg (5 ml IV, 1 ml IM).

CHLORPHENIRAMINE

Chlorpheniramine is used as a second-line drug in the management of anaphylactic reactions, and as the first-line treatment of less severe allergic reactions, such as severe itching.

Main prehospital use

Management of anaphylactic and allergic reactions

Other uses

None in the prehospital setting

Action

Chlorpheniramine blocks the action of histamine released as part of the body's response to allergens

Preparation

10 mg/ml 1 ml ampoule

Indications

Severe anaphylactic reactions (after administration of adrenaline)
Allergic reactions causing distress (e.g. severe itching)

Cautions

Hypotension
Epilepsy
Glaucoma
Hepatic disease

Contraindications

Hypersensitivity
<1 yr of age

Side effects

Hypotension if administered rapidly

Administration

Slow IV injection over 1 minute

Dosage

Adult >12 yrs 10 mg
Child 6–12 yrs 5 mg
Child 1–5 yrs 2.5 mg

COMPOUND SODIUM LACTATE (HARTMANN'S/ RINGERS LACTATE)

Main prehospital uses

Fluid replacement therapy

Other uses

None

Action

As an infusion, transiently increases intra-vascular volume

Preparations

500 and 1000 ml bags
5 and 10 ml ampoules

Indications

Status asthmaticus (to limit formation of dry mucous plugs)
Hypovolaemic shock in the absence of a radial pulse
Burns
Anaphylaxis
Hyperthermia
Dehydration

Cautions

None

Contraindications

Hyperglycaemic ketoacidosis
Crush injury

Side-effects

Fluid overload in patients with uncontrolled haemorrhage can cause clot disruption and increased bleeding
Fluid overload causing heart failure (particularly in the elderly)
Exacerbation of pre-existing acidosis

Administration

IV infusion or bolus

Dose

Adults with dehydration, status asthmaticus, hyperthermia:

– Give 500 ml infusion in 20 mins repeated to effect (maximum dose 2000 ml).

Children with dehydration, status asthmaticus, hyperthermia:

– Give 20 ml/kg bolus repeated once to effect.

Adults and children with hypovolaemic shock or burns:
See Figure 10.1 in Normal saline section of this chapter.
N.B. Do *not* give compound sodium lactate to patients with crush syndrome

DIAZEPAM

Diazepam is the benzodiazepine which has been most commonly used in the management of seizures and status epilepticus. It is ideally given intravenously in someone who is actively fitting at the scene or is having repeated fits. It is given IV as the emulsion Diazemuls to reduce the risk of venous thrombophlebitis. Rectal diazepam is given when IV access cannot be obtained.

Main prehospital use

Management of seizures

Other uses

Cocaine toxicity

Action

CNS depressant and anticonvulsant

Preparations

Rectal tubes containing 5 mg or 10 mg
2 ml ampoule (diazepam emulsion) containing 10 mg (5 mg/ml)

Indications

Prolonged or repeated seizures such as may occur in:

– status epilepticus
– convulsions secondary to infections
– alcohol withdrawal seizures
– convulsions due to poisoning
– eclampsia
– head injury (rule out hypoxia).

Symptomatic cocaine toxicity

- sever hypertension
- chest pain
- fitting.

Cautions

Respiratory disease/depression
History of drug or alcohol abuse
Reduce dose in elderly and debilitated
Facilities for ventilatory support should be immediately available
Consider doses previously administered by carers
Use of CNS depressants

Contraindications

Known hypersensitivity
Respiratory failure

Side-effects

Respiratory depression (especially with opioids and alcohol)
Apnoea
CNS depression and loss of consciousness
Cardiovascular depression and postural hypotension
Amnesia

Administration

IV through a large proximal vein at a rate of 3 mg/minute
Rectal via a tube which should be inserted no more than 2 cm in children and 3–4 cm in adults (tubes have markers)
Rectal tubes should be held in place for a few moments after expelling the contents and the patient's buttocks held together to reduce seepage from the rectum.

Dose

Age	IV	Rectal
>12 yrs	10 mg, repeated once	10 mg repeated once
6–12 yrs	300 µg/kg	10 mg repeated once
1–5 yrs	300 µg/kg	5 mg repeated once
<1 yr	300 µg/kg	2.5 mg repeated once

If a single dose of diazepam has been given rectally, the second dose may be given IV.

ENTONOX

Nitrous oxide is an anaesthetic gas which is rapidly absorbed by inhalation. A mixture of nitrous oxide and oxygen containing 50% of each gas (Entonox) is used in prehospital care to gain rapid control of pain without loss of consciousness. It is administered by the casualty via a demand valve.

Slow, deep breaths are required. The casualty must be conscious, cooperative and have sufficient respiratory excursion to operate the demand valve. Nitrous oxide is extremely soluble and will diffuse rapidly into any gas-filled cavity; it may thus increase the size of a pneumothorax. At temperatures below $-7°C$, nitrous oxide may liquefy and the oxygen and nitrous oxide will separate. The patient may then inhale pure oxygen followed by pure nitrous oxide. It is not adequate to simply shake the cylinder in these situations. Cylinders need to be kept at temperatures above freezing.

Main prehospital use

Rapid control of pain

Action

Anaesthetic agent

Preparations

A mixture of 50% nitrous oxide and 50% oxygen in a blue cylinder with a white shoulder

Indications

Acute pain

Cautions

Chest injuries
Head injuries
Cold weather
Alcohol/drug intoxication
Sickle cell crisis
>50% oxygen indicated

Contraindications

Pneumothorax
Gastrointestinal obstruction
Decompression sickness ("bends")
Reduced GCS
Disturbed psychiatric patients

Side-effects

Decreased level of consciousness
Nausea and vomiting
Confusion +/− distress

Administration

Inhalation via demand valve with onset of action within 3–5 minutes

Dose

As required to relieve pain

EPINEPHRINE (ADRENALINE)

Epinephrine is a sympathomimetic drug which stimulates both α and β receptors. α receptor activity increases peripheral vascular resistance without constricting coronary and cerebral vessels. This raises systolic and diastolic pressures during CPR which makes CPR more effective. β receptor activity increases myocardial contractility in cardiac arrest and relieves bronchospasm in acute severe asthma. Epinephrine also reverses the allergic manifestations of acute anaphylaxis. If epinephrine has already been self-administered by the patient (e.g. Epipen 0.3 mg for adults or 0.15 mg for children) this should be taken into account when determining the timing and dosage for administration.

Main prehospital use

Cardiac arrest
Acute anaphylaxis

Other uses

Nebulized in severe croup

Action

Increases heart rate
Increases blood pressure
Increases myocardial contraction force
Bronchodilation
Vaso-constriction

Preparations

10 ml disposable syringe with 0.1 mg/ml (1:10 000)
1 ml disposable syringe with 1 mg/ml (1:1000)

Indications

Cardiac arrest
Acute anaphylaxis
Severe croup

Cautions

Hypothermia (give single dose only)

Contraindications

None in cardiac arrest

Side-effects

Tachycardia
Angina and arrhythmias
Hypertension
Anxiety
Headache

Administration

IV, IM, endotracheal or nebulized
IV administration is far better in cardiac arrest
IM administration should be used in anaphylaxis

Dose

In cardiac arrest, 1 mg (10 ml of 1:10 000) every 3 mins or 2 mg (20 ml 1:10 000) via ETT (follow with five ventilations) In children, initial dose 0.01 mg/kg IV (0.1 ml/kg of 1:10 000) repeated every 3 mins subsequent doses may be increased to 0.1 mg/kg (0.1 ml/kg of 1:1000) in presence of cardiovascular collapse. Use 0.1 mg/kg via ET tube (0.1 ml/kg of 1:1000) in children. In anaphylaxis, if stridor, wheeze, respiratory distress, upper airway or oral swelling or hypotension are present:

– adults (>12 years of age) 0.5 mg IM (0.5 ml of 1:1000) repeated after 5 mins if necessary (halve dose in prepubertal children)
– child 6–11 yrs 250 μg (0.25 ml 1:1000) repeat after 5 mins if necessary
– child 6 months–5 yrs 120 μg (0.12 ml 1:1000) repeat after 5 mins if necessary
– child <6 months 50 μg (0.05 ml 1:1000) repeat after 5 mins if necessary.

In *severe* croup

– 1 mg (1 ml of 1:1000 diluted to 5 ml with normal saline) via nebulizer.

FUROSEMIDE (FRUSEMIDE)

Furosemide is a potent loop diuretic with a rapid onset used in pulmonary oedema due to left ventricular failure. IV administration produces rapid relief of breathlessness.

Main prehospital use

Acute left ventricular failure

Action

Reduces preload
Inhibits reabsorption from the ascending limb of the loop of Henle in the kidney

Preparations

5 ml ampoule with 50 mg (10 mg/ml)
2 ml ampoule with 40 mg (20 mg/ml)
Minijet containing 80 mg in 8 ml (10 mg/ml)

Indications

Pulmonary oedema due to left ventricular failure

Cautions

Patients with long-standing heart failure
Pregnancy
Hypokalaemia

Contraindications

Liver failure with pre-comatose state
Renal failure with anuria

Side-effects

Hypotension
GI disturbance

Administration

Slow IV injection over 2 mins

Dose

40 or 50 mg initially (halve dose in elderly)
Repeat to a maximum of 120 mg (3 × 40 mg) or 100 mg (2 × 50 mg)

GLUCAGON

Glucagon is an alternative to IV glucose in hypoglycaemia. It increases plasma-glucose concentration by mobilizing glycogen stored in the liver. It is therefore less effective in hypoglycaemia associated with malnutrition and chronic illness. It can be injected IM in a dose of 1 mg (1 unit) in circumstances when IV glucose would be difficult or impossible to administer. Note that IV glucose is the preferred treatment.

Main prehospital use

Treatment of hypoglycaemia

Other uses

Poisoning with β-blockers

Action

Breaks down glycogen (a reserve form of glucose found in the liver and other tissues)
Increases heart rate
Increases myocardial contractility

Preparations

Vial with 1 mg powder for reconstitution with sterile water

Indications

Blood glucose level is <3.0 mmol/l *or*
Suspected hypoglycaemia where oral glucose cannot be administered *or*

Unconscious patient, where hypoglycaemia cannot be excluded

Cautions

Starvation and malnutrition (ineffective)
Adrenal insufficiency
Chronic alcoholism (ineffective)

Contraindications

None

Side-effects

Nausea and vomiting
Hypersensitivity reactions

Administration

IM
The IV route should not be used because it is associated with nausea and vomiting

Dose

1 mg in adult and child over 20 kg, 0.5 mg in children under 20 kg, age <1 month 100 μg
If not effective in 10 minutes IV glucose should be given
Any patient receiving glucagon must be given oral carbohydrates when they are fully conscious. If this is not possible the patient must be hospitalized as blood sugar levels will fall significantly

GLUCOSE

Main prehospital use

Hypoglycaemic states

Action

Reverses hypoglycaemia

Preparations

500 ml bags of 10% (100 mg/ml) glucose solution

Indications

Blood glucose level <3.0 mmol/l *or*
Suspected hypoglycaemia where oral glucose cannot be administered *or*
Unconscious patient, where hypoglycaemia cannot be excluded

Cautions

Use large-bore cannula in largest available vein to minimize risk of thrombophlebitis

Contraindications

None

Side-effects

Tissue necrosis following extravasation

Administration

IV via a large-bore, free-flowing proximal vein

Dose

5 ml/kg of 10% glucose solution in children (max 50 ml bolus at once)
50 ml of 10% glucose solution (5 g) in adults repeated at 5 mins intervals to effect.

GLYCERYL TRINITRATE

Glyceryl trinitrate may be given as tablets to be dissolved under the tongue (sublingual), modified-release tablets to be dissolved inside the lip (buccal) or as an aerosol spray. The spray has a much longer shelf-life and is therefore more often carried by patients with angina for use when they have symptoms. It is one of the most effective drugs for rapid relief of angina.

Main prehospital uses

Management of ischaemic chest pain associated with acute coronary syndromes

Acute cardiogenic pulmonary oedema

Other uses

None in the prehospital setting

Action

Vasodilator which dilates coronary arteries and reduces cardiac preload by dilating systemic veins

Preparations

Sublingual tablets, 300 µg
Aerosol spray, 400 µg/metered dose
Modified-release buccal tablets 2 mg and 5 mg (Suscard)

Indications

Cardiac chest pain due to angina and myocardial infarction
Severe breathing difficulty due to left ventricular failure (acute cardiogenic pulmonary oedema)

Cautions

None

Contraindications

Hypotension – do not give if systolic BP <90 mmHg
Concomitant use of Viagra (sildenafil) or similar drugs. Risk of profound hypotension – do not give within 24 hours
Hypovolaemia
Head trauma
Cerebral haemorrhage

Side-effects

Postural hypotension (remove tablet and flush mouth with water)
Headache
Flushing
Dizziness
Tachycardia

Administration

Sublingual or buccal

Dose

Sublingual tablet, 300 µg repeated as required
Aerosol, 1–2 sprays under the tongue or into the open mouth and then close the mouth. Repeat after 5 minutes if required
Buccal tablet, 2 mg between gum and inner cheek replaced by 5 mg if symptoms not relieved in 3–5 minutes

HEPARIN (UNFRACTIONATED HEPARIN)

Main prehospital uses

Given with thrombolytic agents in ST segment elevation myocardial infarction to prevent thrombus reforming (thrombolytic agents are also platelet activators)

Other uses

None in the prehospital setting

Action

Heparin is a short-acting anticoagulant

Preparations

1000 units/ml, 5 ml ampoule

Indications

Immediately following administration of tenecteplase or first bolus of reteplase

Cautions

Hepatic and renal impairment
Pregnancy

Contraindications

Haemophilia and other bleeding disorders
Thrombocytopenia
Peptic ulcer
Recent cerebral haemorrhage
Severe hypertension
Recent major trauma or surgery
Recent spinal or epidural anaesthesia
Hypersensitivity to heparin

Side-effects

Haemorrhage
Skin necrosis
Thrombocytopenia
Hyperkalaemia
Hypersensitivity reactions

Administration

IV bolus

Dose

Tenecteplase: 4000 units
Reteplase: 5000 units
Note: a Patient Group Directive is required for paramedics to administer heparin

HYDROCORTISONE

Hydrocortisone is administered to help prevent the response to secondary mediators in anaphylaxis of severe asthma. Although its onset of action may be delayed by several hours, it should be given as a second-line treatment in pre-hospital care to avoid unnecessary delays.

Main prehospital use

Severe/life-threatening asthma
Anaphylaxis

Other uses

None in prehospital care

Action

Limits the effect of secondary mediators (such as kinins) and atopic response

Preparations

Ampoule with 100 mg in 1 ml

Indications

Severe or life-threatening asthma
Anaphylaxis

Cautions

None for these indications/doses

Contraindications

Allergy to the diluent

Side-effects

Burning or itching sensation in the groin
Hypotension if administered quickly

Administration

Slow IV injection over 2 mins

Dose

Adult/Child >12 yrs 200 mg
Child 1 month–12 yrs 4 mg/kg
Child <1 month 2.5 mg/kg

HYPOSTOP

Hypostop is a 40% glucose gel containing 23 g of glucose per dose.

Main prehospital use

Management of conscious hypoglycaemic patients able to cooperate and with intact swallow and gag reflexes

Other uses

None

Action

Reverses hypoglycaemia

Preparations

Box containing three single dose tubes of 40% glucose (23 g per tube)

Indications

Hypoglycaemia in conscious cooperative patients with intact swallow and gag reflexes
May be used following glucogen administration when GCS is normal

Cautions

None

Contraindications

Reduced level of consciousness

Side-effects

Aspiration
Airway obstruction

Administration

Smear onto gums for most rapid effect

Dose

Titrated to effect against blood glucose measurements – no upper limit, but if ineffective use 10% glucose IV

IPRATROPIUM BROMIDE

Main prehospital uses

Management of acute severe or life-threatening asthma in adults
Management of acute asthma unresponsive to beta-2 agonist therapy in children
Management of acute exacerbations of COPD

Other uses

Short-term relief of chronic reversible airways obstruction

Action

Ipratropium is an antimuscarinic (atropine-like) drug that causes bronchodilation

Preparations

Ipratropium bromide nebulizer solution presented in unit dose vials of 250 μg in 1 ml or 500 μg in 2 ml

Indications

Life-threatening asthma in adults (mix with first dose of salbutamol)
Acute severe asthma in adults (mix with first dose of salbutamol)
Acute exacerbation of COPD in adults that is unresponsive to the first dose of salbutamol (mix with second dose of salbutamol)
Acute episode of asthma in children that is unresponsive to the first dose of salbutamol (mix with second dose of salbutamol)

Cautions

Glaucoma (protect patient's eyes from nebulizer mist)
Prostatic hyperplasia and bladder outflow obstruction

Contraindications

None

Side-effects

Dry mouth
Nausea
Headache
Acute angle-closure glaucoma (see Cautions)
Constipation
Tachycardia and atrial fibrillation (rare)
Paradoxical bronchospasm (rare)

Administration

Via nebulizer

Dose

Adults and children >5 years: 500 μg, once only
Children 1 to 5 years: 250 μg once only
Infants (<1 year): 125 μg once only

LIDOCAINE (LIGNOCAINE)

Lidocaine is a local anaesthetic drug used in the management of wide-complex tachycardia and ventricular fibrillation. It is effective in suppressing ventricular tachycardia and reducing the risk of ventricular fibrillation (especially after myocardial infarction). It has not been shown to reduce mortality when used prophylactically in myocardial infarction.

Main prehospital use

Treatment of refractory VF, pulseless VT, or symptomatic VT (Amiodarone is now the preferred treatment)

Other uses

Local anaesthetic

Action

Suppresses ventricular ectopic activity and decreases ventricular automaticity
Raises threshold for VF (by depressing conduction in ischaemic areas or improving conduction in normal areas)
Slows conduction of impulses through the Purkinje system
Raises defibrillation threshold

Preparations

10 ml disposable syringe containing 100 mg (10 mg/ml)

Indications

Ventricular fibrillation or pulseless VT refractory to 3 shocks especially after myocardial infarction
Symptomatic ventricular tachycardia
N.B. Amiodarone is now the preferred treatment

Cautions

Reduce dose in congestive cardiac and liver failure

Contraindications

Patients in heart block
Premature ventricular contraction with bradycardia
SBP <90 mmHg (VT with a pulse)

Side-effects

Central nervous system toxicity with confusion, nausea, vomiting, drowsiness, seizures
Dizziness and paraesthesia (if injection too rapid)
Hypotension and bradycardia

Administration

IV and endotracheal

Dose

VF/pulseless VT, 100 mg IV bolus, repeated once if necessary (200 mg if given by endotracheal route repeated once if necessary)
Symptomatic VT, 50–100 mg given slowly, repeat if necessary after 15–20 minutes to a maximum of 200 mg

METOCLOPRAMIDE

Metoclopramide is an antiemetic drug which is currently used to reduce the risk of nausea and vomiting following intravenous morphine and to treat severe nausea and vomiting.

Main prehospital use

Reduce risk of nausea and vomiting following administration of morphine sulphate

Action

Central effects on chemoreceptor trigger zone
Peripheral effects on gut

Preparations

2 ml ampoule with 10 mg (5 mg/ml)

Indications

Nausea or vomiting in adults
Concomitant administration with morphine sulphate and other opiates

Cautions

Hepatic and renal impairment
Elderly

Contraindications

Avoid in first 12 weeks of pregnancy
Renal failure
Patients under age of 20
Gastro-intestinal obstruction
Phaeochromocytoma

Side-effects

Acute dystonic reactions with facial and skeletal muscle spasms. These are more common in the young (especially girls and young women) and the very old.
Drowsiness
Rarely, cardiac dysthythmias

Administration

IV over 2 minutes or IM
Monitor ECG, pulse and BP before, during and after administration

Dose

10 mg

MORPHINE SULPHATE

Morphine sulphate is the standard opioid analgesic against which all others are judged. It is used for the treatment of severe pain including myocardial infarction, major limb injuries or burns. It produces sedation and euphoria as well as its analgesic effect. Onset of action is within 2–3 minutes if given intravenously with the peak effect in 10–20 minutes. In medical cases, smaller doses may be effective (2.5–5 mg) whereas in injured patients, much larger doses may be needed to achieve effective analgesia.

Prehospital use of opioids has been shown to be safe and effective when used appropriately and titrated to effect according to pain scores. Nevertheless, prehospital practitioners must be able to recognize and deal with the three most important side-effects: respiratory depression, systemic vasodilation and nausea and vomiting. Naloxone should always be available whenever opioids are used.

Morphine is a controlled drug under Schedule 2 of the Misuse of Drugs Regulations 1985. It must be stored and its use documented in accordance with these regulations.

Main prehospital use

Severe pain associated with myocardial infarction, fractures and burns, and other causes

Other uses

Left ventricular failure

Action

Acts on μ opioid receptors in the spinal cord and brain

Preparations

1 ml ampoule with 10 mg (10 mg/ml)

Indications

Severe pain

Cautions

Recent alcohol use
Respiratory depression/disease
Chest injuries
Hypotension
Elderly and debilitated
Antidepressant use
Pregnancy

Contraindications

Acute respiratory depression (adult <10 bpm)
Coma or impaired level of consciousness (GCS < 12)
Infants <1 yr
MAOIs
Phaeochromcytoma
Hypersensitivity
Hypotension: SBP
Adults <90 mmHg
5–16 yrs <80 mmHg
1–4 yrs <70 mmHg

Side-effects

Respiratory depression
Cardiovascular depression
Nausea and vomiting
Pupillary constriction

Administration and dose

Adults: IV bolus of 2.5 to 5 mg followed by 1 mg increments titrated against pain score over 10 mins. Give further 5 mg increments at 5 mins intervals, titrated to effect (max. dose 20 mg)
Best achieved by diluting 10 mg (1 ml) in 9 ml of water or 0.9% saline to make a 1 mg/ml solution
Children: use 10 mg in 10 ml solution to administer 0.05 mg/kg (0.05 ml/kg) over 2–3 mins. Repeat dose at 5–10 mins intervals titrated to effect (max. dose 0.2 mg/kg)

NALOXONE

Naloxone is the specific antidote to opioid-induced coma or respiratory depression. Since naloxone has a shorter duration of action than many opioids, close monitoring and repeated injections are necessary according to the respiratory rate and depth of coma.

Main prehospital use

Reversal of respiratory depression associated with opioid excess

Action

Competitive antagonist at opioid μ receptors
In the context of opioid excess, will increase respiratory rate and level of consciousness

Preparations

1 ml ampoule with 400 μg

Indications

Reversal of opioid-induced respiratory, cardiovascular and CNS depression
Overdose with opioids and opioid-containing medicines
Unconsciousness associated with respiratory depression or arrest where opiate or opioid overdose is a possibility

Cautions

Pain
Short duration of action
May precipitate a withdrawal syndrome in those dependent on opiates

Contraindications

Known hypersensitivity
Neonates with opioid-dependent mother

Side-effects

Nausea and vomiting
Tachycardia
Withdrawal symptoms in opioid dependency

Administration

IV or IM
Where rapid reversal is undesirable (e.g. acute pain or risk of withdrawal) then dilute 2 ml (0.8 mg) in 8 ml of water or 0.9% saline and titrate to effect

Dose

0.4 mg repeated every 2–3 minutes up to maximum 10 mg in adults
0.01 mg/kg in children followed once by 0.1 mg/kg
0.1 mg (0.25 ml) in neonates IM once only
Patients who are opioid-dependent are at risk of absconding on recovery. Because IV naloxone has shorter half-life than most opioids, respiratory depression may recur. Consider giving a "depot" IM injection of 0.8 mg in this group before any IV dose.

NORMAL SALINE

Main prehospital uses

Fluid replacement

Other uses

Flush to keep intravenous cannula patent
Flush to "push" IV drugs into the circulation

Action

As an infusion, transiently increases intravascular volume

Preparations

500 and 1000 ml bags
5 and 10 ml ampoules

Indications

Hyperglycaemic ketoacidosis
Status asthmaticus (to limit formation of dry mucous plugs)
Hypovolaemic shock in the absence of a radial pulse
Burns
Crush injury
Anaphylaxis
Hyperthermia
Dehydration
Post-cannulation flush
Post-IV drug administration flush

Cautions

None

Contraindications

None

Side-effects

Fluid overload in patients with uncontrolled haemorrhage can cause clot disruption and increased bleeding
Fluid overload causing heart failure (particularly in the elderly)

Administration

IV infusion or bolus

Dose

As a post-drug flush: 10–20 ml (adults and children)
As a post-cannulation flush: 2 ml (adults and children)
Adults with dehydration, status asthmaticus, diabetic ketoacidosis, hyperthermia:
Give 500 ml infusion in 20 mins repeated to effect (maximum dose 2000 ml)

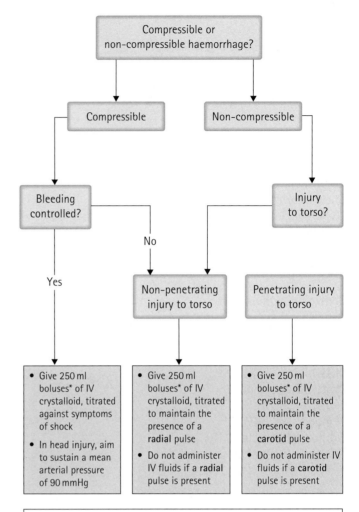

Figure 10.1　Intravenous fluid therapy in hypovolaemic shock, burns, and crush injury

Children with dehydration, status asthmaticus, diabetic ketoacidosis, hyperthermia:
Give 20 ml/kg bolus repeated once to effect
Adults and children with hypovolaemic shock, burns, or crush injury:
See Figure 10.1.

OXYGEN

Under normal conditions the main stimulus to breathe is the amount of carbon dioxide in the blood and not a deficit of oxygen. In some patients with chronic obstructive pulmonary disease (COPD), the stimulus to breathing is a deficit of oxygen (hypoxic drive) as the poor function of their lungs has produced high levels of carbon monoxide in the blood for a long period of time. There has been considerable anxiety in prehospital care about the risks of giving these patients high concentrations of oxygen. The risk is that they will lose some of their hypoxic drive, develop worsening respiratory failure and retain even more carbon dioxide. Excess carbon dioxide makes the blood more acid and is associated with CNS depression and cardiac arrhythmias.

Although some patients with COPD will certainly retain carbon monoxide if given high-concentration oxygen, it is important to realize that the far greater risk to the acutely unwell patient is from hypoxia. Hypoxic patients need oxygen regardless of whether they are at risk of retaining carbon monoxide. Even among those who retain carbon monoxide, it is unlikely that they will develop respiratory depression (lose their hypoxic drive) if they are already profoundly hypoxic because of respiratory failure.

Regardless of whether a patient is known to have COPD, if they are acutely unwell (pulse oximetry under 90% on room air or low respiratory rate, severe dyspnoea and abnormal respiratory pattern) they should be given high-concentration oxygen via a non-rebreathing mask with a flow rate set at 10–15 l/min.

Main prehospital use

Supplemental oxygen in trauma and acute medical emergencies

Action

Essential component of the chemical reaction that occurs in all cells and supports life
Combines with glucose to liberate energy and carbon dioxide

Preparations

Oxygen cylinders are black with a white shoulder
New light-weight cylinders do not follow this convention

Indications

Hypoxia from any cause
Cardiorespiratory arrest
Significant trauma
Pulmonary disease

Cautions

Patients with COPD

Contraindications

Paraquat poisoning

Side-effects

Respiratory depression in COPD
Dry mouth

Administration

Inhalational via non-rebreathing or fixed concentration masks

Dose

100% (practically approximately 85%) via non-rebreathing reservoir masks usually 10–15 l/min: A sufficient flow rate should be used to keep the reservoir bag inflated in all acutely hypoxic or injured patients
24% to 40% via fixed flow mask in patients with COPD who are not acutely hypoxic (may require more to maintain pulse oximetry in the region of 90–93%)

PARACETAMOL

Paracetamol is a simple and safe pain-relieving and temperature-reducing drug which is widely available. In prehospital emergency care, administration of paracetamol in children can control pain and rapidly reduce temperature.

Main prehospital use

Pain relief and temperature control in children

Action

Simple analgesic and antipyretic (temperature-reducing) drug

Preparations

Syrup containing 120 mg/5 ml of solution or 250 mg/5 ml of solution

Indications

Mild to moderate pain
Pyrexia

Cautions

Hepatic and renal impairment

Contraindications

Paracetamol overdose
Previous administration. Within 4 hours or maximum. Cumulative dose given

Side-effects

Rare

Administration

Orally as a single dose using a 5 ml syringe without needle or a measuring spoon

Dose

3 months–1 year, 60–125 mg (repeat at 4 hour intervals to max. 500 mg)
1–5 years, 120–250 mg (max. dose in 24 hrs = 1 g)
6–12 years, 250–500 mg (max. dose in 24 hrs = 2 g)
Adult 1 g (max. dose in 24 hrs = 4 g)
Each dose repeated every 4–6 hours as necessary (maximum of 4 doses in 24 hours)

SALBUTAMOL

Salbutamol is used in the management of uncontrolled, acute severe and life-threatening asthma and other causes of reversible airways obstruction.

Main prehospital use

Treatment of acute asthma

Other uses

Bronchospasm from any other cause (COPD, anaphylaxis, LVF)

Action

Sympathomimetic
Selective β-2-adrenoreceptor stimulant which reverses bronchospasm

Preparations

Nebules containing either 2.5 mg or 5 mg
Metered dose inhaler (various doses)

Indications

Acute asthma attack where normal inhaler therapy has failed to relieve symptoms
Wheezing associated with allergy, anaphylaxis or smoke inhalation
Exacerbation of COPD
Second-line treatment for LVF

Cautions

Hypertension
Angina
Hyperthyroidism
Hypokalaemia
Late pregnancy

Contraindications

None

Side-effects

Tremor
Palpitations
Tachycardia
Headache
Peripheral-vasodilation

Administration

Inhaled as nebulized solution or as an aerosol via a spacer device if the patient has one

Dose

Adults and children >5 yrs:
5 mg via nebulizer repeated to effect or side-effects are intolerable
12 months–5 yrs 2.5 mg repeated to effect at 15 mins intervals
<12 months 2.5 mg once only
In severe or life-threatening asthma, continuous nebulization is required.

SYNTOMETRINE

Oxytocic (uterus-stimulating) drugs are used to minimize blood loss from the placental site during the routine management of the third stage of labour. The combination of ergometrine 500 μg with oxytocin 5 units is given by IM injection with or after delivery of the shoulders.

Main prehospital use

Management of third stage of labour

Other uses

Postpartum haemorrhage within 24 hrs of delivery
Control of bleeding in incomplete miscarriage

Action

Stimulates contraction of the uterus within 7 minutes of IM injection

Preparations

1 ml ampoule containing ergometrine 500 μg and oxytocin 5 units

Indications

Active management of the third stage of labour
Following delivery of the placenta to prevent or treat postpartum haemorrhage
Control of bleeding in incomplete miscarriage

Cautions

Cardiac disease
Hepatic and renal impairment

Contraindications

Known hypersensitivity
First or second stage of labour
Severe cardiac, liver or kidney disease
Hypertension
Eclampsia/pre-eclampsia
Multiple pregnancy (foetus still in utero)

Side–effects

Nausea and vomiting
Abdominal pain
Headache
Hypertension
Cardiac arrhythmias (bradycardia)
Chest pain
Anaphylactic reactions (rare)

Administration

IM with or after delivery of the shoulders

Dose

1 ml

TENECTEPLASE AND RETEPLASE

Tenecteplase and reteplase are thrombolytic drugs which are indicated for myocardial infarction due to their ability to break up thrombus and permit return of blood supply. The benefits of treatment must be considered to outweigh the risks (hence the specific indications and contraindications given below). Trials have shown that the benefit is greatest in those with ECG changes that include ST segment elevation (especially in those with anterior infarction) and in those with *new* bundle brand block.

Main prehospital use

Treatment of acute myocardial infarction with pain of >15 mins and <6 hours duration

Other uses

None prehospital

Action

Activates the fibrinolytic system, inducing the breaking up of intravascular thrombi and emboli

Preparations

Tenecteplase
Powder for reconstitution 40 mg (8000 units), or 50 mg (10 000 units)

Reteplase
Powder for reconsitution 10 units to be dissolved in 10 mls of water for injection
Both with prefilled syringe of water for injection

Indications

Acute myocardial infarction, where pain has been present continuously for at least 15 minutes and less than 6 hours
Patient must fulfill all JRCALC guideline criteria

JRCALC criteria for paramedic-administered thrombolysis (version 3)

Primary assessment

1. Can you confirm that the patient is conscious, coherent, and able to understand that clot-dissolving drugs will be used?

2. Can you confirm that the patient is aged 75 or less?

3. Can you confirm that the patient has had symptoms characteristic of a heart attack (i.e. continuous pain in a typical distribution and of 15 minutes duration or longer)?

4. Can you confirm that the symptoms started less than six hours ago?

5. Can you confirm that the pain built up over seconds and minutes rather than starting totally abruptly?

6. Can you confirm that breathing does not influence the severity of the pain?

7. Can you confirm that the heart rate is between 50 and 140 beats per minute?

8. Can you confirm that the systolic blood pressure is more than 80 mmHg and less than 160 mmHg and that the diastolic blood pressure is below 110 mmHg?

9. Can you confirm that the electrocardiogram shows abnormal ST segment elevation of 2 mm or more in at least two standard leads or in at least two adjacent precordial leads, not including V_1 (ST elevation can sometimes be normal in V_1 and V_2)?

10. Can you confirm that the QRS width is 0.16 mm or less, and that left bundle branch block is absent from the tracing? (Note: RBBB permitted only with qualifying ST segment elevation)

11. Can you confirm that there is NO atrio-ventricular block greater than 1st degree? (If necessary after treatment with IV atropine)

Secondary assessment

12. Can you confirm that the patient is not likely to be pregnant, nor has delivered within the last two weeks?

13. Can you confirm that the patient has not had a peptic ulcer within the last 6 months?

14. Can you confirm that the patient has not had a stroke of any sort within the last 12 months and does not have permanent disability from a previous stroke?

15. Can you confirm the patient has no diagnosed bleeding tendency, has had no recent blood loss (except for normal menstruation), and is not taking warfarin (anticoagulant) therapy?

16. Can you confirm the patient has not had any surgical operation, tooth extractions, significant trauma, or head injury within the last 4 weeks?

17. Can you confirm that the patient has not been treated within the last three months for any other serious head or brain condition? (This is intended to exclude patients with cerebral tumours)

18. Can you confirm that the patient is not being treated for liver failure, renal failure, or any other severe systemic illness?

Contraindications

Does not meat JRCALC guideline criteria

Side-effects

Elevation of body temperature
Nausea and vomiting
Haemorrhage, including stroke
Hypotension
Reperfusion arrhythmias
Anaphylaxis (rare)
Allergic responses including urticarial rash and low back pain

Administration

Tenecteplase: slow IV bolus
Reteplase: slow IV bolus repeated after 30 mins

Dose

Tenecteplase
Single intravenous dose according to the patient's weight

<60 kg	6000 μ
60–69 kg	7000 μ
70–79 kg	8000 μ
80–89 kg	9000 μ
>90 kg	10 000 μ

Reteplase
10 units repeated exactly 30 minutes later

TETRACAINE 4% GEL (AMETOP)

Main prehospital uses

Use to provide local anaesthesia prior to non-urgent venepuncture

Other uses

None in the prehospital setting

Action

Local anaesthetic agent designed to penetrate intact skin to provide local numbing prior to venepuncture

Preparations

1.5 g tubes of white semitransparent gel

Indications

Patient requiring non-urgent venepuncture after 30 to 45 minutes and at risk of distress from the procedure

Cautions

Check for allergy to occlusive dressing of choice

Contraindications

Venepuncture required in less than 30 to 45 minutes.
Do not apply to open wounds, broken skin, lips mouth, eyes, ears, anal or genital region or mucous membranes
Known allergy to tetracaine, any of its constituents or other local anaesthetic agents Infants less than 1 month old
Pregnancy or breastfeeding

Side-effects

Inappropriately rapid absorption from mucous membranes, wounds or inflamed tissue
Hypersensitivity reactions

Administration

Topical application at proposed venepuncture site(s). Cover with transparent occlusive dressing. Wait for 30 to 45 minutes before removing dressing and cream and attempting venepuncture.

Dose

Apply sufficient cream to cover intended venepuncture site(s)

Chapter **11**

Respiratory emergencies

INTRODUCTION

Respiratory emergencies arise frequently and all paramedics should be able to deal with them quickly and effectively. Delays in diagnosis and treatment can lead to the patient's death.

The most common life-threatening problems affecting the respiratory system are:

- asthma
- airway obstruction
- chronic obstructive pulmonary disease (COPD)
- pulmonary oedema
- anaphylaxis.

ANATOMY OF THE RESPIRATORY TRACT

AIR PASSAGES

The anatomy of the upper airway has already been described in Chapter 6. Below the level of the cricoid cartilage, the airway continues as the *trachea*, a flexible tube which is strengthened by incomplete hoops of cartilage and lined with mucous membrane. In the chest the trachea divides into two main *bronchi*, one going to each lung (Figure 11.1). The right one lies more vertically and so receives most of the foreign objects that manage to overcome all the defences in the upper airway. The bronchi subsequently divide, much like a tree, into smaller and smaller branches, the smallest of which are known as respiratory *bronchioles*.

The respiratory bronchioles, and the alveoli and ducts they give rise to, are known as the respiratory portion of the lung. They are so named because they are the only places in the lungs where oxygen is taken up from the inspired air and carbon dioxide released from the blood. As this gas exchange occurs by diffusion, the walls of the airways and blood vessels have to be extremely thin, closely applied to one another and have a large surface area.

CHEST WALL

The lungs lie in the thorax (chest cavity) on either side of the heart, trachea, oesophagus and great vessels. The lungs and chest wall are both lined by a tough tissue layer (the *pleura*) with a potential cavity between the layers known as the intrapleural space.

It is important to realize that both the lung and chest wall are made up of elastic tissue which is pulling in opposite

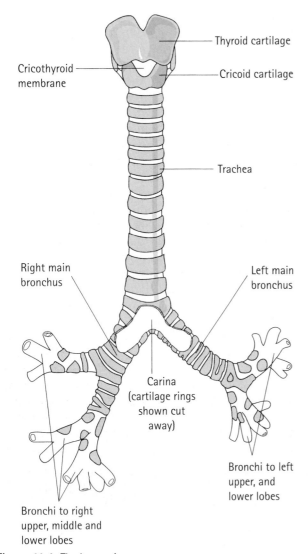

Figure 11.1 The lower airways

Labels: Thyroid cartilage; Cricothyroid membrane; Cricoid cartilage; Trachea; Right main bronchus; Left main bronchus; Carina (cartilage rings shown cut away); Bronchi to left upper, and lower lobes; Bronchi to right upper, middle and lower lobes

directions: the chest wall is trying to open out and the lungs are trying to collapse. The interface between these two opposing forces results in a vacuum (negative pressure) in the intrapleural space. This stretches the lungs so that their outer surfaces are closely applied to the chest wall.

During inspiration the muscles lying between each rib (intercostal muscles) contract and move the ribs upwards and outwards. At the same time the muscular floor of the thorax (the *diaphragm*) contracts and moves downwards. These actions cause the volume inside the chest to increase and the intrapleural pressure to fall. As a result the lungs are stretched even further and air is drawn in. The opposite process occurs in expiration.

MEDIASTINUM

The trachea, oesophagus, heart and major blood vessels lie in close proximity to one another in the centre of the chest. They are collectively named the *mediastinum*.

RESPIRATORY PATHOPHYSIOLOGY

The main functions of the lungs are oxygen uptake and carbon dioxide elimination. To achieve this, air (or, more accurately, oxygen) has to flow to the alveoli (ventilation), blood has to flow to the pulmonary capillaries (perfusion) and oxygen (O_2) and carbon dioxide (CO_2) have to move between the alveoli and blood in the pulmonary capillaries (*diffusion*). Finally, the balance between ventilation and perfusion has to be correct. Impairment of any of these processes can lead to a low level of oxygen in the blood (*hypoxaemia*) and a high level of carbon dioxide in the blood (*hypercarbia*) (Figure 11.2).

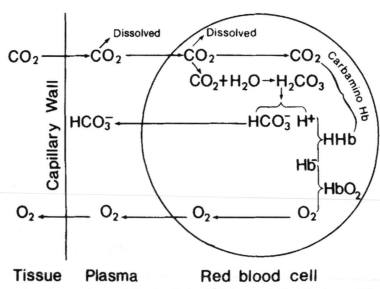

Figure 11.2 Schematic representation of gas exchange at the alveolar level (Hb haemoglobin; H hydrogen; CO_2 carbon dioxide; H_2O water)

VENTILATION

The amount of air breathed in (or out) with each breath is called the *tidal volume*. It is normally equal to 7–8 ml/kg body weight (approximately 500 ml in a 70 kg patient). The volume of air inspired (or expired) each minute is the *minute volume* and can be calculated by multiplying the tidal volume by the respiratory rate. For a 70 kg patient, this gives a value around 5 litres per minute at rest.

Not all of the air breathed in reaches the point where oxygen and carbon dioxide exchange takes place (the respiratory portion of the lung). Approximately 150 ml of each breath remains in the conducting airways and this area is known as the *anatomical dead space* because the gases within it take no part in gas exchange. In some circumstances (e.g. following blood loss), the volume of this space is increased by the addition of areas of lung which are ventilated but not perfused with blood.

DIFFUSION

Blood with low levels of oxygen is pumped by the right ventricle through the pulmonary circulation. Gas exchange between the alveoli and blood takes place across the pulmonary membrane in the alveoli and occurs by passive diffusion. The lung is ideally suited for diffusion as the pulmonary membrane has a large surface area and is very thin. It is not surprising, therefore, that a reduction in surface area (e.g., from a pneumothorax) or an increase in thickness (e.g., from fluid in the alveoli) will reduce gas exchange. The rate of diffusion will also fall if the concentration of oxygen (or, more accurately, the partial pressure) in the alveoli falls, as a result of either decreased ventilation or a lowering of the inspired oxygen concentration.

ASTHMA

PATHOPHYSIOLOGY AND PRESENTATION

Asthma is a common condition from which approximately 10% of the population, in all age groups, suffer. The prevalence appears to be rising and approximately 1000 people die in the UK each year from this condition. The young and the elderly are particularly vulnerable. Effective and rapid treatment is therefore vital.

There are three factors that lead to the generalized airway obstruction characteristic of asthma:

- mucosal inflammation in the airway passages, leading to oedema and swelling of the tissues
- increased production of thick mucus, leading to plugging of bronchioles
- generalized bronchial smooth muscle constriction, leading to bronchospasm.

In the early stages of an attack the obstruction is reversible. However, as the attack progresses it becomes increasingly difficult to reverse the process.

Precipitating causes of an acute exacerbation of asthma include:

- exercise
- infection
- allergy to drugs or other substances
- emotional upset.

However, in many cases there is no obvious cause. Individuals susceptible to other atopic disorders such as eczema are more prone to developing asthma. There also appears to be a familial element.

Mild attacks are normally dealt with by the patient's general practitioner and it is usually severe attacks with which ambulance staff become involved. As a result, the patient is likely to be very aware of the severity of his symptoms. His concerns should be heeded. The early symptoms include exercise-induced and nighttime cough. As an attack progresses, the patient becomes increasingly breathless and starts to wheeze. The wheeze is usually expiratory, but may also be inspiratory. The patient may have visible indrawing in the intercostal spaces with recession subcostally. In severe cases patients may be seen to fix the chest by splaying their arms out firmly, allowing the accessory muscles of respiration to be used. The accessory muscles are those not normally used in respiration and are principally the sternomastoids. The patient is usually anxious and cyanosis may be present in a severe attack. It should be remembered that a *minor attack may develop into a life-threatening situation in a very short time*.

> **Life-threatening deterioration of an asthma attack may be very rapid**

Clinical examination will show the patient to have a tachycardia, resonant chest on percussion and reduced air entry. A polyphonic (more than one musical note) expiratory wheeze will be heard on auscultation. The peak flow rate is characteristically reduced in asthma: this is a measure of the maximum expiratory rate. The rate is measured using a peak flow meter (Figure 11.3); the patient makes three attempts to breathe into the meter and the best result is compared with a standard chart of predicted values for individuals of the same sex, height, age and race. Each attempt must be a sudden, short, hard blow into the meter using maximal effort.

The signs of severe and life-threatening asthma are shown in Boxes 11.1 and 11.2.

In extreme cases the patient may have a "silent chest". This is a most ominous sign as it means that there is not enough air entry to generate a wheeze. Oximetry will show a reduced S_PO_2. In rare cases asthmatic patients develop spontaneous pneumothorax as a result of a ruptured bulla (lung cyst). They may also develop subcutaneous emphysema in the neck and anterior chest wall.

The differential diagnosis of a severe asthma attack includes pulmonary oedema, anaphylaxis, pneumothorax and airway obstruction (Chapter 11).

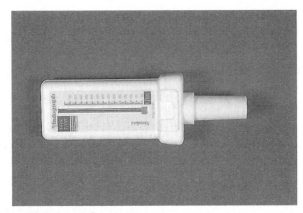

Figure 11.3 A peak flow meter

Box 11.1 Features of severe asthma

Adults	*Children*
Cannot complete sentences	Cannot talk or feed
Pulse >110 per minute	Pulse >140 per minute
Respiratory rate ≥25 per minute	Respiratory rate >50 per minute
Peak flow rate 33–50% of predicted	

Box 11.2 Features of life-threatening asthma

Adults	*Children*
Exhaustion	Reduced conscious level
Cyanosis	Agitation
Bradycardia	Cyanosis
Hypotension	Silent chest
Silent chest	Coma
Peak flow <33% of predicted	
Coma	
SpO$_2$ < 92% on air/95% on oxygen	
Reduced respiratory effort	

Beware the asthma patient with a silent chest

MANAGEMENT

It is essential not to panic but to maintain an air of calm, no matter how worrying the situation is. Panic is rapidly transmitted to the patient and will only make a difficult situation worse. A rapid history, including recent episodes and current treatment, should be obtained from the patient (if possible) or witnesses. An inability to give a history due to shortness of breath is a very worrying sign and in such a situation, attempts to alleviate breathlessness which delay potentially life-saving treatment should not be continued.

The signs of severe or life-threatening asthma (Boxes 11.1 and 11.2) must be sought and other diagnoses considered, treated if present or excluded. The peak flow rate should be

measured and the predicted figure calculated if it is not known to the patient. With experience, very poor results will often be recognized without comparison to normal values. Emergency treatment should be commenced at the earliest opportunity.

It is essential that the patient is transported to hospital as quickly as possible. There can be no exceptions to this rule. It is helpful to advise the receiving hospital of impending arrival especially if there is no response to treatment or the clinical situation is serious.

Patients with severe or life-threatening asthma may not appear distressed or have all of these features. Make the diagnosis if any feature is present

Prehospital treatment of severe and life-threatening asthma

The aim of emergency treatment is to reverse hypoxia with oxygen and reduce bronchospasm using β$_2$-adrenoreceptor agonists. Oral or intravenous steroid therapy has no effect for at least 4 hours.

Adults

- Oxygen, high flow via a reservoir mask (10–15 l/min)
- Salbutamol 5 mg via an oxygen-driven nebulizer, repeated as necessary
- Intravenous access (consider crystalloid infusion if dehydrated)
- Hydrocortisone 200 mg IV
- ECG monitoring
- Immediate evacuation to hospital.

If the asthma is severe or life threatening, ipratropium 0.5 mg should be added to the nebulizer.

Children

- Oxygen, high flow via a reservoir mask (10–15 l/min)
- Salbutamol 5 mg via an oxygen-driven nebulizer (the dose should be halved in children under 6 years old), repeated as necessary
- Intravenous access (consider crystalloid infusion if dehydrated)
- Hydrocortisone 200 mg IV
- ECG monitoring
- Immediate evacuation to hospital.

If the attack is severe or life threatening, ipratropium 0.25 mg should be added to the nebulizer (0.125 mg in children under 1 year).

Unnecessary time should not be lost, in either adults or children, whilst intravenous access is obtained.

Transport to hospital

It is essential that time is not wasted in repeatedly attempting to perform clinical interventions that are not going according to plan. If problems are encountered, the patient should be immediately transferred to hospital. All of the above procedures can be carried out in the back of a moving ambulance. It is important to be prepared to intubate the patient if respiratory arrest occurs; airway pressures are likely to be high and ventilation will therefore be difficult. Cardiac arrest may ensue and the standard protocols should be followed (see Chapter 14).

Paramedics are well placed to deal with severe and life-threatening asthma, but they must act with speed and foresight to ensure a satisfactory outcome.

PULMONARY OEDEMA

PATHOPHYSIOLOGY AND PRESENTATION

Pulmonary oedema is usually caused by acute left ventricular failure (LVF) and is a very common cause of death in the elderly. Fluid collects in the interstitial tissues of the lung (the tissues between the alveoli), usually because of the heart's inability to pump properly. Ultimately, fluid leaks into the alveoli themselves, causing marked interference with oxygenation. Hypoxia rapidly develops and cardiac arrest follows soon afterwards. It is unlikely that ambulance staff will be expected to deal with patients with mild LVF as they usually present to their general practitioner. Paramedics will, however, have to deal with severe cases on a regular basis.

The causes of "pump failure" include:

- acute myocardial infarction (AMI)
- dysrhythmias
- antiarrhythmic drug overdose
- inadequate heart rate (β-blocking drugs or post infarction)
- chronic valvular heart disease (usually aortic or mitral valve)
- cardiac tamponade
- fluid overload.

Cardiac tamponade occurs when fluid builds up around the heart within the pericardial sac, preventing the proper mechanical action of the heart. The differential diagnosis of pulmonary oedema includes asthma COPD and bronchopneumonia. All conditions may coexist.

The early symptoms of pulmonary oedema are breathlessness on exertion, paroxysmal nocturnal dyspnoea (waking at night with severe shortness of breach, which often resolves after sitting or standing) and orthopnoea (breathlessness on lying down). Wheeze and cough are often reported. In severe cases acute respiratory distress is present and the patient often coughs up pink froth or blood. If AMI is the cause the patient may have chest pain, but it is essential to be aware that a "silent infarct" may present as acute pulmonary oedema.

Clinical examination in severe cases will often reveal an anxious, pale, cold and clammy patient, who will be cyanosed and tachypnoeic and have a tachycardia. The patient is likely to be hypotensive. Electrocardiographic monitoring *may* reveal the injury pattern of AMI (ST elevation) or a

> ### Box 11.3 Symptoms of acute pulmonary oedema
>
> - Breathlessness on exertion
> - Paroxysmal nocturnal dyspnoea (waking at night with severe shortness of breath, which often resolves after sitting or standing)
> - Breathlessness on lying down (orthopnoea)
> - Wheeze and cough
> - Pink frothy sputum or haemoptysis
> - Chest pain in (AMI)

> ### Box 11.4 Signs of acute pulmonary oedema
>
> - Anxiety
> - Pallor
> - Coldness
> - Clamminess
> - Cyanosis
> - Tachypnoea
> - Tachycardia
> - Hypotension
> - "Crackles" on auscultation (occasionally wheeze)

dysrhythmia. Fine crepitations ("crackles") may be heard on auscultation of the chest, and occasionally wheeze. When there is wheeze, there may be diagnostic confusion with asthma or chronic obstructive pulmonary disease (COPD); wheeze in a cold, clammy, sweaty patient is usually due to LVF while asthmatic and bronchitic patients are generally warm and well perfused. If pulmonary oedema is severe the patient may be unconscious and may progress to cardiac arrest.

TREATMENT

Treatment is aimed at improving oxygenation, reducing the volume of blood returned to the left ventricle and treating the underlying cause. Definitive treatment of acute pulmonary oedema requires in hospital care. However, there is a great deal that the paramedic can do.

It is important to keep calm but to act swiftly. The patient should be sat up, if he has not already sat up, with his feet or legs dependent. If the patient is able to provide one, a rapid history of events should be taken, noting the patient's current medication. Information may be available from witnesses or relatives. High-flow oxygen should be given via a reservoir mask, even if there is a history of severe underlying lung disease, in which case the respiration should be carefully monitored. Two puffs of glyceryl trinitrate (GTN) spray should be given under the patient's tongue. It is helpful to warn of headache as a side-effect (although regular users will be aware of this) and to be vigilant for the development of hypotension. The spray should not be shaken before use (mixing the propellant with the drug reduces the

Box 11.5 Treatment of acute pulmonary oedema

- Sit the patient up with feet or legs dependent
- Establish the history and current medication
- Give high-flow oxygen via a reservoir mask
- Give two puffs of GTN spray
- Establish intravenous access
- Give intravenous frusemide. Give salbutamol 5 mg via nebulizer
- Monitor the three-lead ECG
- Treat dysrhythmias and cardiac arrest as necessary
- Transfer the patient to hospital as rapidly as possible
- Consider morphine and aspirin if chest pain present

metred dose). The blood pressure should be checked and should be at least 90 mmHg before giving this drug.

Intravenous access should be established and IV frusemide (a diuretic) given. The three-lead ECG should be monitored and any dysrhythmia or cardiac arrest treated appropriately. The patient should be transferred to hospital as rapidly as possible, warning the hospital of the impending arrival. If symptoms are unrelieved, give salbutamol 5 mg via nebulizer. Consider morphine and aspirin if chest pain is present. A 12-lead ECG should be recorded en route.

AIRWAY OBSTRUCTION

HYPOXIA KILLS
An obstructed airway is a dire emergency
Evaluation of the airway is ALWAYS the first step in the primary survey of EVERY patient

PATHOPHYSIOLOGY AND PRESENTATION

Airway obstruction and the resultant hypoxia is the most fundamental and preventable cause of death in trauma and medical collapse. It is a tragedy if simple airway obstruction, causing hypoxia, is the sole cause of death, as it is so readily treated. The maintenance of the airway is central to both basic life support (Chapter 5) and advanced life support (Chapter 14). The aggressive resuscitation of a bleeding multiple trauma victim may be futile if the airway is not secured and adequate oxygenation maintained.

There are many causes of airway obstruction, but perhaps the most common is the tongue falling back onto the posterior pharyngeal wall. Others include a foreign body (for example, food or false teeth); severe facial injury (Chapter 24); acute anaphylaxis resulting in airway oedema; and burns with inhalation of hot gases, which can similarly lead to laryngeal oedema and airway obstruction (Chapter 31). Medical conditions such as epiglottitis are a rare cause of acute obstruction.

TREATMENT

The treatment of airway obstruction is aimed at removing the cause of obstruction and maintaining a secure airway thereafter. The essential features of treatment of a simple obstructed airway and choking are covered fully in Chapter 6. Advanced airway techniques may be required if the patient does not recover consciousness (Chapter 7). Expeditious treatment and transportation are essential if casualties are to have the best chance of survival.

The use of simple airway techniques, augmented with 100% oxygen, is often all that is required as prehospital treatment, although advanced techniques such as intubation are within the scope of paramedic staff when the need arises. If difficulty with airway management is encountered, medical help should be sought *quickly*. This means that crews should be ready to move immediately. Alternatively, if rapid evacuation is not possible because of entrapment, they should call on the expertise of their local Immediate Care scheme or hospital mobile medical team. Paramedics should be able to anticipate problems and lay plans to prevent them, rather than simply responding to problems when they do occur.

EPIGLOTTITIS

Epiglottitis warrants special mention since injudicious examination can precipitate complete airway obstruction. Epiglottitis is a bacterial infection of the epiglottis, seen most often in children. It leads to marked swelling of the epiglottis, with a typical "cherry red" appearance. It is usually associated with fever and malaise. The patient will often be grey, distressed, drooling at the mouth and leaning forward. There is severe continuous stridor.

Examination of the mouth and pharynx must not be attempted in suspected epiglottitis

Complete airway obstruction can develop within minutes. Any procedure that can cause crying or gagging, including simple examination of the throat, can precipitate laryngeal spasm and airway obstruction. *Although most children will need intubation, it should only be attempted by a senior anaesthetist in hospital if the child is breathing spontaneously.* If the condition is suspected the patient should be calmed, given high-concentration oxygen, sat forward and transported quickly to hospital. A paediatric team and senior anaesthetist should be requested to stand by. If airway obstruction occurs before arrival at hospital intubation or needle cricothyroidotomy may be required (Chapter 7).

ANAPHYLAXIS

Anaphylaxis is an acute hypersensitivity (allergic) reaction to foreign protein. True anaphylaxis does not occur on the first exposure to a substance; it occurs only in patients who have been previously exposed, or "sensitized", to that protein. Repeated exposure leads to outpouring of histamine and histamine-like substances that mediate the acute reaction, with each subsequent attack often being worse than the last. *Anaphylactoid* reactions can occur with first exposure to certain severe stimuli, such as insect stings and snake bites (including the British adder). *Anaphylactic* reactions involve the release of the immunoglobin IgE, *anaphylactoid* reactions do not.

Common triggers for anaphylaxis are exposure to antibiotics (particularly the penicillins), insect stings, shellfish, strawberries and nuts (e.g., peanuts). Colloid intravenous fluids (such as Haemaccel and Gelofusine) have also been identified as a rare cause. In essence, *any* substance can cause a reaction, although some are much more common than others. Many patients will be aware of their own triggers and will avoid them wherever possible but in many cases, and especially in first attacks, the cause is unknown. Some hypersensitive patients carry their own adrenaline injection or nasal spray.

Allergic responses vary in severity, from a simple urticarial rash ("nettle rash") to a full-blown acute anaphylactic reaction with cardiorespiratory arrest. The symptoms are very variable and include itchy skin, running eyes and nose, and urticarial rash in the early stages. As the process develops, there is swelling of the face, eyes and lips and occasionally the tongue and fauces also become swollen. Laryngeal oedema leads to airway obstruction. Bronchospasm and wheeze may be noted. In severe attacks tachycardia, tachypnoea and hypotension can be expected – indeed, all the signs of profound shock (Chapter 22). The speed of onset is variable and patients with marked sensitivity can progress to a severe reaction in a matter of minutes.

MANAGEMENT

A calm atmosphere must be maintained as the patient is likely to be very anxious. The history and the precipitating cause should be established. Having checked what treatment has been taken (antihistamines, adrenaline), the treatment of anaphylaxis should be commenced (see below). The patient should be transported to hospital as soon as possible and the hospital advised of the impending arrival.

Treatment of acute anaphylaxis

The airway must be opened, cleared and secured. If it is obstructed, immediate intubation is required. If intubation fails, a surgical airway is required: either way, immediate medical support will be necessary and the patient will need to be moved rapidly to hospital. Oxygen 100%, 15 litres per minute via reservoir mask, should be administered and adrenaline 1:1000 IM should be given immediately. It may be necessary to repeat this. For children, see Table 11.1. Intravenous access should be established and crystalloid given rapidly according to the patient's requirements and local protocols. If bronchospasm is present, this should be treated as asthma (see above).

Box 11.6 Signs and symptoms of anaphylaxis with increasing severity of attack

- Urticarial rash ("nettle rash")
- Itchy skin
- Running eyes and nose
- Swelling of the face, eyes and lips, and occasionally the tongue
- Laryngeal oedema leading to airway obstruction
- Bronchospasm
- Tachycardia
- Tachypnoea
- Hypotension
- Cardiac arrest

Table 11.1 Paediatric doses of adrenaline solutions (1:1000 contains 1 mg/ml)

Age	Adrenaline 1:1000 (ml)
<6 months	0.05
6 months–5 yrs	0.12
6–11 yrs	0.25
>12 yrs	0.5

Box 11.7 Treatment of anaphylaxis

- Open, clear and secure the airway
- If the airway is obstructed, intubate immediately
- If intubation fails, a surgical airway is required
- Give 100% oxygen (15 litres per minute via reservoir mask)
- Give 0.5–1.0 ml of adrenaline 1:1000 IM or 5–10 ml of adrenaline 1:10 000 IM. For children the dose of adrenaline should be 0.01 ml/kg IM or IV
- Repeat either IM or slow IV adrenaline as required
- Establish IV access
- Give crystalloid rapidly according to the patient's requirements and local protocols
- If bronchospasm is present, treat as asthma (see above)
- Give hydrocortisone 100–200 mg IV (children 100 mg)
- Give chlorpheniramine 10 mg IV

Hydrocortisone 200 mg IV (children 4 mg/kg) and chlorpheniramine 10 mg IV should be given. Neither hydrocortisone nor chlorpheniramine (Piriton) is effective immediately in the treatment of anaphylaxis but if given early, both will subsequently be useful in reducing the anaphylactic response. Both must be given slowly to avoid hypotension.

CHRONIC OBSTRUCTIVE PULMONARY DISEASE

Chronic obstructive pulmonary disease (COPD) is also commonly referred to as chronic obstructive airways disease (COAD) and is often known to the public as chronic bronchitis and emphysema. COPD results in chronic airflow limitation which some asthmatics may also suffer. Chronic bronchitis is clinically defined as the production of sputum for at least 3 months each year in two consecutive years. It causes obstruction by plugging the airways (bronchioles) with mucus, and by inflammation and thickening of the airway mucosa. Emphysema is the dilation of alveolar airspaces by the destruction of their walls. The elastic recoil that holds the airways open in expiration is lost and obstruction to airflow occurs. Both conditions usually coexist to some degree. The main cause of COPD is smoking, although some cases are attributable to a rare inherited enzyme (α1-antitrypsin) deficiency.

The patient with chronic bronchitis will usually present with an acute exacerbation of breathlessness, often precipitated by infection. The complexion may be bluish due to cyanosis – hence the description *"blue bloater"*. There is generally a moist, productive cough, severe dyspnoea and wheeze. Auscultation may reveal reduced air entry, scattered wheezes and coarse crepitations (crackles) throughout the lung fields. The patient may have associated heart disease and right heart failure (*cor pulmonale*).

A patient with emphysema tends to have fewer symptoms and is able to maintain reasonably normal blood gas levels. The chest is often barrel shaped. The patient will be breathless and will often purse the lips on expiration; the term *"pink puffer"* is sometimes used but, like "blue bloater", is unhelpful (and offensive) and should not be used.

The pure bronchitic and the pure emphysematous patient represent opposite ends of a clinical spectrum. The majority of patients demonstrate features of both.

Patients with COPD rely on hypoxia as their drive to breathe because their respiratory centre, driven by a high carbon dioxide concentration in people without this condition, becomes relatively insensitive to carbon dioxide due to chronic exposure to elevated levels.

PREHOSPITAL MANAGEMENT

Patients with acute exacerbations of COPD are hypoxic. Emergency treatment is aimed at general supportive measures and relief of hypoxia. Rapid transport to hospital is mandatory. The preemptive siting of an IV cannula may be helpful in case of cardiorespiratory arrest.

Hypoxia kills

Patients with acute respiratory decompensation need supplemental oxygen. However, it is potentially dangerous to give supplemental oxygen to these patients *unless* they are carefully observed and the paramedic is prepared to assist ventilation if required. It is possible that administering oxygen will raise the oxygen concentration in the blood (PO_2) to a level at which the hypoxic drive is switched off, resulting in hypoventilation or apnoea. Patients can be verbally instructed to take additional breaths and can be assisted with a bag and mask with oxygen reservoir if necessary. The risk of shutting off hypoxic drive can be minimized by adjusting oxygen delivery to maintain S_PO_2 at the patient's usual level or at 90–92% if unknown.

Never withhold oxygen from a patient who needs it

Patients who die, do so from *hypoxia,* either because oxygen therapy is withheld or because paramedic staff fail in their duty to support ventilation when the hypoxic drive is lost.

HYPOXIA KILLS QUICKLY
HYPERCARBIA KILLS SLOWLY
So give oxygen and support ventilation if the "hypoxic drive" is lost

Give salbutamol 5 mg via nebulizer, repeated to effect. Mix 500 μg ipratropium with first dose of salbutamol.

CONCLUSION

Respiratory conditions are extremely common. Deaths still result all too frequently when these conditions are inadequately managed. Many of these deaths are those of young asthmatics, the severity of whose symptoms was all too tragically underestimated by themselves or their carers. It is imperative that all clinicians are aware of the potential seriousness of these conditions and fully conversant with their emergency management. Simple protocols and an appropriate sense of urgency will ensure the optimum outcome for these patients.

Chapter 12

The heart: anatomy, physiology and the ECG

The heart is required to provide the body with an adequate supply of oxygenated blood during all bodily functions. It must be able to increase its output from a resting level of approximately 5 litres per minute (in adults) to levels of about 15 litres per minute during exercise. In 70 years of life the human heart beats well over 3 billion times and propels in excess of 300 million litres of blood. In addition to its mechanical properties, the heart has a role in the maintenance of fluid balance and blood pressure via neurohormonal mechanisms. A thorough knowledge of the anatomy (structure and design) and physiology (function) of the human heart and circulatory system enables the paramedic to understand and manage cardiovascular emergencies.

ANATOMY

LOCATION AND SIZE

The heart is a muscular, hollow organ located within the thorax (Figure 12.1). It is enclosed in the pericardial sac (or pericardium) in a space called the mediastinum. The mediastinum is sandwiched between the lungs, with the sternum and its connecting costal cartilages in front and the ribs and the thoracic spinal column behind. The base of the heart rests on the diaphragm and its apex points towards the left nipple, under which a cardiac pulsation (the apex beat) may be seen or felt in thin individuals. The heart thus lies obliquely in the mediastinum with two-thirds of the muscle to the left of the midline of the sternum and is about the same size as the person's clenched fist.

THE PERICARDIUM

The pericardial sac (Figure 12.2) consists of a tough fibrous outer coat and a deeper double-layered secretory membrane, the serous pericardium, which surrounds the heart and extends to the great blood vessels – the aorta and pulmonary trunk.

Between the outer (*parietal*) and inner (*visceral*) layer of the serous pericardium is the pericardial cavity which contains a slippery secretion, the pericardial fluid. This fluid

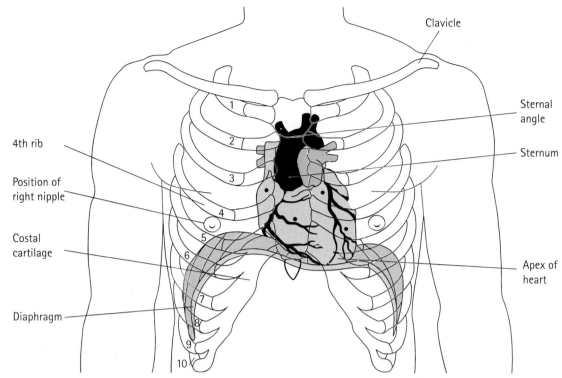

Figure 12.1 The anatomical location of the heart

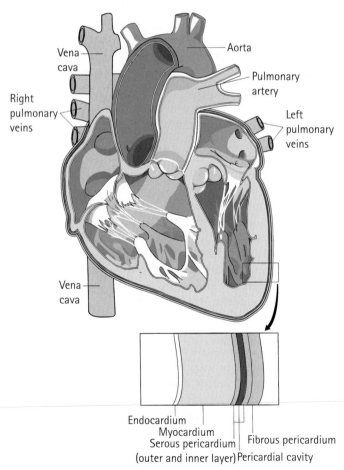

Figure 12.2 Pericardium and myocardium

reduces friction between the membranes as the cavities of the heart fill and then empty. The pericardium has no direct influence on the systolic (emptying) function of the heart but does prevent excess filling of the heart chambers, thus influencing diastolic function (see below). The pericardium also has a role in prevention of spread of infection from adjacent structures. It is particularly relevant to prehospital care because acute inflammation, pericarditis, can cause chest pain and because a collection of fluid within the pericardial cavity may so restrict cardiac filling as to present with cardiac tamponade (see Chapter 14).

THE MYOCARDIAL WALL

The wall of the heart is formed by three layers: the outer layer of the serous pericardium, also called the epicardium, the myocardium and the inner endocardium.

The myocardium is the cardiac muscle tissue itself. It makes up most of the wall thickness of the heart and is responsible for its pumping function. Cardiac muscle consists of an organized network of muscle fibres, branching and connecting with each other. In this way electrical activity, and corresponding mechanical activity, can spread throughout the entire network of cardiac muscle cells in an organized manner.

Blood vessels and lymphatic vessels, nerves and specialized cardiac conduction fibres lie within the myocardial muscle bulk. Fibrous cells and collagen are also found between the muscle cells and provide a basic "skeleton" for the shape of the heart chambers, as well as establishing the atrioventricular (AV) ring. This ring ensures electrical "insulation" between the atria and ventricles and competence of the AV valves. Excess fibrosis within the myocardium, as seen in hypertension or as part of normal ageing, leads to impaired pumping: predominantly impairment of filling. Because of the combination of specialized conduction fibres and the particular alignment of myocardial muscle fibres, muscular contraction is organized and efficient rather than haphazard and inefficient.

The endocardium provides a smooth lining inside the heart and covers the heart valves. It is continuous with the innermost layer of the great blood vessels and the rest of the cardiovascular system. It may play an important role as an endocrine organ, releasing various chemicals into the blood in response to increased stretch. Being in contact with the bloodstream, the endocardium also has a role as a barrier to infection. Infective endocarditis occurs when areas of the endocardium, especially over the heart valves, are colonized by bacteria.

THE CHAMBERS AND VALVES OF THE HEART

The heart consists of four chambers: right atrium and left atrium (plural "atria") separated by the AV ring from the right and left ventricles (Figure 12.3). The atrial septum and ventricular septum divide the right side of the heart from the left side. During intrauterine growth there is rotation of the heart such that the right heart chambers eventually lie in front of the left chambers and the septa tend to face forwards. For this reason it is the right ventricle that is most often damaged during blunt or sharp anterior chest trauma.

Each ventricle ejects the same quantity of blood, but they are not equal in either the pressure they generate or their muscle mass. The left ventricle is circular in cross-section with a myocardial thickness of about 1 cm, while the right ventricle is relatively thin walled and "wraps itself" around the left in a crescent shape.

The right atrium opens into the right ventricle through an atrioventricular (AV) valve called the *tricuspid* valve. Similarly, the left atrium opens into the left ventricle through an AV valve called the *bicuspid* or *mitral* valve. The pulmonary artery arises from the right ventricle and has a *pulmonary* valve. The aorta arises from the left ventricle and has an *aortic* valve. The valves open and close in response to pressure differences that develop between the various heart chambers and great blood vessels. A series of tendinous cords connect the tricuspid and mitral valve leaflets to the inner walls of the appropriate ventricle via papillary muscles (Figure 12.2) and serve to ensure competent closure of the valves.

PACEMAKER CELLS AND THE CONDUCTION SYSTEM OF THE HEART

Resting myocardial cells are polarized (i.e. electrically charged) such that there is a relative negative potential between intracellular and extracellular spaces. This is achieved and maintained by the cell membrane and is described in more detail later. Stimulation of the cell allows abrupt and transient reversal of polarity (*depolarization*) and results in activation of the contractile proteins within the myocardial cell. Thus electrical activation is the trigger for mechanical activity. A wave of depolarization will spread to neighbouring myocardial cells. In order for the heart to pump effectively, depolarization must excite the cardiac chambers in a coordinated manner. This is facilitated by the conduction system (Figure 12.4) which consists of five specialized components.

- The sinoatrial (SA) or sinus node
- The atrioventricular (AV) node

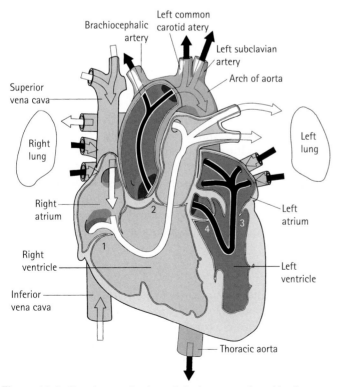

Figure 12.3 Chambers and valves of the heart: 1, tricuspid valve; 2, pulmonary valve; 3, bicuspid valve; 4, aortic valve

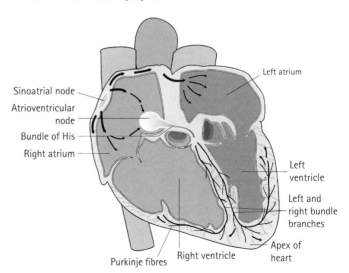

Figure 12.4 The conducting system of the heart

- The atrioventricular bundle (bundle of His)
- The right and left bundle branches
- The Purkinje fibres.

The SA node, a group of cells in the right atrium, has an intrinsically unstable membrane potential. Even without the influence of circulating hormones or the autonomic nervous system, the SA node will rhythmically and spontaneously depolarize and normally acts as the primary pacemaker of the heart. Heart rhythms that are governed by the SA node are termed *sinus rhythm*.

The depolarization wave spreads outwards through the atria and reaches the AV node located in the septum between the two atria. Conduction between atria and ventricles is normally only possible through the AV node and is relatively slow. This has the effect of protecting the ventricles from rapid atrial rhythms (such as flutter and fibrillation) and ensuring that atrial contraction (and therefore ventricular filling) is complete before ventricular emptying starts. The cardiac impulse continues to spread through the bundle of His and the right and left bundle branches within the interventricular septum towards the apex of the heart. Purkinje fibres (muscle fibres specialized for conduction) rapidly excite the muscle bulk of the left and right ventricle.

MYOCARDIAL BLOOD SUPPLY

The arterial supply of the myocardium is in the form of two coronary arteries that arise from the ascending aorta just above the aortic valve and pass along the epicardial surface within pericardial fat, accompanied by the venous drainage (Figure 12.5). The *left main coronary artery* divides into the *left anterior descending artery* and the *circumflex artery.* Together these supply the left atrium and most of the left ventricular muscle bulk as well as a small part of the right ventricle. The

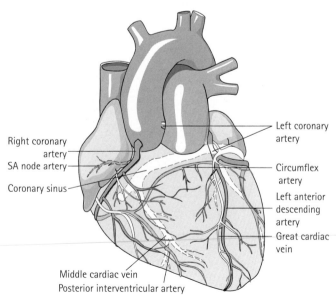

Figure 12.5 Myocardial blood supply

Right coronary artery
SA node artery
Coronary sinus
Middle cardiac vein
Posterior interventricular artery
Left coronary artery
Circumflex artery
Left anterior descending artery
Great cardiac vein

right coronary artery supplies the right atrium, right ventricle and lower part of the ventricular septum. It also gives off an important small branch to supply the SA node and commonly supplies the AV node. It is for this reason that a right coronary artery occlusion is more likely to lead to a myocardial infarction that is complicated by (electrical) heart block. Anatomically, the myocardial blood supply does vary between individuals.

Most venous blood is drained via the cardiac veins into the *coronary sinus* which opens directly into the right atrium. Some of the smaller veins empty directly into the heart chambers.

CIRCULATORY SYSTEM

A complex system of branching arteries arises from the left ventricle. The arterial system carries blood away from the heart through arteries and smaller arterioles into the capillary network of body tissues. The capillary network is responsible for the exchange of nutrients and waste products at tissue level and is often referred to as the *microcirculation*. From there the circulating blood returns through venules and the venous system to the right side of the heart.

Arteries

The aorta arises from the left ventricle and gives off important main branches to the head, neck and arms within the chest, before passing into the abdomen where it ultimately divides into the two common iliac arteries (Figure 12.6a). The larger arteries have walls rich in elastic fibres, whereas medium-sized arteries and arterioles (the smallest arteries) have predominantly muscular walls. The muscle layer may contract to cause vasoconstriction or relax to allow vasodilation. This leads to changes in the calibre of these arteries and consequent changes in regional blood flow.

Capillaries

Capillaries are very small, thin-walled vessels which connect arterioles to venules (Figure 12.6b). They often form extensive branching networks, particularly in body tissues with high metabolic activity, for example the liver, kidney or central nervous system. The capillary walls are a single layer of cells with a basement membrane to anchor these cells. Their structure allows a rapid exchange of nutrients and waste products with surrounding tissue cells.

Veins

Several capillaries unite to form *venules* or small veins which drain into the veins carrying blood from the tissues to the heart. The veins become progressively larger in diameter and ultimately drain into the right atrium via the superior and inferior vena cavae (Figure 12.6c). In order to aid blood flow towards the heart, veins contain valves, particularly in dependent tissues, which prevent the backflow of blood. Compared with the arteries, blood within veins does

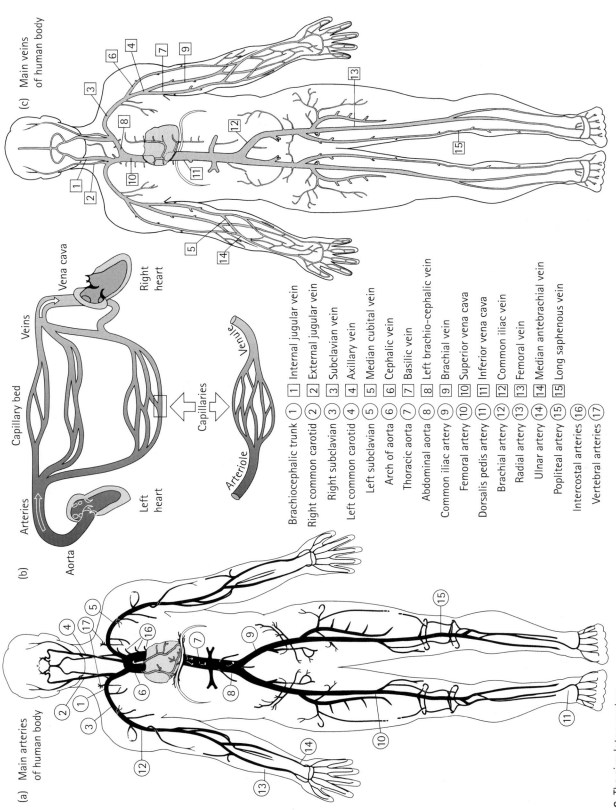

(c) Main veins of human body

(b)

Vena cava

Veins

Capillary bed

Arteries

Aorta

Right heart

Left heart

Venule

Capillaries

Arteriole

Brachiocephalic trunk ① Internal jugular vein ①
Right common carotid ② External jugular vein ②
Right subclavian ③ Subclavian vein ③
Left common carotid ④ Axillary vein ④
Left subclavian ⑤ Median cubital vein ⑤
Arch of aorta ⑥ Cephalic vein ⑥
Thoracic aorta ⑦ Basilic vein ⑦
Abdominal aorta ⑧ Left brachio-cephalic vein ⑧
Common iliac artery ⑨ Brachial vein ⑨
Femoral artery ⑩ Superior vena cava ⑩
Dorsalis pedis artery ⑪ Inferior vena cava ⑪
Brachial artery ⑫ Common iliac vein ⑫
Radial artery ⑬ Femoral vein ⑬
Ulnar artery ⑭ Median antebrachial vein ⑭
Popliteal artery ⑮ Long saphenous vein ⑮
Intercostal arteries ⑯
Vertebral arteries ⑰

(a) Main arteries of human body

Figure 12.6 The circulatory system

Table 12.1 Circulating blood volume in relation to age

Age group	Blood volume (ml/kg body weight)
Adult	70
Child	80
Neonate	90

not exhibit pulsatile flow, is under far lower pressure and is at greater risk of coagulating (venous thrombosis). On the other hand, atheroma develops in arterial walls rather than the walls of veins.

Content of the circulatory system

The normal circulating blood volume is variable but in a 70 kg adult it is about 5 litres (equivalent to about 70 ml/kg body weight) (Table 12.1).

Blood consists of a fluid component (plasma) and a particulate component: red blood cells (erythrocytes), white blood cells (leucocytes) and platelets (thrombocytes). The plasma accounts for about 55% of total blood volume.

Haemoglobin within red blood cells is the main transporter of oxygen and carbon dioxide. White blood cells are involved in immunity from infection and rejection of foreign tissues. Platelets primarily stop bleeding by adhesion to damaged blood vessel surfaces and aggregation with other activated platelets and various clotting factors. Such platelet activity is partially inhibited by aspirin.

Proteins in the plasma include albumin, α- and β-globulins and fibrinogen. Plasma proteins play an important role in maintaining *homeostasis* within the body – a constant, stable internal environment – which is essential for optimal tissue function. Fibrinogen helps to form a web of protein fibres when blood-clotting mechanisms are activated. Albumin and α- and β-globulins assist in transporting other proteins and lipids. γ-Globulins provide immunity and defence against infection.

NERVE SUPPLY TO THE HEART

In laboratory conditions the heart can beat even if it is removed completely from the body, owing to the inherent pacemaker function of the SA node. However, the heart receives nerve impulses from the cardiovascular regulatory centres in the midbrain and medulla oblongata (Figure 12.7). These are transmitted via sympathetic and parasympathetic nerve fibres. These tend to cause an increase or decrease in the heart rate and the strength of the pumping action of the heart respectively.

There are also sensory nerve fibres allowing the recognition of the pain of ischaemia (angina). It is likely that these

nerve endings are stimulated by adenosine. Angina-like chest pains may be experienced when adenosine is given to terminate a supraventricular tachycardia. Abnormalities of such nerve supply may account for the absence of characteristic pains in some diabetic individuals who suffer myocardial infarction.

The atria and ventricles also contain sensory fibres that respond to stretch and contractility, as part of the baroreceptor reflex controlling systemic blood pressure. Stretch due to increased atrial and ventricular volume also stimulates release, from these chambers, of natriuretic peptides that have a role in sodium and fluid balance. Higher circulating levels of such peptides are seen in patients with heart failure.

The pericardium also has a nerve supply, which is why pericarditis is characteristically painful.

PHYSIOLOGY

CARDIAC PUMP

The heart is a double pump which serves two circulations: the pulmonary and the systemic (Figure 12.8). The right ventricle pumps blood at lower pressure (about 25 mmHg) into the lungs via the pulmonary trunk, while the left ventricle pumps blood at higher pressure (about 120 mmHg) into the aorta.

The right atrium receives deoxygenated blood (blood that has lost oxygen to the cells and taken on carbon dioxide) from the systemic circulation via the superior and inferior vena cavae and from the coronary circulation via the coronary sinus. From the right atrium the deoxygenated blood crosses the tricuspid valve into the right ventricle and thence through the pulmonary valve into the pulmonary trunk and consequently into the left and right lungs. Reoxygenation occurs in the pulmonary capillary bed and oxygenated blood then flows via four pulmonary veins back into the left atrium, through the mitral valve into the left ventricle and finally is pumped out of the aortic valve.

CARDIAC CYCLE

The adult human heart beats about 70 times per minute at rest. One heartbeat within a single cardiac cycle therefore lasts about 0.8 seconds or 800 milliseconds (ms). During a cardiac cycle the atria and ventricles alternately contract and relax (Figure 12.9). The phase of contraction is called *systole*, the phase of relaxation is called *diastole*. Blood movement through the heart is caused by pressure changes within the heart chambers. During atrial diastole, which lasts approximately 700 ms, both atria fill with blood from the superior and inferior vena cavae on the right and the pulmonary veins on the left.

The two atria contract for about 100 ms during atrial systole while the two ventricles are still relaxed. Thus the right and left atria actively support filling of the ventricles by

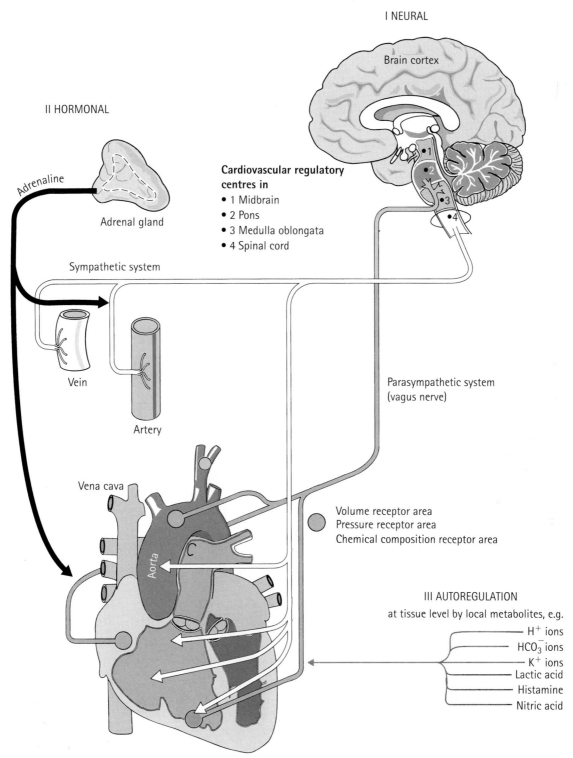

I NEURAL

Brain cortex

Cardiovascular regulatory centres in
- 1 Midbrain
- 2 Pons
- 3 Medulla oblongata
- 4 Spinal cord

II HORMONAL

Adrenaline

Adrenal gland

Sympathetic system

Vein

Artery

Vena cava

Aorta

C

Parasympathetic system (vagus nerve)

Volume receptor area
Pressure receptor area
Chemical composition receptor area

III AUTOREGULATION

at tissue level by local metabolites, e.g.

- H$^+$ ions
- HCO$_3^-$ ions
- K$^+$ ions
- Lactic acid
- Histamine
- Nitric acid

Figure 12.7 Regulatory control of the cardiovascular system

squeezing approximately 20–30% of the blood into the ventricular chambers; 70–80% of the blood contained in the atrial reservoirs flows passively down a pressure gradient through the opened atrioventricular valves into the ventricles before atrial contraction.

As the ventricles begin to contract during ventricular systole, the pressure in the ventricles rises above the pressure in the atria and the AV valves shut. Ventricular pressure continues to rise until it exceeds pressure in the pulmonary trunk of the right side of the heart and in the aorta on the left side. The pulmonary and aortic valves are forced open and blood is ejected from the ventricles into the pulmonary and systemic circulation respectively. As the ventricular volumes decrease owing to outflow of blood after 300 ms,

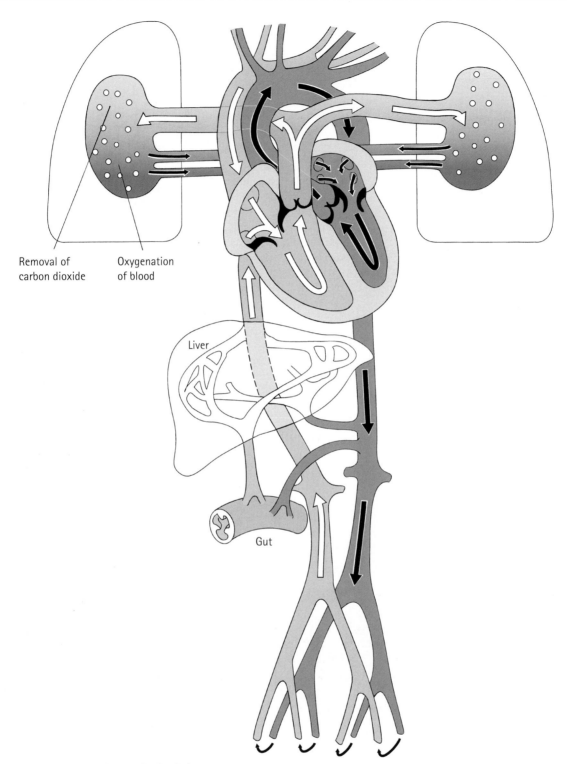

Removal of carbon dioxide

Oxygenation of blood

Liver

Gut

Figure 12.8 The pulmonary and systemic circulations

ventricular diastole or relaxation begins. Ventricular pressure now falls below pressure in the pulmonary trunk or aorta and the pulmonary and aortic valves close. Once ventricular pressure is lower than atrial pressure, the tricuspid and mitral valves open and blood flows from both atria into the ventricles.

Heart sounds are due to closure of the heart valves at different phases of the cardiac cycle. The first heart sound is caused by the closure of the mitral and tricuspid valve and is soft in character ("lub"). The second is a higher-pitched sound ("dup") and is due to the closure of the aortic and pulmonary valve. Hence: *lub-dup–lub-dup–lub-dup*. In most

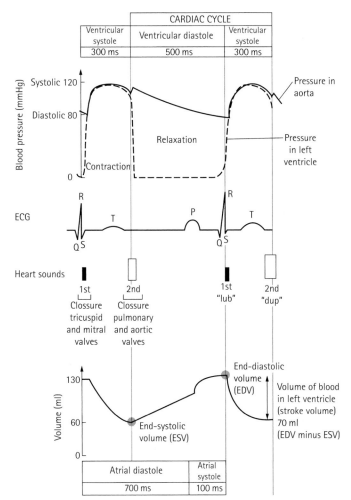

Figure 12.9 The cardiac cycle

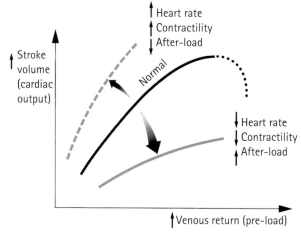

Figure 12.10 Starling's law

STROKE VOLUME

The stroke volume is the amount of blood ejected from each ventricle during a single contraction during the cardiac cycle. It amounts to 70–80 ml at rest but can be doubled with exercise. The heart rate, on the other hand, can treble with exercise. Thus cardiac output can be varied by changing the heart rate, the stroke volume or both. Three factors determine stroke volume.

- *Preload* – the filling of the heart during diastole
- *Afterload* – the resistance in the arterial circulation against which the heart has to pump
- *Contractility* – the intrinsic performance of the heart muscle at a given preload and afterload

adults the sound of blood flow around the heart is inaudible, even with a stethoscope. However, when flow is turbulent, due to high cardiac output or valve disease, an added sound, or *murmur*, is heard between the closure sounds.

Coronary blood flow into the cardiac muscle takes place almost exclusively during diastole or relaxation of ventricular muscle. During systole coronary blood flow is very limited owing to compression of the intramyocardial coronary artery branches. As the heart rate rises, the duration of diastole is shortened whereas the ejection phase remains relatively constant.

CARDIAC OUTPUT

Cardiac output is defined as the volume of blood ejected by each ventricle per minute. At rest the cardiac output amounts to 5000 ml (5 litres) per minute. During severe exercise the cardiac output can be increased up to sixfold to reach 30 litres per minute. Cardiac output is calculated by multiplying the heart rate by the *stroke volume* (volume ejected per heartbeat).

Cardiac output = stroke volume × heart rate

Preload

The degree of filling of the heart determines preload. Ventricular performance depends on the preload. Within certain limits, the higher the degree of venous filling of the heart, the higher its stroke volume and therefore cardiac output (Figure 12.10). In other words, the more myocardial fibres are stretched, the more forcefully they contract. However, if the load increases beyond physiological limits, the heart begins to fail owing to overstretching of myocardial fibres. The degree of venous filling depends on the venous return or the amount of circulating blood volume entering the right side of the heart.

Afterload

Afterload is the resistance against which the heart has to pump during ejection. This opposing force to ejection depends on the pressure in the systemic arterial circulation. Afterload is increased in a patient with hypertension (high blood pressure) due to arteriosclerosis; as a result, stroke volume and therefore cardiac output decrease. If afterload is reduced, the left ventricle is able to contract more quickly and forcefully and therefore the stroke volume and cardiac output increase.

Myocardial contractility

Myocardial contractility is defined as the strength of contraction of myocardial fibres at any given stretch or preload. Naturally produced hormones and drugs such as adrenaline (epinephrine) and noradrenaline (norepinephrine) increase myocardial contractility and are called *positive inotropes*. They increase the stroke volume and cardiac output. Hypoxia and acidosis have a negative inotropic effect on the myocardium.

In common clinical usage, left ventricular performance is often expressed as the *ejection fraction*. This is defined as the proportion of the left ventricular end-diastolic volume that is ejected with each heartbeat and is expressed as a percentage. It may be measured by echocardiography. It is a more sensitive measure of systolic ventricular performance than stroke volume. At rest, the ejection fraction is approximately 50%.

REGULATION OF HEART RATE

As mentioned above, the ability to change heart rate is of great importance in the regulation of cardiac output in response to increased requirements during arousal (primitive flight/fight response) or where stroke volume falls (e.g. in hypovolaemic shock). Rates above 100 per minute are described as *tachycardia* while those below 60 per minute are termed *bradycardia*.

> Heart rate < 60 bradycardia
> Heart rate > 100 tachycardia

Autonomic nervous system control of heart rate

Both sympathetic and parasympathetic fibres of the autonomic nervous system innervate the heart (Figure 12.11). There is a balance between these two systems, although at rest the parasympathetic system tends to dominate, slowing the intrinsic SA node discharge to about 60–70 beats per minute. Parasympathetic fibres reach the heart via the right and left vagus nerves, which supply the SA node, AV node and both atria. Excessive vagal nerve activation may have profound slowing effects and even lead to sinus arrest and asystole. Vagal nerve activity may be blocked by administration of atropine. This is the rationale for the use of atropine in asystolic cardiac arrest.

Sympathetic fibres reach the SA node, AV node, atria and ventricles, where activation tends to increase heart rate. Activity of the sympathetic nervous system is blocked by β-blockers (e.g. propranolol or atenolol), which is why patients taking β-blockers for the management of angina or hypertension may fail to develop a tachycardia in response to significant haemorrhage. Sympathetic and parasympathetic parts of the autonomic nervous system receive input from higher brain centres such as the cerebral cortex. Through this mechanism the heart rate can increase in anticipation of exercise.

Regulation of heart rate by hormones and ions

The catecholamine hormones adrenaline and noradrenaline are released from the adrenal glands in the "fight or flight" response. They increase both heart rate (positive chronotropism) and contractility (positive inotropism), though these effects are not as abrupt as those caused by changes in autonomic nervous system activity. The heart is also sensitive to levels of thyroid hormone, an underactive thyroid being associated with bradycardia and an overactive thyroid with tachycardia or even atrial fibrillation.

Myocardial cells are surrounded by extracellular fluid which is composed of water containing small electrically charged particles called ions, for example sodium (Na^+), potassium (K^+) and calcium (Ca^{++}). For optimal cell function (Table 12.2) a balance is essential between intracellular (inside the cell) and extracellular (outside the cell) fluid composition. Any electrolyte or ion imbalance will compromise cardiac function. Elevated levels of K^+ or Na^+ will decrease the heart rate and contractility. Increased Ca^{++} in the extracellular fluid speeds up the heart and strengthens its pumping action. In clinical practice such effects on heart rate are unimportant.

Increases of body core temperature will increase the rate of depolarization of the SA node, so fever is associated with tachycardia while hypothermia causes bradycardia.

HAEMODYNAMICS OF THE CIRCULATION

The systemic circulation is responsible for supplying all organs and tissues with oxygen and nutrients according to their needs. Blood flow is determined by a number of factors:

- cardiac output (heart rate/stroke volume)
- blood pressure
- total peripheral resistance in the systemic circulation
- characteristics of arterial wall.

BLOOD PRESSURE

Blood pressure (BP) is the pressure that the blood exerts upon a vessel wall. In the systemic circulation the term refers to the pressure generated by contraction of the left ventricle in the aorta. In the aorta the BP rises during systole to about 120 mmHg (equivalent to 16 kilopascals) and falls to about 80 mmHg (11 kPa) during diastole (Table 12.3). The rate of rise of systolic pressure will depend on myocardial contractility and on the elasticity of the large artery walls. In older individuals and those with atheromatous disease, the arteries are relatively stiff, leading to higher systolic

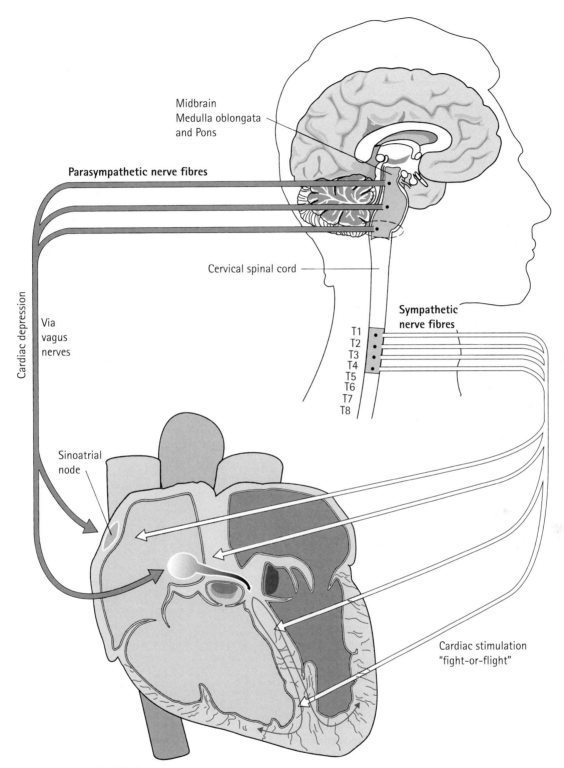

Figure 12.11 Autonomic control of the heart

pressure. The diastolic pressure is important because it determines the perfusion pressure of the coronary arteries. It is maintained by energy from the elastic recoil of the large artery walls and a wave of pressure reflected from more distal arteries. As the arteries decrease in calibre, the velocity of blood flow increases and systolic blood pressure may be higher in the peripheries than centrally.

TOTAL PERIPHERAL RESISTANCE

Total peripheral resistance refers to the sum of all vascular resistances of the systemic blood vessels. The smaller the radius of a blood vessel and the longer its length, the greater the resistance it offers to blood flow. Through changes in cross-sectional area, arterioles are able to modify blood

Table 12.2 Role of electrolytes in cardiac function

Electrolyte	Symbol	Role
Sodium	Na^+	Initiates depolarization of myocardial cell
Potassium	K^+	Initiates repolarization of myocardial cell
Calcium	Ca^{++}	1. Initiates depolarization of pacemaker cells 2. Sustains cardiac action potential 3. Increases myocardial contractility

Table 12.3 Normal blood pressure in healthy, young adults

	Normal blood pressure		Range
	(mmHg)	(kPa)	
Systolic	120	16	±10%
Diastolic	80	11	±10%

flow. The velocity of blood flow is therefore lowest in the capillary beds. This principle is important as it enables capillary exchange of oxygen and carbon dioxide, nutrients and waste products to take place (Figure 12.12).

CIRCULATION TIME

It takes about 1 minute in a resting adult for an intravenous drug in the bloodstream to travel from the right atrium through the pulmonary circulation, to the left ventricle and onward into the systemic circulation, then back to the right atrium.

ELECTRICAL ACTIVITY OF CARDIAC CELLS

Cardiac cells, like all other cells in the body, are electrically charged. In its resting state the interior of a myocardial cell is negatively charged in comparison to the outer surface of the cell membrane. This resting cell membrane potential is caused by the uneven distribution of ions in the extracellular and intracellular fluid. Ions are small particles that are either negatively or positively charged. Potassium (K^+) is the main intracellular ion and would tend to escape to the outside of the cell membrane down a concentration gradient. Sodium (Na^+) is the main extracellular ion and would similarly tend to move along a concentration gradient to intrude into the cells. At rest, energy-consuming exchange pumps keep potassium ions inside the cell and sodium ions outside.

Once a cardiac cell is stimulated, ionic channels within the cell membrane open and the electrical charges inside and outside the cell change. The inside becomes positively charged due to a large influx of sodium ions through special cell membrane channels. Potassium ions flow out of the cell.

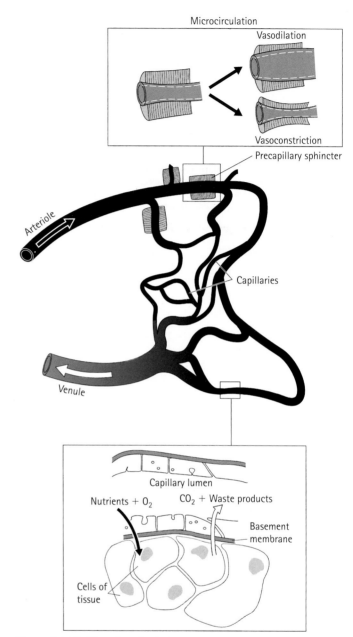

Figure 12.12 The microcirculation

Positively charged calcium ions (Ca^{++}) also travel into the cells. The resting membrane potential thus becomes positive: a cardiac action potential has been generated (Figure 12.13). A *depolarization* has taken place, lasting for about 200 ms. After this time the resting membrane potential is restored by the opening of special potassium channels and potassium ions diffuse out of myocardial cells along their concentration gradient. Simultaneously Na^+ and Ca^{++} channels start closing and fewer and fewer sodium and calcium ions enter the cells. Recovery of the resting membrane potential is called *repolarization*.

It is important to realize that events described above do not just apply to a single myocardial cell. Electrical depolarization is "contagious" (Figure 12.14). Owing to close

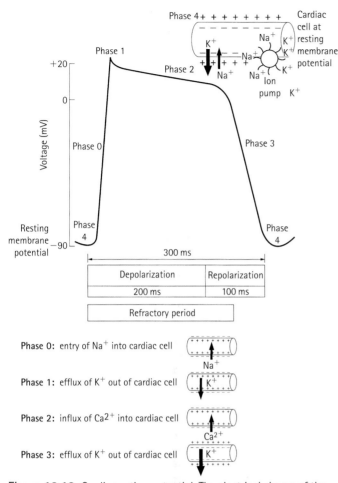

Figure 12.13 Cardiac action potential. The electrical charge of the muscle fibre membrane is denoted by plus or minus signs

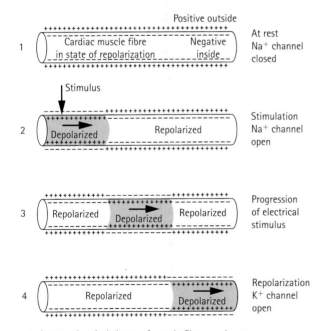

± denotes electrical charge of muscle fibre membrane

Figure 12.14 Progression of the cardiac action potential along cardiac muscle fibre. Plus or minus signs denote the electrical charge of the muscle fibre membrane

contact of all myocardial cells with each other an electrical wave sweeps rapidly through the myocardium. Electrical excitation must always occur before mechanical contraction of myocardial cells can take place, although the two processes are closely coupled with each other except during true electromechanical dissociation (EMD).

Following depolarization, cardiac muscle cells are refractory to a subsequent electrical stimulation for a period of 250 ms. The refractory period allows the heart to alternate between contraction and ejection of blood and relaxation with refilling.

The ability of a particular muscle cell spontaneously to initiate depolarization is known as *automaticity*. The cells of the SA node tend to initiate the wave of depolarization because they have the most rapid automaticity. In complete heart block (see below) the depolarization wave from the SA node does not reach the ventricles and a focus in the AV node or ventricle becomes responsible for electrical activation of the heart. Because these areas have a slower automaticity the heart rate will fall to about 30–50 beats per minute.

OVERALL REGULATORY CONTROL OF THE CARDIOVASCULAR SYSTEM

The entire body must be supplied with enough blood containing oxygen and nutrients to meet tissue demands either at rest or under stress. All organs need a minimum blood flow. Active tissues, for example muscles in severe exercise, require more blood, which is therefore redistributed at the expense of other resting organs, for example the gastrointestinal tract.

The cardiovascular centre for overall regulatory control of the cardiovascular system is situated in the medulla oblongata and pons in the brain (see Figure 12.7). Peripheral receptors in the heart chambers, aortic arch and carotid arteries send signals to these specialized brain regions. Baroreceptors provide a constant feedback of blood pressure and stretch and chemoreceptors are sensitive to the chemical composition of the blood. The cardiovascular centre integrates this information and sends nerve impulses back to the heart and blood vessels via the vagus nerves and nerve fibres of the sympathetic nervous system. These nerve impulses regulate heart rate, cardiac contractility and the vasomotor tone of blood vessels, which is reflected in their degree of vasodilation or vasoconstriction.

Apart from the nervous system control of the cardiovascular system, blood pressure and blood flow are affected by several hormones circulating in the blood, for example adrenaline, noradrenaline, angiotensin and antidiuretic hormone.

A third factor which adjusts blood flow in organs is local control or *autoregulation*. Autoregulation is particularly important in the brain, kidney and heart. Local metabolites (hydrogen ions, carbon dioxide and potassium ions), lactic acid, hypoxia and vasoactive substances such as histamine and nitric oxide produce a local vasodilation of arterioles.

This results in an increased flow of blood into the tissue which restores tissue oxygen supply.

ELECTROCARDIOGRAPHY

At any moment there are numerous wavefronts of depolarization travelling in various directions within the heart. The electrocardiogram (ECG) is a graphical representation of the sum of these wavefronts recorded on the skin surface using a variety of electrodes (Figure 12.15). The ECG does not enable conclusions to be made about mechanical events taking place in the heart, the force of contraction or the blood pressure. It serves as a tool to diagnose abnormalities of rate, rhythm and conduction. Furthermore, it serves to locate ischaemic areas of cardiac muscle or an acute myocardial infarction. It may also provide indirect clues to electrolyte abnormalities, hypothermia and drug intoxication. It is essential in good paramedic practice to evaluate ECG findings in conjunction with a thorough clinical history and assessment of the patient.

UNDERSTANDING THE ECG

The shape of the surface ECG is determined by the sequence of depolarization and repolarization within the specialized conducting system and the myocardium, the proximity of the electrode to the heart, the mass of the heart muscle and the position of the electrode with respect to the heart. Because the left ventricle has greater muscle mass than the right, the surface ECG is most influenced by left ventricular activity.

Electrocardiograms are conventionally recorded from 12 leads. This is achieved by placing electrodes on the right arm, left arm and left leg, as well as six electrodes in predefined locations on the chest and a ground reference on the right leg. Bipolar leads record changes in electrical potential between two electrodes and are represented as follows.

- Lead I: potential at the left arm minus that at the right arm
- Lead II: potential at the left leg minus that at the right arm
- Lead III: potential at the left leg minus that at the left arm.

Unipolar leads record electrical potential at the site of an exploring electrode with respect to the average potential of all three limb electrodes. The exploring electrode may itself be placed on a limb or on the chest wall and such unipolar leads are by convention labelled with the letter "V".

The standard leads ("viewing" the heart in the vertical plane) are named I, II, III, aVR, aVL and aVF and the chest leads ("viewing" the heart in the horizontal plane) V_1, V_2, V_3, V_4, V_5 and V_6 (Figures 12.16 and 12.17).

- aVR may be remembered as the **R**ight (a**VR**) arm lead
- aVL may be remembered as the **L**eft (a**VL**) arm lead
- aVF may be remembered as the **F**oot (a**VF**) lead.

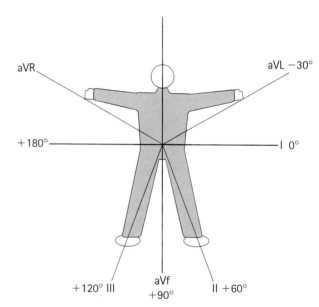

Figure 12.16 The standard leads

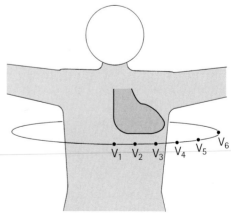

Figure 12.17 The chest leads

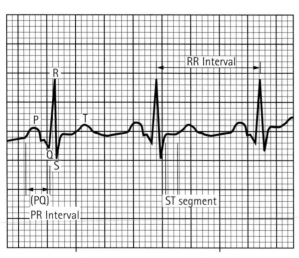

Sinus rhythm: heart rate 80/min

Figure 12.15 An ECG trace (rhythm strip)

The position of these leads is described in degrees clockwise from lead I (0°); thus lead aVF is 90°, lead III is 120° and lead aVR is 210°. It is apparent therefore that leads II, III and aVF "look at" the undersurface of the heart – these are the *inferior* leads – whereas lead aVL "looks at" the heart from "above" (i.e. from the left shoulder). The chest leads (Figure 12.17) form an incomplete arc around the chest.

In the prehospital setting accurate 12-lead ECG recording with or without transmission is an important part of the management of patients with suspected acute myocardial infarction if prehospital administration of thrombolytic therapy is contemplated. However, it is standard to monitor rate and rhythm using a single lead – lead II. This is because the P wave of atrial depolarization is usually best seen in this lead.

Only three electrodes are required:

- right arm/shoulder electrode
- left arm/shoulder electrode
- left lower anterior chest wall electrode.

ECG RECORDING PAPER

In order to allow ECG analysis and comparison of ECGs recorded at different times for the same patient, the paper used is standardized. The ECG machine, or the printer of a defibrillator or ECG monitor, runs with a paper speed of 25 mm per second (Figure 12.18).

The graph paper is divided into small squares of side 1 mm. A large square consists of five small squares and measures 5 mm × 5 mm. At the standard paper speed each small square (1 mm) represents 0.04 seconds and each large square (5 mm) represents 0.20 seconds. The amplitude of the electrical impulse is indicated along the vertical axis. A 10 mm deflection (two large squares) represents a 1 mV electrical signal provided that the ECG machine is properly calibrated.

> The horizontal axis of the ECG trace is time

COMPONENTS OF THE ECG

The ECG machine is "wired" so that it records a positive deflection when electrical charge is flowing towards it (Figure 12.19) or a negative deflection when electrical charge flows away (Figure 12.20). When current is flowing at 90° to the electrode (Figure 12.21), either no deflection or, more commonly, equal negative and positive deflection (Figure 12.22), is produced.

Depolarization of the heart begins at the SA node in the right atrium and spreads through the atria (Figure 12.23); this produces the P wave. From the atria the depolarization

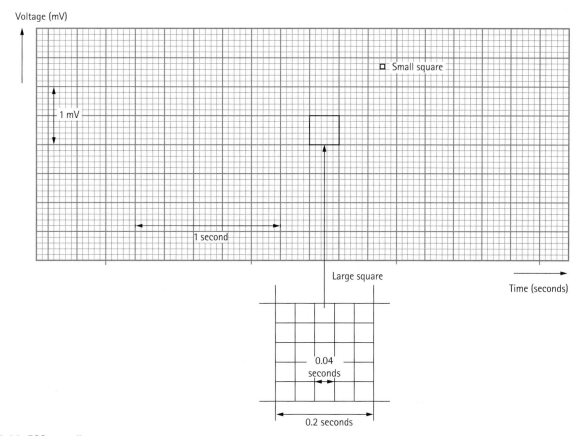

Figure 12.18 ECG recording paper

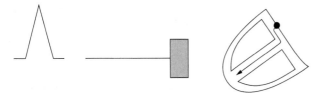

Figure 12.19 Trace recorded when electrical charge flows towards the ECG machine

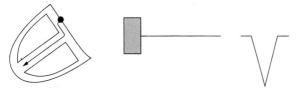

Figure 12.20 Trace recorded when electrical charge flows away from the ECG machine

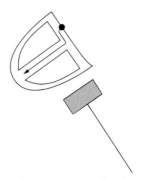

Figure 12.21 Current flowing at 90° to the electrode

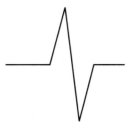

Figure 12.22 Trace recorded when current flows at 90° to the electrode

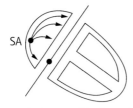

Figure 12.23 Atrial depolarization; SA, sinoatrial node

passes to the atrioventricular node, then down the bundle of His, and then simultaneously up the left bundle (to the left ventricle) and the right bundle (to the right ventricle) (Figure 12.24). Depolarization of the ventricles produces

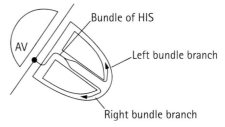

Figure 12.24 The conducting pathway in the ventricles; AV, atrioventricular node

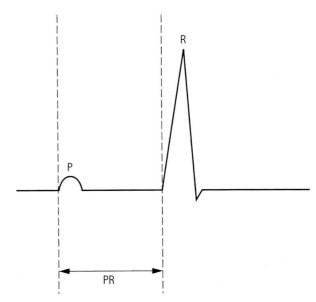

Figure 12.25 The P wave and QRS complexes and the PR interval

the QRS complex on the ECG. Any depolarization of the ventricle that does not follow the normal depolarization pathway will take much longer to occur as it does not utilize the His-Purkinje system. This will produce a wide, abnormal QRS complex on the ECG.

The time from the beginning of atrial depolarization to the beginning of ventricular depolarization is the PR interval (Figure 12.25). It is normally 0.12–0.20 seconds, i.e. 3–5 small squares on the ECG paper, and is mainly due to delay of transmission at the AV node.

Following depolarization (and contraction) of the ventricles, they repolarize and return to their resting electrical state to await the next depolarization. This is represented on the ECG as the T waves.

Thus the normal ECG trace consists of a series of waves: the P wave, the QRS complex and the T wave (Figure 12.26). Other components of importance include the PR interval and the ST segment (Table 12.4).

One small square equals 0.04 seconds
One large square equals 0.20 seconds

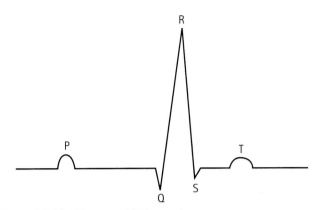

Figure 12.26   The normal ECG complex

Table 12.4   Cardiac events related to ECG components

Cardiac event	ECG component	Normal value (s)
Electrical activation of atria	P wave	0.10
Electrical activation of ventricles	QRS complex	<0.12
Repolarization of ventricles and return to resting membrane potential	T wave	0.15–0.25
Spread of excitation from SA node through AV node to ventricular muscle	PR interval	0.12–0.20
Early part of repolarization of ventricles	ST segment	0.20
Time between two successive ventricular depolarizations	RR interval	

SUMMARY

P wave

The P wave represents depolarization of the atria and in lead II is a small positive (upward) deflection. It lasts normally less than 0.10 seconds, is less than 2.5 mm in height and precedes each QRS complex.

QRS complex

The QRS complex represents depolarization of the ventricles. It consists of one or more waves.

- R wave: any positive deflection
- Q wave: any negative deflection preceding an R wave
- S wave: any negative deflection following an R wave.

A QRS complex that consists of a single, large negative deflection is called a QS wave. The duration of a normal QRS complex is less than 0.12 seconds (less than three small squares) in adults. The height or amplitude is variable from 2 mm to 15 mm. The QRS complex in lead II usually shows a large positive (upward) R wave.

T wave

The T wave represents repolarization of the ventricles and is positive (upright) in lead II. Its duration is variable (0.10–0.25 second) and its amplitude is less than 5 mm. Note that there is no recognizable wave equivalent for atrial repolarization which occurs physiologically during ventricular depolarization. Thus the atrial "T wave" is hidden in the QRS complex.

PR interval

The PR interval represents the time it takes for an electrical impulse generated in the SA node to reach the ventricles via the AV node and bundle branches. The PR interval begins with the onset of the P wave and terminates at the onset of the QRS complex; strictly speaking, the PR interval should be called a PQ interval. The duration of the PR interval is normally 0.12–0.20 seconds (3–5 small squares). A normal PR interval indicates that no conduction delay has occurred between the SA node through the AV node and bundle of His.

ST segment

The ST segment represents the interval between ventricular depolarization and repolarization of the ventricles. It stretches from the end of the S wave or QRS complex to the beginning of the T wave. It lasts for 0.20 seconds (five small squares) or less, although its length is dependent on the heart rate – the ST segment shortens with faster heart rates. Normally the ST segment is flat or identical with the isoelectric line.

SYSTEMATIC ANALYSIS OF THE ECG IN SEVEN STEPS

The main purpose of a systematic approach to analysing a patient's ECG is to be able to recognize a heart rhythm disorder or *arrhythmia*. Furthermore, it may be possible for the paramedic to suspect myocardial ischaemia, acute myocardial infarction or an electrolyte imbalance. However, the patient's overall condition – not just isolated ECG findings – will determine diagnosis and further management.

Step 1: Determine the heart rate

The heart rate is most easily calculated by dividing 300 by the number of large squares between two consecutive R waves of QRS complexes, the RR interval (Table 12.5).

This method is accurate if the heart rhythm is regular. If the rhythm is irregular, the rate can be calculated by measuring the number of large squares between 5 or 10 R waves, dividing by 5 or 10, and then dividing into 300.

Table 12.5 Calculation of heart rate

Number of large squares between two adjacent R waves	Heart rate (beats/min)	
1	300/1	300
2	300/2	150
3	300/3	100
4	300/4	75
5	300/5	60
6	300/6	50
7	300/7	43
8	300/8	37
9	300/9	33
10	300/10	30

Step 2: Determine the heart rhythm

The heart rhythm is determined by comparing the length of several RR intervals on a sufficiently long strip of the ECG trace. The heart rhythm is regular if the distances between R waves counted in large or small squares are equal. Irregular rhythms can be either "regularly irregular" or "irregularly irregular". The latter describes a rhythm where the QRS complexes occur in totally haphazard fashion.

Step 3: Analyse the P waves

In sinus rhythm there is a P wave before each QRS complex. In atrial fibrillation P waves are absent. In atrial flutter the P wave rate is about 300 per minute and appears as a "saw-tooth" pattern. If there are more P waves than QRS complexes, an atrioventricular block may be present.

Step 4: Analyse the QRS complex

The QRS complex may exhibit up to three waveforms (see above) and normally lasts less than three small squares or 0.12 second. If the QRS duration is greater than this, conduction through the ventricle is abnormally slow, either because one of the bundles of His is not functioning or because the origin of depolarization is within the ventricle.

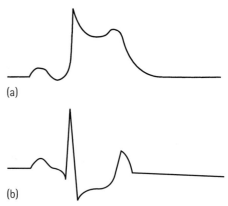

(a)

(b)

Figure 12.27 ST segment elevation (A) and depression (B)

Step 5: Measure the PR interval

If the PR interval is less than 0.12 seconds (three small squares) the electrical impulse has not progressed from the atria to the ventricles via the normal conduction pathway. A prolonged PR interval, greater than 0.2 seconds (five small squares), occurs in "first-degree" heart block.

Step 6: Analyse the T wave

A normal T wave is upright and oriented in the same direction as the R wave of the QRS complex in that lead. Inversion of the T wave may indicate that an acute myocardial infarction has occurred in the past or that the myocardium is currently ischaemic. The T wave may also be inverted or flattened when the left ventricle is thickened (*hypertrophy*) or if the patient's serum potassium level is low (*hypokalaemia*). The T wave appears tall and symmetrically peaked if the patient has a high serum potassium level (*hyperkalaemia*).

Step 7: Analyse the ST segment

ST segment abnormalities are seen in acute coronary syndromes, pericarditis, ventricular hypertrophy and as an effect of some drugs (e.g. digoxin). Elevation of the ST segment can signify an acute myocardial infarction, especially if it is greater than two small squares above the isoelectric line. An ST segment depression can occur in acute cardiac ischaemia but should only confidently be diagnosed on a 12-lead ECG (Figure 12.27). In terms of treatment, ST segment elevation is particularly important because it is an indication for administration of thrombolytic therapy in cases of suspected acute myocardial infarction.

ANALYSIS OF RHYTHM

Heart rhythms can be divided into three groups:

- normal sinus rhythm
- slow rhythms (bradyarrhythmias)
- fast rhythms (tachyarrhythmias).

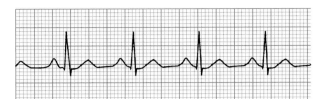

Figure 12.28 Sinus rhythm

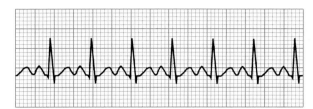

Figure 12.29 Sinus tachycardia

Box 12.2 Summary of tachycardias

Narrow complex and regular (supraventricular tachycardia – SVT)
Sinus tachycardia
True atrial tachycardia
AV nodal reentrant (junctional) tachycardia
Atrial flutter with fixed AV relationship (e.g. 2:1, 3:1 conduction)
AV reentrant tachycardia (accessory pathway)

Narrow complex and irregular
Atrial fibrillation
Atrial flutter with variable conduction
Frequent atrial ectopic beats

Broad complex and regular
Any cause of SVT with coexisting bundle branch block
Ventricular tachycardia

Broad and irregular
Atrial fibrillation with bundle branch block
Polymorphic ventricular tachycardia (torsades de pointes)

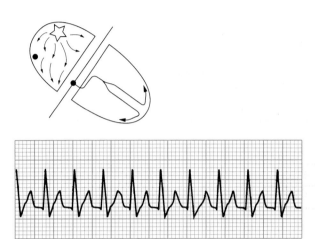

Figure 12.30 Atrial tachycardia: p waves are not visible

Sinus rhythm

Sinus rhythm (Figure 12.28) is defined as a rhythm where each P wave is followed by a QRS complex, with an equal number of P waves and QRS complexes. In young people in particular this is not absolutely regular, SA node discharge varying slightly with each breath via an intact autonomic nervous system. This minor irregularity can be detected at the pulse or on ECG as "sinus arrhythmia". Sinus rhythm greater than 100 beats/min constitutes sinus tachycardia and less than 60 beats/min is sinus bradycardia.

Tachycardias

Any rhythm with a rate exceeding 100 beats/min is a tachycardia. Such rhythms can be simply described in terms of their regularity and the width of the QRS complex (Box 12.2). More specific electrophysiological diagnosis may be attempted to shed more light on the aetiology of the arrhythmia.

Regular narrow complex

If the rhythm originates in the SA node, it is a *sinus tachycardia* (Figure 12.29). Sinus tachycardia is unlikely with a heart

rate of greater than 150 beats/min. It is frequently seen as a response to anxiety, fever, blood loss and pain. If a discharging focus occurs in the muscle of the atria (Figure 12.30), depolarization passes through the atria following an abnormal pathway before traversing the AV node and passing down the normal ventricular conduction pathways. The P wave is therefore abnormally shaped while the QRS complex looks normal. This is a true *atrial tachycardia* and is a very rare cause of supraventricular tachycardia (SVT). This rhythm is often so fast that the abnormal P waves cannot be seen. An isolated complex arising from an abnormal atrial focus is called an *atrial premature beat* or *atrial ectopic* (Figure 12.31). In most cases of narrow complex regular tachycardia the abnormal focus is within the AV node (Figure 12.32) or involves the combination of the AV node and an accessory pathway (or muscle bridge) capable of allowing retrograde conduction of activity from the ventricle to the atria (Figure 12.33). In both these situations, drugs that block AV nodal transmission (adenosine or verapamil) will stop the tachycardia.

Atrial tachycardia: abnormal P wave, normal QRS

Irregular narrow complex

In some people, particularly the elderly, there is no coordinated atrial activity because of the presence of multiple micro-wavelets of depolarization. Atrial activity is usually seen as a fine baseline fibrillation, with irregular QRS

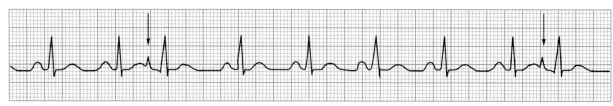

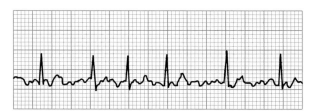

Figure 12.31 Atrial ectopics

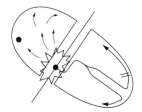

Figure 12.32 Simultaneous retrograde and normal depolarization of the ventricles

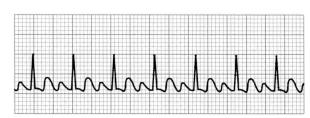

Figure 12.34 Atrial fibrillation

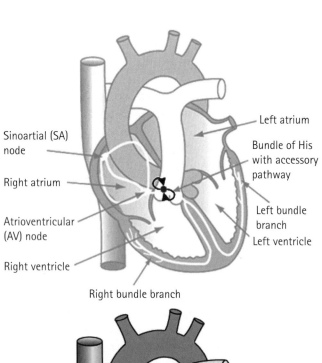

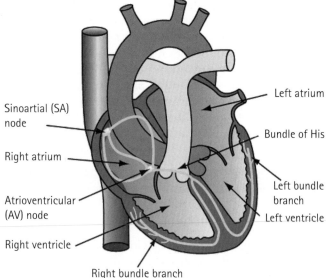

Figure 12.33 SVT utilizing both AV node and accessory pathway

Figure 12.35 Atrial flutter with 3:1 block (every third flutter wave hidden in QRS)

complexes. This is *atrial fibrillation* (Figure 12.34). Atrial fibrillation is often described as "fast AF". In fact, the speed refers to the ventricular activation rate, *not* the speed of activity in the atria.

> **Atrial fibrillation: no P wave, normal QRS**

Atrial flutter occurs when atrial depolarization is "driven" by a wave of electrical activity, independent of SA node activity, passing in a large continuous circuit around the right atrium. The frequency of this circuit is usually about 300 per minute and leads to the presence of "flutter waves" on the surface ECG. These appear as rapid rhythmic oscillations about the isoelectric line (a "saw-tooth" appearance). A proportion of these flutter waves are followed by QRS complexes. If there is a fixed ratio of flutter waves to QRS complexes, the ECG and the pulse will be regular (Figure 12.35). Where such a fixed ratio is 2:1 the ECG will show an SVT at a rate of about 150 per minute. When the ratio of flutter waves to QRS complexes is variable the tachycardia is irregular.

> **Atrial flutter: abnormal (saw-tooth) P wave, normal QRS**

Regular broad complex

An abnormal rhythm may arise from a focus in the ventricles (Figure 12.36). Depolarization therefore follows an

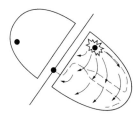

Figure 12.36 An abnormal rhythm arising from a focus in the ventricles

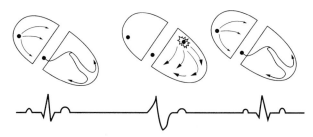

Figure 12.37 Ventricular ectopic beat between normal beats

abnormal path through the ventricle, ignoring the normal His-Purkinje system, producing a wider, abnormal QRS complex. When a single complex arises from a ventricular focus, it is known as a ventricular ectopic (Figures 12.37 and 12.38). Repetitive ventricular activation is a cause of an idioventricular rhythm or, when the rate is greater than 100 per minute, *ventricular tachycardia*. If such a tachycardia persists for longer than 30 seconds it is defined as "sustained". Ventricular tachycardia may be the primary arrhythmia in sudden cardiac arrest (Figure 12.39), but some individuals can tolerate this arrhythmia surprisingly well. A similar ECG appearance will be seen if any of the causes of SVT coexist with failure of conduction through one of the branches of the bundle of His (i.e. bundle branch block).

Bradycardia and heart block

Sinus bradycardia occurs when the pulse is less than 60 beats/min, but the ECG is otherwise normal (Figure 12.40).

The PR interval (0.12–0.20 seconds, 3–5 small squares) indicates the time taken for depolarization to pass from the

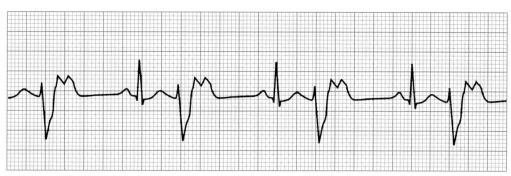

Figure 12.38 Ventricular ectopic beats

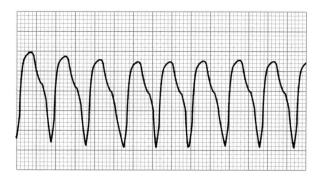

Figure 12.39 Ventricular tachycardia

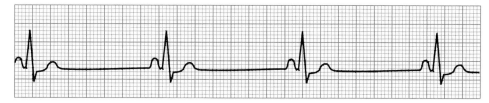

Figure 12.40 Sinus bradycardia

SA node through the atria to the ventricles. When sinus rhythm is present but the PR interval is longer than 0.2 s it is termed *first-degree heart block* (Figure 12.41). Treatment is rarely required. Nevertheless, whilst first-degree block can be seen in normal individuals, it may also be a manifestation of excess vagal nerve activity, ischaemia and the effects of various drugs.

> **In first-degree heart block atrial depolarization is always transmitted to the ventricles**

If some waves of atrial depolarization fail to be transmitted to the ventricles, *second-degree heart block* has occurred. Because atrial depolarization has occurred normally, the P wave is normal whether or not it is followed by a QRS complex (Figure 12.42).

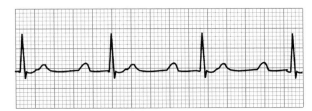

Figure 12.41 First-degree heart block

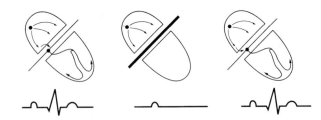

Figure 12.42 Second-degree heart block

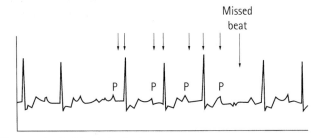

Figure 12.43 Wenckebach phenomenon

Second-degree (Mobitz) type I heart block (also known as the Wenckebach phenomenon) occurs when there is progressive prolongation of the PR interval, until a P wave occurs without a following QRS complex (Figure 12.43). The P wave is usually normal as normal atrial depolarization has occurred. The abnormality is the increasing time taken for transmission of atrial depolarization to the ventricles. This only rarely causes haemodynamic compromise.

Alternatively the PR interval may remain constant with occasional depolarizations failing to transmit to the ventricles. The missed (or dropped) beat may be regular (e.g. every third or fourth beat) or irregular (random) (Figure 12.44). This is *(Mobitz) type II second-degree heart block*. This is a more significant abnormality and may progress to complete heart block (see below) or ventricular standstill. Causes include ischaemia, fibrosis of the AV node, connective tissue disorders and some drugs.

> **In second-degree heart block some atrial depolarizations are not transmitted to the ventricles**

Sometimes no atrial depolarizations at all are transmitted to the ventricles and there is complete dissociation between atrial and ventricular activity (Figure 12.45). This produces isolated regular P waves on the ECG and unless an *escape rhythm* occurs from a ventricular focus, *ventricular standstill* occurs and may be rapidly fatal. When a ventricular rhythm is present the QRS complexes may be narrow if the focus is at the lower part of the AV node, bundle of His or the septum or, more characteristically, broad. The ventricular rhythm and pulse, are slow and usually regular. P waves and QRS complexes appear independently on the ECG, with some P waves hidden by QRS complexes. This is *third-degree* or *complete heart block* (Figures 12.46 and 12.47). Because there is no relationship between the electrical activity of the atria and the ventricles, this is also known as complete atrioventricular dissociation.

> **In third-degree heart block there is no transmission of depolarization from atria to ventricles**

To the lay person terms such as "first-degree heart block" imply a mechanical obstruction within the heart rather than an innocent slowing of electrical activation. Care should be

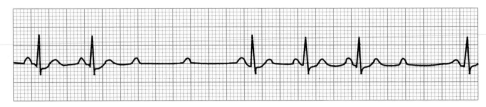

Figure 12.44 Mobitz type II second-degree heart block

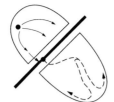

Figure 12.45 Third-degree heart block

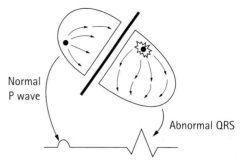

Normal P wave

Abnormal QRS

Figure 12.46 Spontaneous ventricular depolarization in third-degree heart block

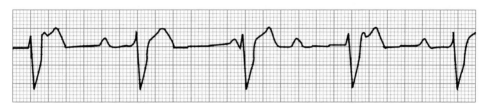

Figure 12.47 Complete (third-degree) heart block

taken when discussing ECG findings in the presence of the patient.

The treatment of arrhythmias is discussed in Chapter 13.

CONCLUSION

Coronary heart disease is the most common cause of death in the UK. The paramedic will frequently encounter cardiac arrest and cardiac emergencies (see Chapters 13 and 14). Knowledge of the anatomy and physiology of the cardiovascular system and of the ECG will enable the paramedic to strengthen the *chain of survival*, by recognizing the mechanism of cardiovascular dysfunction and commencing definitive and life-saving treatment at the scene and en route to hospital.

FURTHER READING

Anderson JE 1983 Grant's atlas of anatomy, 8th edn. Williams and Wilkins, Baltimore

Epstein O, Perkin CD, de Bono DP, Cookson J 1992 Clinical examination. Gower Medical Publishing, London

Hampton JR 1992 The ECG made easy, 4th edn. Churchill Livingstone, Edinburgh

Lamb JF, Ingram CG, Johnston IA, Pitman RM 1991 Essentials of physiology, 3rd edn. Blackwell, Oxford

Lumley JSP 1990 Surface anatomy: the anatomical basis of clinical examination. Churchill Livingstone, Edinburgh

Weston CFM 1999 Understanding the electrocardiogram. In: Greaves I, Porter K (eds) Prehospital medicine. The principles and practice of immediate care. Arnold, London

Chapter 13

Monitoring and defibrillation

Sophisticated monitoring of patients outside hospital is now commonplace. In spite of the availability of "hi-tech" equipment, clinical assessment of the patient's pulse, blood pressure, cardiorespiratory status and cerebral function (assessed, for example, by using the Glasgow Coma Scale) remains as important as ever. In fact, the experienced paramedic soon becomes adept at assessing whether a patient is well or ill!

This chapter considers both formal clinical assessment and the monitoring techniques available to the paramedic. Defibrillators are also considered here because most cardiac monitors used by the ambulance service also serve this function; furthermore, the use of defibrillators is dependent on the results of cardiac monitoring. The actual technique of defibrillation is discussed in Chapter 14.

CLINICAL ASSESSMENT

COLOUR

The presence of *pallor* may signify anaemia and is best seen by examination of the mucous membranes, particularly the conjunctivae or the mouth. It is, however, an unreliable physical sign, being seen also in the presence of vasoconstriction due to hypotension, hypothermia and intense emotion such as fear or pain. It may be difficult to assess outside hospital because of poor light, the influence of ambient temperature or the presence of dirt, grease or other contaminants. The skin is especially difficult to assess because of varying pigment and thickness – some people always appear pale – and should not be relied upon to diagnose anaemia.

Flushing or redness is caused by cutaneous vasodilation and may be a sign of fever or extreme exertion. The term *cyanosis* refers to the bluish-grey discolouration of the skin or mucous membranes that results from an excess of reduced haemoglobin. Two types are recognized:

- central cyanosis
- peripheral cyanosis.

In *central cyanosis* inadequate oxygenation of the blood occurs because of imperfect oxygenation of blood in the lungs or, rarely, a mixing of oxygenated and deoxygenated blood in the heart (deoxygenated blood may bypass the lungs with AV septal defects in the heart). It is, for example, seen in patients with heart failure due to chronic airways disease. The condition is assessed by examination of the oral mucosa. Traditionally, cyanosis is seen when there is greater than 5 g per 100 ml of deoxygenated haemoglobin in capillary blood.

Peripheral cyanosis occurs when increased extraction of oxygen occurs in the periphery, usually due to slow blood flow; it is most readily recognized in the fingers, particularly in the nail beds. The important differentiating feature from central cyanosis is that in peripheral cyanosis blood is oxygenated normally so that the oral mucosa is a normal colour. Peripheral cyanosis may be recognized in the hands when the peripheral circulation is slowed; this may be caused by cold and its presence does not necessarily indicate disease.

PULSE

In the collapsed patient a pulse in a prominent artery should be palpated. In most cases the carotid artery will be used; the femoral pulse is also suitable, although less accessible. The role of pulse assessment during the management of cardiac arrest is covered in Chapter 2. Valuable information may be obtained from the rate, strength and character of a central (carotid or femoral) pulse. Assessment of a peripheral pulse (radial, brachial or foot pulse) is less reliable, although the brachial pulse is recommended for palpation in cardiac arrest in infants (see Chapter 37). The heart rate may be assessed by counting the pulse. The radial pulse in the wrist is most commonly used for this purpose. It is unreliable in atrial fibrillation, where not every heart beat causes a pulse at the wrist, and in conditions of reduced cardiac output – in this situation a central pulse should always be employed. In many cases the ECG or the pulse oximeter will be used to document the heart rate.

RESPIRATORY RATE

The respiratory rate, depth and regularity should be assessed in all cases where cardiac or respiratory function is compromised or where central control of respiration may be reduced – for example, after head injury or drug overdose. The respiratory rate is usually expressed in breaths per minute. The normal rate is highest in neonates and babies and falls progressively with age until the adult range of 12–18 breaths per minute is reached. More rapid respiratory rates are described as *tachypnoea* and may be associated, in the breathless patient, with use of the accessory muscles of respiration in the neck. In severe breathlessness there is drawing in of the spaces between the ribs (*intercostal recession*). Some patients with heart failure, neurological disease or drug intoxication demonstrate varying respiratory rate and depth known as *Cheyne-Stokes respiration*.

BLOOD PRESSURE

The accurate measurement of blood pressure is an important part of the assessment of the patient. Successive readings may be compared and allow the patient's progress and response to treatment to be monitored. The mercury sphygmomanometer is being phased out of use because of worries concerning mercury toxicity and certainly is not robust enough for field use. It is also difficult to read in adverse lighting conditions. For these reasons aneroid sphygmomanometers (Figure 13.1) or electronic methods are usually employed in prehospital medicine. It is more important to practise correct technique and to ensure adequate maintenance.

Regardless of the type of measurement device employed, it should be remembered that blood pressure

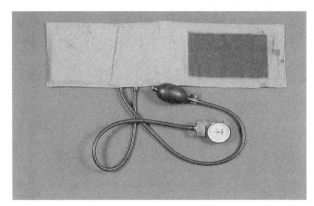

Figure 13.1 An aneroid sphygmomanometer

varies significantly with state of arousal, posture and exertion, as well as with disorders of the cardiovascular system. When possible (and this is not always the case in prehospital care) the pressure should be recorded with the patient seated comfortably with the arm supported so that the humerus is at the level of the heart.

Manual methods

The sphygmomanometer cuff should be the correct size for the patient's arm if accurate readings are to be obtained. Smaller cuffs are appropriate for children while larger cuffs should be employed for obese adults. The ideal size of cuff is equal in width to approximately two-thirds of the length of the upper arm. This may not always be available with the restricted equipment carried on an ambulance but where an inappropriate cuff size has been used, the cuff size should be recorded.

The blood pressure cuff is applied to the upper arm, in the absence of intervening clothing. Most modern cuffs have a method of indicating the correct position of the cuff over the brachial artery. The cuff is inflated above the systolic blood pressure; this point may be determined by palpating the radial pulse while inflating the cuff. An estimate of systolic blood pressure may be obtained by determining the point at which the radial pulse returns when the cuff is subsequently deflated. This may be the only measurement possible if the Korotkoff sounds (those sounds heard with a stethoscope over the artery distal to the cuff) are difficult to hear when the blood pressure is low or because of adverse circumstances in prehospital care. The blood pressure is best determined by slowly deflating the cuff while listening for the return of Korotkoff sounds through a stethoscope diaphragm placed over the brachial artery in the antecubital fossa. The systolic blood pressure is taken at the point when the sounds return (that is, when systolic blood pressure exceeds the pressure in the cuff). The diastolic pressure is measured at the point of disappearance of the sounds.

Electronic blood pressure monitoring

Electronic devices that measure blood pressure noninvasively are available; sometimes this facility is incorporated

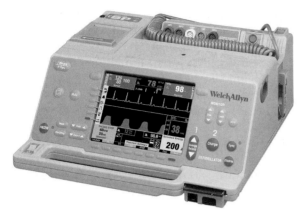

Figure 13.2 Robust non-invasive prehospital monitoring

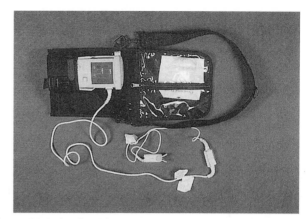

Figure 13.3 A pulse oximeter

into other monitoring equipment, for example a cardiac monitor. In most cases a blood pressure cuff is applied to the upper arm in the conventional manner and connected to the monitoring unit through tubing that permits inflation and deflation of the cuff. The circuit incorporates a sensor (microphone or oscillotonometer) that monitors brachial artery pulsation, thereby allowing the systolic and diastolic pressure to be determined. The blood pressure reading obtained is displayed digitally on a screen. Most modern units also display the pulse rate. The frequency with which the blood pressure is measured can be preset according to the patient's requirements and allows progress to be monitored. Although these units offer convenience (particularly where limited help is available or access to the patient is difficult), it is essential that the manufacturer's instructions are followed precisely if consistently accurate readings are to be obtained. The units require regular checking and standardization to ensure accuracy. Systematic errors are often seen when the pulse is irregular, such as in atrial fibrillation.

Intraarterial blood pressure monitoring

Intraarterial measurement is performed when continuous monitoring of arterial pressure is required, most often in the operating theatre or intensive therapy unit. A catheter is inserted directly into an artery and the pressure wave is monitored by a transducer connected to the catheter. Such intraarterial monitoring lines may be in situ when a patient is transferred between hospitals; paramedics should be aware of their presence and clarify any precautions necessary during the journey with the appropriate staff.

PULSE OXIMETRY

In recent years pulse oximetry has become established as the most convenient non-invasive method of monitoring arterial oxygen saturation (Figure 13.3). It is widely used outside hospital and is particularly useful where there is delay in moving a patient (e.g., in cases of entrapment) or for monitoring the patient during transport. It offers many advantages over clinical methods of assessing oxygenation, though there are a number of potential pitfalls in its use.

The majority of oxygen is carried in the blood in loose attachment to haemoglobin within red blood cells. Pulse oximeters express the saturation of the blood with oxygen in terms of the ratio of oxygenated haemoglobin to the total haemoglobin (which includes the oxygenated and non-oxygenated or reduced haemoglobin). All tissues, including oxygenated and reduced haemoglobin, absorb or attenuate differing wavelengths of light. Pulse oximeters use these principles and the pulsatility of arterial blood flow.

A probe containing a light source is attached to a finger or the earlobe. The light source emits two wavelengths of red light in short, rapid (600 per second) bursts. The light traverses the tissue and is monitored on the opposite side by a photodetector that is therefore exposed to alternating bursts of attenuated transmitted light and ambient light. By integrating this with changes in pulse wave, a computer microprocessor determines the average arterial blood saturation.

As a pulsatile blood flow is required, problems may arise when the peripheral circulation is impaired. Rapid fluctuations in ambient light levels may produce false signals and movement during patient transport may also cause inaccurate readings. Carboxyhaemoglobin, present in cases of carbon monoxide poisoning, may cause a pulse oximeter to overestimate the true oxygen saturation: in carbon monoxide poisoning, pulse oximetry will measure the total percentage saturation of haemoglobin with oxygen (oxyhaemoglobin) and carbon monoxide (carboxyhaemoglobin). Dirt, grease and nail varnish (dark and metallic colours only) also lead to inaccurate measurements. Skin colour has no effect on oxygen saturation recording.

Incorrect pulse oximeter readings may be caused by

- poor circulation
- fluctuating light levels
- carbon monoxide poisoning
- skin, dirt and grease
- nail varnish (dark and metallic colours only).

The relationship between arterial oxygen tension (PaO_2) and arterial oxygen saturation is described by the oxyhaemoglobin

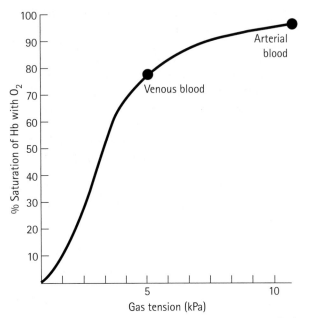

Figure 13.4 The oxygen dissociation curve for haemoglobin (Hb)

Box 13.1 Arterial oxygen saturation values on air	
Normal range	97–100%
Mild hypoxia	90–97%
Moderate hypoxia	85–90%
Severe hypoxia	<85%

dissociation curve (Figure 13.4). The relationship between arterial oxygen tension (content) and the oxygen saturation forms an S-shaped curve, which implies that there may be a marked drop in arterial oxygen content before this is reflected in a fall in oxygen saturation. Normal values when breathing room air are shown in Box 13.1.

The most serious pitfall of pulse oximetry arises when alveolar hypoventilation causes respiratory failure; this may arise from lung disease, muscular weakness or central respiratory depression. A rise in arterial and alveolar carbon dioxide tension (PCO_2) occurs and alveolar PO_2 falls with resultant arterial hypoxaemia. If a patient is breathing air the oxygen saturation will fall quickly and provide a reasonably early warning of hypoventilation. If, however, the patient is receiving supplementary oxygen the alveolar PO_2 will be much higher and the alveolar PCO_2 will have to rise much further before hypoxaemia sufficient to produce measurable desaturation occurs. *It must be stressed that a normal oxygen saturation in the presence of an increased inspired oxygen concentration gives no information about the adequacy of ventilation.*

Pulse oximetry does not measure carbon dioxide

Pulse oximetry has been used to assess the vascular supply to a limb when arterial trauma is thought to be present but has proved to be unreliable and even misleading when used

for this purpose. A trend of falling oxygen saturation readings is likely to be more valuable than an isolated reading and several readings should therefore be recorded if used for this purpose. Alternatively the saturation values in an injured and an uninjured limb can be compared.

Despite these limitations, the pulse oximeter is a valuable development in the monitoring of arterial oxygen saturation which allows the detection of the presence of serious hypoxaemia easily and non-invasively. *A sustained trend of falling oxygen saturation is always a clinically important observation, despite doubts about the precision of individual readings.*

ELECTROCARDIOGRAPHIC MONITORING

Electrocardiographic (ECG) monitoring is undertaken to define the cardiac rhythm. Documentation of an abnormal cardiac rhythm may play a vital part in the patient's subsequent management, particularly in cases of chest pain, collapse, syncope, palpitation or shock.

In some circumstances treatment of an abnormal cardiac rhythm will be instituted by the paramedic before arrival at hospital. Accurate rhythm monitoring and interpretation are especially important in the management of cardiac arrest (described in Chapter 14).

CARDIAC MONITORS

Many types of cardiac monitoring system are available but in the ambulance service the cardiac monitor is usually an integral part of the defibrillator. Manual defibrillators and cardiac monitors feature a screen for displaying the cardiac rhythm and usually incorporate an arrangement for obtaining a printout of the ECG. Automated external defibrillators (AEDs) often store the ECG electronically and a hard copy is obtained from the appropriate playback device.

Many cardiac monitors incorporate a heart rate meter which is triggered by the QRS complex of the ECG. An alarm will sound automatically should the heart rate fall outside preset limits; lights and audible signals may also provide additional indications of the heart rate. Traditional (analogue) monitors display the ECG on a cathode ray oscilloscope screen. Many modern cardiac monitors convert the electronic signals into a digital form; the rhythm may then be displayed on a liquid crystal screen and computer-aided rhythm analysis of the ECG becomes possible. Digital signals are also easier to store electronically for subsequent playback and analysis.

MONITORING ELECTRODES

In most circumstances paramedics will instigate ECG monitoring by attaching (may be 3 or 4) adhesive electrodes to the patient's chest. The positions illustrated in Figure 13.5 will allow records that approximate to leads I, II or III of the conventional ECG. The configuration that displays the most prominent P wave (if organized atrial activity is present)

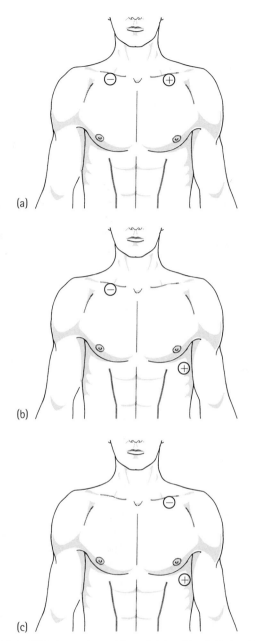

Figure 13.5 ECG electrode positions. (a) (positive left shoulder, negative right shoulder) equivalent to lead I; (b) (positive left lower chest, negative right clavicle) equivalent to lead II; (c) (positive left lower chest, negative left clavicle) equivalent to lead III. The electrodes are applied simultaneously, selection of the lead to be recorded by the machine determines which pair of leads are used to record the trace

with sufficient QRS amplitude to trigger the rate meter should be adopted; this will usually be lead II. A variety of other systems of electrode placement have been suggested and vests exist with sewn-in electrodes for ease of use. However, these more novel systems have not been widely adopted.

Electrical interference may be minimized by applying the electrodes over bone rather than muscle; the precordium should be left unobstructed so that chest compression and defibrillation may be carried out if necessary. Occasionally,

hair may need to be shaved from the areas where the electrodes are to be attached and the skin should where possible be cleaned with alcohol to remove skin oil. Some adhesive electrodes incorporate a wrapping on the electrode which is used to abrade the skin and improve electrical contact. Movement artefact will be minimized in conscious, cooperative patients by keeping them warm and asking them not to move their arms.

MONITORING AFTER CARDIAC ARREST

It is important to obtain a readout of the cardiac rhythm as soon as possible after cardiac arrest. Modern monitor-defibrillators enable the cardiac rhythm to be monitored through large defibrillator electrodes (semi-automatic) or paddles (manual) applied to the chest wall. If ventricular fibrillation is present, defibrillation can be carried out immediately, while if the original rhythm appears to be asystole different paddle positions may be employed to exclude fine ventricular fibrillation.

Defibrillator paddles do not make ideal monitoring electrodes: they need to be kept in position by hand and are really only suitable for a quick look at the rhythm, otherwise chest compression will be interrupted for an unacceptable time. A better ECG signal is obtained from adhesive electrodes which should be applied as soon as convenient, so that continuous monitoring and recording of the rhythm may take place.

> Ensure that your defibrillator is changed to read from leads when the electrodes have been attached

DIAGNOSIS FROM CARDIAC MONITORS

The displays and printouts from cardiac monitors are suitable only for rhythm recognition and not for analysis of ST segment changes or more sophisticated ECG morphology interpretation. The printout of the ECG should be inspected carefully to diagnose the cardiac rhythm and retained for transfer to the patient's records on arrival at hospital. The time when the trace is recorded is essential information and should be added manually at the start of the record if this is not done automatically by the monitor. It is also good practice to write on the printed rhythm strip other relevant clinical information such as symptoms or blood pressure.

DEFIBRILLATORS

External defibrillation of the human heart was first reported in the 1950s. During defibrillation sufficient electrical energy is delivered to the surface of the chest to enable a current of electricity to depolarize a critical mass of the fibrillating myocardium, in the hope that orderly cardiac depolarization ensues. The amount of energy that reaches the heart is dependent on both the delivered energy and the resistance to (or, more accurately, the *impedance* to) electrical flow

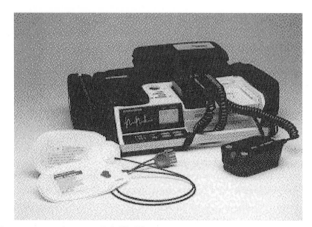

Figure 13.6 A manual defibrillator

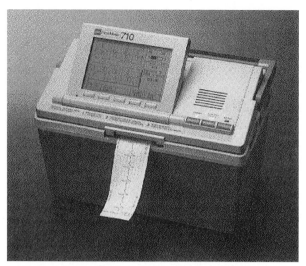

Figure 13.7 A semi-automatic external defibrillator (SAD)

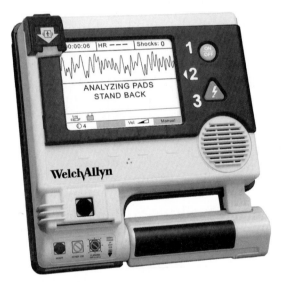

Figure 13.8 An automated external defibrillator

between the two electrodes or paddles. Impedance is itself determined by the size of the electrodes/paddles, the surface properties of the skin/electrode interface, the number of previous shocks delivered over the same area and properties of the underlying subcutaneous tissues including the amount of air in the lungs. Most defibrillators deliver a predetermined energy, measured in joules. Some, however, assess impedance and deliver variable energy based on that.

All frontline ambulances in the UK are now equipped with defibrillators. Defibrillators are of three types:

- manual
- semi-automatic (advisory)
- fully automated.

With manual defibrillators (Figure 13.6) the operator interprets the cardiac rhythm, decides whether a defibrillatory countershock is required, charges the machine and administers the shock. Experience in ECG interpretation is required and training in the use of such devices is therefore more prolonged. With the semi-automatic defibrillator (Figure 13.7) the processes of rhythm recognition and charging for defibrillation are automated. All that is required of the operator is to recognize that cardiac arrest may have occurred, to attach two electrodes to the patient's chest and to follow the instructions from the defibrillator if these seem appropriate. The electrodes serve the dual purpose of cardiac rhythm monitoring and delivery of the direct current (DC) countershock. During the analysis period (which in most models is less than 10 seconds) no contact must be made with the patient to avoid the chance of movement artefact. Many models incorporate written on-screen instructions and some models also feature synthesized voice instructions to guide the operator. They also offer the advantage of "hands-free defibrillation".

The AED (Automated External Defibrillator Figure 13.8) is accurate in the interpretation of shockable rhythms and only rarely is a DC shock advised inappropriately.

Fully automated defibrillators administer a DC shock on recognition of a shockable rhythm without involvement of the operator. An override key can be used to convert an automated external defibrillator into a manual one.

DEFIBRILLATOR BATTERY CARE

Two types of battery are in widespread use: the lead-acid battery and the nickel-cadmium cell. The lead-acid battery works on the same principle as the accumulator used in the motor car; however, the acid is present as a gel and these units are less susceptible to the effects of movement and position. Lead-acid batteries hold their charge for prolonged periods, losing approximately 1% per month. They can be recharged rapidly after use and may be left on charge when already fully charged without the problems caused by similar treatment of nickel-cadmium cells.

Nickel-cadmium cells have been widely used in defibrillators. They are designed for regular use and ideally should be fully discharged before recharging. Regular charging when fully charged or when the cells are not greatly depleted reduces the efficiency of the battery and must be avoided. Regular reconditioning cycles (where the battery is fully discharged before being recharged) are required to maintain optimal battery condition and should be performed in accordance with the maker's recommendations. Nickel-cadmium cells lose approximately 1% of their charge per day and are less suitable than lead-acid cells for equipment that is used infrequently.

Dry batteries have a prolonged shelf-life and are used in certain types of first-responder defibrillator. They are replaced when the machine is used or if their shelf-life is exceeded before use.

DEFIBRILLATION WAVEFORM

The majority of defibrillators in use deliver a *monophasic* energy wave, where the energy flows in one direction between the two electrodes. There is evidence that a more effective defibrillation can be achieved by a discharge of energy that reverses direction. This has lead to the development of *biphasic* wave defibrillators, with the added advantage of reduced size and weight. These are gradually replacing the older monophasic devices.

DEFIBRILLATOR SAFETY

Defibrillators are potentially dangerous pieces of equipment. A high-energy shock of several thousand volts is administered to the patient. It is essential that no part of the operator or any assistant is in electrical contact with the patient when the shock is administered. The operator must shout "Stand clear!" and visually check that no person is touching the patient. There are hazards for the unwary, particularly where the patient is lying on a metal table or when the surroundings are wet. Intravenous fluid giving sets may act as a potential conductor and helpers should not be holding these while a shock is administered. Defibrillation in the rain is normally safe unless the rain is torrential, providing the chest is wiped dry first. Patients lying in a pool of water should be moved before defibrillation and the carers must ensure they are not connected to the patient by standing in water. Nitrate patches should be removed to reduce the risk of them igniting and causing severe burns.

Oxygen presents an important hazard during defibrillation as it produces a highly combustible environment. A number of cases have been reported of patients suffering severe burns following fires started by a spark from a defibrillator in an oxygen-rich environment. It is therefore essential that any oxygen source (for example, bag–valve–mask) is removed at least three feet from the patient before administering each shock.

DEFIBRILLATION IN PATIENTS WITH PACEMAKERS

Increasing numbers of patients are now fitted with permanent pacemakers. A generator is implanted in the chest wall, usually below the clavicle and between the skin and the pectoral muscle, and an electrode leads from the generator to the right side of the heart. In dual-chamber systems (that pace both atria and ventricles) two electrodes are employed.

Occasionally the pacing electrodes may be inserted into the heart from the epicardial surface; these are connected to a generator often implanted into the upper abdominal wall.

Modern pacemaker generators incorporate protection circuits that prevent the discharge from a defibrillator damaging the pacemaker. An electric current may, however, travel through the pacing electrode and cause an electrical burn at the point of contact with the myocardium. This may cause a subsequent rise in pacemaker threshold with loss of pacing. When defibrillation is successful this rise in threshold may not be apparent until some weeks later and to minimize the chances of this occurring, defibrillator electrodes should be placed as far away from the generator as possible – at least 12 cm whenever possible.

With temporary pacing, an external generator is connected to a temporary pacing electrode (usually inserted through the subclavian or jugular vein). Paramedics may encounter these during the transfer of patients between hospitals. Should defibrillation be necessary, the same precautions that apply to permanent pacemakers should be followed, placing the defibrillator electrodes as far away as possible from the point where the temporary pacing wire enters the skin. Increasing numbers of patients are being fitted with internal implanted defibrillators. If an external shock is required, manage these patients in the same manner as those with an implanted pacemaker.

> Glyceryl trinitrate patches must be removed prior to defibrillation to avoid the risk of explosion

FURTHER READING

Austin R, Snow A 2000 Defibrillation. In: Chellel A (ed.) Resuscitation: a guide for nurses. Churchill Livingstone, Edinburgh

Beevers D 1988 The ABC of hypertension. BMJ Books, London

Colquhoun MC, Handley AJ, Evans TR 1995 The ABC of resuscitation, 3rd edn. BMJ Books, London

Gwinnutt CL 1999 Advanced life support. In: Greaves I, Porter KM (eds) Pre-hospital medicine. The principles and practice of emergency care. Arnold, London

Hutton P, Clutton-Brook T 1994 The benefits and pitfalls of pulse oximetry. British Medical Journal 307: 457–458

Chapter **14**

Cardiac arrest in adults: Advanced life support

INTRODUCTION

Cardiac arrest is the most serious emergency confronted by paramedics. It is the final common pathway for death in the prehospital environment from medical illness or trauma. The chances of a patient surviving a prehospital arrest and reaching hospital alive are about 15%; however, only one-third of this number are likely to leave hospital alive. This presents the paramedic with two challenges.

- To recognize and intervene appropriately in the care of the critically ill patient in order to prevent a cardiac arrest occurring.
- To respond promptly and skilfully to patients in cardiac arrest in order to optimize their chance of survival.

CARDIAC ARREST: A DEFINITION

For advanced life support providers, including paramedics, cardiac arrest may be defined as the absence of a palpable pulse in an unresponsive patient. Recent evidence has shown, however, that the pulse check is an unreliable sign if used in isolation from the clinical setting. Lay rescuers are no longer taught to use a pulse check to verify cardiac arrest. Instead, they start chest compressions, after giving rescue breaths, if there are no *signs of circulation* (in other words normal breathing, coughing or movement). Similarly, paramedics should not rely solely on the pulse check to diagnose cardiac arrest, but should look for other indicators that the circulation has failed.

Box 14.1 Risk factors for cardiac arrest

- Obstructed airway
- Myocardial infarction, unstable angina
- Periarrest arrhythmia
- Status asthmaticus
- Status epilepticus
- Uncontrolled haemorrhage
- Anaphylaxis

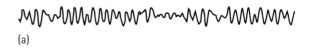

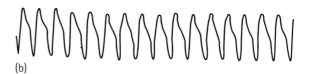

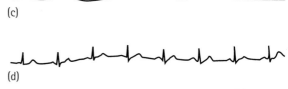

Figure 14.1 Rhythms associated with cardiac arrest. (a) Ventricular fibrillation; (b) ventricular tachycardia (pulseless); (c) asystole; (d) pulseless electrical activity

CAUSES AND PREVENTION OF CARDIAC ARREST

The majority of cardiac arrests occur as a consequence of ischaemic heart disease, due to either an acute obstruction of a coronary artery with infarction of cardiac muscle (myocardial infarction) or critical coronary ischaemia which disturbs electrical activity within the heart and produces a potentially lethal arrhythmia (*ventricular fibrillation*). Cardiac arrest may also occur as a secondary result of respiratory arrest or from other causes such as hypothermia, electrolyte imbalance, poisoning, electrocution or anaphylaxis.

Recognition and early intervention in the acutely ill patient may avert the development of a cardiac arrest. In order to identify the compromised patient, the paramedic must make a thorough but rapid assessment of the airway, breathing and circulation whilst simultaneously obtaining a history from the patient (if possible) and bystanders.

Where appropriate, early interventions, such as airway management, oxygenation, analgesia, correction of arrhythmias and haemorrhage control, may prevent an arrest occurring.

Box 14.1 lists conditions which are associated with an increased risk of cardiac arrest.

CARDIAC ARREST RHYTHMS

Electrocardiogram (ECG) monitoring in cardiac arrest will establish the initial rhythm, which will be one the following (Figure 14.1).

- Ventricular fibrillation (VF)
- *Pulseless* ventricular tachycardia (VT)
- Asystole
- Pulseless electrical activity (previously called electromechanical dissociation).

For treatment purposes, these rhythms are divided into:

- VF/pulseless VT
- non-VF/pulseless VT.

The initial rhythm of a patient in cardiac arrest will determine which treatment algorithm is used first. Patients in VF/VT are treated according to the VF/VT protocol and patients in asystole or pulseless electrical activity (PEA) are treated according to the non-VF/VT protocol.

The individual components of this algorithm will be discussed in the relevant sections below.

CHAIN OF SURVIVAL

Basic life support and early defibrillation are the most important interventions in the management of a cardiac arrest. Most cardiac arrests in the prehospital environment result initially from the development of ventricular fibrillation or ventricular tachycardia. These arrhythmias are amenable to treatment with a defibrillator. The time between the onset of VF to the first defibrillatory shock is critical and directly associated with survival. Early defibrillation leads to the greatest chance of success. Emergency medical systems should aim to provide rapid defibrillation within minutes of a cardiac arrest as after 8–10 minutes, the frequency of significant persistent neurological damage or fatal outcome becomes unacceptably high. The chain of survival is a system of care designed to optimize outcome in a prehospital cardiac arrest.

EARLY ACCESS

Early access emphasizes the importance of the public calling for help immediately on discovering an apnoeic patient. This allows the activation of the ambulance service and despatch of a paramedic crew with a defibrillator.

EARLY CPR

Effective CPR prior to the arrival of the paramedic is associated with improved survival. This may either be initiated by

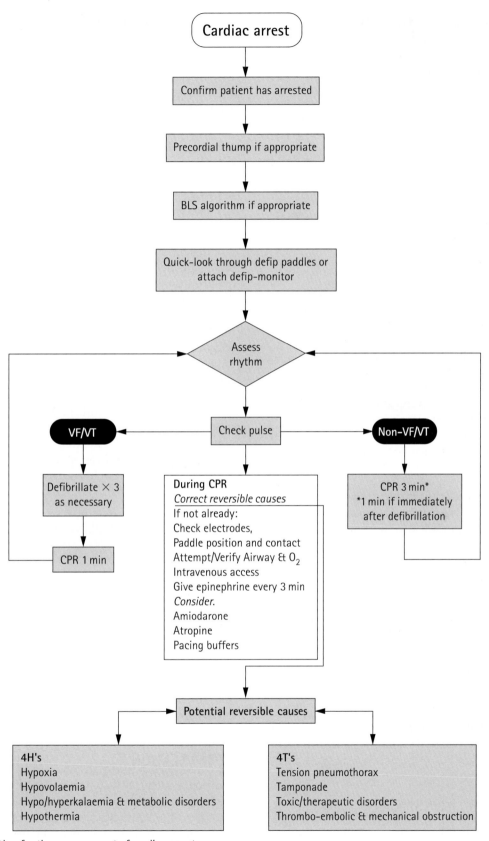

Figure 14.2 Algorithm for the management of cardiac arrest

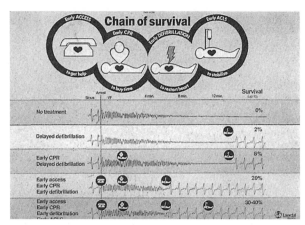

Figure 14.3 The chain of survival

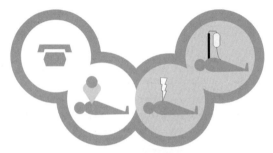

Figure 14.4 Early CPR and defibrillation at an out-of-hospital cardiac arrest

a trained bystander or following instructions from the ambulance service operator (despatcher-assisted CPR). Basic life support increases the window of opportunity for defibrillation by prolonging the time during which a patient remains in a shockable rhythm (VF/VT).

EARLY DEFIBRILLATION

The earlier that defibrillation can be undertaken, the greater the chance of survival. A first responder or member of the public using an automated external defibrillator may in some cases perform defibrillation prior to the arrival of the paramedic. However, in most cases it will not be performed until after the arrival of the ambulance service. Rapid, safe defibrillation, where indicated, is the first priority of the paramedic when attending a patient in cardiac arrest.

EARLY ADVANCED LIFE SUPPORT

This involves endotracheal intubation, obtaining intravenous access and administering cardiac drugs such as adrenaline (epinephrine). The paramedic usually performs this after the initial assessment of the patient, having given defibrillatory shocks if necessary.

THE ADVANCED LIFE SUPPORT APPROACH

When arriving at the scene of a suspected cardiac arrest, the paramedic should follow the standard assessment sequence for a collapsed patient. Care should be taken to ensure the safety of both paramedics and bystanders during the initial approach and subsequent management of the cardiac arrest.

- Safe approach
- Establish unresponsiveness
- Open the airway
- Assess breathing
- Attach monitor and assess the circulation.

If a defibrillator is not immediately available for cardiac monitoring then basic life support should be commenced while the defibrillator is brought to the scene. If good-quality bystander CPR is in progress then the paramedic should encourage them to continue whilst the resuscitation equipment is assembled. The defibrillator should be attached to the patient using either adhesive defibrillating gel pads or paddles and gel pads as this allows the underlying rhythm to be rapidly established. Attaching ECG leads first delays early defibrillation and should generally be avoided for the initial monitoring of the collapsed patient.

Once the patient is confirmed to be in cardiac arrest, he should be treated according to the initial rhythm. Patients with VF or pulseless VT are treated according to the VF/VT algorithm and patients in asystole or PEA are treated according to the non-VF/VT algorithms as described below.

VENTRICULAR FIBRILLATION OR PULSELESS VENTRICULAR TACHYCARDIA (VF/VT)

PRECORDIAL THUMP

If the paramedic witnesses the cardiac arrest before a defibrillator is attached (or monitors the onset of VF/pulseless VT) then a precordial thump may be administered. This is equivalent to a low-energy defibrillatory shock and may revert a patient in the early stages of VF or VT to a perfusing rhythm. The thump should be given in the normal position for chest compression from a height of approximately 15 cm above the chest, using a closed fist (Fig. 14.6).

DEFIBRILLATION

Ventricular tachycardia without cardiac output usually rapidly degenerates into ventricular fibrillation as electrical activity in the ventricles becomes more disorganized. The treatment, defibrillation, is therefore the same for both conditions. The chances of successful defibrillation are greatest if the shock can be delivered within the first 90 seconds of the cardiac arrest. After this time the biochemical composition within the cells starts to change as the cells become

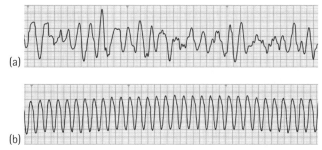

(a)

(b)

Figure 14.5 (a) Ventricular fibrillation; (b) ventricular tachycardia

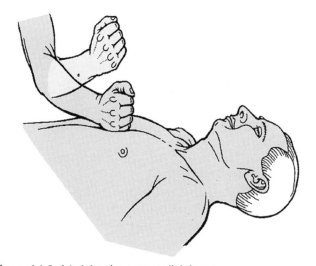

Figure 14.6 Administering a precordial thump

deprived of oxygen and nutrients and the chance of successful defibrillation declines by about 7–10% per minute.

Once the decision to defibrillate is taken, up to three shocks should be administered in rapid succession at 200 J, 200 J and then 360 J. The reason for this is that the *impedance* (resistance to current flow) through the chest wall is reduced by each shock given in close succession, and the current flow is correspondingly increased. As only approximately 5% of the current passing between the paddles actually goes through the heart, the prospect of successful defibrillation is increased when shocks are given in close succession. The rapid sequence also serves to maximize the number of attempts at defibrillation during the most receptive phase of early resuscitation. Time should not be wasted repeating pulse checks if the patient remains unresponsive and there is no change in the underlying rhythm (VF or VT).

In the event of the rhythm changing from VF to a potentially perfusing rhythm (VT or PEA) or the morphology of a pulseless VT complex changes, then a reassessment for signs of a circulation should be undertaken. Only if the patient remains in a shockable rhythm with no signs of circulation are further shocks undertaken. With modern defibrillators, three shocks can be administered within 45 seconds (and often in less than 30 seconds); BLS is only necessary during this period if the shocks are delayed by technical or practical difficulties.

If defibrillation has resulted in the return of a spontaneous cardiac output, attention should be paid to postresuscitation care. If defibrillation has led to a non-shockable rhythm (asystole or PEA) then the paramedic should withhold further drug administration and perform CPR for 1 minute before rechecking the pulse and cardiac rhythm. This is recommended as the shock may on some occasions lead to a period of myocardial stunning, where the patient has returned to a perfusing rhythm but the effect of the shock has stunned the heart such that a pulse is not palpable. After 1 minute the effects of myocardial stunning will have diminished and the true cardiac rhythm and pulse may be determined. If at this stage the patient remains in PEA or asystole then the paramedic should switch to the non-VF/VT protocol, administer adrenaline and continue CPR for another 2 minutes.

If after three shocks the patient remains in VF/VT then CPR should be performed for 1 minute and the paramedic should attempt to obtain intravenous access, intubate and administer 1 mg adrenaline intravenously followed by an intravenous flush. There is now evidence that the early (after the third shock) intravenous administration of the antiarrhythmic amiodarone 300 mg may improve short-term survival to hospital admission in patients with shock-refractory VF. Drug administration should not, however, delay the delivery of subsequent shocks.

Venous access is normally obtained in a peripheral upper limb vein. If permitted, the external jugular vein (ideally on the right) may be cannulated as it is superficial, often distended in cardiac arrest and closer to the heart than the forearm veins. Tracheal intubation is undertaken to protect the airway and optimize oxygenation. Certain drugs may be administered via the endotracheal tube to the bronchial tree at double the intravenous dose (for example, adrenaline and atropine). However, absorption is erratic, especially if pulmonary oedema is present, and endotracheal administration can also cause transient hypoxia.

Endotracheal intubation should be achieved within 30 seconds, otherwise further spells of ventilation with a bag and mask should be undertaken to avoid excessive hypoxaemia. In order to maintain coronary perfusion pressures, once endotracheal intubation is achieved, chest compressions may continue uninterrupted (except for defibrillation or pulse checks) with asynchronous ventilation at a rate of approximately 12 breaths per minute. The use of a mechanical ventilator may assist the paramedic in performing this task.

During the first minutes of CPR, an ambulance crew of two will not normally have time to intubate, establish venous access and administer drug therapy. Generally intravenous access and drug administration should take priority and subsequent periods of CPR allow these tasks to be completed. None of these tasks should, however, delay the primary treatment of VF/VT which is defibrillation.

Adrenaline is a vasopressor with α- and β-adrenergic activity and the first-line drug in cardiac arrest in the UK. In

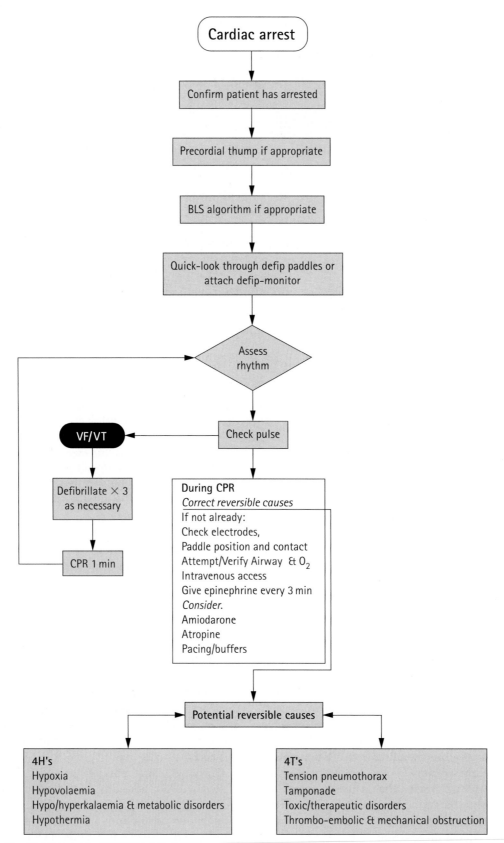

Figure 14.7 Algorithm for the treatment of VF/pulseless VT

cardiac arrest its greatest effect is through peripheral vaso-constriction (mediated by α-receptors) which raises the systemic vascular resistance, hence increasing cerebral and coronary perfusion during CPR.

After 1 minute of CPR the rhythm is reassessed and further defibrillatory shocks are given as indicated. If after a further three shocks the patient is still in VF then a further minute of CPR is undertaken and 1 mg of IV adrenaline administered.

PERSISTENT VF

After three triplets of shocks different strategies for defibrillation should be considered. The paramedic should consider changing the paddle position (to anterior/posterior) or using a different defibrillator if one is available. An anti-arrhythmic drug (amiodarone 300 mg IV) may be used if it has not already been given. Paramedics should avoid administering more than one type of antiarrhythmic drug to the same patient as these drugs in combination may paradoxically make the arrhythmia more difficult to treat.

A greater amount of time can justifiably be spent at the scene when the patient is in ventricular fibrillation, since the only treatment for this condition is defibrillation which cannot be administered safely in a moving ambulance. At *least* three sequences of three shocks are recommended before transfer to hospital is considered. Resuscitation must not be abandoned in the presence of ventricular fibrillation.

SPURIOUS ASYSTOLE

Spurious asystole is the rare phenomenon that can occur when monitoring through paddles and gel pads. Following the delivery of a shock, apparent asystole may appear on the defibrillator monitor despite the patient remaining in a shockable rhythm (so-called spurious asystole). This occurs because the retention of some electrical charge in gel pads masks the true rhythm. The true underlying rhythm can be demonstrated by attaching standard ECG leads.

Spurious asystole is more likely to occur after several successive shocks have been applied through a set of gel pads and in the presence of high transthoracic impedance. If asystole is seen following a shock whilst using gel pads/paddles then the rhythm should immediately be confirmed by attaching standard ECG electrodes/leads. The problem may be avoided if hands-free adhesive electrodes are used, as spurious asystole has not been described with this equipment.

The small chance of spurious asystole occurring should not, however, deter the use of gel pads and paddles (or preferably adhesive electrode patches) as the method of choice for the rapid, initial monitoring of a collapsed patient. The routine attachment of ECG leads for initial monitoring can lead to significant delays in the delivery of a shock. After the delivery of the first three shocks (or the occurrence of asystole) then ECG leads should be attached and used for monitoring from that point onwards.

NON-VF/VT

Patients in a rhythm other than VF and pulseless VT (in other words, asystole or PEA) are treated according to the non-VF/VT algorithm. The management of a non-VF/VT cardiac arrest shifts from rapid defibrillation to undertaking CPR, endotracheal intubation and intravenous adrenaline whilst seeking to identify and treat any reversible causes of the cardiac arrest.

CPR is performed in cycles lasting 3 minutes during which time the paramedic will attempt to obtain intravenous access and perform an endotracheal intubation. At the end of each 3-minute cycle CPR is stopped and the rhythm and pulse are checked for 10 seconds. Adrenaline 1 mg IV (or 2 mg via the endotracheal tube) is administered during each cycle. During resuscitation the paramedic should attempt to identify and treat any reversible causes of the cardiac arrest.

ASYSTOLE

Although asystole carries with it an adverse prognosis in adults (overall survival rate approximately 5%), this is partly because it tends to be the terminal stage of primary cardiac arrest. However, when asystole is secondary to other causes such as respiratory arrest or drug intoxication, the prognosis may be more favourable.

The diagnosis of asystole is confirmed by the presence of an almost flat ECG trace in a pulseless patient. Asystole rarely produces a completely flat (isoelectric) line. In all cases of presumed asystole, a rapid check must be made to confirm that:

- the leads are connected correctly
- the defibrillator is set to read through the leads
- the chest electrodes remain attached
- the amplitude setting (*gain*) on the monitor has not been set too low.

If there is any doubt that the underlying rhythm may be fine VF rather than asystole then the patient should be managed as for VF.

Adrenaline 1 mg IV should be given as soon as intravenous access is achieved. Atropine is considered a second-line drug for the treatment of asystole; it accelerates the spontaneously beating heart by depressing parasympathetic tone. Anecdotal reports of benefit in apparent asystole due to excessive parasympathetic stimulation (for example, the diving reflex in near drowning, suction of the pharynx or intubation) mean that it is still included in treatment protocols for asystole. Atropine is given as a single dose of 3 mg intravenously (or 6 mg endobronchially in concentrated solution, 10–20 ml); 60 ml of atropine (1 mg in 10 ml) is too large a volume and not appropriate for endobronchial use.

The JRCALC guidelines now state that the paramedic may consider discontinuing resuscitation in the presence of persistent asystole (longer than 20 minutes)

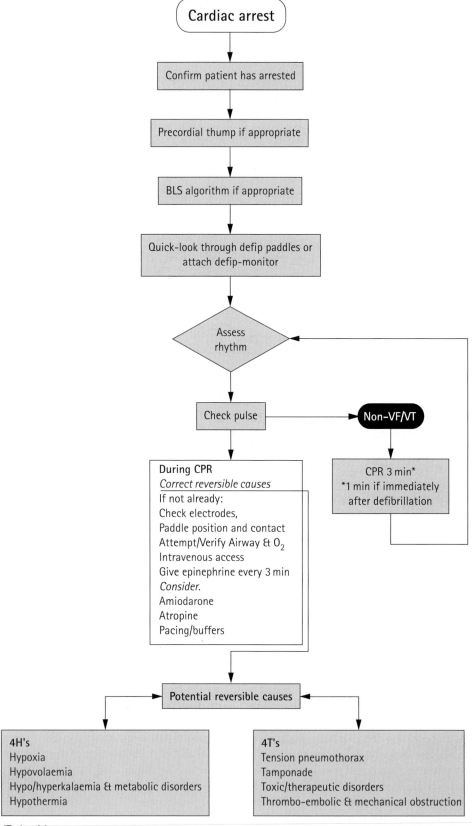

Figure 14.8 Non-VF/VT algorithm

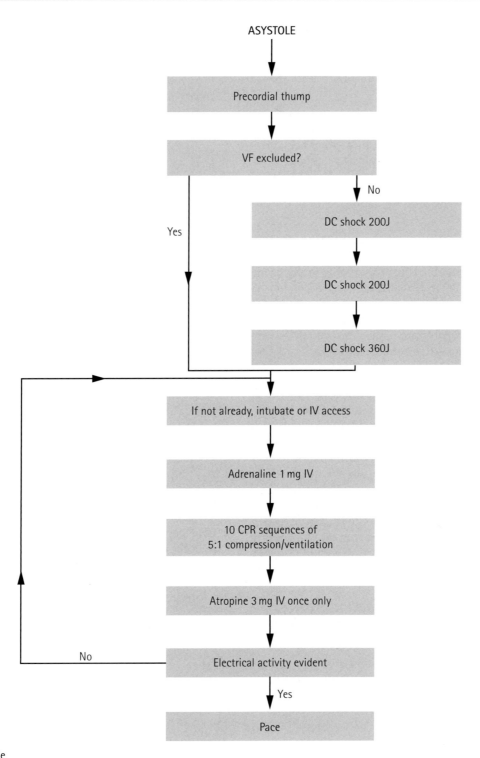

Figure 14.9 Asystole

provided that no exclusion criteria are present (children and young adults, pregnant females, electrocution, drowning, trauma, suspected hypothermia and overdose). The importance of documenting the presence of asystole for at least 30 seconds is emphasized in these guidelines. Paramedics should be guided by their own local protocols in this regard.

If patients fall into the exclusion groups listed above then they should be rapidly transported to hospital with ongoing attempts at resuscitation whilst en route.

VENTRICULAR STANDSTILL

Ventricular standstill is the presence of isolated *P* waves or the occasional ventricular complex on the ECG trace and should

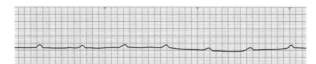

Figure 14.10 Ventricular standstill

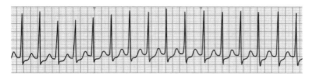

Figure 14.11 Pulseless electrical activity

be treated with atropine as above and temporary external pacing (if available) whilst the patient is rapidly transferred to the nearest A&E department. If a temporary pacing facility is not available on the defibrillator then attempts at fist pacing (repetitive thumps every 1 second at the cardiac apex) may be tried. If these manoeuvres fail to produce a cardiac output (measured by the presence of a palpable pulse) then CPR should be continued whilst the patient is transferred to hospital.

PULSELESS ELECTRICAL ACTIVITY

PEA may be defined as the presence of an ECG trace compatible with but not producing any detectable cardiac output. It is diagnosed on the basis of clinical signs of cardiac arrest (unconsciousness and an absent major pulse) in the presence of QRS complexes on the monitor. Treatment again focuses on the identification and treatment of reversible causes, and resuscitation with CPR, endotracheal intubation and intravenous adrenaline. If PEA is associated with a bradycardia (<60/min) then atropine 3 mg IV (or 6 mg via the tracheal tube) should be given. Patients with PEA should be rapidly transported to hospital.

REVERSIBLE CAUSES OF CARDIAC ARREST

There are a number of potentially reversible causes of cardiac arrest which should be excluded or identified whenever possible, especially in patients with non-VF/VT rhythms. These include the four "Hs":

- Hypoxia
- Hypovolaemia
- Hypothermia
- Hypo/hyperkalaemia (electrolyte imbalance).

and the four "Ts":

- Tension pneumothorax
- cardiac Tamponade
- Thromboembolic (pulmonary embolism)
- Toxic (drug overdose or intoxication).

At present, paramedics can only intervene to a limited degree in the treatment of these conditions (Box 14.2). Cardiac

---

> **Box 14.2 Treatable causes of cardiac arrest**
>
> *Hypoxia*
> **Recognition:** Obstructed airway, severe asthma, drowning
> **Treatment:** Endotracheal intubation and ventilation with high-concentration oxygen
>
> *Hypovolaemia*
> **Recognition:** History/evidence of trauma, internal or external bleeding
> **Treatment:** Control external bleeding, fluid protocols for shock. Aggressive fluid therapy is likely to be needed
>
> *Tension pneumothorax*
> **Recognition:** History of asthma or penetrating chest injury, high inflation pressures required to ventilate the patient, trachea deviated away from the pneumothorax, reduced breath sounds on the side of the pneumothorax
> **Treatment:** Needle thoracocentesis

tamponade and pulmonary embolism are difficult to diagnose, even in hospital, and the emergency treatment of these conditions requires special skills. If tamponade secondary to penetrating cardiac trauma is suspected, the outlook is extremely poor and if a doctor capable of performing a thoracotomy cannot be brought rapidly to the scene, the only alternative is immediate transfer to hospital. However, in pulmonary embolism, chest compressions may help to dislodge the clot.

Vigilance at the scene may alert the paramedic to an overdose or drug misuse, information that may be invaluable upon arrival in hospital but of little significance in the prehospital setting. A diagnosis of electrolyte imbalance is extremely rare in the prehospital environment but is occasionally possible, for example when the patient is suspected of having taken an overdose of a calcium blocker such as nifedipine.

However, hypoxia, hypovolaemia and tension pneumothorax are all eminently treatable in the prehospital environment and hypothermia should be recognized and actions taken to initiate recovery and prevent deterioration.

HIGH-DOSE ADRENALINE

In the non-VF/VT algorithms, the use of an intravenous bolus of 5 mg adrenaline was previously recommended after three loops (3 minutes of CPR each loop) had been performed. However, survival has not been shown to improve with this regime and it no longer forms part of the Resuscitation Council UK guidelines.

RESUSCITATION IN SPECIAL CIRCUMSTANCES

HYPOTHERMIA (SEE ALSO CHAPTER 40)

Hypothermia can be difficult to diagnose and treat in the prehospital environment. Severe hypothermia may cause bradycardia and reduced respiratory effort and therefore the initial breathing and circulation check should be undertaken for up to 1 minute before cardiac arrest is confirmed. Attempts should be made to prevent further heat loss and the patient should be rapidly transported to hospital where active rewarming can take place. Warm intravenous fluids may be given but it should be remembered that if outdoors, these may rapidly become cold intravenous fluids! Whilst a hypothermic patient in VF with a core temperature of less than 30°C rarely responds to defibrillation, the paramedic is unlikely to be able to reliably record the temperature in the prehospital environment. Such patients should receive up to three shocks followed by rapid transportation to hospital if VF persists.

Patients in cardiac arrest due to hypothermia should not be declared dead in the prehospital environment. It is important to differentiate patients in cardiac arrest due to hypothermia from those that have died and subsequently become cold. For example, patients found in a cold environment (water, snow, wind, freezing conditions) who are likely to have been hypothermic at the time of arrest should be resuscitated. However, resuscitation of a cold patient found with postmortem staining and rigor mortis in a warm environment (for example, a house) is inappropriate. Local protocols should help to guide the paramedic in these difficult decisions. If in doubt the paramedic should not withhold resuscitation.

DROWNING (SEE CHAPTER 41)

Cardiac arrest in drowning may be primary (e.g. secondary to an acute myocardial infarction causing ventricular fibrillation whilst swimming) or secondary (hypoxia from the submersion causing cardiac arrest). Attempts to retrieve the casualty from water must ensure that the rescuer's personal safety is paramount. There is a high incidence of spinal injury associated with drowning and appropriate steps to protect the spinal cord should be taken unless the history of the incident makes a spinal injury unlikely.

Treatment follows standard ALS protocols, but with increased emphasis on early ventilation and endotracheal intubation in order to correct hypoxia and protect the airway. Survival following prolonged immersion (>45 minutes) and resuscitation has been recorded and therefore attempts at resuscitation should not be abandoned in the prehospital environment.

ASTHMA (SEE CHAPTER 11)

Cardiac arrest in asthma invariably arises due to hypoxia caused by severe bronchospasm and mucous plugging. Standard ALS algorithms should be followed with emphasis being placed on early intubation and ventilation. Tension pneumothorax may be difficult to diagnose but should always be considered in the rapidly deteriorating asthmatic. The diagnosis is based on physical examination.

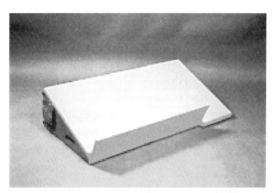

Figure 14.12 An improvised wedge for resuscitation of a pregnant woman

PREGNANCY (SEE CHAPTER 51)

Cardiac arrest during pregnancy is fortunately a rare event. Unlike the usual adult cardiac arrest scenario, there is a patient and an unborn baby to resuscitate. Standard ALS protocols should be followed with the addition of manual displacement of the pregnant uterus to the left. Alternatively a wedge (pillows, blanket or rescuers' thighs) should be placed under the patient's right side in order to improve venous return (Figure 14.12). The best chance for both the patient and the unborn baby is if an emergency caesarean section is undertaken within 5 minutes of the arrest, hence rapid transport to hospital is essential.

ANAPHYLAXIS (SEE CHAPTER 11)

Cardiac arrest due to anaphylaxis is usually caused by a combination of profound hypotension (secondary to vasodilation) and hypoxia due to acute airway obstruction and severe bronchospasm. Resuscitation should aim to achieve early control of the airway and ventilation using a bag and mask followed by rapid intubation. Attempts at endotracheal intubation may fail due to upper airway swelling and if permitted, paramedics may need to consider an emergency needle cricothyroidotomy. The circulation should be supported with a rapid infusion of intravenous fluids and adrenaline. High-dose adrenaline should be considered after 5 minutes of advanced life support. Intravenous steroids and antihistamines may be given although there is little evidence to support their use in cardiac arrest.

As anaphylaxis often occurs in younger patients with an otherwise healthy heart, prolonged attempts at resuscitation are often appropriate. The paramedic should consider early evacuation to hospital where specialist facilities and personnel are available for the management of these difficult patients.

TRAUMA

The aetiology of cardiac arrest in traumatic circumstances is likely to be due to hypovolaemia due to massive haemorrhage, organ disruption, airway obstruction and massive head or spinal injuries. These patients commonly present in PEA or asystole and the approach to the resuscitation of these patients follows the standard algorithms detailed above. Attention to cervical spine care is important during rapid evacuation to hospital but must not cause delays. Where possible, airway and breathing should be secured on scene but intravenous access and fluid administration can be secured en route to hospital and should not delay the transfer of these patients.

ADDITIONAL SUPPORT

It is not always necessary for a paramedic to request additional assistance at the scene of a cardiac arrest. However, the volume of equipment used nowadays is such that the assistance of a second crew is invariably welcome. If another crew cannot be obtained, an Immediate Care doctor or nurse can be extremely helpful. Control of the scene, removal to hospital and the care of relatives can all be achieved more effectively if additional support is recruited.

Paramedics will on occasion encounter doctors and other healthcare professionals at the scene of a cardiac arrest. They may at times feel compromised by instructions or information given to them by such personnel. It can take confidence, tact and experience to reason with doctors and nurses, some of whom will have less up-to-date training in resuscitation than they do. Whilst the doctor at the scene of a cardiac arrest will carry overall responsibility for any actions or omissions in their care of the patient, it may be necessary for paramedics to remind doctors of local resuscitation protocols. Doctors unfamiliar with current resuscitation techniques will often welcome the arrival of the paramedics, recognizing their expertise in prehospital resuscitation.

POSTRESUSCITATION CARE

Following the return of a spontaneous circulation after a resuscitation attempt, the paramedic should focus on the postresuscitation care of the patient. The priority now shifts from on-the-scene resuscitation to rapid transportation to hospital. However, the patient must be kept alive during the transfer. Airway and breathing care should be performed on scene whilst circulation and disability assessment and treatment are performed in the ambulance whilst en route to hospital.

ON SCENE

The following actions should be completed before leaving the scene.

- *Airway:* a patent airway must be established and high-flow oxygen administered.
- *Breathing:* adequate respiratory effort and symmetrical chest movement must be ensured and air entry to both lungs and

tracheal position checked. An SpO_2 monitor must be attached and the patient ventilated if he is in respiratory arrest. Both hypo- and hyper-ventilation must be avoided. If available, an end-tidal CO_2 monitor is invaluable in confirming ET tube placement and to ensure normo-capnià.

EN ROUTE TO HOSPITAL

The following actions should be carried out en route to hospital.

- *Circulation:* cardiac monitoring must be continued and the blood pressure recorded. Intravenous access should be obtained if it is not already in place.
- *Disability:* neurological status should be recorded using the AVPU score. (plus ECS if time permits).

ETHICAL MATTERS

WITHHOLDING CPR

The paramedic's safety is paramount in all resuscitation attempts. In certain situations, for example high-voltage electrical injury or chemical spillage, commencing resuscitation may place the paramedic in undue danger. In this event the paramedic should first try to make the scene safe. If it is not possible to make the scene safe then resuscitation should not be attempted until such time that additional help arrives and the scene is made safe.

There are a limited number of other occasions when it is considered inappropriate to commence resuscitation. These situations include those in which there is no possibility of survival such as when there is decapitation, rigor mortis, decomposition, incineration or massive cranial destruction. These cases are clear-cut and will usually be addressed by local protocols. The absence of bystander CPR for 15 minutes or more from cardiac arrest in a patient subsequently found in asystole may be another indication for withholding resuscitation.

Certain patients may have an active do not attempt resuscitation (DNAR) order. In these cases the doctor in charge of the patient's care will have made a DNAR order usually after discussion with the patient and next of kin. Such patients might include those with malignant or end-stage disease being transferred from hospital to hospice for palliative care. Local protocols should address how this decision is communicated to the ambulance service. Paramedics should ensure that they establish whether a DNAR order is in place prior to transfer of such patients and that they receive written confirmation of the valid DNAR order.

Living wills or advance directives are written instructions prepared in advance by a patient about his wishes should he later be unable to communicate them. Local protocols may address how to respond at a cardiac arrest if presented with an advance directive. Generally speaking, accepted practice is to withhold resuscitation provided that the paramedic believes the living will is genuine and relates to the patient he is treating. Ignoring a valid living will may place the paramedic and the ambulance trust in a vulnerable position legally, since acting against a person's wishes may constitute assault.

With the exception of the examples stated above, resuscitation should generally be started in all other cases of cardiac arrest. Judgements about the present or future quality of life made at the time of cardiac arrest are frequently inaccurate. Similarly, perceptions of a prolonged downtime before the commencement of CPR/ALS do not reliably predict a poor outcome and should not be criteria for withholding resuscitation in the prehospital environment. If in doubt, resuscitation should be commenced. The decision to terminate resuscitation attempts or withdraw further treatment can then be made in a more considered manner after full assessment in hospital. Further discussion on this complex topic can be found in the Ethical Aspects of CPR and ECC chapter of the CPR 2000 guidelines (see Further reading).

RELATIVES OBSERVING RESUSCITATION

The pros and cons of relatives in the resuscitation room has been a hotly debated topic in hospital medicine over the past 10 years. Resuscitation is a traumatic and invasive procedure and can be quite distressing for relatives to witness. On the other hand, some people feel that knowing they "were there" for their loved one, it can help them through the grieving process. Unlike in-hospital resuscitation attempts, the paramedic rarely has any choice over the presence or absence of relatives during a resuscitation attempt, particularly when the arrest occurs in the patient's own home or a public place. The relatives will often decide for themselves if they will be present during the resuscitation. The paramedic's primary responsibility remains with the patient with whom he is dealing and relatives should not be permitted to interfere with the resuscitation attempt. However, a moment's thought and a brief explanation to a relative about what is happening will not detract from the resuscitation attempt and can be comforting to the relative. It may also help with the grieving process later if the resuscitation attempt turns out to be unsuccessful.

It is unusual for relatives to be obstructive whilst resuscitation is ongoing, particularly if the paramedic has explained to them what is happening. In the rare event that the paramedic feels that the resuscitation attempt is being compromised by the presence of a relative or bystander then either they should be asked to leave or, alternatively, the resuscitation can be carried out in the back of the ambulance.

DISCONTINUING RESUSCITATION EFFORTS

The chance of survival from a non-VF/VT cardiac arrest after 20 minutes of advanced life support is negligible. Some ambulance services have developed protocols that permit paramedics to discontinue resuscitation attempts in the presence of persistent asystole. This approach has recently been endorsed by the publication of the JRCALC guidelines. In these circumstances, if a patient remains in asystole after full advanced life support for 20 minutes, resuscitation may be discontinued provided that there are no signs of life:

- no heart or breath sounds
- no palpable pulse over 30 seconds
- no movement or response to pain
- fixed and dilated pupils.

In these circumstances a 30-second rhythm strip should be recorded and attached to the patient's report form when confirming death.

It is important to remember that certain groups of patients may have a potentially reversible cause for asystole. Examples of such conditions include near drowning, pregnancy, hypothermia, electrocution, trauma, poisoning and anaphylaxis. These patients are often younger and treatment should be continued even if the initiation of basic life support was delayed. Every attempt must be made in these circumstances to restore cardiac output and the decision to terminate resuscitation should only be made in hospital.

CONTINUITY OF CARE

PATIENT TRANSPORTATION

The decision to transport a patient in cardiac arrest to hospital will depend on the location of the cardiac arrest, the distance from the nearest A&E department, the underlying rhythm and any special circumstances surrounding the arrest. More time can justifiably be spent at the scene when the patient is in ventricular fibrillation, since the only treatment is defibrillation which cannot be safely undertaken in a moving ambulance. At least three sequences of three shocks are recommended before transfer to hospital is considered. No such delay is necessary in cases of asystole or electromechanical dissociation and the patient can be moved once CPR and adrenaline administration are under way.

PATIENT HANDOVER

Advance warning should be given to the receiving hospital that you will be arriving with a patient in cardiac arrest. Local protocols will outline the mechanisms for alerting the receiving hospital. Consideration should be given to the essential information required by hospital staff. This includes:

- approximate time from collapse to arrival at scene
- administration and efficiency of any bystander CPR
- paramedic interventions so far (e.g. cannulation, defibrillation, intubation)
- any available medical history
- likely cause and any complications that have arisen
- response to resuscitative efforts.

The enthusiasm to convey this information may distract the ambulance crew from their main responsibilities, which are to transfer the patient rapidly on to the resuscitation trolley or coronary care bed and allow hospital staff to gain control of the airway, breathing and circulation as priorities.

BEREAVEMENT

Although the problems of ethics and bereavement mainly involve medical and nursing staff in the community or at hospital, consideration must be given to the paramedic's obligations in these areas. As with all healthcare workers, emotional stress can be underestimated and paramedics should always have an opportunity to receive feedback and debrief following a stressful incident (see Chapter 57).

CONCLUSION

The paramedic represents the arm of acute medical care reaching out to those who collapse with sudden illness. As such, paramedics are better placed than any other healthcare provider to administer promptly the most effective lifesaving skills. General practitioners are not so well equipped and hospital staff cannot be present at the critical moment when therapeutic interventions have the greatest chance of success. The role of the paramedic in the timely provision of advanced life support in the community is therefore paramount and the application and retention of up-to-date knowledge and skills are constant challenges.

It must be appreciated that cardiac arrest is not a homogeneous entity so its cause, presentation and prognosis will differ from one individual to another. To afford the patient the best chance, the paramedic must understand the scientific principles underlying the advanced life support protocols, be fully familiar with them and regularly review the theoretical and practical aspects of resuscitation. Difficult decisions often have to be faced and efforts do not terminate on arrival at hospital when, after an efficient handover, feedback and support may be needed from other members of the emergency team.

FURTHER READING

Colquhoun MC, Handley AJ, Evans TR 2003 ABC of resuscitation, 5th edn. BMJ Books, London

Resuscitation Council UK 2000 Advanced life support provider course manual, 4th edn. Resuscitation Council UK, London

Websites

Resuscitation Council UK: www.resus.org.uk

European Resuscitation Council: www.erc.edu

Chapter 15

Cardiovascular emergencies

INTRODUCTION

Diseases of the cardiovascular system account for the majority of medical emergencies encountered by paramedics. In the UK the picture is dominated by ischaemic heart disease and in particular manifestations of acute coronary syndrome (acute myocardial infarction and unstable angina). Therefore ischaemic heart disease is considered in detail in this chapter, although reference will also be made to other cardiovascular emergencies.

The optimal early treatment of patients with myocardial infarction may prevent subsequent more serious complications. Arrhythmias causing cardiopulmonary arrest are the subject of Chapter 13, but it is important to realize that the appropriate treatment of other arrhythmias may prevent subsequent cardiac arrest. The principles of their treatment are discussed in this section, which should be read in conjunction with the section on electrocardiography in Chapter 11.

Cardiorespiratory arrest due to lethal cardiac arrhythmias is the most dramatic medical emergency and many studies in both the USA and Europe have reported successful treatment of the condition by ambulance personnel.

ISCHAEMIC HEART DISEASE

Ischaemic or *coronary heart disease* (IHD, CHD) accounts for more deaths in the UK than any other condition. Approximately one in four men and one in five women die from the disease: this represents around 170 000 deaths per year. Approximately 1.4 million patients suffer from angina and there are in excess of 300 000 episodes of myocardial infarction per year.

The economic consequences of IHD are staggering, with an estimated 5 million working days lost every year in the UK, costing industry £3 billion in lost production. Recognizing that there is wide variation in access to good-quality care

---

Box 15.1 Some major risk factors for IHD

- Cigarette smoking
- High blood cholesterol levels
- Hypertension
- Diabetes
- Family history

throughout the United Kingdom, a National Service Framework for Coronary Heart Disease has been published for England and similar documents are available in the other home countries. These outline effective interventions in many aspects of cardiac care and suggest mechanisms by which they may be delivered.

Several important factors have been identified that contribute to IHD, though the exact mechanism by which each factor causes coronary disease is poorly understood. Some factors are unalterable, such as age, gender, ethnic group and family history while others are, at least theoretically, modifiable: these include cigarette smoking, a high blood cholesterol level, hypertension, obesity and diabetes mellitus. The association of two or more risk factors greatly increases the chance of developing ischaemic heart disease. However, while individuals at higher risk can be identified by analysis of their risk factor profile, it is important to realize that cardiovascular events may still occur in individuals without identifiable risk factors. It follows, therefore, that the absence of risk factors in an individual patient does *not* help exclude the diagnosis of IHD outside hospital.

PATHOLOGY

The term *ischaemic heart disease* describes a condition characterized by an imbalance between the supply of oxygenated blood to, and the requirements of, the myocardium. The usual cause is a reduction in supply due to the development of coronary artery stenosis (narrowing), though it is also possible to experience symptomatic IHD due to excessive demand, for instance in the presence of severe left ventricular hypertrophy due to aortic stenosis or hypertension. Occasionally coronary stenosis may be due to transient muscular spasm of the arterial wall. However, by far the commonest cause is coronary atheroma – an accumulation of lipid-rich deposits in the wall of the coronary arteries. Atheroma may develop diffusely, affecting the artery in a generalized fashion, or may affect localized segments of the artery, leading to the concept of a "plaque" of atheroma. Such plaques may expand outwards (away from the centre of the artery) without leading to significant reduction in coronary blood flow and may thus be present in the absence of symptoms. If the plaque intrudes into the coronary artery lumen the fixed narrowing restricts blood and leads to exertional angina (Figure 15.1).

Under certain circumstances the fibrous cap that separates the atheromatous plaque from the bloodstream tears or ruptures. The contents of the plaque are a strong stimulant to platelet aggregation and thrombus formation. Coronary artery thrombosis occurs, leading to an abrupt change in plaque shape and clinical condition. Rupture of the cap of a previously insignificant plaque can lead to sudden severe coronary stenosis or even total coronary occlusion. In this way, patients who are well enough to play vigorous sport (or have a normal exercise ECG test) may present with an acute coronary event the next day. Total coronary occlusion leads to myocardial cell death (infarction) within the territory

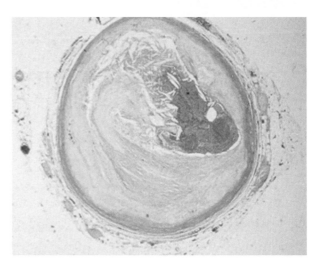

Figure 15.1 Coronary atheromatous plaque rupture

supplied by the affected artery. Such cell death frequently also occurs, albeit to a lesser degree, when small thrombotic fragments embolize from subtotal occlusive thrombosis. If an alternative source of blood supply is available – coronary collaterals – some episodes of coronary occlusion do not result in myocardial damage.

ISCHAEMIC CARDIAC PAIN

Angina pectoris

The discomfort of angina is caused by reversible myocardial ischaemia and usually occurs during conditions of increased oxygen demand in the presence of a fixed supply, most typically during physical exertion or mental and emotional stress. When the patient ceases the activity and rests the discomfort passes off rapidly (within 2–3 minutes), as myocardial oxygen requirements fall. Patients with angina often describe a feeling of tightness in the chest ("like a tight band") or liken the discomfort to a weight on the chest; sometimes it is described as a squeezing sensation. The pain is felt retrosternally (behind the sternum) and may radiate across the chest, spreading into the arms. In some patients the pain may also radiate into the throat or jaw and occasionally through to the back. The characteristic relationship to exertion is the cardinal feature in the diagnosis of angina. Patients may volunteer that the discomfort is provoked more easily on activity after heavy meals, when walking up hill or into the wind and in the early morning. A feeling of breathlessness is common, as is perspiration.

Where there is doubt about the origin of a patient's pain, because possible ischaemic pain is atypical in site or nature, it is the characteristic relationship to exertion that may provide the clue to its nature. Approximately 20 000 patients develop angina for the first time every year and there is a high incidence of infarction in the first few months after its appearance.

Unstable angina

The term *unstable angina* is used to describe a rapidly progressive, deteriorating pattern of angina often occurring in patients whose angina has been previously stable. The patient's exercise tolerance is reduced and ischaemic pain occurs more frequently. The consumption of glyceryl trinitrate is often increased. Ischaemic pain occurring at rest or on only minor exertion is a particularly worrying feature. Unstable angina is a medical emergency and most patients are admitted to hospital for investigation and treatment, as there is a high instance of subsequent myocardial infarction. The difference between unstable angina and myocardial infarction is becoming increasingly blurred. Both are characterized by plaque rupture and thrombus formation but the simplistic idea that evidence of significant myocardial cell death is the hallmark of myocardial infarction and is not seen in unstable angina has been challenged. Newer highly sensitive enzyme markers have demonstrated that cell death does indeed occur in many who would have been labelled as unstable angina by older diagnostic criteria.

Myocardial infarction

The pain of myocardial infarction is similar in nature, site and distribution to that of angina, though it usually persists longer and is associated with more profound extra effects, such as profuse perspiration, dizziness and nausea. The intensity of the pain is not a reliable indicator of the immediate risk to the patient, nor even a reliable method of diagnosing myocardial infarction, though patients with preexisting angina often describe the pain of infarction as being similar, although much more severe. It is not usually relieved by glyceryl trinitrate. Only about half those with acute myocardial infarction will have a history of previous heart disease.

To complicate matters further, pain (particularly in elderly people) may be a minor feature or absent altogether: the diagnosis will then only be made if a high index of suspicion is maintained.

MYOCARDIAL INFARCTION

Abrupt loss of functioning myocardium due to coronary thrombosis has mechanical and electrical effects, as well as peripheral effects mediated via hormonal and autonomic nervous reflexes.

The mechanical effects depend on the extent and location of the muscle loss, as well as on the preexisting state of the myocardium. The loss of even a small volume of muscle may be tolerated badly in a patient whose ventricle has been damaged by previous episodes of infarction. Both the filling capacity (diastolic function) and the ability to eject blood (systolic function) are impaired and left ventricular failure results. In the acute phase this is characterized by breathlessness due to pulmonary oedema. If systolic function is severely impaired, cardiac output falls to such low levels that reflex mechanisms can no longer maintain the blood pressure. Perfusion of the skin and major organs is reduced and urine output is attenuated – *cardiogenic shock*. Other mechanical effects include *mitral regurgitation* due to infarction or ischaemia of the papillary muscles of the mitral valve, *cardiac tamponade* due to rupture of the free wall of the infarcted myocardium and resultant loss of blood into the pericardium, *ventricular septal defect* due to rupture of an infarcted intraventricular septum leading to shunting of blood from left to right ventricle. These mechanical complications usually become obvious in hospital. Diagnosis in the prehospital phase is difficult, although cardiogenic shock and cardiac tamponade are causes of electromechanical dissociation.

Electrical effects are easier to diagnose using prehospital cardiac monitoring and indeed, are more commonly seen early in the course of the acute coronary event. Ischaemic and infarcted myocardial segments are electrically unstable and prone to ventricular fibrillation or tachycardia, both causes of cardiac arrest and sudden cardiac death (see below). Atrial fibrillation also may occur, due to either atrial myocardial infarction or acute atrial dilation consequent on abnormal ventricular filling. This irregular and usually rapid rhythm leads to a further reduction in cardiac output and an increase in risk of intracardiac thrombosis and peripheral embolization. Interruption in the blood supply of the sinus node or atrioventricular node is a cause of bradycardia and degrees of heart block. The same effects are sometimes seen due to excess vagal nerve (parasympathetic) discharge, the importance being that reversal of these bradycardias can lead to significant improvement in clinical condition. The pain and anxiety of myocardial infarction may, conversely, be associated with excess sympathetic tone, causing sinus tachycardia and hypertension (and increasing the potential for ventricular arrhythmias), both of which, by increasing myocardial oxygen demand, are likely to lead to more rapid and extensive infarction.

CLINICAL FEATURES

A patient with acute myocardial infarction is usually middle-aged or elderly and may have a history of preceding angina or previous infarction. Risk factors for the development of ischaemic heart disease (e.g., cigarette smoking, hypertension, diabetes or hypercholesterolaemia) may be present but the absence of these features should not prevent the diagnosis.

Box 15.2 Complications of myocardial infarction

- Cardiogenic shock
- Mitral regurgitation
- Cardiac tamponade
- Ventricular septal defect

Box 15.3 Symptoms of myocardial infarction

- Chest pain
- Fear and anxiety
- Nausea
- Vomiting
- Sweating
- Shortness of breath
- Palpitation

The dominant symptom of myocardial infarction is chest pain, the characteristics of which are discussed above. The patient is usually apprehensive, in pain and appears distressed. Nausea, vomiting and sweating are commonly associated features and shortness of breath is present particularly when pulmonary oedema occurs. The blood pressure should be recorded in all cases: it may be high in patients with pre-existing hypertension or in the presence of severe pain. A low blood pressure with reduced cardiac output occurs in cardiogenic shock and is an ominous sign but may also be seen in association with more easily reversible electrical complications (see above).

A presumptive diagnosis of myocardial infarction can be made from the history and associated clinical features. Other conditions, for example dissecting aortic aneurysm or pulmonary thromboembolism (PE), may produce a similar clinical picture and are very difficult to distinguish from myocardial infarction (without further investigation in hospital). This should not concern ambulance personnel unduly, unless administration of thrombolytic therapy is being considered outside hospital, as the principles of treatment before hospital admission are broadly similar.

TREATMENT

General

The management path involves: early recognition (by patients/relatives), rapid response (by health services), rapid assessment, resuscitation where appropriate, accurate diagnosis, prompt reperfusion (either by thrombolytic drugs or by primary angioplasty – balloon dilation), correction of complications, rehabilitation, education, secondary prevention and reassurance. Although it is not immediately apparent, the ambulance paramedic may have opportunities to influence the latter phases of this management pathway, either officially within cardiac rehabilitation programmes or unofficially through contacts with acquaintances who have suffered heart disease.

The British Heart Foundation (BHF) recommends that the optimal early treatment involves a combined response from the patient's general practitioner and the ambulance service – the GP to provide diagnostic expertise, knowledge of the patient's past history and access to morphine and the ambulance service to provide resuscitation skills and equipment and rapid transport to hospital. In practice, this has lead to many GPs either advising patients to phone 999 or activating the ambulance service directly. Practice varies greatly, though in general the ambulance services have shouldered an increasing responsibility for the early management of acute myocardial infarction. The BHF also recognized the importance of early thrombolytic treatment and encouraged prehospital administration of such agents as a way of achieving short "call-to-needle times" (see below). The need for early thrombolytic therapy has been confirmed by the various National Service Framework documents and such time intervals will be assessed as indicators of good-quality care.

The patient will usually be most comfortable sitting upright and *high-concentration oxygen* should be given. The patient and any relatives/bystanders will be anxious and a professional, reassuring efficient approach is essential. Cardiac monitoring should start as soon as possible and venous access should be obtained at an early stage, usually with an intravenous cannula placed in a forearm vein and flushed with heparinized saline to prevent clotting. If a cardiac arrest should occur it is a great advantage if an intravenous cannula is already in situ and monitoring already instituted. The cardiac rhythm should be recorded as well as 12-lead ECG, heart rate and blood pressure, prior to hospital transfer.

Analgesia

The relief of pain is a major priority in the treatment of patients with infarction. Diamorphine or morphine are the agents of choice. General practitioners attending the patient will usually administer one of these drugs. Ambulance services now have protocols for paramedics to administer morphine for treating the severe pain of myocardial infarction. Morphine should be given by slow intravenous injection, with careful observation of its effect. Opiate analgesics not only relieve the pain of myocardial infarction, and in this way tend to reduce abnormalities of autonomic balance, but also have beneficial effects on ventricular filling pressures, acting to reduce myocardial workload and oxygen requirements. In the absence of any other analgesic, nitrous oxide inhalation (Entonox) is effective against the pain of myocardial infarction.

Of course, anything that reduces ischaemia is likely to relieve pain, so glyceryl trinitrate and β-blockers have been shown to be effective in this regard, as has successful thrombolytic therapy.

Aspirin

A daily dose of soluble aspirin (75–300 mg) has been shown to have beneficial cardiovascular effects by reducing platelet aggregation (one of the major components of thrombus formation). In the early days after myocardial infarction aspirin reduces mortality, in addition to any effects of thrombolytic treatment. Although there is no convincing evidence that the benefit of aspirin administration is as time dependent as that of thrombolytic treatment, most local protocols allow aspirin to be given outside hospital. Active peptic ulceration and bleeding disorders are contraindications. The recommended first dose is 300 mg, which should be chewed.

Antiemetic drugs

Opiates and related analgesics will worsen the nausea that frequently accompanies myocardial infarction and produce vomiting. An antiemetic drug should therefore be administered intravenously; metoclopramide (Maxolon) is licensed for use in this fashion. Drugs with vasoconstrictor properties, for example cyclizine, may increase myocardial workload and are not recommended for use in patients with myocardial infarction.

Glyceryl trinitrate

Nitrates cause relaxation of the smooth muscle layer of blood vessel walls and therefore venous and arterial dilation. Venous dilation leads to a reduction in ventricular preload (see Chapter 11), cardiac workload and oxygen consumption. The benefit of the drug in angina, during myocardial infarction and in acute heart failure is largely due to this action, although coronary vasodilation may be relevant in some cases, as may a reduction in blood pressure due to arterial vasodilation. Some patients may be particularly sensitive to nitrates and administration may be associated with profound hypotension. This is another cause of "collapse" in patients with acute coronary events. Sublingual administration of 0.4–0.8 mg is either by tablet or spray. Whilst the spray has a long shelf-life and is easy to administer, the tablet has the advantage that it can be removed if side-effects occur or when relief is obtained.

Atropine

Atropine reverses vagal nerve overactivity. Where bradycardia with hypotension or other evidence of reduced cardiac output persists, atropine should be given intravenously with continuous ECG monitoring. Comparatively small doses (0.5 mg) may be adequate to increase the heart rate with significant improvement in cardiac output and blood pressure. Local protocols should be followed in all cases.

Diuretic drugs

Intravenous diuretic agents are employed in acute heart failure in the presence of pulmonary oedema. Frusemide (40–120 mg) given intravenously is the agent most frequently employed. Its effects are mediated initially via venodilation and later by salt and water excretion.

Antiarrhythmic drugs

The prehospital use of antiarrhythmic drugs such as lignocaine to prevent potentially lethal arrhythmias has not been supported by clinical research and the role for such agents is in the management of cardiac arrest. Early intravenous administration of β-blockers has been shown to reduce infarct size, the frequency of ventricular rupture and the risk of ventricular fibrillation. However, the prehospital use of such drugs in the early stages of acute coronary syndromes has not been widely established.

Thrombolytic therapy

Thrombolytic agents activate the natural mechanism for producing clot breakdown (*lysis*). Dissolution of the obstructing thrombus occurs with reperfusion of ischaemic myocardium. Several large trials have clearly demonstrated reduced mortality in cases of myocardial infarction treated with intravenous thrombolytic agents. A variety of such agents are now available, including those given by continuous infusion, requiring electric pumps, and those given by single and double bolus injection. Drugs in the latter group are more convenient for prehospital use. Treatment is most effective when given as soon as possible after the onset of symptoms. Unfortunately for prehospital practitioners, diagnosis is most difficult in the early stages when the benefit of treatment is at its greatest. Accurate diagnosis, usually requiring recording (and transmission) of an electrocardiogram, is particularly important because thrombolytic agents have potentially dangerous side-effects, the most severe being intracerebral haemorrhage occurring some hours after administration. Those at highest risk of complications can be identified using a simple checklist and these individuals may be considered for emergency angioplasty (balloon dilation) of the occluded artery as an alternative after arrival in hospital.

The time intervals between calling for help and receiving thrombolytic therapy (*call-to-needle time*) and between arriving in hospital and receiving such therapy (*door-to-needle time*) can be measured quite easily. These intervals form auditable performance indicators of the quality of care provided to patients with coronary disease. Methods to reduce delay to treatment include prehospital treatment by GPs or ambulance paramedics, direct admission of patients to the coronary care unit for rapid diagnosis and institution of therapy and the "fast-tracking" of patients with possible infarction through rapid assessment and treatment in the accident and emergency department.

In an increasing number of areas paramedics administer thrombolytic agents autonomously, having independently made the clinical judgement that a patient with an ST segment myocardial infarction meets the relevant criteria for prehospital treatment. In other areas, paramedics are required to transmit a 12-lead ECG using telemetry equipment to a receiving hospital (usually the coronary care unit or emergency department) for approval by a doctor before commencing treatment. It is likely that, as the confidence of paramedics grows, autonomous decision-making by paramedics will become the norm.

Tenecteplase and reteplase are the preferred thrombolytic agents for prehospital use, as each is administered in

Box 15.4 Primary treatment of myocardial infarction

- Oxygen
- Analgesia
- Antiemetic
- Glyceryl trinitrate
- Thrombolysis
- Aspirin

Box 15.5 Treatment of complications

- Treatment of arrhythmias
- Treatment of heart failure

bolus doses rather than as an infusion. Tenecteplase is given in a single dose adjusted according to the patient's weight. Reteplase is given as two bolus doses that must be administered 30 minutes apart.

Adverse events following thrombolytic therapy include ventricular fibrillation, ventricular tachycardia and other arrhythmias. Hypotension and shock may also occur. However, these events are often of short duration and may be self-terminating. They are also common complications of myocardial infarction and paramedics are skilled in their management. Treatment is no different, regardless of whether a thrombolytic agent has been given. Rarely, anaphylaxis may occur, and is also treated according to standard protocols, ensuring that administration of the thrombolytic agent is discontinued immediately signs or symptoms become evident.

The adverse event that is specific to thrombolytic agents is an increased risk of bleeding. Haemorrhage from cannulation sites and other wounds should be controlled by sustained direct pressure. Patients who have received thrombolytic drugs should be moved from house to ambulance and from ambulance to hospital trolley with great care to minimize the risk of accidental injury. The incidence of haemorrhagic stroke (through disruption of an existing intracerebral clot) is 1 per 200 patients thrombolysed, and half of these cases will result in death. Stroke usually occurs more than an hour after the initiation of thrombolytic therapy, and is therefore rarely encountered in the prehospital setting. If it does occur, patients should be managed in accordance with the usual ABC priorities and be transferred rapidly to hospital. Whilst the risk of stroke following thrombolysis is alarming, this must be offset against the considerably greater reduction in mortality and morbidity achieved by the early administration of these drugs to appropriate patients.

In order to ensure that the benefit of prehospital thrombolysis outweighs the risk of adverse events, only patients meeting the criteria established by the Joint Royal Colleges Ambulance Liaison Committee (JRCALC) should be administered thrombolytic agents by paramedics. These are detailed in the table below.

JRCALC criteria

Primary assessment

1. Can you confirm that the patient is conscious, coherent and able to understand that clot-dissolving drugs will be used?
2. Can you confirm that the patient is aged 75 or less?
3. Can you confirm that the patient has had symptoms characteristic of a heart attack (i.e. continuous pain in a typical distribution and of 15 minutes duration or longer)?
4. Can you confirm that the symptoms started less than 6 hours ago?
5. Can you confirm that the pain built up over seconds and minutes rather than starting totally abruptly?
6. Can you confirm that breathing does not influence the severity of the pain?
7. Can you confirm that the heart rate is between 50 and 140 beats per minute?
8. Can you confirm that the systolic blood pressure is more than 80 mmHg and less than 160 mmHg and that the diastolic blood pressure is below 110 mmHg?
9. Can you confirm that the electrocardiogram shows abnormal ST segment elevation of 2 mm or more in at least two standard leads or in at least two adjacent precordial leads, not including V_1? (ST elevation can sometimes be normal in V_1 and V_2)
10. Can you confirm that the QRS width is 0.16 mm or less, and that left bundle branch block is absent from tracing? (Note: RBBB permitted only with qualifying ST segment elevation)
11. Can you confirm that there is NO atrioventricular block greater than 1st degree? (If necessary after treatment with IV atropine)

Secondary assessment

12. Can you confirm that the patient is not likely to be pregnant, nor has delivered within the last two weeks?
13. Can you confirm that the patient has not had a peptic ulcer within the last 6 months?
14. Can you confirm that the patient has not had a stroke of any sort within the last 12 months and does not have permanent disability from a previous stroke?
15. Can you confirm the patient has no diagnosed bleeding tendency, has had no recent blood loss (except for normal menstruation), and is not taking warfarin (anticoagulant) therapy?
16. Can you confirm the patient has not had any surgical operation, tooth extractions, significant trauma or head injury within the last 4 weeks?
17. Can you confirm that the patient has not been treated within the last three months for any other serious head or brain condition? (This is intended to exclude patients with cerebral tumours)
18. Can you confirm that the patient is not being treated for liver failure, renal failure or any other severe systemic illness?

Patients who do not meet the criteria for prehospital thrombolysis should be admitted urgently to hospital for treatment. Transmission of pre-alert message identifying the impending arrival of a patient with an acute coronary syndrome has been shown to reduce door-to-treatment times.

In some areas, primary coronary intervention (PCI or angioplasty) is being increasingly used as the first-line treatment of myocardial infarction in preference to thrombolysis. Paramedics should refer to local protocols to determine if this is the case for their area of practice.

HEPARIN

In addition to their fibrinolytic properties, tenecteplase and reteplase are potent platelet activators, and heparin should therefore be administered concurrently to reduce the risk of re-occlusion of the coronary arteries.

SUDDEN CARDIAC DEATH

Sudden, apparently unheralded cardiac death remains a distressingly common occurrence. It has been recognized for many years that the majority of patients who die from coronary heart disease do so outside hospital, very often before medical help arrives. Ventricular fibrillation complicating the early stages of acute myocardial infarction is responsible for many cases, while a lethal arrhythmia complicating episodes of ischaemia due to severe coronary disease, without actual evidence of acute infarction at postmortem, accounts for many more. Non-coronary disease may also cause sudden cardiac death: valvular heart disease (especially aortic stenosis), arrhythmias complicating cardiomyopathy, metabolic, iatrogenic or inherited conditions explain some cases.

THE DEVELOPMENT OF OUT-OF-HOSPITAL CORONARY CARE

With the realization that the majority of deaths from myocardial infarction occur in the early stages (around half of all patients who die do so in the first hour after the onset of symptoms), special cardiac arrest teams became part of the routine hospital management of patients at high risk of developing cardiac arrest. These teams provided basic cardiopulmonary resuscitative methods, defibrillation and more advanced drug treatments. Once the effectiveness of resuscitation in hospital became established, attempts were made to provide similar skills in the community. Frank Pantridge, in Belfast, set up a mobile coronary care unit staffed by a doctor and a nurse. Early experience confirmed the high incidence of lethal arrhythmias at the onset of myocardial infarction and many patients attended by mobile units were successfully resuscitated from cardiac arrest before hospital admission. Pantridge and his co-workers also drew attention to the value of cardiopulmonary resuscitation (CPR) initiated by a bystander when cardiac arrest occurred before the arrival of medical help.

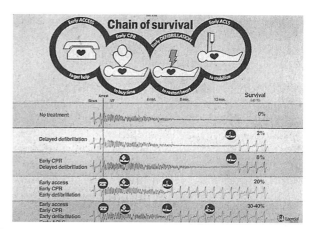

Figure 15.2 The "chain of survival"

In the early 1970s, Leonard Cobb, in Seattle, was inspired by these results and equipped paramedics with defibrillators and also trained fire-fighters to perform basic life support. The fire service in Seattle was highly coordinated and a standard fire appliance could reach any part of the city within 4 minutes, enabling CPR to be started before the arrival of the more highly trained ambulance crew. The most crucial determinant of survival from cardiac arrest was found to be the speed with which defibrillation was performed. To accelerate this further, the fire-fighters were equipped with defibrillators, a process facilitated by the development of the semi-automatic advisory model that requires less training to use.

Community CPR schemes were inaugurated. Later research has confirmed the importance of rapid access to the emergency medical services, the rapid institution of basic life support together with early defibrillation and the early application of advanced life support techniques, including advanced airway management and the use of drugs, in determining survival from cardiac arrest occurring outside hospital. These stages should be seen as an interrelated sequence of events, each one constituting a link in the *chain of survival* (Figure 15.2). Intensive efforts to reduce delays to the minimum have resulted in survival rates from cardiac arrest of 40% being reported from that part of the USA. British results have been less impressive and there remains controversy regarding the added benefit of paramedics' advanced life support skills over defibrillation alone.

DISSECTING AORTIC ANEURYSM

A dissecting aortic aneurysm is one of the most serious cardiovascular emergencies. The condition is more common in men and hypertension is an important predisposing factor. However, the patient may not have been known to be hypertensive. The condition starts with a tear in the intima of the aorta, usually in the ascending part of the arch of the aorta. Blood dissects a pathway between the layers of the aortic wall, extending proximally to the aortic valve and running distally for a variable distance. On occasions "reentry" may occur, when the distal part of the dissection reestablishes continuity with the lumen forming a "double-barrelled" aorta. The dissection may involve one or more major branches of the aorta, including the coronary arteries. The proximal dissection around the root of the aorta may distort the aortic valve and cause aortic regurgitation. Rupture of the aorta into the pericardium or pleura may occur and is usually rapidly fatal (Figure 15.3).

The clinical manifestations of dissecting aortic aneurysm include severe chest pain, aortic regurgitation, restriction of blood flow through branches of the aorta and the consequences of the aortic rupture. The pain of dissecting aneurysm is similar to that of myocardial infarction, though perhaps a little more abrupt in onset. It is sometimes described as having a "tearing" quality and often radiates into the back between the scapulae. It may also be felt in other parts of the chest or in the lumbar area and on occasions in the abdomen; the site of the pain may change as the aneurysm extends. The most frequent clue that a dissecting aneurysm is the cause of the patient's pain (as opposed to myocardial infarction or other causes of severe chest pain) is evidence of obstruction to blood flow in the major branches of the aorta caused by the dissection. This is sometimes manifested as a discrepancy in the pulses in the arms or a marked difference in blood pressure on the two sides. The same may occur with the carotid or femoral vessels: disturbance of consciousness occurs with interruption of cerebral blood supply. Myocardial infarction (from obstruction of the coronary arteries) or paraplegia (from obstruction to spinal blood flow) may be seen, while gastrointestinal symptoms and haematuria may also occur when the mesenteric or renal vessels are involved. The administration of thrombolytic drugs for myocardial infarction due to aortic dissection will seriously jeopardize the outcome.

The occurrence of severe chest pain, often reaching a rapid peak of intensity, followed within minutes or hours by signs of arterial occlusion as outlined above, should suggest the diagnosis. In practice, the diagnosis is rarely made before hospital admission. The presence of sustained hypertension may occur with dissection but also occurs in patients with myocardial infarction; profound hypotension may also occur in both conditions.

MANAGEMENT

In many cases the patient will be suspected to be suffering from myocardial infarction. ECG monitoring, oxygen therapy and analgesia are equally appropriate in both conditions, while sublingual nitrates will do no harm in dissection. Venous access will be established at an early stage and used to provide effective analgesia.

In summary, if a paramedic mistakes aortic dissection for acute infarction little harm is likely to result, unless prehospital thrombolytic agents are given. Where consciousness is disturbed owing to involvement of the cerebral blood vessels in the dissection, a diagnosis of stroke may be considered, though a preceding history of back or chest pain will usually alert to the correct diagnosis and appropriate treatment for an unconscious patient (with careful attention to airway maintenance and adequate ventilation) becomes an important priority.

PULMONARY EMBOLISM

Pulmonary embolism is a frequent finding at postmortem, the inference being that it frequently contributes to the death of patients. The diagnosis, however, is infrequently made before death, perhaps in only 25% of cases. Pulmonary embolism occurs when a thrombus that has formed in a large vein in the leg or pelvis becomes dislodged and is carried through the venous system and right ventricle into the pulmonary circulation. Venous thrombosis differs from arterial thrombosis in being formed in the absence of atheroma. Three main factors have been identified in the cause of such thrombi: abnormalities in the blood vessel, blood that clots more easily and obstruction to venous flow resulting in stasis. Conditions associated with a high risk of thromboembolism include pregnancy, recent operations (particularly orthopaedic and gynaecological procedures), chronic heart failure or pulmonary disease, fractures and other injuries of the legs, chronic venous insufficiency affecting the lower leg, prolonged immobility and the presence of carcinoma.

The immediate result of pulmonary thromboembolism is obstruction of all or part of the pulmonary arterial bed and the consequences will depend on the size of the area of vascular bed obstructed. The increased resistance to pulmonary blood

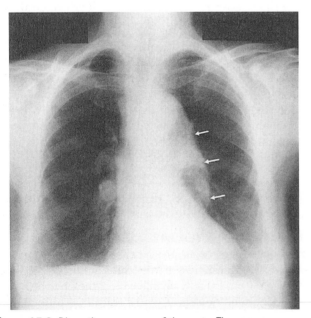

Figure 15.3 Dissecting aneurysm of the aorta. The arrows demonstrate an abnormally large descending aortic silhouette. The definitive diagnosis is usually made by CT scanning, MRI scanning or transoesophageal echocardiography

Box 15.6 Clinical features of pulmonary embolism

- Chest pain
- Central cyanosis
- Tachycardia
- Dyspnoea
- Remember to check for deep vein thrombosis

Box 15.7 Treatment of pulmonary embolism

- Oxygen
- Cardiac monitoring
- Intravenous access
- Opiate analgesia

Box 15.8 Causes of cardiac tamponade

- Trauma
- Following myocardial infarction
- Following surgery
- Malignancy
- Infection

flow that results from obstruction, when severe, will lead to pulmonary hypertension with acute right ventricular dilation and failure, tachycardia and a decline in cardiac output. Pulmonary embolism can therefore present with collapse due to electromechanical dissociation.

DIAGNOSIS

In milder cases examination findings may be entirely normal. With more severe emboli, pleuritic chest pain (pain made worse by breathing), central cyanosis, tachycardia and dyspnoea occur. The presence of deep vein thrombosis (DVT), usually in the legs, provides an excellent clue to diagnosis but is often absent. Similarly, the presence of any of the risk factors mentioned above make the diagnosis more likely. However, diagnosis on clinical grounds is difficult and many of the diagnostic features are beyond the scope of the paramedical examination. Detailed hospital investigation is often necessary, the results of which determine the most appropriate treatment.

TREATMENT

Outside hospital, treatment will centre on emergency resuscitation where appropriate, the administration of oxygen, instituting cardiac monitoring and securing intravenous access. Where a strong analgesic is required, the same agents recommended for the treatment of myocardial infarction may be employed, although it is unusual for a pulmonary embolism to cause the same severe pain.

CARDIAC TAMPONADE

Cardiac tamponade occurs when fluid collects in the pericardial cavity in quantities sufficient to interfere with cardiac filling and obstruct venous return. If the condition develops rapidly (as may occur with the collection of blood following trauma), 250 ml may be sufficient to produce severe consequences. Where fluid accumulates more slowly and the pericardium has time to stretch and adapt to the accumulation of fluid, up to 1000 ml may be present. Tamponade occurs most commonly from bleeding into the pericardial space as a result of trauma, surgical procedures or cardiac rupture following myocardial infarction. Tumours invading the pericardium (most commonly from the bronchus or breast) may also cause the accumulation of fluid. Bacterial infection occasionally causes purulent fluid to accumulate in the pericardium, particularly in immunocompromised patients. A pericardial effusion may follow acute pericarditis from viral or other causes and produce similar mechanical effects.

DIAGNOSIS

The cardinal diagnostic feature of cardiac tamponade is a reduction in cardiac output associated with systemic venous congestion. With rapidly developing effusions, as may occur with cardiac trauma, quiet heart sounds occur but the recognition of this sign is difficult outside hospital. Electromechanical dissociation may occur. When tamponade develops slowly, the clinical features may resemble heart failure: dyspnoea, tachycardia, congestion of the neck veins, hepatic engorgement and peripheral oedema. Immediate treatment may be life-saving and in most cases will be undertaken in hospital after confirmation of the diagnosis by echocardiography. Only very rarely is pericardial aspiration by medical staff performed before hospital admission. Treatment by the paramedic will be the provision of oxygen, establishment of intravenous access and cardiac monitoring. Where trauma is responsible, the treatment of associated injuries may dominate the picture.

CARDIAC ARRHYTHMIAS

The treatment of asystole, pulseless ventricular tachycardia and ventricular fibrillation is considered in Chapter 13: these arrhythmias are not considered further in this chapter.

All arrhythmia patients require oxygen

In prehospital care, treatment of arrhythmias is relatively simple. The golden rule is to treat the patient and not the arrhythmia.

Treat the patient, not the arrhythmia

TREATMENT OF TACHYCARDIA

All treatments for tachycardia have their own risks and are therefore most safely undertaken in hospital. Prehospital treatment should therefore only be undertaken if the arrhythmia presents a significant threat to the patient's cardiovascular status or life and wherever possible during ECG monitoring, with a paper record made of the initial tachycardia and any response to treatment.

Tachycardias may be classified as regular or irregular with narrow or broad (>120 ms) QRS complexes (see also Chapter 11).

Sinus tachycardia

Treatment should be directed towards the cause of the tachycardia (e.g. hypovolaemia due to haemorrhage).

Atrial tachycardia and atrial flutter

Drug treatment may be considered during rapid transfer to hospital. Carotid sinus massage (Figure 15.4) or the Valsalva manoeuvre ("*Take a huge breath in and strain as if you were on the toilet*") may increase the degree of atrioventricular block, but is most unlikely to terminate the arrhythmia. Rather, by transiently slowing AV conduction such methods may abolish ventricular activity long enough for the underlying atrial abnormality to be recognized and the correct diagnosis made. Both of these are "vagal manoeuvres" and are *more effective in the younger patient and when lying flat*. Carotid sinus massage (massage over the carotid artery level with the upper border of the larynx) should not be performed for more than 5–10 seconds. Vagal stimulation with a Valsalva occurs on *release* of the manoeuvre. The patient with acute paroxysmal cardiovascular compromise is best treated by synchronized cardioversion after arrival in hospital. Amiodarone (150 mg IV given over 10 minutes, repeated once) may be administered by paramedics.

Atrial fibrillation

Atrial fibrillation with a moderate ventricular response (pulse rate <120/min) usually responds to a course of oral digoxin. In the patient with pronounced tachycardia, intravenous digoxin, verapamil or β-blocker may slow the ventricular rate. More advanced drugs or synchronized defibrillation (if there is haemodynamic compromise) may restore regular sinus rhythm; treatment is best undertaken in hospital.

Junctional tachycardia

Junctional tachycardia (or AV nodal reentrant tachycardia – AVNRT; Figure 15.5) may be terminated by vagal manoeuvres (carotid sinus massage or the Valsalva manoeuvre) and these should be tried first. If vagal manoeuvres fail, the first-line treatment is adenosine 3 mg by rapid IV injection,

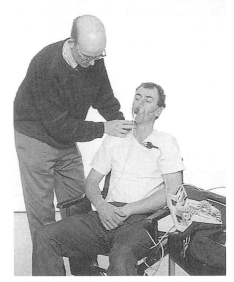

Figure 15.4 Treatment of supraventricular tachycardia by carotid sinus massage

Box 15.9 Types of tachycardia

- Regular narrow complex
  Sinus tachycardia
  AV nodal tachycardia
  Macrorentrant AV tachycardia (in Wolff–Parkinson–White syndrome)
  Atrial tachycardia with fixed AV conduction
  Atrial flutter with fixed AV conduction
- Irregular narrow complex
  Atrial fibrillation
  Atrial flutter with variable AV conduction
  Atrial tachycardia with variable AV conduction
- Regular broad complex
  Ventricular tachycardia
  Any cause of regular narrow complex with coexistent bundle branch block
- Irregular broad complex
  Atrial fibrillation with coexistent bundle branch block

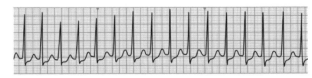

Figure 15.5 Junctional tachycardia (AVNRT)

followed if unsuccessful after 1–2 minutes by 6 mg and followed again if unsuccessful by 12 mg. Paramedics are not currently licensed to administer adenosine. Immediate evacuation for treatment in hospital is appropriate. Cardiac monitoring must be maintained during the treatment. Adenosine has been used successfully outside hospital.

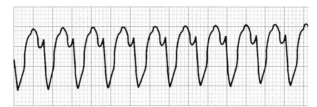

Figure 15.6 Ventricular tachycardia

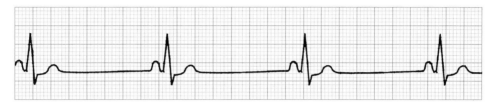

Figure 15.7 Sinus bradycardia

Verapamil 5 mg IV (and repeated once if necessary) is also effective in the treatment of junctional tachycardia, but is *absolutely contraindicated* if the patient is taking oral β-blockers and must be given by a doctor.

Direct current (DC) cardioversion is effective in terminating junctional tachycardia, but should be undertaken after transfer to hospital. Amiodarone (150 mg IV given over 10 minutes repeated once) may be administered by paramedics.

> **Remember to print a rhythm strip**

Ventricular tachycardia

If ventricular tachycardia (Figure 15.6) is pulseless the resuscitation algorithm for ventricular fibrillation should be followed. If a pulse is present, oxygen should be given, followed by immediate rapid transfer to hospital. Administration of intravenous amiodarone is indicated, subject to local protocol, followed if necessary after arrival in hospital by DC cardioversion.

Isolated ventricular complexes (ventricular premature beats) do not require treatment unless they occur in salvos in which case 150 mg of amiodarone should be given IV.

TREATMENT OF BRADYCARDIA

First- and second-degree heart block rarely require treatment. Very occasionally, enough complexes fail to be transmitted in second-degree heart block to cause bradycardia with cardiovascular compromise. Atropine 0.5 mg (repeated if necessary to a maximum dose of 3 mg) should then be given.

If third-degree heart block ("complete heart block") is accompanied by an adequate cardiovascular status, it may be appropriate to delay treatment until arrival in hospital. Otherwise treatment is with intravenous atropine (0.5 mg, repeated if needed to a maximum dose of 3 mg). If this is unsuccessful, external pacing (if available) should be attempted. It is important to remember, however, that this is uncomfortable in the conscious patient.

In summary, bradycardia or heart block requires the following treatment.

- First-degree block – none
- Second-degree block – none or atropine
- Third-degree block – none, external pacing or atropine
- Sinus bradycardia (Figure 15.7) – none or atropine.

FURTHER READING

Colquhoun MC, Handley AJ, Evans TR (eds) 1995 The ABC of resuscitation, 3rd edn. BMJ Books, London
Weston CFM 1999 Cardiac emergencies. In: Greaves I, Porter KM (eds) Prehospital medicine. The principles and practice of immediate care. Arnold, London

Chapter 16

The unconscious patient

CHAPTER CONTENTS

INTRODUCTION

The unconscious patient is a patient in danger. Unconscious individuals cannot actively protect themselves from the environment and many of the normal protective reflexes are lost. Paramedic staff who attend an unconscious casualty have several roles: they must assess and treat any potentially or immediately life-threatening conditions; they must ensure that the patient comes to no further harm; and finally they must transfer the patient safely to the nearest appropriate care facility and communicate their findings to the receiving medical personnel.

DEFINITIONS

Consciousness is best thought of as a scale. At the highest level, a patient is fully aware of the environment and can be described as "alert". Patients who have lost all awareness of their surroundings can be described as "unconscious". As the conscious level falls the eyes close, speech may become confused or cease and motor responses change. An individual who is not rousable from unconsciousness is said to be in coma. At the deepest levels of coma the patient will be totally unresponsive to any stimulus.

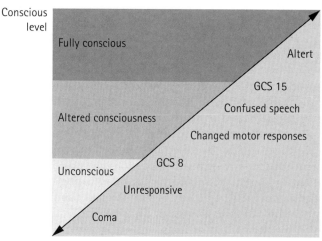

Figure 16.1 Consciousness is a scale

MANAGEMENT OF THE UNCONSCIOUS PATIENT

The initial assessment of the unconscious patient should follow the standard system of the ABC.

APPROACH TO THE PATIENT

The first priority is to ensure safety before approaching the patient. The victim of an assault may still be surrounded by assailants who present a danger to the paramedic. There may be other potential risks such as noxious fumes or smoke and invisible dangers such as carbon monoxide. An approach to the patient should only be made when it is clear that there is no risk.

> Use the SAFE approach
>
> SHOUT for help (when necessary)
> APPROACH with care
> FREE from danger
> EVALUATE the ABCs

ASSESSMENT

Response

The next stage is to see if the patient is conscious. Questions such as *"Can you hear me?"* should be used and the patient's shoulders gently rocked whilst the forehead is stabilized to see if the patient is rousable (it is important to be wary of rocking if the patient is a victim of trauma). If the patient responds by speaking, then there is no immediate airway problem. If there is no verbal response, the next step is to check the airway.

Airway

The unconscious patient is at risk of airway obstruction from the tongue falling back into the oropharynx. A patient with a partially obstructed airway will make grunting or snoring noises in an effort to overcome the obstruction. The patient may also have lost normal protective reflexes and may aspirate food or vomit into the lungs, so it is vital to make sure that there is no debris in the upper airway. This should be sought by direct inspection, looking into the mouth and removing any obvious foreign body. If vomit or blood is present, it should be aspirated, using a portable suction device. The airway is then opened using the head tilt or chin lift manoeuvres as described in Chapter 5, but avoiding head tilt in patients who are known to be victims of trauma. If the airway cannot be maintained with simple manoeuvres it may be necessary to introduce a correctly sized oropharyngeal (Guedel) or nasopharyngeal airway (Chapter 6). It is important to be careful if inserting an oral airway into a patient who is only lightly unconscious: it may promote gagging and vomiting.

Once the airway has been opened, cleared and secured, it is time to move on to assess the patient's breathing. If there is any suspicion that the patient may have been a victim of trauma, the neck is immobilized in a rigid cervical collar whilst the airway is being assessed.

Breathing

The first stage in the breathing assessment is to look, listen and feel for signs of breathing. The respiratory rate may be very slow if the patient has taken an overdose of an opiate. Abnormal breathing patterns are seen in some patients with head injuries. If the patient is breathing, supplemental oxygen should be administered via a face mask as soon as possible. After assessment of breathing, the next step is to assess the circulation.

> Always give high-concentration oxygen

Circulation

The next stage is to check that the patient has a pulse. If both spontaneous breathing and the pulse are absent, it will be necessary to proceed with cardiopulmonary resuscitation. If the patient is not breathing but has a pulse, ventilation using a bag and mask will be needed.

If the patient has a pulse, the blood pressure should be measured and an intravenous cannula inserted (unless there is time-critical trauma in which case this should be done en route).

Diabetes and disability

If there is any evidence that the patient may be a diabetic suffering from hypoglycaemia, intravenous glucose should be given. It is important to look for a diabetic warning bracelet or insulin syringes in the patient's pocket. A finger-prick blood sample (or blood from the cannula) is tested for glucose with a reagent strip. A result of 3.0 mmol/l or below supports the diagnosis of hypoglycaemia, but the patient should be treated even if the result is normal and there is a strong suspicion of the diagnosis as the tests can be inaccurate at very low and very high values.

The next stage is to perform the rapid neurological checks – AVPU (see Chapter 2) and assessment of pupillary responses. If both pupils are constricted (like pinpoints) the diagnosis of opiate overdose is a possibility. Other signs of opiate overdose are needle marks from previous injections (Figure 16.2) and slow, shallow respiration. If local protocols allow the use of naloxone (Narcan), then 0.4–10 mg should be given intravenously and the patient observed for a response. Otherwise, the patient's airway must be protected, respiration supported as necessary with a bag and mask and the patient transported as quickly as possible to hospital.

Further information

Whilst the patient's condition is being stabilized, it is essential to try to obtain more information about the collapse. The unconscious patient will be unable to offer any history, so any details obtained from relatives and witnesses may be

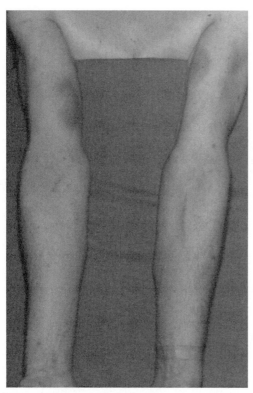

Figure 16.2 Needle marks in an intravenous drug user

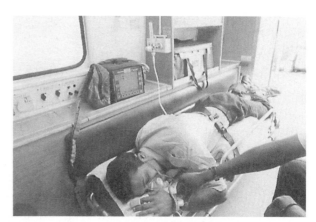

Figure 16.3 Transporting a patient in the recovery position

crucial. Important questions to ask can be remembered using the mnemonic AMPLE:

> **A**llergies
> **M**edication
> **P**ast illnesses
> **L**ast ate
> **E**vent

The patient may have suffered an allergic reaction and collapsed with anaphylactic shock; a relative may be aware of an allergic history or the patient may be wearing a warning bracelet or carrying a treatment pack of injectable adrenaline.

Knowledge of the patient's medication may indicate a likely cause of the collapse. It is vital to ask about the use of recreational drugs and alcohol. Medicines may be found near the patient or in a pocket. Relatives should be asked if the patient has had any previous episodes of collapse or serious illness.

It is important to know when the patient last ate. Someone who has recently had a meal presents a much higher risk of aspiration of food into the airway.

Questions such as *"Please describe exactly what happened"*, *"Did the patient collapse suddenly?"* or *"Was he assaulted?"* will aid in the gathering of information. However, the collection of this information should not delay transport of the patient

to hospital. The definitive diagnosis of the cause of collapse will in many cases not be made until the patient has had extensive further investigation in hospital. The unconscious patient who is breathing, has a pulse and is not a victim of trauma should be transferred to hospital in the recovery position in order to protect the airway (Figure 16.3). Alternatively the patient can be managed on his back as long as suction is available and the patient can be put into the recovery position immediately if it is required. The unconscious trauma victim patient should be immobilized on a long spinal board with a rigid collar.

> **Suction must be immediately available in case of vomiting**

During transport the patient's condition should be reevaluated. Routine observations and neurological checks should be regularly repeated. If there is time, further neurological checks (Glasgow Coma Scale and lateralizing neurological signs, see Chapter 2) should be performed and the patient's temperature can be taken. A limited secondary survey may help to determine the cause of the collapse. Signs to look for include:

- "raccoon eyes" (base of skull fracture – Battle's sign is usually late)
- a bitten tongue and urinary incontinence (epileptic fit)
- pyrexia and rash (meningococcal septicaemia).

> **Always go back to A then B then C ...**

If any of the patient's routine observations change, the airway, breathing and circulation must be reassessed and any problems which are identified treated as necessary. Deterioration in the neurological status (decreasing AVPU score, decreasing Glasgow Coma Score or development of lateralizing signs) is ominous: the patient MUST reach the definitive care centre as soon as possible.

The management of the unconscious patient is summarized in Figure 16.4.

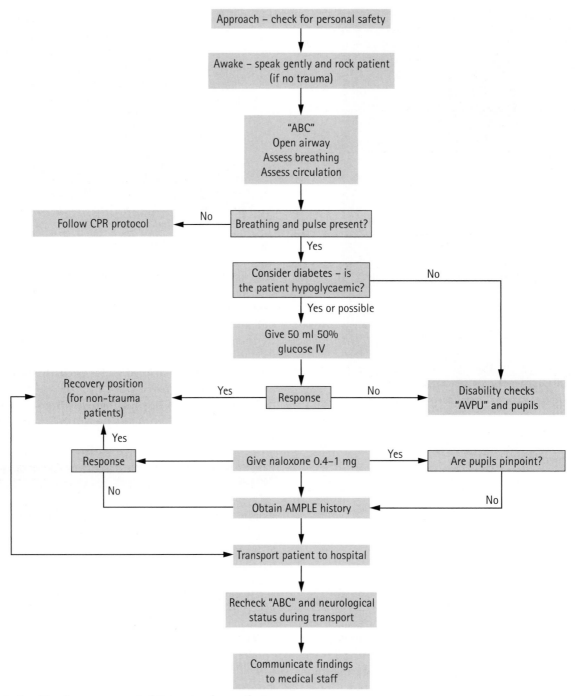

Figure 16.4 Algorithm for management of the unconscious patient

ASSESSMENT OF NEUROLOGICAL STATUS IN THE UNCONSCIOUS PATIENT

The assessment of the airway, breathing and circulation should always take priority. After A, B and C, the next step is assessment of disability, D, the preliminary examination of the patient's neurological status. This is an important part of clinical assessment and allows the determination of the patient's conscious level. The more deeply unconscious the patient, the more he is at risk from the environment. The assessment may indicate possible causes of the unconscious state and serves as a baseline so that progress of the patient's condition can be monitored.

There are two neurological checks that should be performed when assessing disability: assessment of conscious level and of the pupillary reactions. These checks should be repeated regularly to look for any changes in the patient's neurological state.

CONSCIOUS LEVEL

Conscious patients are alert and aware of their surroundings. As the level of consciousness falls, individuals may respond to vocal stimuli and then only to painful stimuli. Finally they may be totally unresponsive. The first letter of each of these responses spells the mnemonic AVPU, used to describe a simple tool to assess conscious level.

> **A**lert
> Responds to **V**ocal stimuli
> Responds to **P**ainful stimuli
> **U**nresponsive

On initial assessment, the patient who is awake, knows his name and is aware of the surroundings scores "A". This is usually noted down in this format:

> A V P U

The next step is to talk to a patient who does not speak spontaneously. A response by speech or movement scores "V". If there is no response, a painful stimulus is applied. The best stimulus to use is pressure over the supraorbital ridge, above one of the eyes (see Figure 16.5). A response to this stimulus scores "P", no response scores "U". Using a painful stimulus below the neck (for example, a "sternal rub") runs the small risk of a patient failing to respond in the trauma scenario because of sensory loss due to a spinal injury.

The assessment must be repeated regularly. A change in conscious level is the most important single sign in the assessment of the unconscious patient with a head injury.

PUPILLARY RESPONSES

The state of the pupils can provide important information which may help to determine the cause of collapse. Causes of pupillary changes are noted in Table 16.1. Bilateral pinpoint pupils are a particularly valuable sign, since they virtually always indicate opiate overdosage (although a brainstem stroke can produce the same appearance). Bilateral dilated pupils are less helpful because there are many potential causes. It must be remembered that patients with fixed dilated pupils are not necessarily dead and this sign is not an indication to terminate cardiopulmonary resuscitation. Pupils of different sizes may be highly significant. A person with a head injury, for example a subdural or extradural haematoma (see Chapter 23), may initially have normal pupils. As the haematoma expands, pressure increases inside the head and presses on one of the third cranial nerves, which will cause the pupil *on that side* to dilate. As intracranial

---

Box 16.1 Basic neurological checks

- Conscious level
- Pupillary responses

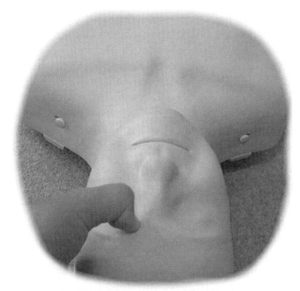

Supra orbital pressure

Figure 16.5 Applying a painful stimulus (pressure on the supraorbital nerve)

Table 16.1 Pupillary changes and possible diagnosis (Adult)

Pupillary signs	Possible diagnosis
Bilaterally fixed and dilated	Death; hypovolaemic shock; drugs such as atropine, adrenaline and Ecstasy
Unilaterally fixed and dilated	Head injury; stroke
Bilateral pinpoint constriction	Opiate overdose
Bilateral constriction	Brainstem stroke
Irregular pupil	Trauma; previous eye operation

Box 16.2 Pupillary assessment

- Size
- Shape
- Comparison with other pupil
- Reaction to light

Box 16.3 Further neurological checks

- Glasgow Coma Scale
- Focal neurological deficit

pressure increases further, the third nerve on the opposite side will be affected and the other pupil will dilate.

To assess the pupils, the first step is to gently open the eyelid. Signs of local trauma such as haemorrhage under the conjunctiva may be present. The pupillary size and shape should be noted (an irregular pupil may indicate local trauma or previous surgery to the eye). The two pupils should be compared to see if they appear the same and a light shone in each eye in turn to see if the pupils show the normal reflex constriction.

The most important sign of deterioration in neurological status is a change in the clinical signs. This can only be determined if the conscious level and the pupillary signs are repeatedly checked.

FURTHER NEUROLOGICAL EXAMINATION

An important priority with the unconscious patient is early transfer to hospital for further assessment and management. A more extensive neurological evaluation can usually be deferred until the patient has arrived at the receiving medical facility. However, if there is time during transport, two other useful neurological checks can be performed: a more detailed assessment of the conscious level of the patient using the Glasgow Coma Scale, and a brief neurological examination to determine if the patient has any areas of localized weakness or paralysis (focal neurological deficit).

GLASGOW COMA SCALE

The Glasgow Coma Scale uses three areas of patient response to determine a score that indicates coma level: these are *eye opening, speech* and *best motor response*. Eye opening is scored from 1 to 4, speech from 1 to 5 and best motor response from 1 to 6. The highest score (the alert patient) is therefore 15 and the lowest (in deep coma or dead) is 3. The scoring system is shown in Table 16.2. "Coma" is officially recognized as a score of 8 or less.

The components of the system can be incorporated into the ambulance service initial assessment sheet (report form) as an aid to remembering the individual scores. A patient in "coma" will give no verbal responses (scores 1), the eyes will remain closed (scores 1) and the patient will at best localize to pain (scores 5) – that is, a maximum score of 7. The best response is recorded if it differs between the two sides.

When assessing the ability to obey commands in a trauma setting, it is essential that the requested task is not rendered impossible by the patient's other injuries: *"Put your left hand on your head"* is not appropriate if the patient has a compound forearm fracture of the left arm.

A painful stimulus is best applied by pressure over the supraorbital nerve (Figure 16.5).

> The patient's numerical result on the Glasgow Coma *Scale* is their Glasgow Coma *Score*

Table 16.2 The Glasgow Coma Scale

Component	Response	Score
Best motor response	Obeys commands	6
	Localizes to pain[a]	5
	Withdraws from pain[b]	4
	Flexor response to pain[c]	3
	Extensor response to pain[d]	2
	No motor response to pain	1
Best verbal response	Oriented	5
	Confused conversation[e]	4
	Inappropriate speech[f]	3
	Incomprehensible speech[g]	2
	No speech	1
Eye opening	Spontaneous	4
	In response to speech	3
	In response to pain	2
	No eye opening	1

[a]Moves hand towards pain; [b]moves away from pain; [c]bends arm at elbow and wrist in response to a painful stimulus; [d]straightens at elbow and knee in response to a painful stimulus; [e]disorientated in time, person and place; [f]inappropriate response to question; [g]moans and groans.

FOCAL NEUROLOGICAL DEFICIT

A full neurological assessment is inappropriate in the prehospital care of the unconscious patient. However, useful information can be obtained by close observation. On close examination of the face, note should be made of a drooping of the smile on one side, indicating a facial paralysis (Figure 16.6), common in patients who have had a cerebrovascular accident (stroke).

After a painful stimulus, movement of the patient's limbs should be observed and may reveal paralysis in one or more of the limbs. Weakness and paralysis are signs of focal neurological deficit and should be recorded and communicated to the receiving doctor at the medical facility.

COMMON CAUSES OF COMA

The causes of collapse can be remembered with the mnemonic CID, CID (think of who investigates – the CID). The two Cs stand for *Cerebral causes* (such as cerebrovascular accident, subarachnoid haemorrhage and epilepsy) and *Cardiac causes* (including the simple faint, myocardial infarction and cardiac arrhythmias). The Is stand for *Injury* to the head and major trauma elsewhere and for *Infection* (for example, meningitis). The Ds refer to *Diabetes* and other

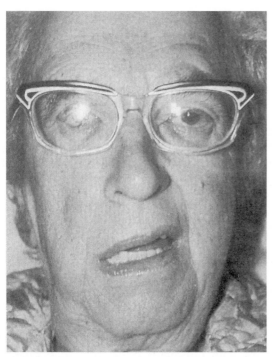

Figure 16.6 Facial signs following a cerebrovascular accident

metabolic emergencies and to *Drugs*, poisons and alcohol. A final rare cause of unconsciousness that can be added to this mnemonic is *Failure* – both of organs (such as respiratory, cardiac or renal failure) and failure to maintain normal body temperature. If CID will not give the answer, think of failure.

> Cerebral
> Injury to the head
> Diabetes and metabolic
>
> Cardiac
> Infection
> Drugs, poisons and alcohol
>
> Failure of organs

CID   CID   F

CEREBRAL CAUSES OF UNCONSCIOUSNESS

The most common cerebral causes of unconsciousness are epilepsy, cerebrovascular accident (stroke) and subarachnoid haemorrhage. Head injury and meningitis are considered later in the chapter.

Cerebrovascular accident

Cerebrovascular accidents (CVAs) or strokes have two basic causes. They may result from haemorrhage from a cerebral blood vessel – a *haemorrhagic stroke* – or from blockage of the blood supply to part of the brain – a *cerebral infarction*.

> **Box 16.4 Cerebral causes of Unconsciousness**
>
> * Epilepsy
> * Cerebrovascular accident
> * Subarachnoid haemorrhage

A blood vessel can become blocked by atheroma (fat deposits that build up on the vessel wall with increasing age) or by an embolus (a clot of blood or other material that has come from another part of the body, often the heart or neck, and lodged in the brain).

The two types of stroke cannot be distinguished clinically and present with the same features. The patient's conscious level may be decreased and there will be localizing neurological signs, such as paralysis on one side, facial asymmetry and dysarthria (difficulty articulating speech). If the features are transient and resolve completely over the space of several hours then the episode is known as a *transient ischaemic attack* (TIA). TIAs are often precursors of full-blown strokes.

Little treatment is available at present for people who have cerebrovascular accidents. Close attention should be paid to ABCs to ensure that the airway is protected and the patient is well oxygenated. A cannula should be sited so that emergency drugs can be given. The patient should then be transferred to hospital so that a definitive diagnosis can be made and treatment started.

> The term "right–sided stroke" implies right-sided weakness:
> A "right–sided CVA", however, implies involvement of the
> right side of the brain and hence *left-sided* weakness

Subarachnoid haemorrhage

Subarachnoid haemorrhage is a bleed into the fluid that surrounds the brain. It is usually caused by the sudden bursting of a small swelling (an aneurysm) of a cerebral vessel. The results of the haemorrhage can be rapidly fatal. The condition affects all ages and may be precipitated by a sudden rise in blood pressure.

The characteristic history is of a patient who develops a sudden headache (often described as "like being hit on the back of the head with a hammer") and who then collapses. Subarachnoid haemorrhage may occur during sexual intercourse. The patient may develop focal neurological signs and convulse. The airway should be secured, ventilation assisted as necessary, a cannula sited and rapid transfer arranged to the nearest hospital with emergency facilities.

Epilepsy

Epilepsy is a condition of abnormal brain activity which presents with convulsions or "fits". Any associated decrease in conscious level is transitory, although full recovery may take several hours or even longer. The most common type of epilepsy is "grand mal" epilepsy. The patient may present in one of three phases. A paramedic should be able to recognize these phases and be able to treat the patient appropriately.

Initially the patient collapses and the whole body contracts – the *tonic phase*; this usually lasts for a period of up to 30 seconds. There then follows a period of generalized contractions and relaxations, the *tonic-clonic phase* (the "fit"), the duration of which can be very variable. If the tonic-clonic phase continues for more than 15 minutes the patient is said to be in *status epilepticus*. Finally, the convulsion stops and consciousness slowly returns: this is the *postictal phase*. The patient may at first be confused before gradually returning to full awareness.

If the patient is still convulsing, the first task is to ensure that he comes to no further harm. A bite guard may be inserted into the mouth to prevent damage to the lips and tongue but this is rarely possible and under no circumstances should the mouth be forcibly opened. An oxygen mask should be placed on or near the face of the patient. If the convulsion shows no sign of ceasing give diazepam 10–20 mg IV and transport, the patient rapidly to the nearest available hospital with resuscitation facilities. Care should be taken to ensure that the individual is protected from self-injury during the ambulance journey. The patient's blood glucose level must be checked with a reagent strip to exclude hypoglycaemia as the underlying cause of the fitting (see below).

Most diagnostic difficulty is encountered when a patient is found in the postictal state. An epilepsy warning bracelet may be worn or antiepileptic medication found in the patient's pocket. Witnesses should be asked for a description of the event. The recovering patient should be examined for signs of a bitten tongue or urinary incontinence. The patient who is immediately alert after an episode of collapse is unlikely to have had a grand mal fit.

Neurological abnormalities (for example, unequal pupils or focal weakness) may not be of significance after a fit and can only be properly assessed once the patient has fully recovered, when many such abnormalities will have resolved.

Other forms of epilepsy may occasionally be seen. The patient with temporal lobe epilepsy often experiences a warning "aura" prior to the fit. This may take the form of an unusual smell or taste. Focal fits occur when only one area of the body is involved. Some forms of epilepsy can be triggered by flashing lights or repetitive patterns. "Petit mal" fits are otherwise known as "absence" attacks, because the patients appear not to be listening and are unaware of their surroundings for a short time. There is no tonic or tonic-clonic phase. These types of epilepsy are commoner in the younger patient and may disappear with age. It is extremely unlikely that paramedical assistance will be requested for a patient having a petit mal seizure.

INJURY

Head injury

The diagnosis of head injury should not be overlooked, particularly in the drunk or intoxicated patient. Signs of trauma such as a head wound or palpable depressed fracture may be present. Other, more subtle signs that indicate a base of skull fracture are bruising around both eyes ("raccoon eyes"), bruising over the mastoid process (Battle's sign, which usually takes a number of hours to develop) and blood or cerebrospinal fluid leaking from an ear. However, the patient with a head injury may have no external signs at all.

Patients with more severe head injuries may have areas of haemorrhage inside the skull. An extradural haemorrhage occurs when blood leaks out of a ruptured artery outside the covering of the brain (the *dura mater*). Characteristically this occurs with trauma to the temporoparietal region and damage to the middle meningeal artery. Initially, the patient may fall unconscious but then recover for a short time. As the bleed enlarges the patient becomes unconscious again and may then develop localizing neurological signs. Unless the blood is evacuated urgently the patient is likely to suffer permanent disability or death.

A bleed inside the dura mater but surrounding the brain is known as a subdural haemorrhage. This usually results from bleeding from ruptured small veins and can develop suddenly or gradually. A subdural haemorrhage is associated with more extensive injury to the brain (and a worse prognosis) than an extradural haemorrhage. Subdural haemorrhages are common in alcoholic patients who have impaired blood clotting and who suffer frequent head injuries (Figure 16.7).

Trauma can also occur to the brain tissue itself. If blood leaks into the brain tissue it is known as an intracerebral haemorrhage. If it extends into the fluid surrounding the brain it can be described as a traumatic subarachnoid haemorrhage. Sometimes the brain swells without any bleeding, with resultant damage to the brain cells.

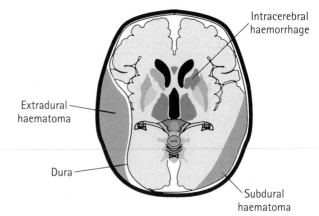

Figure 16.7 The anatomy of intracranial bleeding

None of these diagnoses can be confirmed before hospital admission. Attention should be aimed at ensuring that A, B and C are fully assessed and treated. Of particular importance is the patient's breathing: the underventilated patient retains carbon dioxide, which dilates the cerebral blood vessels and results in a rise in the intracranial pressure.

When adequate ventilation has been achieved and any other immediately life-threatening problems recognized and dealt with where possible, the patient should be transported to the nearest unit capable of offering definitive neurological care. This should be a hospital that offers diagnostic CT scanning and access to neurosurgical facilities.

Injury elsewhere

Cellular hypoxia of the brain will result in unconsciousness. Hypoxia can be caused by obstruction of the airway, breathing difficulty (for example, a tension pneumothorax) or mechanical obstruction from cardiac tamponade or from fluid loss (the human body requires 50% of its normal circulating blood volume to be able to maintain consciousness). The treatment of hypoxia and hypovolaemia during the initial assessment using the ABC method is therefore vital in the management of the unconscious trauma victim.

> It is essential not to assume that coma is due to a head injury and so neglect management of the airway, breathing and circulation

Any immediately life-threatening injury should be assessed and where possible treated, the patient's cervical spine stabilized and the patient transported to the nearest available centre capable of treating major trauma.

C I Ⓓ CID F

DIABETES AND OTHER METABOLIC EMERGENCIES

Hypoglycaemia

A low blood glucose level is one of the most common causes of coma found in the community. It is seen most often in diabetic patients who have taken too much insulin in relation to their food intake and activity level. However, it can occasionally also occur in non-diabetic patients. People who are chronic alcoholics have very low sugar stores and may develop acute hypoglycaemia after a bout of drinking. A patient debilitated by malignancy or chronic liver disease may be similarly affected.

The features of hypoglycaemia develop rapidly, usually over a period of a few minutes. The first symptoms may be of dizziness and light-headedness. Profuse sweating often occurs. As the condition worsens changes of behaviour are seen. The patient may become confused and aggressive and appear as if drunk. Weakness and incoordination develop. With further progression the patient's level of response will reduce and the patient is likely to be cold and clammy. Unless treatment is given rapidly, convulsions will ensue, with potential secondary brain damage.

Hyperglycaemia

A very high blood glucose level can also result in loss of consciousness. This can occur in patients who are developing diabetes or in those in whom the established condition is out of control, for instance if they have a coincidental infection. This is known as diabetic ketoacidosis. The patient may have complained of thirst, weight loss and passing large amounts of urine prior to his collapse. On examination the patient will look dehydrated, with dry skin and sunken eyes. It may be possible to detect a sweet smell of ketones on his breath (not everyone can smell ketones). These patients may also have a characteristic respiratory pattern with deep, sighing breaths, known as Kussmaul's respiration.

If the diagnosis of diabetic ketoacidosis is suspected, a quick assessment of ABC and transfer of the patient to hospital is appropriate giving 250–2000 ml of normal saline IV en route to facilitate rehydration. A glucose testing strip will read high. If a diabetic patient has collapsed and it is unclear whether the cause is hypo- or hyperglycaemia then *hypoglycaemia* should be assumed and the patient should be given glucose. Untreated hypoglycaemia can kill, whilst hyperglycaemia will not worsen significantly with a single injection of intravenous glucose.

Other metabolic emergencies

Other metabolic emergencies are rare and difficult to diagnose out of hospital. Addison's disease is a failure of the patient's adrenal gland, responsible for secreting the body's natural steroids. This results in an electrolyte imbalance, a low blood pressure and collapse. Patients who have been on high doses of steroids that are suddenly stopped can develop a similar condition. Hypotension is treated with a normal saline fluid infusion and transfer of the patient to the nearest emergency department.

CID Ⓒ I D F

CARDIAC CAUSES OF UNCONSCIOUSNESS

Cardiac arrhythmias

Major cardiac arrhythmias such as ventricular fibrillation result in collapse and should be treated using the cardiac arrest protocols (see Chapter 14). Non-arrest arrhythmias may only cause transitory upset in cardiac output and result in a brief loss of consciousness. The most common of these episodes are known as Stokes–Adams attacks, when a patient (who is usually elderly) has a short run of a haemodynamically compromising arrhythmia. Patients have no warning symptoms of the collapse and recover quickly. They may report previous similar episodes. On examination, the presence of any irregularity of the cardiac rhythm or slowness of the pulse rate should be noted. A cannula should be inserted and the patient transported to hospital (with ECG monitoring) for cardiological investigation.

Simple faint

The simple faint or syncope is characterized by a sudden transient loss of consciousness. It is caused by a temporary decrease of blood flow to the brain. This may be precipitated by a number of factors: emotional triggers include fright, sexual desire and the sight of blood; physical triggers such as pain, drugs (such as glyceryl trinitrate), standing up too quickly or for prolonged periods (especially in hot weather) and anaemia may also be responsible.

The patient should be laid flat with the feet raised or in a head-down position. If he does not recover rapidly, an alternative diagnosis should be suspected. When the patient awakens, he should be asked about any possible precipitating causes of the faint. If there is any suspicion that there may be underlying disease, if the patient does not recover fully or if there is concern about his safety alone at home, he should be taken to hospital for further investigation.

CID   C①D F

INFECTION

Infection is a rare but serious cause of collapse. It is most commonly encountered in the young child who develops meningococcal septicaemia. The child rapidly becomes unwell with a high fever. There may be the symptoms of meningitis with a stiff neck and photophobia (light hurting the eyes) before the collapse, but the septicaemia can occur without meningitis. On examination, the characteristic non-blanching purpuric rash which resembles widespread bruising should be sought (Figure 16.8). These children should be administered benzyl penicillin without delay and transported to hospital as rapidly as possible. Any delay in giving them antibiotics can be fatal (from onset of symptoms to death is often less than a day and sometimes only a matter of a few hours).

Other infections of the brain such as encephalitis (infection of the tissues of the brain) and, very rarely, cerebral abscess can also cause collapse. These patients are likely to exhibit abnormal neurological signs.

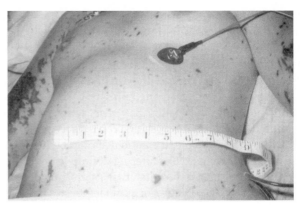

Figure 16.8 The rash of meningococcal septicaemia

Overwhelming septicaemia, whatever the organism, may cause unconsciousness. The diagnosis should be considered in an unconscious patient who is tachycardic with a low blood pressure and no signs of blood loss. Intravenous fluids should be started and the patient transferred to hospital as soon as possible.

CID   CI ⑩   F

DRUGS, ALCOHOL AND POISONS

Alcohol

Alcohol is the great deceiver when assessing the unconscious patient. A drunk patient is not necessarily unconscious because of the alcohol; the cause may be a head injury, hypoglycaemia or an overdose. Furthermore, the drunkard has the same risk (if not a greater risk) of respiratory obstruction and of aspiration of fluid and food into the lungs as any other unconscious patient.

> When a drunk patient is unconscious
> THINK:
>   HEAD INJURY
>   HYPOGLYCAEMIA
>
> ONLY THEN THINK:
>   ALCOHOL
> as the cause of the loss of consciousness

When attending a collapsed drunk it is essential to remember to check the blood glucose level with a reagent strip. Hypoglycaemia may be present and should be treated with intravenous glucose. The patient should be transported to hospital for further assessment to exclude other pathological conditions and in order to monitor recovery. It is important to be wary of leaving an apparently drunk patient in police custody when other possible causes of decreased consciousness have not been excluded.

Opiate poisoning

Intravenous drug abuse with opiate drugs such as morphine, diamorphine (heroin) and pethidine is an increasing problem. Opiates are also contained in tablets such as co-proxamol (Distalgesic) and may be taken in overdose. The features of opiate overdose are pinpoint pupils, respiratory depression and coma. The diagnosis should be suspected in any collapsed patient who has pinpoint pupils.

Management should follow the ABC routine. If opiate overdose is suspected, the opiate antagonist naloxone (Narcan) should be considered but if the patient is breathing adequately, reversal is usually best delayed until after arrival in hospital. Prehospital reversal may result in the newly awake patient absconding, only to collapse again elsewhere. Naloxone reverses all the side-effects of the opiate, in particular the respiratory depression and the coma. However, it is short-acting, with a half-life of about 40 minutes. All patients with overdose must therefore be transported to hospital for further assessment and observation. Naloxone is given intravenously in a dose of 0.4–10 mg. Response to the drug is rapid, with wakening within a minute. If intravenous access is not possible, naloxone can be given intramuscularly. If naloxone is not available, the patient should be transported to hospital as quickly as possible while respiration is assisted as necessary.

Other drugs that can cause coma

The next most common group of drugs causing coma is the antidepressants, particularly tricyclic antidepressants such as amitriptyline and mianserin. Signs that may indicate tricyclic overdose include dilated pupils, convulsions and respiratory depression. These overdoses can also cause severe cardiac arrhythmias. The patient's cardiac rhythm must be monitored during transport to hospital.

The benzodiazepines are a group of drugs that are used to relieve anxiety. They include such drugs as diazepam, temazepam and nitrazepam. When taken in overdose they can cause drowsiness, but only very rarely result in coma.

The complete list of drugs that can cause coma is long. Drugs are often taken in combination with alcohol. The effects of the drugs may then be additive. However, the principles of management remain the same: protect the airway, ensure good ventilation, stabilize the circulation and transport the patient to hospital.

A final agent that should be considered when thinking of poisoning as a cause of coma is the gas carbon monoxide. Poisoning can result from faulty gas fires and central heating boilers and major fires, as well as attempted suicides from car exhaust fumes. The toxic effects are due to hypoxia. The patient should be removed from the source of carbon monoxide and given high-concentration oxygen via a face mask. It is important to remember that carbon monoxide is odourless and invisible and may endanger the safety of rescuers.

CID   CID   (F)

FAILURE

Organ failure

The failure of major body organs can result in coma. Organ failure can be acute, for example the respiratory failure that occurs with a severe asthma attack, or chronic as in chronic obstructive pulmonary disease. Chronic organ failure is usually accompanied by other signs of disease which indicate the responsible organ. The patient who is suffering hepatic failure and is in coma is likely to be jaundiced, the patient in respiratory failure may be cyanosed, and the patient with cardiac failure will have a weak, thready pulse. Renal failure can be more difficult to diagnose clinically. Patients with severe renal disease usually have a sallow complexion or a dialysis fistula or abdominal CAPD catheter. AB and C should be stabilized as far as possible and the patient taken to the nearest appropriate hospital.

Failure to maintain body temperature

Hypothermia, a core body temperature of less than 35°C, can be a cause of or a result of coma. As body temperature falls, the conscious level deteriorates. At first, patients are listless and drowsy. The diagnosis should be suspected in the collapsed elderly patient or in anyone who has been unconscious for a long period or has been exposed to the environment (such as the entrapped trauma victim). The diagnosis is best confirmed with a low-reading rectal thermometer, but this should not be performed in the prehospital environment. No attempt should be made to intubate these patients unless it is absolutely necessary as fatal cardiac arrhythmias can be provoked. Any wet clothes must be removed and the patient wrapped in warm blankets and transported to the nearest hospital.

CONCLUSION

There are many possible causes of unconsciousness, but the vast majority of patients will have sustained trauma or be suffering from one of a relatively small range of common conditions. In all cases, the approach is the same: scrupulous attention to airway, breathing and circulation and a systematic attempt to identify the cause of the problem. Although it may not always be possible to identify a cause, management of ABC and rapid transfer to hospital will always be appropriate and in many cases there *will* be evidence suggesting the likely diagnosis. Some of these causes will respond rapidly to simple treatment, others will require further investigation and treatment in hospital.

Chapter 17

The acute abdomen

CHAPTER CONTENTS

INTRODUCTION

Abdominal emergencies usually present with acute abdominal pain in association with other symptoms and signs. The causes range from life-threatening conditions that require immediate resuscitation and laparotomy to those that require more conservative management.

Even in a hospital with ample facilities it can be difficult to assess and diagnose an abdominal emergency. It is therefore particularly difficult to carry out this task in the prehospital environment. Consequently the paramedic should concentrate instead on assessing the severity of the patient's condition and on managing it appropriately. In particular it is important to detect patients who require immediate resuscitation and urgent transfer.

This chapter discusses the essential parts of the medical history and examination that will enable the paramedic to assess the severity of the patient's condition. In doing this it is important that the clinically relevant aspects of abdominal anatomy are understood.

APPLIED ANATOMY

BOUNDARIES

The abdomen is a bony and muscular cavity supported by the lumbar and sacral elements of the spine and the pelvis.

The back wall is a semi-rigid structure, consisting of the spine and paraspinal muscles. In contrast, the flanks and anterior abdominal wall are formed by deformable layers of muscles and sheet-like fibres; these musculotendinous layers are hung from the costal margins of the thoracic cage above and are attached to the bones and ligaments of the upper aspect of the pelvic girdle below (Figure 17.1).

The abdomen's internal boundaries are defined by two other sheets of muscle. The diaphragm divides the upper abdomen from the thoracic cavity. As this major muscle of respiration moves down with inspiration, it alters the relationship of the thoracic and abdominal contents. The lower boundary is formed by the more rigid pelvic floor muscles. These separate the abdomen from the buttocks, the perineum and the genital areas of the external pelvis. However, this lower boundary does allow access of the femoral vessels and nerves anteriorly into the bulk of the thigh muscles. The former represent the main blood supply and drainage of the lower limbs.

PERITONEUM

The internal aspect of the abdominal cavity is lined by a thick, double-layered sheet of peritoneum (Figure 17.2), which divides the abdominal organs into those that are inside the peritoneum (intraperitoneal) and those that are outside the peritoneum (retroperitoneal and extraperitoneal). The outermost layer (the parietal peritoneum) is

(a)

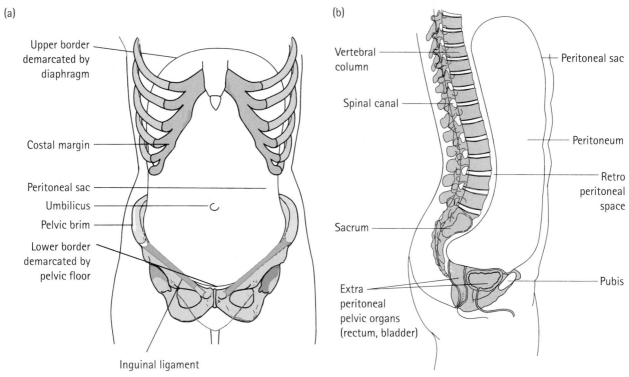

Upper border demarcated by diaphragm

Costal margin

Peritoneal sac

Umbilicus

Pelvic brim

Lower border demarcated by pelvic floor

Inguinal ligament

(b)

Vertebral column

Spinal canal

Sacrum

Extra peritoneal pelvic organs (rectum, bladder)

Peritoneal sac

Peritoneum

Retro peritoneal space

Pubis

Figure 17.1 The abdomen. (a) front view; (b) side view

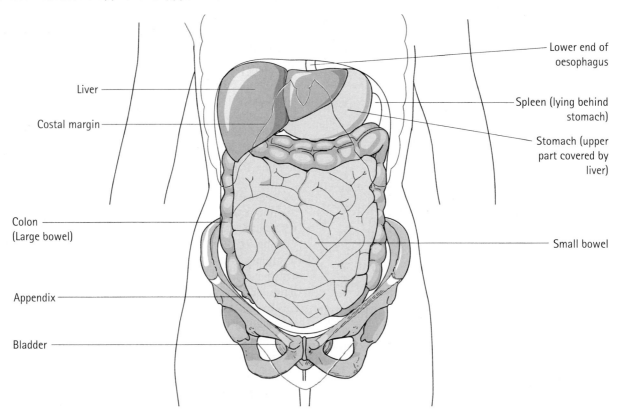

Liver

Costal margin

Colon (Large bowel)

Appendix

Bladder

Lower end of oesophagus

Spleen (lying behind stomach)

Stomach (upper part covered by liver)

Small bowel

Figure 17.2 Anatomy of the peritoneal cavity. The upper surface of the bladder forms a border of the peritoneal cavity

supplied by nerves which also supply the skin overlying that area of peritoneum, making it possible to localize accurately areas of injury and inflammation. In contrast, the internal layers (the visceral peritoneum) have a different nerve supply that does not allow precise localization of pathological problems. The peritoneal cavity is a potential space between the layers that normally contains small amounts of fluid and cells.

The layers of peritoneum covering the intraperitoneal structures provide not only structural support but also vascular and nervous access to and from the abdominal organs. The majority of the small bowel is intraperitoneal and is mobile. Consequently the blood supply of the small bowel may be interrupted if its mobile vessels are sheared from the immobile aorta as well as from the caval and portal venous systems.

The liver, spleen and stomach normally lie behind the protection of the lower ribs. Fractures of these ribs may therefore injure the underlying organs. During deep inspiration, they may be pushed into the more exposed areas of the abdomen by movement of the diaphragm. The liver and spleen have limited motion due to strong ligamentous attachments. Consequently, this may lead to shearing injuries occurring along the line of the attachments. Both liver and spleen are highly vascular organs and therefore injury may lead to life-threatening blood loss.

RETROPERITONEUM AND EXTRAPERITONEUM

Several structures lie behind the peritoneum (retroperitoneally) on the semi-rigid posterior abdominal wall and in the pelvis (see below). The pelvis forms a firm support for the major vessels and branches of the abdominal aorta and inferior vena cava (IVC) which are adherent to it. Distally the aorta and IVC supply both the pelvic contents and lower limbs via the internal and external iliac vessels respectively.

As the retroperitoneal structures have limited mobility they cannot move out of the way following penetrating injury. Consequently viscera such as the ascending and descending parts of the large bowel are more likely to be damaged following this mechanism of injury than the small bowel and transverse colon.

The duodenum lies coiled around the pancreas high up in the retroperitoneal space. These organs can therefore be damaged together following significant blunt trauma or penetrating injury. In either case the leakage of pancreatic and duodenal contents presents late because of the deep location of these structures within the abdomen.

The mobility of the kidneys and ureters is closely related to diaphragmatic movement during respiration. In general these organs are well protected by the lower ribs and lumbar musculature, but are prone to direct blunt trauma and shearing forces acting through its vascular connection with the aorta.

Box 17.1 Retroperitoneal structures

- Aorta
- Inferior vena cava
- Large bowel (ascending and descending parts)
- Duodenum
- Pancreas
- Kidneys and ureters

HERNIAS

The abdominal muscle layers are designed to allow structures to pass through at certain levels. Here, potential weaknesses occur through which abdominal contents may protrude. These *hernias* may cause discomfort or may lead to obstruction of the bowel or trapping of the omentum, which carries the blood supply to the bowel (Box 17.2).

> HERNIA: a protrusion of an organ or tissue out of the body cavity in which it normally lies

ASSESSMENT

When this knowledge of applied anatomy is combined with the important aspects of the medical history and examination (Box 17.3) a reliable assessment of the severity of the patient's condition can be made.

Pain

Pain is the major symptom of abdominal emergencies. It also has characteristics that can provide a clue to the underlying problem. It is important to ask the following questions.

- Where is the pain?
- What type of pain is it (i.e. inflammatory, colicky or ischaemic)?
- Does the pain move?
- What makes the pain better?
- What makes the pain worse?
- How long has the pain been present?
- How rapid was the onset of pain?
- Have you had this pain before? If so, what happened?

The nerve fibres of the outer peritoneal layer also supply the skin overlying that area of peritoneum. This enables any

---

Box 17.2 Types of hernia

- Inguinal
- Femoral
- Hiatus
- Epigastric
- Lumbar
- Incisional

Box 17.3 Important aspects of the medical history and examination

History	
Pain	Altered bowel habit
Vomiting	Examination
Bleeding	Shock
	Distension

Box 17.4 Signs of peritonitis

- Patient can localize the area of tenderness precisely (early)
- Coughing precipitates abdominal pain in the area of tenderness (early)
- There is rebound tenderness in the painful area (intermediate)
- No abdominal movement with expansion of the chest on inspiration (late)
- Generalized rigidity of the abdominal wall (very late)

---

pathological condition to be precisely located by the site of the pain the patient is experiencing or by eliciting tenderness and guarding by pressing on the inflamed area. If the pressing hand is suddenly withdrawn, the patient will experience an increase in pain as the stretched, inflamed peritoneum springs back into place. This is known as *rebound tenderness*. This local area of peritonitis gives rise to inflammatory pain that is usually throbbing and persistent but may also increase in intensity as the disease develops.

This type of pain can be eased by intravenous opiate analgesia. Before it is given, however, the patient will tend to lie still and be unwilling to move since movement aggravates the pain. Occasionally this can lead to splinting of the diaphragm and elimination of abdominal breathing. Toxins are released into the general circulation from the inflamed area and this leads to the patient becoming pyrexial. In extreme cases general peritonitis develops and there is involuntary spasm of the abdominal muscle with "board-like" rigidity of the abdominal wall.

The inner layer of peritoneum and its contents have nerve fibres that cannot localize injuries or inflammation precisely. Nevertheless, these deep nerves are particularly sensitive to stretching or spasm of tissue. This gives rise to colicky pain whereby the intensity of the discomfort increases and decreases intermittently. During these attacks of pain the patient is usually very restless in an attempt to find a position of comfort. This type of pain is also usually eased with intravenous opiate analgesics.

In contrast, ischaemic pain can be a mixture of both inflammatory and colicky pain and usually requires larger amounts of intravenous opiate analgesia. The important factor in this type of pain is the time from onset to restoration of normal blood flow, because this affects the degree of necrosis with consequent life-threatening or organ-dependent damage. Therefore if a condition giving rise to this pain is suspected (see below), urgent transfer to the emergency department is required and the staff must be warned of the patient's imminent arrival.

Some areas of the abdomen have a nerve supply that also supplies distant areas of skin. For example, the nerve supplying the diaphragm comes from an area of the spinal cord that also gives rise to the innervation of the skin overlying the ipsilateral shoulder. This conjoint nerve supply can lead to pain occurring at a site distant from its cause, a phenomenon

Table 17.1 Sites of referred pain from abdominal pathological conditions

Site of referred pain	Site of abdominal disease
Shoulder tip	Diaphragm
Retrosternal	Oesophagus and upper stomach
Epigastrium	Distal stomach to the second part of the duodenum
Periumbilical	Second part of the duodenum to the mid-transverse colon
Hypogastrium	Mid-transverse colon to the rectum
Left loin and back	Abdominal aortic aneurysm
Flank and genital pain	Ureter
Back	Pancreas
Back	Duodenum
Hip and knee	Pelvic organs

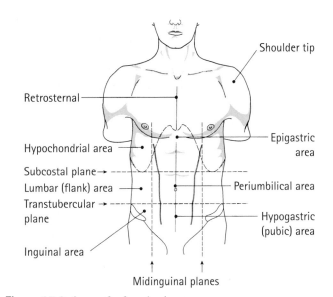

Figure 17.3 Areas of referred pain

known as *referred pain*. There are several examples specific to the abdomen (Table 17.1 and Figure 17.3).

Awareness of this phenomenon can help reduce the chances of making an incorrect diagnosis. In particular, retrosternal chest pain should not be automatically assumed to be due to a myocardial infarct or angina. Instead the paramedic must look for further clues in the patient's history or examination to support or disprove this conclusion.

If the intraperitoneal disorder develops it may eventually impinge on the outer peritoneal surface. To the patient, it seems that the pain has moved. A good example of this is seen when a patient develops appendicitis. Initially the intraperitoneal nerves are involved and pain is referred to the periumbilical area. Eventually, however, the inflamed appendix begins to irritate the overlying outer peritoneal surface. Consequently, as far as the patient is concerned, the pain has "moved" to the right iliac fossa.

Vomiting

Vomiting may accompany severe pain or be directly caused by the abdominal disease. It is a common presentation in most acute abdominal conditions.

Intestinal obstruction is one of the causes of vomiting, but the timing of its onset is dependent upon the site of the obstruction. Vomiting will present early with a proximal obstruction (e.g., in the oesophagus, stomach, duodenum and jejunum). Proximal obstruction can result in significant loss of water and electrolytes.

Vomiting blood indicates disease of the upper gastro-intestinal tract. Unaltered, bright red blood suggests an oesophageal lesion, whereas altered blood, resembling "coffee grounds", due to partial digestion, indicates a gastric or duodenal site.

Upper gastrointestinal bleeding can also give rise to *melaena*, altered blood being lost as sticky, black, "tarry" stools with a characteristic smell. In contrast, bleeding from the lower gastrointestinal tract is seen as altered blood if the lesion is in the proximal part of the large bowel (e.g. caecal or small bowel carcinoma) or as bright red blood if it lies more distally (e.g. haemorrhoids or rectal carcinoma).

Shock

Hypovolaemic shock associated with an abdominal emergency is indicative of severe acute disease or less severe disease with sustained haemorrhage or electrolyte loss.

Shock can also result from an uncontrolled release of digestive juices into the peritoneal cavity following pancreatitis or perforation of the stomach or duodenum. In addition, shock may be secondary to sepsis in fulminant peritonitis when it has reached a premorbid stage.

Altered bowel habit

Diarrhoea and constipation are two very common presentations with abdominal emergencies, but are not very specific for any abdominal disorder. Altered bowel habit is a characteristic sign of intestinal obstruction and the chances of it being an early sign are higher if the site of the obstruction is in the large bowel. These distal obstructions also allow greater retention of gas and fluid and are therefore associated with intestinal distension.

Abdominal distension

Abdominal distension is a common presentation that again is non-specific. However, when it is associated with severe, colicky abdominal pain, vomiting and absolute constipation

Box 17.5 Abdominal causes of hypovolaemic shock

- Acute gastrointestinal bleeding
- Ruptured abdominal aortic aneurysm
- Trauma leading to abdominal vessels or organs being torn or ruptured
- Intestinal obstruction
- Mesenteric infarction
- Continuous vomiting or diarrhoea without fluid replacement
- Ectopic pregnancy (ruptured)

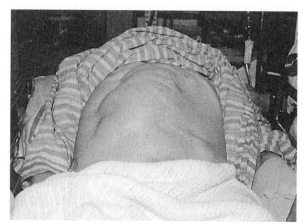

Figure 17.4 Intestinal obstruction secondary to intestinal adhesion from previous surgery. Loops of distended bowel and previous abdominal scars are seen

(i.e. failure to pass faeces, fluid or flatus) it is pathognomonic (absolutely diagnostic) of intestinal obstruction (Figure 17.4).

COMMON EXAMPLES OF ABDOMINAL EMERGENCIES

STOMACH AND PROXIMAL DUODENUM

Mild cases of gastritis and duodenitis lead to epigastric or retrosternal inflammatory pain and mild epigastric tenderness. This is frequently associated with nausea and haematemesis. Gastroenteritis presents as mild to severe, colicky abdominal pain which is poorly localized. It is commonly associated with vomiting, especially initially, and this may be followed, or replaced by, diarrhoea. Depending upon the duration of the disease, and its causative agent, this can lead to dehydration. The patient usually has a raised temperature and diffuse, mild abdominal tenderness. Guarding and rebound tenderness are uncommon findings.

Severe tenderness with localized signs of peritonitis (guarding and rigidity) suggests that the bowel may have perforated. If this is left untreated, the area of tenderness and pain increases as more of the gastric contents leak into the peritoneal cavity. Ultimately the patient will become shocked and critically ill and may die from overwhelming septic shock.

BILIARY TREE

Biliary tract obstruction presents initially as epigastric colicky pain and may be provoked by eating fatty meals. Nausea, vomiting and belching are also common associated features and occasionally the patient is jaundiced. Later, when the inflamed gallbladder touches the outer peritoneum, tenderness and inflammatory-type pain are localized to the right hypochondrium. This pain may radiate to or from the right shoulderblade on the back. Occasionally, when the inferior surface of the diaphragm is also involved in this inflammatory process, right shoulder tip pain occurs.

Secondary infection is common in the stagnant bile trapped in the biliary tree proximal to the obstruction. This increases the local inflammation and can give rise to pyrexia, tachycardia, tachypnoea and, in severe cases, rigors.

INTESTINES

Colic from small and large bowel obstruction is usually localized to the periumbilical and hypogastric regions respectively. The pain is not commonly related to any specific trigger and the patient may be comfortable between bouts, while remaining apprehensive about a subsequent spasm. As described previously, the frequency of vomiting and dehydration as an early associated feature increases with the more proximal location of the intestinal obstruction. Conversely, obstruction of the large bowel is associated with an early presentation of an altered bowel habit, including absolute constipation and later, abdominal distension. There may be passage of blood per rectum from an obstructing lesion.

APPENDICITIS

The initial presentation and the change in characteristics of the site of the pain in appendicitis have been described above. Appendicitis is usually associated with poor appetite, vomiting and a mild pyrexia. As with all inflammatory conditions, if it is left untreated the patient's condition will become more pyrexial and toxic as infection and necrosis develop.

PANCREAS

Patients with pancreatitis have epigastric tenderness and severe inflammatory pain. The latter gradually increases in intensity and may radiate into the back. There are many causes, but it is frequently associated with a history of either gallstones or the recent excessive intake of alcohol. In order to gain some relief, the patients will either sit and lean forward or lie curled up on their side. Nausea and vomiting are common. Severe cases are associated with dehydration and a major metabolic disturbance due to the release of pancreatic enzymes, resulting in the digestion of the pancreas itself. Bruising of the flanks and abdomen indicates a more fulminant presentation with internal haemorrhage.

KIDNEYS AND URETERS

Obstruction in the kidneys or ureters presents as ipsilateral colicky pain localized to the posterior aspect of the flank (renal angle). This is typical of renal and proximal ureteric obstruction. With a more distal ureteric location, however, pain may radiate anteriorly and distally from the flank to the ipsilateral iliac fossa and even into the testis or labia majora. Severe pain is commonly associated with vomiting. In addition, urinary symptoms of frequency and dysuria can accompany lower ureteric problems, especially when the obstruction lies near the junction with the bladder. Occasionally the ureteric obstruction is complete and permanent, enabling infection to develop proximally. In these serious cases pyrexia, rigors and other signs of sepsis can occur and can progress to a fulminant form of septic shock if the obstruction is not relieved quickly.

Pathological lesions at any site in the urinary tract can give rise to dark urine owing to the presence of blood in the urine. However, provided there is no torrential bleeding source, a good rule of thumb is the more red the blood looks, the more distally the lesion is located. Renal or ureteric colic associated with visible blood or clots is a common presentation of a renal tumour.

BLOOD VESSELS

Aortic aneurysm

Aortic aneurysms develop progressively with age and enlargement may be relatively painless until catastrophic haemorrhage occurs following rupture or dissection. Commonly an aneurysm presents as collapse, sweating and abdominal ischaemic pain. However, because of its retroperitoneal position, this pain can be referred to the back or even the left flank and consequently can be misinterpreted, with disastrous consequences. An abdominal pulsatile mass may be palpable but tenderness and the patient's respiratory and circulatory problems make this examination difficult. Occasionally there is vomiting, haematemesis, lower limb pain and neurological deficit. A brachiofemoral pulse delay or asymmetrical femoral pulses will indicate a dissection and may herald ischaemic problems for the intestines, kidneys, lower limbs and spinal cord.

Patients with aortic aneurysms giving rise to abdominal pain require an urgent operation. It is therefore essential that they are rapidly transferred to hospital and that time is not wasted attempting to insert intravenous lines. Indeed, overzealous fluid resuscitation may actually be detrimental, as the tamponade effect of any clot that forms at the site of rupture will be lost.

Mesenteric artery embolus

Mesenteric artery embolism has a sudden onset. Initially there is colicky abdominal pain, which after about an hour becomes unrelenting and poorly localized. With the exception of nausea and vomiting there may be very few signs and symptoms in the initial stages. The hallmark of this condition therefore is severe pain with very few signs on abdominal examination. Occasionally shock develops early on. With subsequent progression localized peritonitis and dehydration develop, the latter being due to impaired absorption, vomiting and fluid becoming trapped in the atonic bowel. Later, when the bowel wall becomes gangrenous and necrotic, generalized peritonitis and septic shock occur.

GENITAL TRACT

Pelvic inflammatory disease

Pelvic inflammatory disease is a blanket term used to cover inflammation of the female upper genital tract and the adjacent peritoneum and bowel. The patient invariably has bilateral inflammatory iliac fossa pain and tenderness. Usually there are also signs of infection such as pyrexia, tachycardia and occasionally rigors. In addition there is frequently a history of menstrual irregularities, abnormal vaginal discharge and dyspareunia (pain on sexual intercourse).

Ectopic pregnancy

Ectopic pregnancy occurs when a fertilized ovum becomes implanted outside the uterus. Usually the patient develops recurrent episodes of inflammatory lower abdominal pain, tenderness and guarding. This is associated with amenorrhoea, transient "fainting" feelings and irregular vaginal bleeding. Occasionally there is rupture of a fallopian tube and significant bleeding. This gives rise to severe inflammatory pain in the iliac fossa or hypogastrium, generalized tenderness and guarding, and syncope due to blood loss. Shoulder tip pain can occur when there is much free intraperitoneal blood and the patient has been lying with her head down. In these circumstances the free blood irritates the inferior surface of the diaphragm and gives rise to the referred shoulder pain described previously.

These patients require immediate resuscitation and urgent transfer to hospital so that haemostasis can be achieved surgically. This must not be delayed.

Ovarian cyst torsion

Ovarian cyst torsion presents as sudden onset of recurrent colicky pain in the ipsilateral iliac fossa. Nausea and vomiting are common associated features. In addition, the abdominal wall overlying the torsion is tender and may be rigid during the attacks.

Testicular torsion

Twisting of the testis on its cord causes intense ischaemic pain localized in the testis. Usually there is localized tenderness and vomiting (which may be the sole presenting feature), but no significant swelling. These patients require urgent surgery to salvage the testis and must be transferred immediately to hospital.

SUMMARY

Paramedics managing a patient with an abdominal emergency must concentrate on assessing the severity of the condition, carrying out appropriate treatment and transporting the patient safely to hospital. All immediately life-threatening conditions must be corrected first. If this is not possible, for example in cases of major haematemesis, then the patient must be rapidly transferred to hospital and the emergency department forewarned. Any further resuscitation can be provided in transit, but must not delay the patient's transfer.

If the immediately life-threatening conditions can be corrected, relevant aspects of the patient's history should be obtained and adequate intravenous analgesia provided. The abdomen can then be examined if the severity of the condition is still unclear. With these two elements completed the paramedic can transport the patient to hospital with the appropriate degree of urgency.

Chapter 18

Poisoning

CHAPTER CONTENTS

INTRODUCTION

Poisoning takes a variety of forms. Harmful substances may be ingested, inhaled or absorbed through the skin. The exposure to the poison may be accidental (as with most childhood poisonings) or deliberate as part of an attempted suicide or following "recreational" activities. The role of the paramedic is crucial in the management of poisonings in the community: without their detailed assessment of the situation and immediate management, the task of the emergency physician is difficult and occasionally futile.

GENERAL CONSIDERATIONS

The assessment of a patient with suspected poisoning is often difficult. The patient found unconscious with a suicide note and an empty bottle of pills poses no problem in diagnosis, but the information at the scene may not be that clear-cut. The patient may be just behaving oddly or have cardiovascular or respiratory problems. In deliberate ingestions, there may be a distinct unwillingness to volunteer any useful information. If there are no witnesses and the patient is unable to give a history, the diagnosis of poisoning becomes increasingly difficult. Fortunately, however, the majority of poisoned patients will require little in the early stages other than standard emergency care consisting of protection of the airway and support of breathing and circulation.

APPROACH TO THE POISONED PATIENT

The patient with suspected poisoning is managed with the "SAFE" approach used for all medical emergencies (see Chapters 2 and 9).

Always use the SAFE approach

The paramedic must remember that the patient may have been poisoned by exposure to dangerous substances which may still be in the immediate environment. It is of benefit to no-one if ambulance crew become secondary casualties. Caution must therefore be exercised in approaching the patient, remaining alert to clues in the environment that may suggest inhalational or dermal exposure to a toxic substance.

If a safe approach is possible, the next task is to ensure that no further harm comes to the patient. If the patient is in a dangerous position, for example lying unconscious in the middle of the road, then he should be moved immediately. Similarly, a patient who has been exposed to an inhalational poison and is still in the poisoned atmosphere, for example a smoky room in a house fire or a garage full of carbon monoxide, again needs to be moved immediately. If access is not possible, it may be necessary to advise the fire service regarding appropriate action.

Once the patient is in a place of safety, an assessment of his clinical state needs to be made and a history taken. If the situation permits, these tasks should be undertaken simultaneously. If this is not possible then it is for the paramedic to decide which of these tasks takes priority. If the patient is extremely ill or unconscious, the first priority is to secure and maintain the airway and support the breathing and circulation whilst preparing for immediate transfer to hospital. If the patient is stable, a history should be taken, both from the patient and from any witnesses.

HISTORY

When taking the history, four crucial questions must be asked.

- What was taken?
- How much was taken?
- When was it taken?
- What was taken with the overdose (for example, alcohol)?

Without a knowledge of the nature of the substance, the quantity taken and the time elapsed between ingestion and presentation, it is extremely difficult to assess the severity of the poisoning or to make any predictions as to the patient's subsequent course.

If possible, the paramedic should take any medicine containers found at the scene to the hospital along with the patient. The presence of any additional substances such as alcohol, which may contribute to the patient's condition, must also be noted. In up to 30% of cases of deliberate ingestion of a poison, two or more substances have been taken. If the patient has vomited, there is no value in taking samples of vomit to hospital, although it should be noted if the patient has vomited back any recognizable tablets.

> Always consider the possibility of alcohol consumption

EXAMINATION

The immediate examination of the patient should aim to establish the stability of the vital signs. Many poisons depress the level of consciousness and adults who deliberately ingest poisons have often also taken alcohol. In many of these cases the actual poison will not cause serious harm to the patient other than by endangering the airway as a result of the altered mental state. Simple attention to the airway may be all that is needed to ensure a good prognosis but if omitted, a relatively "harmless" poisoning may be fatal.

As a general rule, most cases of poisoning require no treatment other than maintenance of the vital signs. If this is achieved, the majority of patients will have a favourable outcome.

Once the airway, breathing and circulation have been assessed a more focused examination should follow, both to give an indication of the patient's general state and also hopefully to obtain information relating to the nature of the poisoning (Table 18.1). This examination is intended to identify signs which suggest a specific diagnosis amenable to treatment in the prehospital situation and must not delay the transfer of a seriously ill patient to hospital.

Table 18.1 Diagnostic clues following drug overdose

Clinical sign	Drug
Tachycardia	Tricyclic antidepressants, antihistamines, amphetamines
Increased respiratory rate (tachypnoea)	Salicylates (aspirin), substances causing shock
Decreased respiratory rate	Opiates
Hypotension	Anticholinergic drugs, vasodilators, alcohol
Pupillary dilation	Tricyclic antidepressants, amphetamines
Pupillary constriction	Opiates
Nasal bleeding or perioral sores	Solvent abuse ("glue sniffing")

A rapid pulse rate may indicate ingestion of substances such as tricyclic antidepressants, antihistamines, amphetamines or other arrhythmogenic agents. Similarly, a low blood pressure may result from ingestion of anticholinergic medications or vasodilators such as alcohol. An increased respiratory rate is associated with substances that cause shock, but it also occurs in the early stages of salicylate overdose. A decreased respiratory rate occurs with opiate ingestion. The pupils may be dilated (tricyclic antidepressant and amphetamine ingestion) or constricted (opiate ingestion). The presence of nasal bleeding or perioral sores suggests solvent abuse.

It should again be emphasized that the gathering of this information should in no way delay the stabilization and transport of the patient to the nearest hospital. As noted earl-ier, most cases of poisoning require little other than maintenance of the airway breathing and circulation. Unfortunately, this may require skills and techniques only available in the hospital setting.

Similarly, in cases where further absorption of the poison can be prevented or where there is a specific antidote to the poison, any delay in hospitalization will decrease the chances of a successful outcome.

POISONING IN CHILDREN

Poisoning in children is common, but not commonly serious. A typical case of poisoning in childhood is the accidental ingestion of a mildly toxic substance by a child aged 1–3 years. Most incidents are minor.

In the UK, the majority of children ingest therapeutic agents: paracetamol, iron, benzodiazepines, tricyclic antidepressants and the contraceptive pill are the most common.

The remainder are usually poisoned by a variety of household products (p. 199). The accidental ingestion is usually noticed rapidly by the parents and the children often present very soon after ingestion (unlike the situation in many adult poisonings).

Some parents keep syrup of ipecacuanha in the house for use as an emetic in case of accidental poisoning. The use of this substance is controversial, as it can result in aspiration pneumonitis and gastrointestinal haemorrhage. In addition, it is only effective in removing the poison if given within 5 minutes of ingestion. As a general rule, however, it should not be used in the prehospital setting. If ipecacuanha has been given, the paramedic needs to be aware that up to 15% of children will develop prolonged vomiting, diarrhoea and drowsiness. Because its effects are delayed, the child may become drowsy as a result of the poisoning before the ipecacuanha induces vomiting, increasing the risk of aspiration.

The vast majority of poisoned children can be expected to recover if vital functions are preserved. Aspiration pneumonitis is far more dangerous to the patient than most poisons.

SPECIFIC POISONS

MEDICATIONS

Almost any medication can be harmful if taken in excess. Unfortunately, members of the public often perceive a difference in the toxicity of prescription medications compared with over-the-counter medications, believing the former to be more dangerous than the latter. This leads to the tragic consequence of a patient "crying for help" by taking an overdose of paracetamol, believing it to be of limited toxicity, with a fatal outcome. Conversely, the patient who takes a relatively innocuous overdose of benzodiazepines may genuinely believe that the drug may be toxic enough to be fatal, as it is only available on prescription.

Benzodiazepines

The prescription medications most commonly taken in overdose in the UK are the benzodiazepines. These usually just cause drowsiness or unconsciousness, although if taken with alcohol they may cause respiratory depression. The management of these patients consists of clearing and maintaining the airway and supporting the breathing with bag–mask ventilation if required. Although there is a specific antidote to benzodiazepines (flumazenil), there are dangers with its use in the prehospital setting. The patient may develop seizures as a result of benzodiazepine withdrawal or because other medications (e.g. tricyclic antidepressants) may also have been ingested. Should this happen, the seizures are extremely difficult to treat as the usual anticonvulsant in this situation – diazepam – will not work in the presence of the flumazenil. A further problem arises with the patient who revives following the administration of flumazenil, refuses further treatment and leaves

the scene; because the effects of the flumazenil are short-lived, unlike the effects of the benzodiazepines, the patient may succumb again to the overdose, possibly when no witnesses are present to call for help.

Paracetamol

The most common over-the-counter medication taken in overdose is paracetamol. As noted previously, the great danger of this drug is that it is perceived as harmless. Because there are often no immediately felt ill-effects after taking this drug, there may be a prolonged delay in seeking treatment. The tragedy is that such a delay may be fatal. Paracetamol is an extremely toxic drug when taken in overdose and although there is a specific antidote, it is most effective if given within 15 hours of ingestion. A delay in presentation, therefore, may render the antidote ineffective and lead to a preventable death. For the paramedic, the management of such cases is usually just transporting the patient to hospital for specific treatment. However, it should be remembered that the patient may perceive the overdose to be harmless and may decide to refuse treatment or transport to hospital. The paramedic must use all his powers of communication and persuasion in these cases, as the patient may die if he is not treated.

It should be remembered that drowsiness is not a feature of early paracetamol poisoning. If the patient is drowsy, he is likely to have taken a second medication or alcohol. He may, alternatively, have taken a compound analgesic such as co-codamol (paracetamol and codeine), co-dydramol (paracetamol and dihydrocodeine) or co-proxamol (paracetamol and dextropropoxyphene).

Tricyclic antidepressants

Tricyclic antidepressants are commonly prescribed to the patients who are most at risk of attempted self-harm. It is unfortunate that this group of drugs are amongst the most toxic medications when taken in overdose.

Poisoning by these drugs affects the central nervous system, causing depressed consciousness followed by seizures. They also affect the cardiovascular system, producing cardiac arrhythmias ranging from sinus tachycardia in the early stages of poisoning to ventricular tachycardia in the later stages of severe poisoning. The patient usually has a degree of vasodilation, which causes hypotension. Together with the impaired function of the heart, this leads to poor perfusion of organs and a metabolic acidosis. With the depressed conscious level impairing ventilation, respiratory acidosis is also a common finding in these patients.

The management of these patients can be very challenging; however, the ABC approach will provide sufficient prehospital care for most of them. The airway should be cleared and protected and oxygen given via a face mask. Ventilation may be needed and this should initially be via a bag–valve–mask system. Hyperventilating the patient will

Box 18.1 Tricyclic antidepressant poisoning – clinical features

- Depressed consciousness
- Seizures
- Cardiac arrhythmias
- Hypotension
- Tachypnoea
- Impaired ventilation

Box 18.2 Tricuclic antidepressant poisoning – management

- Airway and oxygen
- Breathing – support ventilation
- Circulation – maintain circulation, rapid transfer, monitor ECG
- Control seizures with diazepam

help correct both metabolic and respiratory acidosis. Hypotension should be treated with an intravenous fluid challenge and an ECG monitor should be applied to determine and monitor the cardiac rhythm.

Should seizures occur, these can be treated in the normal manner with intravenous or rectal diazepam, remembering that this may well depress respiration further. Cardiac arrhythmias such as sinus tachycardia need no specific treatment. If the patient develops a ventricular arrhythmia with a pulse, specific urgent in-hospital investigations and treatment will be required, including repeated boluses of sodium bicarbonate until the rhythm normalizes or the pH reaches 7.55.

The decision to intubate these patients is fraught with difficulties. Although intubation will protect the airway from vomit and facilitate ventilation, the procedure can cause marked cardiac stimulation and may precipitate a life-threatening arrhythmia. It is usually safer to use a bag–valve–mask system for ventilation, with the patient in the recovery position and slightly head down. Should the patient need intubation, this can more safely be accomplished in the hospital setting with the aid of sedating and paralysing agents.

β-Blockers

β-Blockers are widely prescribed to the elderly. This section of the population is at risk of poisoning for two reasons: poor vision and impaired memory predispose to accidental overdose of prescription medications; and intentional overdose, although less common in this age group, is usually undertaken with more determination.

The results of β-blocker overdose reflect the *function* of the drug, namely to produce bradycardia and hypotension (unlike tricyclic antidepressants where overdose reflects the *side-effects* of the drug). The patient may also have a depressed conscious level as a result of cerebral underperfusion. The treatment follows ABC principles: the airway is secured and breathing is assessed. Hypotension is treated with intravenous fluid and bradycardia is treated with 0.5 mg atropine intravenously. Further doses (to a maximum of 3 mg) may be given if there is no effect or if the patient deteriorates after transient improvement. Use of an external pacemaker may also be considered. Glucagon 0.5–1.0 mg given intramuscularly or intravenously (and repeated up to 5 mg) has been shown to be of benefit in severe β-blocker poisoning. In such cases the patient may require insertion of an intravenous pacemaker, therefore there should be no delay in taking the patient to the nearest hospital.

Insulin

It is uncommon for insulin to be taken as a deliberate overdose, unless there is a genuine desire to die and steps are taken to avoid discovery, but accidental overdoses occur frequently. The patient may be comatose, in which case the diagnosis and management are paradoxically easy: protection of the airway, breathing and circulation, a simple thumb-prick blood glucose assay to confirm the diagnosis and the administration of intravenous dextrose or intramuscular glucagon will result in a gratifying return to consciousness and normality. The assessment and management of the combative, apparently drunk patient in the early stages of hypoglycaemia is much less straightforward. It should be emphasized that every minute's delay in the treatment of hypoglycaemia will have a cumulative effect. It is important, therefore, to make the diagnosis and institute appropriate therapy as rapidly as possible.

After receiving treatment from the paramedic, with associated clinical improvement, a diabetic patient who has frequent hypoglycaemic episodes may be reluctant to travel to hospital once "cured". In such cases the paramedic will need to be persuasive, for the patient requires careful assessment in hospital to determine the reason for the hypoglycaemic event. The patient's diabetic regimen may need altering, there may be another cause for the hypoglycaemia and, most importantly, if the overdose was of a long-acting insulin, the patient may need a period of observation in order to ensure that the episode does not recur. This is particularly true if glucagen has been administered due to its short half-life.

Opiates

Opiates may be taken in overdose accidentally (in the case of the patient with chronic pain), intentionally, with a view to self-harm, or recreationally, by injecting drug abusers. The effects of opiate poisoning are a depressed level of consciousness, depressed respiration (breathing tends to be slow and deep) and hypotension. The greatest dangers are of aspiration of stomach contents while comatose, hypoxia and respiratory acidosis.

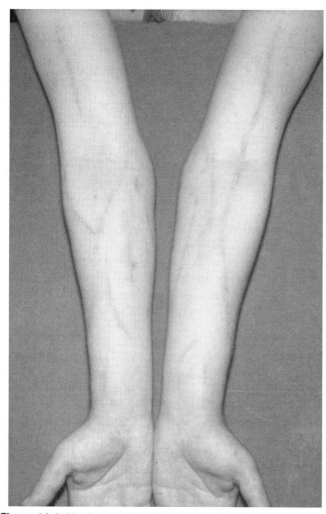

Figure 18.1 Needle marks in an intravenous drug abuser

Table 18.2 Treatment for overdosage of specific drugs

Drug	Effects	Treatment
Tricyclic antidepressants	Heart rate increased Blood pressure lowered Drowsiness Convulsions	ABC IV fluids Diazepam (for fits) Bicarbonate (in hospital)
β-Blockers	Heart rate increased Blood pressure lowered Possible drowsiness	ABC IV fluids Atropine Glucagon May need external pacer
Opiates	Drowsiness Respiration reduced Pinpoint pupils Blood pressure lowered	ABC Naloxone
Insulin	Agitated Conscious level lowered Pale, clammy appearance Low blood glucose level	ABC Dextrose Glucagon

The diagnosis of opiate poisoning may be obvious: witnesses may be aware of the patient's medication or lifestyle, there may be labelled medication nearby or the patient's physical characteristics may suggest opiate abuse (e.g. needle marks – Figure 18.1). On examination, the patient is usually comatose, with pinpoint pupils and sighing respiration. Hypotension may be present. The treatment, fortunately, is simple. After securing the airway, supplying oxygen, assisting breathing and establishing intravenous access, naloxone should be administered intravenously in boluses of 0.4 mg, allowing a few minutes for effect, and repeated to a maximum dose of 10 mg or until the patient begins to recover. Failure to respond to a dose of 2 mg suggests that opiates are not responsible for the loss of consciousness although in some cases larger doses may be necessary.

The danger of using naloxone in these cases, which the paramedic must constantly bear in mind, is that the half-life, and therefore the effect, of naloxone is shorter than the effect of most commonly used opiates. The result of this is that the improvement in the patient's condition may be short-lived and coma may return. Unfortunately, the patient may take advantage of being "cured" to refuse transport to hospital or further treatment. A patient who is allowed to leave the scene may well lapse into another coma, possibly with no witnesses to summon help.

There are practical and medicolegal problems associated with taking such patients to hospital against their will. One method that may be used in such cases is to administer intramuscular naloxone (1 mg) to the poisoned patient before giving the intravenous dose. In this way, if the patient leaves the scene following recovery, naloxone will be slowly released into the circulation from the IM dose and may prevent a relapse.

The specific treatments for overdosage are summarized in Table 18.2.

HOUSEHOLD SUBSTANCES

Almost any product designed for household use can be (and has been – "I've taken the dog's antibiotics!") ingested, whether accidentally or intentionally. This chapter cannot hope to deal with all of them, but some of the more common substances are considered below with the general principles of management.

Most household products in current use are of low systemic toxicity if accidentally ingested. Commonly ingested

Box 18.3 Effects of laburnum ingestion

- Burning mouth and throat
- Nausea
- Abdominal pain
- Vomiting
- Diarrhoea
- Drowsiness
- Incoordination
- Delirium
- Twitching
- Coma

substances include bleaches, turpentine substitute, paraffin and household cleaning products. The treatment of ingestion of these substances is to administer oral fluids (milk) and rapidly transfer the patient to hospital. There may be local irritation of the mouth or oesophagus, but systemic toxicity is unusual. The patient should *not* be encouraged to vomit, as this may lead to a potentially fatal pneumonitis.

PLANTS AND FUNGI

It is unusual for adults to eat poisonous plants, though mistakes occur occasionally. More commonly, it is children who ingest berries, seeds or other parts of plants in the wild, the garden or around the home. Fortunately the quantities involved are usually small because the plant material is sufficiently unpalatable to prevent consumption of more than very minimal amounts.

The most common plant poisoning in Britain is the ingestion of laburnum seeds. If more than 10 seeds have been ingested, the effects listed above may occur. However, fatalities are extremely rare.

The treatment of laburnum poisoning is the same as that for all plant ingestions: evaluation and support of the airway, breathing and circulation and transportation of the patient to hospital. It is of vital importance in all plant poisonings that a sample of the ingested plant is also taken to hospital for identification.

Many poisonous fungi can be mistaken for edible mushrooms, but serious poisoning is rare in Britain. Usually, patients who have ingested fungi have a violent but self-limiting attack of abdominal pain, diarrhoea, nausea and vomiting about 2 hours after the ingestion. Rarely, there may be signs of excessive cholinergic stimulation (bronchospasm, bradycardia, constricted pupils and collapse). This can be treated with boluses of intravenous atropine, but it should be remembered that this may exacerbate any agitation or hallucinations. As with plant ingestion, the patient and the fungi should be taken to the nearest hospital as soon as possible.

> Wherever possible, take a sample of the ingested plant to hospital

OTHER SUBSTANCES

Inhalational agents

A number of substances are harmful if inhaled. The two main groups of inhalational "poisons" are the recreational drugs (opiates, cocaine and solvents – see Chapter 54) and substances inhaled accidentally or for deliberate self-harm (carbon monoxide and other gases). The treatment of the first group is rapid assessment of the airway, breathing and circulation, supportive care, administration of naloxone in the case of opiate poisoning and rapid transport to hospital.

The second group is important because in these cases there is a danger to the paramedic. Care should be taken that the paramedic does not become a secondary casualty by inhaling the toxic fumes. If it is possible to approach safely, the patient should be removed from the environment and given high-concentration oxygen. The patient should then be taken to the nearest suitable hospital.

Recreational drugs

There are unfortunately many harmful substances that are inhaled, ingested or injected for "recreational" purposes. Some of these have already been discussed. The general effect of these drugs is to affect the central nervous system, producing depression (opiates and benzodiazepines) or stimulation (Ecstasy, amphetamines and cocaine). The treatment of poisoning by these substances is the assessment and support of airway, breathing and circulation, the administration of naloxone in opiate poisoning and rapid transport to hospital (see Chapter 54).

CONCLUSION

Poisoning is common and likely to become more common, with the increase in medications being dispensed and the growth of substance abuse. The paramedic has a crucial role in the care of poisoned victims, being in the best position to gather vital information at the scene and provide immediate life-saving treatment.

Immediate evaluation and support of airway, breathing and circulation, the administration of specific antidotes and rapid transport to hospital will ensure that the patient is given the best chance of survival. Most patients will survive with no further treatment, other than a continuation of support of the airway, breathing and circulation. In a number of specific instances, administration of an antidote may be life saving. Under no circumstances should the paramedic put himself at risk and become another victim.

FURTHER READING

Proudfoot Management of poisoning, 2nd edn. Churchill Livingstone, Edinburgh

Chapter 19

Risk of infection

CHAPTER CONTENTS

INTRODUCTION

Healthcare workers will encounter many patients who are suffering from infectious diseases. Only a small minority of these patients present any risk of infection to paramedical, medical and nursing staff. Furthermore, the chances of becoming infected from contact with one of these patients while at work is very small indeed. A basic knowledge of the common causes of infectious diseases and methods of avoiding their spread is necessary to ensure that risk of infection is minimized.

TERMINOLOGY

The two most common causes of infection are bacteria and viruses. Bacteria are small, unicellular organisms that have evolved to live in very specialized environments. Bacterial infections usually respond to antibiotics. Viruses are much smaller organisms that cannot be seen with a normal light microscope. They do not respond to antibiotics and there are few drugs available to treat the illnesses that they cause. Other organisms such as protozoa and fungi can also cause infection. They do not usually represent an infection risk in the prehospital environment.

A person is *infected* if he has an illness caused by a microorganism. The disease is *infectious* if it can be transmitted from person to person. Some people may have harmful organisms in their body and yet not exhibit signs of the infection. These individuals are known as *carriers* and may transmit infection to others The area in which the microorganism grows is known as the *source*, while the vehicle of transport of infection e.g. the hands in a faecal–oral transmitted infection) is known as the *reservoir*. The *incubation period* of a disease is

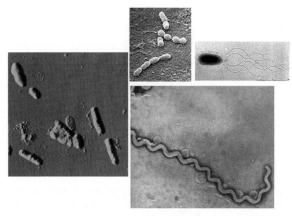

Figure 19.1 A common bacterium and virus

the time during which the microorganism is multiplying in body tissue before the signs and symptoms of illness have developed. The *infectious period* is the time during which the infection may be transmitted to other people.

ROUTES OF INFECTION

Infection can be spread by a number of different routes. Droplet spread is the common route of infection for respiratory disease. Coughing or sneezing propels showers of small fluid droplets through the air. These contain bacteria and viruses which others may inspire, resulting in transmission of the infection.

Many wound infections are caused by direct contact, for instance when an unwashed hand touches a surgical wound. Direct contact may also be a route of transmission of disease during mouth-to-mouth contact in artificial ventilation. If the direct contact actually punctures the skin, for example with a bite or a needlestick injury, the risk of infection is much higher. The risk is highest when foreign material such as blood is injected, for example from a hollow (hypodermic) needle.

Dirty hands can also act as the reservoir for spreading infection from the lower gastrointestinal tract. This occurs when unwashed hands are placed near the mouth. This is known as faecal–oral spread and is the route of infection of many gastrointestinal infections and diseases such as hepatitis A.

Finally, infections can be spread by indirect contact when clothing, dressings or medical equipment contaminated with bacteria or viruses from an infected patient are used for another casualty. For this reason all medical equipment should be kept scrupulously clean.

IMPORTANT INFECTIOUS DISEASES IN THE UK

BACTERIAL INFECTIONS

Tuberculosis

Tuberculosis is a disease that mainly affects the respiratory system, causing shortness of breath and cough. It can also affect the lymph nodes of the neck and may cause discharging sinuses to the skin although this is unusual. It is caused by the bacterium *Mycobacterium tuberculosis* and other related mycobacteria. The incidence of the disease has recently risen in the UK, possibly owing to the increasing number of immigrants, a decrease in the uptake of vaccination and poor living standards in inner cities. The disease is spread by the droplet route and occasionally by direct contact with infected debris from a tuberculous lymph node.

The typical patient is an emaciated homeless person, who presents coughing up small amounts of blood. The incubation period of the disease is 4–8 weeks and patients continue to be infectious until their illness has been treated. All paramedic staff should ensure that they are fully immunized against tuberculosis and have a Heaf test (intradermal tuberculin) every 3 years to check their immunity. Those who do not show a good response to the Heaf test should have a chest radiograph to ensure that they do not have the disease.

If a patient with active tuberculosis has been transported, the ambulance must be thoroughly aired, linen laundered and all contaminated respiratory equipment such as face masks and tubing destroyed. Concerns about staff contacting the disease should be discussed with the occupational health department who will arrange further investigation.

Meningitis

Meningitis is an infection of the membranes that surround the brain. It can be caused by bacteria or viruses. The presenting symptoms are headache, photophobia (light hurting the eyes) and neck stiffness. The common bacteria that cause meningitis are *Haemophilus influenzae*, *Neisseria meningitidis* and *Streptococcus pneumoniae*. Meningitis secondary to *Neisseria* infection (meningococcal meningitis) represents an infection risk to close contacts of the patient. It has an incubation period of 2–3 days and usually presents in young people. *Neisseria meningitidis* infection may cause a meningococcal septicaemia demonstrated by a widespread bruising rash (purpura). The child with meningococcal disease may deteriorate very rapidly and must be administered benzyl penicillin and transported to hospital as soon as possible.

When transporting such a patient, a face mask should be worn and the ambulance and all equipment thoroughly cleaned afterwards. Hand washing is essential. If the final diagnosis is proved to be meningococcal meningitis, the occupational health department will consider giving a course of antibiotics to reduce any possible risk of acquiring the infection, although prophylactic antibiotics are *not* usually given to paramedic or medical staff unless they have been "kissing" contacts (mouth-to-mouth ventilation).

Whooping cough

Whooping cough (pertussis) is a bacterial respiratory infection caused by the bacterium *Bordetella pertussis*. It mainly affects children and is most severe in those under 6 months of age. Characteristically, after an incubation period of 7–10 days the child develops what appears to be a mild cough. This gradually worsens and the child develops a "whooping" noise when coughing (an inspiratory whoop between bouts of coughing). The disease often lasts several months and may be complicated by vomiting, weight loss and pneumonia.

Due to fears about the safety of the MMR (measles, mumps and rubella) vaccine and a consequent decline in uptake by parents, it is possible that whooping cough may increase in incidence. Whooping cough does not represent a great risk to paramedic staff, but an ambulance should be thoroughly cleaned and aired if a child with the illness has been transported.

VIRAL INFECTIONS

Hepatitis

Hepatitis is the name given to infective conditions affecting the liver. There are several different viruses which can cause hepatitis and which present different risks to paramedical staff. *Infectious hepatitis* is caused by the *hepatitis A virus* and is spread by the faecal–oral route. It is common in conditions of poor sanitation and tends to occur in outbreaks, for instance in prisons or mental health institutions. The incubation period of the disease is 2–6 weeks and the patient presents with general malaise, jaundice, nausea and vomiting. The disease tends to run a benign course and usually resolves over a period of 1–2 months.

Infection with *hepatitis B virus* results in a much more serious illness, sometimes known as *serum hepatitis*. This condition is spread by the intravenous route or by sexual contact and causes a much more severe hepatitis which can result in death or the patient being left as a chronic carrier of the disease. It is most common in Britain in injecting drug abusers who share needles. It is much easier to contract hepatitis B than the more widely feared human immunodeficiency virus (HIV) from needle contact with an infected person. An effective vaccine is available for immunization against hepatitis B. All ambulance staff should ensure that they are vaccinated and have their antibody levels checked every 3 years.

Another virus causing hepatitis has recently been discovered. It is called *hepatitis C virus* and causes a very similar condition to hepatitis B. It is also spread by the intravenous or sexual routes. There is no effective vaccine against hepatitis C in clinical use at present.

The paramedic can prevent spread of all these diseases by being extremely careful whenever using sharp instruments or needles. Significant contamination with infected or potentially infected blood or body fluids (e.g. needlestick injury) must be reported immediately. The name of the index patient should be recorded for subsequent serological blood testing subject to the patient's consent. Expert advice should be sought at the earliest opportunity.

HIV infection and AIDS

There have been few diseases that have generated such widespread public interest and dread as the acquired immunodeficiency syndrome (AIDS). It can be caused by either of two viruses, HIV-1 or HIV-2 (human immunodeficiency virus 1 or 2), which are spread by sexual contact or by the intravenous route. The disease causes fear because as yet there is no vaccine and no cure. However, the virus is very fragile when outside the human body and is easy to destroy. The risk of becoming infected from a needlestick injury is 10 times lower for HIV than for hepatitis B virus, taking equivalent inoculating doses of the virus. The chances of acquiring HIV while at work are very small, but disease transmission has occurred in medical and nursing staff through needlestick injury and there are occasional instances of contamination through non-intact skin.

The duty of care to a patient with AIDS remains the same as for any patient. The nature of the illness should not affect the standard of care that is given. If universal precautions are used the infection risk can be minimized. The ambulance should be thoroughly cleaned and disinfected after use and all disposable items placed in labelled double bags and sent for incineration.

If an accident occurs which puts health service personnel at risk of contracting HIV infection, it is essential that medical advice is sought *immediately*. Postexposure prophylactic drug therapy (PEP) is effective in reducing the serum conversion rate from HIV negative to positive but ideally should be started within one hour. Occupational health or the local sexual health clinic or A&E department will offer advice, therapy and access to counselling. The decision regarding postexposure prophylaxis is based on a risk assessment of the index patient and the nature of the potentially infecting accident. In very high-risk cases (known HIV-positive patient and significant inoculating blood volume) treatment will be started with the minimum delay pending blood testing of the index case (with consent), if their status is not already known. In cases with lower risk, the decision to treat will be delayed until the results are known.

Herpes virus infections

The herpes viruses cause a variety of different blistering eruptions. Herpes simplex type 1 causes cold sores on the mouth and on the fingers ("whitlow"). Herpes simplex type 2 causes similar lesions on the genitalia. Type 1 infections are common on the fingers of nursing staff who deal with patients with exposed cold sores. Spread of the infection can be prevented by wearing gloves when dealing with such patients and regularly washing the hands.

The chickenpox virus is another herpes virus. Chickenpox is a widespread blistering eruption which is common in children and is highly infectious. The incubation period of the disease is 14–21 days and the vesicles first appear on the face and scalp before spreading to the trunk and finally the limbs. It remains infectious until the vesicles are dry. Chickenpox can affect adults more seriously, so it is best to avoid carrying an infected patient if any member of the crew has not had the illness as a child. The virus remains dormant in nerve endings and may reactivate at a later date, resulting in "shingles" or herpes zoster (Figure 19.3). This is characterized by vesicles erupting in small areas corresponding to the spinal nerves that supply the skin (dermatomes). It commonly occurs in the elderly, precipitated by stress or underlying

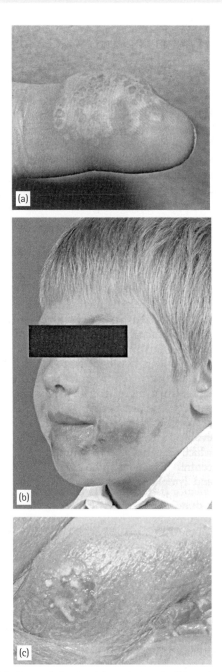

Figure 19.2 Herpes infection (a) on the hands; (b) on the face; (c) on the genitalia

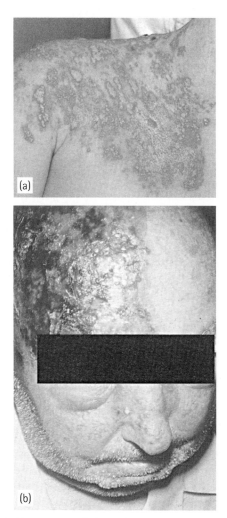

Figure 19.3 Herpes zoster (shingles)

disease, and can be very painful. Chickenpox and shingles are usually self-limiting diseases but both can become severe if the patient is immunosuppressed, for example with AIDS, or if pregnant.

After carrying such a patient, the ambulance should be cleaned thoroughly to avoid the possibility of spreading the infection to other casualties.

Other childhood infectious diseases

There are a number of other childhood infectious diseases caused by viruses, of which the paramedic should be aware.

The incidence of these illnesses has until recently been on the decrease because of the widespread uptake of the vaccination programme. In the light of concern regarding vaccine safety, this may now change.

Measles

Measles is a viral illness transmitted by droplet spread. After an incubation period of 10 days the child develops fever, cough and conjunctivitis. A rash appears 2–4 days later. The disease is infectious from the beginning of symptoms until 4 days after the appearance of the rash. The illness is not always benign and can result in deafness and brain damage. Patients with measles do not present any particular risk to paramedic staff, but the ambulance and equipment should be thoroughly cleaned after use to prevent transmission of infection to others.

German measles (rubella)

Rubella is similar to measles but is a less severe disease, with a transient rash and lymphadenopathy (swelling of the

Table 19.1 Common and serious infectious diseases in the UK

Disease	Mode of transmission	Incubation period	Infectious period	Symptoms and signs
AIDS	Sexual contact, dirty needles	Months to years	Unknown	Unusually susceptible to infections
Chickenpox	Droplet spread, direct and indirect contact	14–21 days	For 2 days before rash until vesicles dry	Fever, blistering rash that comes in crops
German measles	Droplet spread	14–21 days	From 7 days before until 4 days after rash	Fever, rash and sore throat
Glandular fever	Mouth-to-mouth contact	2–6 weeks	Unknown	Generally unwell, swollen lymph glands
Hepatitis A	Faecal–oral	15–40 days		Lethargy, jaundice
Hepatitis B, C	Sexual contact, dirty needles	40–160 days	Variable, beware of chronic carriers	Lethargy, jaundice
Herpes virus	Sexual contact, direct contact	2–10 days	For 2 days before rash until vesicles dry	Blistering eruption
Measles	Droplet spread	10 days	From beginning of symptoms to 4 days after appearance of rash	Fever, cough, conjunctivitis, rash
Meningococcal disease	Droplet spread and contact	2–3 days	Until treated	Fever, stiff neck, haemorrhagic rash
Mumps	Droplet spread	14–21 days	For 2 days before parotid swelling to 5 days after	Malaise, swollen parotid glands, orchitis
Tuberculosis	Droplet spread	4–8 weeks	Until treated	Cough, haemoptysis, weight loss
Whooping cough	Droplet spread	6–10 days	From 7 days after exposure to 21 days after first symptoms	Fever, characteristic cough

lymph nodes). The incubation period is 14–21 days and the disease is infective from 1 week before until 4 days after the onset of the rash. The most important aspect of rubella infection is the potential fetal damage which can result when mothers are exposed to the virus in the early months of their pregnancy. For this reason all British girls are immunized against rubella prior to leaving school. The national immunization programme has now been extended to cover all teenagers, to lower the incidence of the illness in the community. All female ambulance staff should ensure that they are immunized against the disease and if pregnant, should not transport patients who are suspected of having the disease.

Mumps

Mumps is a viral illness which results in swelling of one or both parotid glands (the salivary glands situated near the angle of the jaw). The incubation period of the illness is 14–21 days and the patient is infectious for several days before the parotid gland swells and for the subsequent 5 days. The child with mumps looks exceptionally miserable, with general malaise and parotid swelling. Mumps in adult life can result in inflammation of the testes (orchitis) with subsequent sterility. Adult males who have not had mumps should therefore avoid transporting children who are suspected of having

the illness. Inflammation of the ovaries (oophoritis), thyroid (thyroiditis), brain (encephalitis) and pancreas (pancreatitis) can all result from mumps infection.

The common and serious infectious diseases encountered in the UK are summarized in Table 19.1.

MINIMIZING THE SPREAD OF INFECTIOUS DISEASES

The risk of catching an infectious disease is small and can be minimized further by the observation of some simple precautions.

Box 19.1 Measures to avoid the spread of infectious disease

- Ensuring that one is fully immunized
- Observing good general hygiene
- Using disposable equipment when possible
- Having a regular cleaning schedule for equipment and the ambulance
- Using "universal precautions" (see below)
- Taking extreme care when using sharps

IMMUNIZATION

Paramedical staff should ensure that their immunization schedules are up to date. In addition to routine childhood immunization, the following immunizations are essential.

- Tetanus – a booster should be given every 10 years
- Tuberculosis – a Heaf test is necessary every 3 years to check on immunity
- Hepatitis B – a full course of three injections should be given and then antibody levels checked. If levels are low a further booster dose may be necessary. Antibody levels should be checked every 3 years
- Rubella – antibody titres should be checked and immunization offered to female personnel who are not immune.

GENERAL HYGIENE

All healthcare professionals should observe general standards of personal hygiene. Hands should be thoroughly washed in a surgical scrub solution after each patient. Nails must be kept clean and regularly trimmed otherwise they may act as a reservoir for bacteria. Hair should be kept short or tied back so that it cannot contaminate a wound. A paramedic with any large wound or open weeping areas should not work until the injury has healed. Small lacerations should be cleaned and dressed with a waterproof dressing to decrease the risk of infection.

EQUIPMENT

Medical equipment, particularly items such as airway tubing, can act as a reservoir of infection. Whenever possible, disposable equipment should be used and then replaced. Disposable sharps should be kept in puncture-resistant containers. Other disposables should be placed in plastic bags and clearly marked before being sent to be destroyed.

The ambulance is another potential reservoir of infection. It should be aired regularly and the interior cleaned thoroughly at least once a day. All non-disposable equipment should be scrubbed with an antiseptic solution after each patient. Linen should be changed and sent for cleaning to the laundry. All uniforms should be clean and ideally impermeable to blood and other bodily secretions. If a uniform does become contaminated during use, the paramedic should shower and change to remove any skin contamination which may have occurred through the garment.

UNIVERSAL PRECAUTIONS

A small number of people in the general community may represent an infection risk. Unfortunately, there is no easy way of identifying this group. Therefore all patients should be assumed to represent a potential risk and universal precautions to prevent contact with blood or other bodily fluids should be taken, as described below.

Box 19.2 Universal precautions

- Ensure that protective equipment is always available in the ambulance
- Observe blood and body fluid precautions with ALL casualties
- Wear gloves whenever exposed to blood or other body fluids
- Protect eyes, face and trunk if blood is likely to be splashed
- Wash immediately if blood or body fluid is splashed onto skin

---

- Protective equipment must always be easily available. If it is not immediately to hand it will not be used. The ambulance is well stocked with gloves, masks and aprons and the routine of using them must be developed.
- Latex gloves should be worn whenever contact with bodily fluids is anticipated, for example in venepuncture or in dressing a wound. Hands should be washed thoroughly after the gloves have been removed. Thicker protective gloves should be worn to protect the extremities when there is a likelihood of sustaining an injury, such as when removing an entrapped patient surrounded by broken glass in a road traffic accident.
- If there is a possibility of blood or bodily fluids being splashed over the body, additional protective measures should be taken. A mask and glasses may help to protect the face and eyes. Alternatively a face shield can be worn. A plastic apron may help to prevent seepage of blood through to the skin. Sensible measures such as the use of pressure on bleeding areas should be taken to minimize the spread of body fluids.
- If blood or any other body fluid reaches the skin, it should be washed immediately in order to reduce any possible chance of infection.

SHARPS

Extreme care should be taken when using needles, blades and other sharps. They should be disposed of immediately in a puncture-resistant container, such as the Sharpsafe. Needles should never be resheathed or broken because of the risk of needlestick injury. Ideally, sharps should not be handed from one person to another. It is also important to beware of sharp items such as broken glass or edges of metal which can present a danger when attending accident victims.

HIGH–RISK SITUATIONS

There are several situations in which ambulance staff may be subjected to a higher risk of exposure to an infectious disease. In these situations further precautionary measures may be necessary.

Box 19.3 Sharps

- Use extreme care whenever handling sharps
- Never break needles
- Never resheathe needles
- Dispose of sharps in a puncture-resistant container
- Avoid passing sharps from one person to another

CARDIOPULMONARY RESUSCITATION

There have been no case reports of HIV or hepatitis B infection caused by transmission of the virus during mouth-to-mouth ventilation. However, both viruses are present in saliva so a small risk may be present. In addition, there have been isolated cases of transmission of herpes virus, tuberculosis and meningitis. For these reasons mouth-to-mouth ventilation should be avoided if at all possible. Instead, ventilation should be performed using a Laerdal pocket mask with a one-way valve or a self-inflating bag with mask.

TRANSPORT OF HIGH–RISK PATIENTS

On some occasions an ambulance may be called upon to transport a patient with a known infectious disease. In this case some anticipatory measures can be taken. A crew with known immunity to the disease should be selected where possible. For example, a patient with mumps should be transmitted by a paramedic who has proven immunity or who has previously had the disease. Disposable linen should be used in the ambulance, and gowns and masks should be worn by the crew whenever they examine the patient. After the transfer of the patient all disposables should be placed in plastic bags and sent for incineration.

ACTION TO TAKE IN CASE OF EXPOSURE TO INFECTIOUS DISEASE

Crew members who have been exposed to an infectious disease and are worried that they may have contracted the infection should contact their occupational health department. The occupational health staff will want to know the nature of the illness, the time of exposure and the way in which the exposure occurred. As much information about the infected patient should be obtained as possible. Investigations and treatment will depend on the nature of the disease; for example, antibiotics as prophylaxis against meningococcal meningitis (rarely required), and Heaf testing and chest X-ray for tuberculosis.

Following a needlestick injury, the affected area should be immediately washed in running water (Figure 19.4). The patient should be asked if he is known to have an infectious disease. If possible a blood sample should be taken from the patient to assess the hepatitis and HIV status (*the patient will need counselling before having these investigations and must give informed consent*). The next step is to attend the occupational

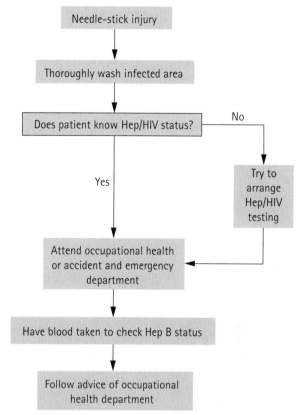

Figure 19.4 Dealing with a needlestick injury (Hep, hepatitis)

health unit or local A&E unit without delay. Blood will be taken for checking hepatitis status and to ensure immunity. Any treatment will depend on one's own hepatitis status and that of the patient. The occupational health department may offer HIV counselling.

INFECTIONS TRANSMITTED FROM PARAMEDIC STAFF TO PATIENT

It should be remembered that a patient can acquire an infection from a paramedic as easily as a paramedic can from a patient. All paramedic personnel therefore have a duty to ensure that they are healthy and are not harbouring any potentially infectious diseases. Any concerns about illness should be discussed with the occupational health department or with a local general practitioner. Similarly, paramedics should not work if they have large open wounds and must ensure that any small cuts or abrasions are covered with waterproof dressings.

CONCLUSION

There is no doubt that the nature of a paramedic's occupation exposes him to certain additional risks of contracting an infectious disease. Fortunately, a few simple measures will significantly reduce these risks. All relevant immunizations must be up to date and appropriate new immunizations received. Sensible precautions must be followed in any situation where there is a risk, however small, of exposure to an infectious condition. Finally when exposure or suspected exposure has occurred, immediate specialist advice should be sought. If all these precautions are followed, the paramedic can be reassured that the chances of any significant problems due to the transmission of an infective agent will be very small.

Section 4

4 TRAUMA

Chapter 20

Obtaining a trauma history

CHAPTER CONTENTS

INTRODUCTION

The trauma patient requires *rapid* assessment and management prior to transport to hospital for definitive care. This early evaluation and resuscitation must be structured and methodical and must identify time-critical cases where patients have life-threatening injuries. These patients can never be fully managed by field resuscitation and need the urgent services of a major receiving hospital, trauma team and trauma surgeons. Prehospital care is only a component of the *golden hour* concept, introduced by the Baltimore Shock-Trauma Unit surgeon Dr R Adams Cowley: this is the target time from injury to definitive surgical treatment. The prehospital phase of the golden hour should ideally not exceed 10 minutes in critical patients (understanding that an entrapment will prevent this) and taking a trauma history must be incorporated within this timeframe.

> The "golden hour" is the time from injury to definitive surgical treatment

The medical history of the patient and the mechanism of the injury are the two essential requirements of the trauma history and must be obtained at a speed appropriate to the clinical state of the patient.

TAKING A HISTORY

After an appropriate introduction, the patient should be asked about what has happened. A positive and appropriate response will also provide the information that the patient is conscious, has a patent airway, sufficient tidal volume to speak and sufficient cardiac output to provide an adequate cerebral circulation. The patient may be unable to give a full account and information from bystanders may be important in influencing the patient's subsequent treatment.

The major complaints and location of pain must be sought next, followed by accompanying symptoms such as breathing difficulty and nausea. Any episode of altered level of consciousness and any events or symptoms preceding the accident, such as chest pain, must be established.

The mnemonic AMPLE is a helpful *aide-mémoire* for the components of the trauma history.

A >	Allergies
M >	Medication
P >	Past medical history
L >	Last ate or drank
E >	Events and environment

The importance of a history of allergy is self-evident. The seriously injured patient will require treatment with a number of medications including antibiotics, analgesics and anaesthetic drugs, all of which have the ability to produce an allergic reaction. A Medic-Alert bracelet or necklace may be worn by those who consider themselves at high risk of an allergic reaction (or who have chronic conditions that are prone to acute complications such as diabetes, epilepsy or a pacemaker).

Certain prescribed medications alter the patient's response to injury. Specifically β-blocker medication will prevent a patient developing a tachycardia in response to haemorrhage. Patients receiving anticoagulant therapy are at increased risk of developing life-threatening haemorrhage. The patient receiving warfarin may develop an intracranial bleed after minor head injury.

The past medical history is important in that patients who have previous significant illnesses (particularly cardiac or respiratory) have a relatively poor prognosis following injury. Knowledge of a patient's existing illnesses also helps explain findings on examination which might otherwise be thought to be the result of injury.

It is always wise to assume that an injured patient has a full stomach and that there is a constant risk of vomiting and aspiration. However, if a patient has not eaten or drunk for several hours prior to the injury the risk is low. Recent ingestion of alcohol or recreational drugs may affect the patient's conscious level, although it should always be assumed that a depressed level of consciousness following trauma is the result of hypoxia, hypovolaemia, or brain injury until proven otherwise.

The events and environment relate to the mechanism of injury (see below) and the environment in which the injury occurred. The environmental factors to consider are temperature, the presence of toxic substances (chemicals and radiation) and material which may contaminate a wound. If a patient has been contaminated with toxic chemicals at the scene it will compound their conventional injuries. Identification of a chemical contaminant is the responsibility of the fire service who have rapid access to information systems, although the medical information provided from these sources is likely to be limited.

History taking must not delay immediate resuscitation within the primary survey where this is clearly required.

THE MECHANISM OF INJURY

Most patients who are the victims of blunt trauma will be delivered to hospital lying on their back on a spinal board with integral head immobiliser. The trauma team has little or no perception of the clues at the scene that relate to the nature, direction and force of injury. Ambulance personnel are the "eyes and ears" of the emergency department and they are privileged to know far more about the mechanism of injury. They are under an obligation to pass on this information and the department staff would be wise to listen with care. Failure on either side will harm only one person – the patient.

ROAD TRAFFIC ACCIDENTS

Certain mechanisms of injury, such as side-impact collisions, can be used to predict the pattern of injury found in an individual patient. The paramedic should therefore assess the pattern of damage to the vehicles – a process known as "reading the wreckage". The so-called "T-bone" type, side-impact vehicle accident with intrusion into the passenger compartment increases the likelihood of pelvic, chest, shoulder and intraabdominal injury on the same side. These

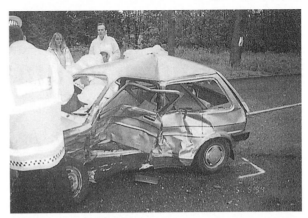

Figure 20.1 A "T-bone" impact

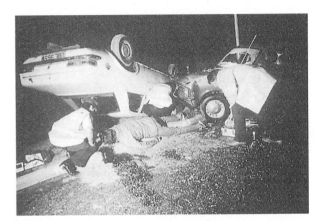

Figure 20.2 Ejection from a rollover accident

injuries tend to be caused by intrusion into the passenger compartment of the vehicle B-post (the post between the side doors) and door structures. Injury to the cervical spine is also possible in this type of incident (Figure 20.1). When examining wreckage, especially when assessing intrusion, it should always be remembered that the elastic nature of metallic structures may allow some rebound of the intruded metal after the impact. This may lead to an initial underestimation of the actual degree of intrusion on impact.

Ejection from the vehicle in a road traffic accident increases the likelihood that the patient has sustained spinal cord and other serious injuries (Figure 20.2) and is associated with a threefold increase in mortality rate. Death of another occupant of the vehicle implies that the live patient has been subject to a high-energy collision and is therefore at risk of major injury even if injuries are not immediately apparent.

> Entrapment for over 15 minutes is associated with an increased magnitude of injury severity

Rollover incidents tend to be associated with an increase in cervical spine injuries. This is consistent with the forceful lateral bending and flexion-extension forces involved and the increased likelihood of axial loading of the spine.

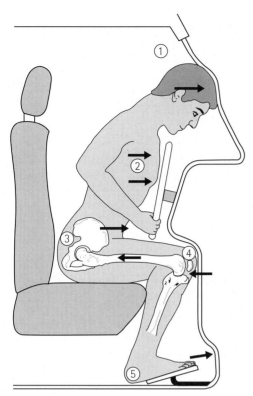

Figure 20.3 Frontal impact injuries. 1, head and neck injuries; 2, chest injuries; 3, posterior hip dislocation; 4, knee injuries; 5, foot and ankle injuries with entrapment

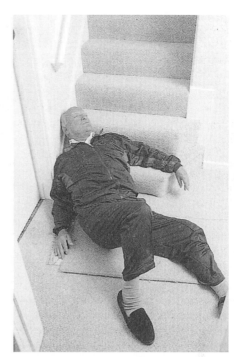

Figure 20.4 The elderly are at risk of significant injury from simple household accidents

In head-on collisions, the unrestrained driver will travel forwards at the same velocity as the vehicle until he impacts the steering column, windscreen and dashboard. The steering column tends to be forced upwards towards the windscreen on impact, so the chest, neck and face are commonly injured. Windscreen impact injuries tend to cause hyperextension to the neck, as well as axial loading to the cervical spine, and dashboard injuries commonly injure the knees, femurs and hips.

The restrained driver will normally be spared the majority of the above injuries but facial injuries from the steering wheel are common, as are "seatbelt injuries" to the clavicles, sternum and ribs. Even with seatbelt restraint, intrusion of wreckage, especially the dashboard and floorpan around the feet, can still cause major lower limb injuries (Figure 20.3). The introduction of driver and passenger airbags has undoubtedly enhanced the protection of vehicle front-seat occupants. Used with seatbelts, airbags will prevent many of the facial and neck injuries mentioned above.

Rear-end collisions are associated with cervical spine injury through the "whiplash" mechanism. Although in impacts at lower speed this is likely to take the form of ligamentous sprain, the possible increased risk of fractures due to forced hyperflexion and extension must be remembered and the spine immobilized.

Pedestrians struck by cars may sustain a variety of injuries. The initial contact is usually with the vehicle's bumper against the patient's knees. This may produce fractures or,

more commonly, ligament injury at the knee. In high-speed collisions the patient may then be thrown onto the bonnet of the car and often extends his arm to protect himself. This results in upper limb injury with fracture or dislocation. Finally, the pedestrian's head may strike the windscreen with resultant major head or cervical spine injury. The degree of injury will be proportional to the speed at which the vehicle was travelling.

> **Consider taking Polaroid photographs of the scene for A&E staff**

FALLS FROM A HEIGHT

Falls from a height inevitably involve sudden deceleration on impact. The distance of the fall, type of surface contacted and anatomical points of impact will determine the injury pattern.

Most adult falls involve lower limb fractures, often including the calcaneum, femur and, by transmitted force, the pelvis. Lower limb injury is commonly bilateral although the patient may only complain of pain in one limb. The spine, in particular the lumbar and thoracic areas, is frequently affected, often with multiple crush fractures of the vertebral bodies. The narrowness of the spinal canal in the thoracic area makes cord injury at this level more likely.

Even trivial falls may cause serious injury in the elderly, particularly where disease has rendered the patient vulnerable to injury. The elderly man who falls down two or three stairs and strikes his forehead on the ground may hyperextend his relatively rigid cervical spine enough to produce a fracture (Figure 20.4).

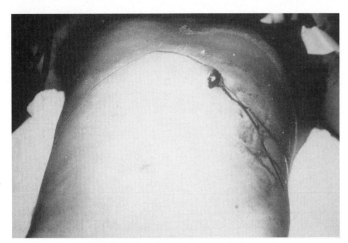

Figure 20.5 An epigastric stab wound

PENETRATING TRAUMA

Penetrating injuries from knife and bullet wounds are becoming more common in UK prehospital care practice.

Knife wounds cause direct injury in the direction of blade penetration. The damage depends on the length of the blade and the degree of penetration. Knife wounds to the neck and chest may be particularly dangerous owing to the presence of important blood vessels and organs. Wounds to the upper abdomen and the lower thorax are of concern, as the diaphragm may be penetrated and intrathoracic or intra-abdominal structures injured, remote from the entry wound. A wound in the epigastrium may penetrate the diaphragm, causing ventricular puncture and pericardial tamponade. A description of the type of knife is important to the hospital team in trying to ascertain the depth of penetration and the potential for injury to internal organs.

Civilian bullet wounds in the main tend to be from either a handgun or a shotgun. Lethal damage from these injuries depends largely on the anatomical area of injury and the type of projectile; for example, if a projectile breaks up during the first few centimetres of penetration it will cause increased tissue injury. The energy transferred from the missile along its wounding path will depend on the density and elasticity of the tissue. High-energy transfer is likely if the missile strikes bone. It is now conventional to talk in terms of high- and low-energy transfer rather than high- and low-velocity injury, as a high-velocity missile may still result in a low-energy transfer wound. With high-energy transfer, injury may occur some distance away from the bullet's entry wound, which is a result of "temporary cavitation" (see Chapter 30).

BLAST INJURIES

Six patterns of injury are commonly associated with explosions (Figure 20.6).

- Primary blast injury: the shock wave
- Secondary blast injury: injuries from flying debris

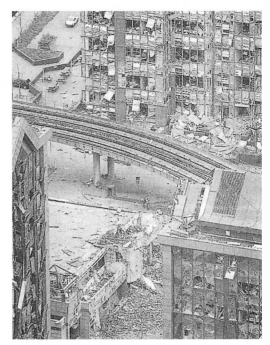

Figure 20.6 A London bomb incident

- Tertiary blast injury: injuries due to the blast wind such as amputations
- Crush injury
- Burns
- Psychological trauma.

Primary blast injuries are those caused by the blast wave arising directly from the explosion. Secondary injuries arise from fragmentation (the bomb casing or environmental fragments carried by the blast wind). Tertiary injuries arise from the direct effect of the blast wind on the body; either the whole body may be projected, striking surrounding furniture or buildings, or exposed parts are amputated. Flash burns arise from the intense, short-lived heat of the explosion. Where there is an explosion in a confined space there may be additional crush injury from falling masonry. Psychological injury should also be anticipated, which may not be confined to those with physical injury or even those exposed to the blast – carers are also vulnerable.

Primary injury commonly causes damage to the ears, lungs and gastrointestinal tract. The injuries to the lung range from pinpoint haemorrhages to massive intrapulmonary haemorrhage ("blast lung"). Secondary blast injuries are directly related to the types of flying debris and the sites of penetration. Tertiary injuries depend on many factors including the position of the casualty in relation to the blast. Flash burns tend to affect those nearest to the site of the explosion and will burn exposed areas of skin (often hands and face). Blast injury can therefore produce a variety of injuries, which are considered in greater detail in Chapter 30.

Chapter 21

The primary and secondary survey

CHAPTER CONTENTS

ASSESSMENT OF THE SCENE

Prior to any assessment of the patient at the accident scene (Figure 21.1), personal safety, scene safety and the availability of sufficient personnel and equipment should be established (see Chapter 1).

- Are additional ambulances required?
- Is the scene safe from hazards, are emergency vehicles parked safely and is the necessary equipment accessible?
- Are the fire and rescue services required?
- Is medical assistance needed?

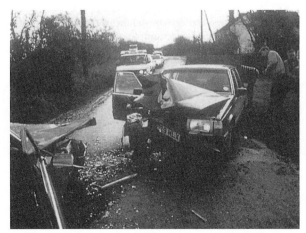

Figure 21.1 A typical road traffic accident

The scene must be assessed in order to determine casualty numbers and to establish the mechanisms involved in the accident, while the casualties are assessed for priority of intervention and evacuation.

ASSESSMENT OF THE PATIENT

The initial assessment requires basic clinical competence and, most importantly, a methodology which can be applied consistently and in priority order.

> Initial patient assessment is the most important clinical skill possessed by an ambulance paramedic or technician

The trauma patient often has more than one immediately life-threatening condition. A structured approach to assessment and management is necessary if injuries are to be detected and treated with the correct priority. The Advanced Trauma Life Support® and Prehospital Trauma Life Support® courses use the simple premise that the condition with the greatest threat to life should be treated first. The initial phase of assessment and management of the patient is termed the *primary survey* and is a primary assessment of vital functions and management of any abnormalities which are found.

> The primary survey is designed to identify life-threatening injuries

The *secondary survey* is a methodical assessment of the patient designed to detect all the patient's injuries, no matter how minor. This component of the initial assessment and management is rarely completed in prehospital care as it is difficult to fully expose and examine a patient and may introduce delays in reaching definitive care which will have an adverse effect on patient survival.

These procedures have their origins in trauma assessment, but the logical approach of the primary survey is equally appropriate to the assessment of the seriously ill as to the seriously injured patient.

The term "survey" wrongly implies assessment only. The primary survey is both an assessment *and* an immediate treatment procedure, assessing for threats to life associated with compromise to the airway, breathing, circulation and impaired conscious level.

> Primary Survey = Assessment + Management

PRIMARY SURVEY

A primary survey may be completed rapidly if there are no life-threatening injuries. The ability to converse normally with a patient demonstrates a normal airway, adequate breathing and circulation to the brain and an alert conscious level. However, the detection of major primary survey abnormalities may mean that it is impossible to complete the primary survey until after the patient arrives in hospital.

The primary survey sequence of airway (A) before breathing (B), which in turn precedes circulation (C), is dictated by the relative speed of the threat to life of each. Airway obstruction will cause death in a few minutes, breathing disruption will usually take a few additional minutes to cause death and circulatory compromise will take longer again. On that basis, immediate assessment and correction of any airway (A) problem, while protecting the cervical spine, is followed by assessment and correction of any breathing (B) compromise. Any circulatory deficit (C) found on circulatory assessment is then rectified. Next, the level of consciousness and pupil signs are assessed (D, disability), before proceeding to E (exposure and environment), once again looking for major injuries.

Thus the full structure of the primary survey is:

- airway, with cervical spine immobilization
- breathing, with oxygen
- circulation, with control of external haemorrhage
- disability – preliminary neurological examination
- expose and environment.

> Trauma patients found to have a major problem in the primary survey require immediate removal to an appropriate hospital facility

Patients with significant trauma require immediate evacuation to hospital. Highly organized on-site care is essential. The aim is to prepare the patient for departure from the scene in *10 minutes* from the ambulance's arrival. This imposes enormous demands on both the paramedic and technician and to achieve this takes teamwork and practice.

"SCOOP AND RUN"

For many years there has been debate over the length of time that should be spent treating a patient at the scene of an accident and the complexity of the treatment that should be given. Research on injured patients has consistently demonstrated that the survival rate is increased if the time taken to reach definitive care in hospital is short. This is reflected in the modern "scoop and run" method which incorporates:

- airway and cervical spine protection
- breathing assessment and support
- arrest of major external haemorrhage
- immobilization on a long spinal board (where appropriate)
- rapid evacuation to an appropriate hospital
- cannulation en route.

This rapid evacuation of critical patients is not to be confused with what has previously been implied by "scoop and run". To succeed, it requires impeccable airway care and ventilatory support. Arrest of major external haemorrhage and basic splintage of major long bone fractures have also to be achieved. If there is evidence of, or the mechanism of injury suggests, the possibility of spinal injury, the patient is then secured, with cervical collar, head restraints and straps, to a long spinal board and removed to the ambulance. Infusion and any further resuscitation measures may be performed en route to hospital *but must not delay evacuation of the patient*. The paramedic should also warn the hospital of the impending arrival of the seriously injured patient so that an appropriate team of medical and nursing staff can be assembled.

Whilst patients with life-threatening injuries need rapid transport to hospital, when no primary survey abnormality is detected a more thorough assessment (secondary survey) and additional treatment prior to transport may be indicated.

> On-site medical support is useful in dealing with entrapped patients with significant injuries in order to supervise difficult patient assessments and to institute analgesia and other therapy

PERFORMING THE PRIMARY SURVEY

The primary survey and resuscitation permit identification of life-threatening conditions and their simultaneous treatment.

AIRWAY AND CERVICAL SPINE

Assessment

Any injury severe enough to compromise the airway may also damage the cervical spine. It should always be assumed that the cervical spine is injured (unless the mechanism of injury clearly and definitively excludes the possibility) and it must be protected from movement during airway interventions and transport. Causes of airway obstruction include:

- tongue prolapse
- foreign bodies
- vomit
- major facial injury.

Obstruction of the airway may be complete or partial and direct, for example by vomit, or secondary to impaired consciousness, for example in head injury. Obstruction may occur at any level from the mouth and nose to the trachea.

Complete obstruction of the airway will manifest as an absence of breathing. Partial obstruction causes noisy breathing with hypoxia being manifested as an alteration in mental state and the late development of cyanosis.

Management

If complete or partial airway obstruction is identified it must be rectified as rapidly as possible without endangering the cervical spine. This involves a series of stepped airway interventions of increasing complexity until obstruction is relieved. The mouth is inspected and any foreign material removed with a finger sweep, suction device or on occasions a Magill's forceps. A simple airway manoeuvre is applied to pull the tongue away from the wall of the pharynx. The jaw thrust is preferred since it produces less cervical spine movement than the chin lift. Head tilt should not be used if there is any risk of cervical spine injury. Next, an airway adjunct such as an oral or nasal airway is inserted. Finally if airway obstruction persists an endotracheal tube should be inserted if possible. Each intervention is followed by reassessment of the airway.

In a small number of patients, an effective airway can only be established by the use of needle cricothyrotomy or a formal surgical airway. Following cricothyrotomy (Chapter 7), high-flow oxygen (15 litres/minute) is directed through the cannula into the trachea. Build-up of carbon dioxide limits the use of this technique to about 20–30 minutes. A formal surgical airway, in which an incision is made into the trachea and an endotracheal tube or tracheostomy tube is inserted, can only be performed by a doctor but with a cuffed tube it provides, like oral endotracheal intubation, a definitive protected airway.

In a small group of patients obstruction will be particularly difficult to relieve. These patients have their jaw clamped tightly shut. In this situation a nasal airway will be of benefit and occasionally the patient will relax after the

---

Box 21.1 Stepped airway care

1. Airway clearance – manual and aspiration
2. Manual airway opening manoeuvres
3. Jaw thrust
4. Oropharyngeal airway
5. Nasopharyngeal airway
6. Orotracheal intubation
7. Cricothyroid transtracheal jet insufflation
8. Definitive surgical airway (performed by a doctor)

---

administration of high-flow oxygen, but relief of obstruction will require the use of muscle relaxant drugs by an anaesthetist in order to allow intubation. Expeditious transfer to hospital is required in these cases.

Once the airway is secure, neck immobilization must continue with the application of a correctly sized semi-rigid cervical collar and head immobilization device. The patient must subsequently be fully immobilized on a long spinal board with at least four body straps. This is best achieved immediately before transfer to the ambulance after the primary survey. Restless patients should only be fitted with a semi-rigid collar, since full immobilization may only exacerbate movement in the cervical spine if the rest of the body is flailing. If the history conclusively excludes the possibility of a spinal injury, immobilization is not necessary. Routine immobilization, whatever the cause of the injury, is inappropriate, wastes time and delays arrival in hospital.

BREATHING

Assessment

Before examining the chest, an examination of the neck is essential. This is best performed before the cervical collar is in place. The following should be sought.

- Swelling
- Surgical emphysema
- Tracheal deviation
- Neck vein distension
- Bruising
- Lacerations.

Limited continuing observation of the neck is possible through the "window" in the front of the collar.

> **Clearing the airway does not assure adequate ventilation**

Breathing must be assessed for rate, adequacy and equal bilateral ventilation of the lungs. The chest must be visualized in order to assess movement, instability, flail segment and any wounds. The chest wall must be felt to detect surgical emphysema, tenderness from rib fractures and paradoxical movement. Percussion bilaterally may reveal one-sided hyperresonance over a large pneumothorax. Finally,

Box 21.2 Life-threatening breathing problems (ATOMIC)

- Airway obstruction (intrathoracic)
- Tension pneumothorax
- Open chest injury
- Massive haemothorax
- Flail chest
- Cardiac tamponade

auscultation for the presence of breath sounds bilaterally must be performed. It is essential to remember that the aim of the primary survey is to identify life-threatening problems.

Distress, confusion and abnormally rapid or slow respiratory rate are alarming signs and the patient may require assisted ventilation.

Management

Management of spontaneous ventilation in any patient with significant trauma requires the provision of supplemental oxygen, with a non-rebreathing reservoir mask and an oxygen flow rate of 10–15 litres per minute.

In adults, a respiratory rate of less than 10/min or more than 30/min suggests significant ventilatory inadequacy. Inadequate ventilation demands assisted ventilation. This is most easily performed using a bag–valve–mask and reservoir device, with oxygen supplied at a minimum of 10 litres per minute.

Explanation to the patient, where appropriate, is followed by supplementing the patient's respiratory rate and volume. The self-inflating bag may be emptied to a maximum of 500–700 ml, preferably with a two-handed technique, and at a rate of 10 breaths per minute. This will achieve an acceptable minute volume of about 5–7 litres.

Formal intermittent positive pressure ventilation with bag and mask or endotracheal tube may be necessary in the event of respiratory arrest. A time-cycled, pressure-limited mechanical ventilator may also be useful, especially for longer transfers. Care must be taken to assess for any indication of airway obstruction or loss of patency in transit. Continued vigilance for adequacy of ventilation is essential.

Displacement of an endotracheal tube in transit, or development of tension pneumothorax secondary to positive pressure ventilation, may occur at any time. The use of pulse oximetry and end-tidal CO_2 monitors can assist greatly in transit but repeated auscultation is essential.

Tension pneumothorax may be present during initial assessment or appear secondary to positive pressure ventilation, where a simple, undetected pneumothorax is expanded by the pressure of the ventilating gases. It is characteristically detected by the combination of rapidly increasing breathlessness and unilaterally absent breath sounds. Hyperresonance on percussion of the affected hemithorax, raised and congested neck veins and hypotension are frequently noted. Finally, cyanosis and tracheal shift away from

the affected side complete the picture of this extreme respiratory emergency.

Increasing resistance to ventilation and unilaterally reduced breath sounds in a ventilated patient should alert the paramedic to a possible tension pneumothorax, once a right mainstem bronchus intubation has been excluded. Immediate decompression using needle thoracocentesis is required. This procedure is discussed in Chapter 24.

Open chest wounds must be covered with an Asherman seal or occlusive dressing sealed on three sides.

Massive haemothorax is best managed in the prehospital environment by expeditious evacuation to hospital where a chest drain can be inserted. Intravenous access can be achieved en route. Needle thoracocentesis is not indicated in haemothorax unless there is a possibility of coincident tension pneumohaemothorax.

Patients with significant flail chest may require ventilatory support; apart from this, simple support to the flail segment is the only treatment necessary pending arrival in hospital. Unless there is a penetrating wound in the appropriate area, cardiac tamponade is extremely difficult to diagnose prehospital. Unless a doctor is present (who may perform an emergency thoracotomy or needle pericardiocentesis), the patient's only hope is rapid evacuation to hospital.

CIRCULATION

The circulatory assessment relies on simple clinical parameters.

- Skin colour
- Skin temperature
- Pulse rate and volume
- Capillary refill time (normal less than 2 seconds)
- Mental state
- Assess the thorax, abdomen, pelvis and femurs for evidence of injury and consequent concealed haemorrhage (think "blood on the floor and four more").

Pale, cool skin, tachycardia, delayed capillary return and altered mental state indicate significant shock. Hypotension frequently is not apparent until at least 30% of the blood volume has been lost.

> Shock is a disorder of the circulation characterized by reduced organ perfusion and tissue oxygenation

Management

Any external blood loss should be arrested by the application of direct pressure. Pelvic and long-bone fractures should be rapidly immobilized. Unless the patient is trapped or the transfer time is likely to be very long, intravenous access should be obtained in transit. In general, there is nothing to be gained from taking blood samples prehospital, although it may occasionally be useful if there is a very prolonged entrapment and specific local protocols involving the hospital laboratories are in place.

Fluid administration in trauma remains a very controversial area. In general, a policy of hypotensive resuscitation should be followed. As long as the patient has a palpable radial pulse (indicative of renal perfusion), fluid should not be given (although access should still be obtained during transit unless the transit time is very short). If the radial pulse is not palpable, small aliquots of 250 ml of normal saline (or a similar crystalloid) should be given until a palpable pulse returns and repeated to maintain it. Under no circumstances, however, should any of these actions delay transfer to hospital since patients who are actively bleeding require urgent life-saving surgical intervention. Elevation of the blood pressure above the level of 90 mmHg may precipitate rebleeding as well as diluting clotting factors and result in a worse prognosis.

DISABILITY

The accident scene rarely provides the opportunity for detailed assessment of neurological status. A quick neurogical examination is used, comprising an assessment of responsiveness and an assessment of pupil size and reactions. The AVPU mnemonic should be used.

A is the patient **a**lert?
V is the patient responding to **v**erbal stimuli?
P is the patient responding to **p**ainful stimuli?
U is the patient **u**nresponsive?

The responses are recorded and form the baseline for ongoing observation. The pupil sizes and their reaction to light should also be assessed.

An initial Glasgow Coma Score (GCS) (see Chapter 22) can be used to provide a similar baseline against which subsequent improvement or deterioration can be judged, but the GCS is complex, less easy to perform and slower. It is best suited for used in the resuscitation room and beyond.

An AVPU response of P or U is an indication for serious concern due to the likelihood of significant intracranial injury.

EXPOSE AND ENVIRONMENT

Complete exposure of the patient is impractical in the pre-hospital environment and will potentially render the patient hypothermic. The chest and neck area are exposed as part of the primary survey. If critical problems are found during the primary survey and not immediately resolved, the patient needs rapid transport to a major receiving hospital unit.

If, during the primary survey, the patient deteriorates, the paramedic must return to airway reassessment and once the airway is cleared proceed to breathing, then circulation. If the paramedic follows this procedure meticulously, no critical cause of sudden deterioration will be missed. If the patient deteriorates at any point, it is *essential* to return to A of the primary survey and to reassess the patient in the normal sequence. The temptation, for example, to *"go directly to B"* if the patient becomes short of breath or C if the patient develops a tachycardia *must* be resisted.

E in the primary survey is a rapid "all-over" assessment for life-threatening or serious injuries. It must not be confused with the secondary survey which is a detailed head-to-toe assessment designed to ensure that *every* injury is identified.

> E picks up life-threatening or serious injuries

THE SECONDARY SURVEY

The secondary survey is the more detailed head-to-toe examination designed, as stated above, to identify every injury the patient has sustained. In the vast majority of cases, the secondary survey will be performed after the primary survey has been repeated in hospital. Under no circumstances should the performance of a secondary survey delay transfer of a patient to hospital. In prolonged transfers a secondary survey may occasionally be appropriate (Figure 21.2). There is an ordered approach to this survey, as in the primary survey, so it can be rapidly performed to minimize time at the scene.

Patients initially assessed as non-critical may deteriorate from occult "primary survey" injury and a degree of urgency must be maintained during the secondary survey.

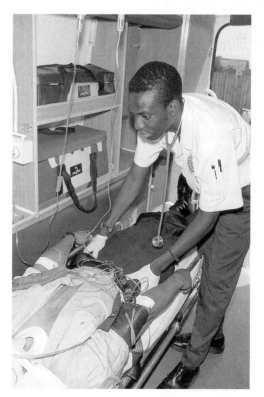

Figure 21.2 The secondary survey

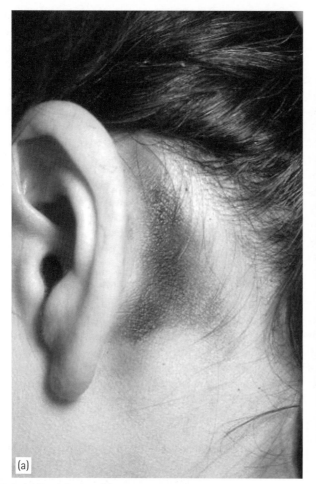 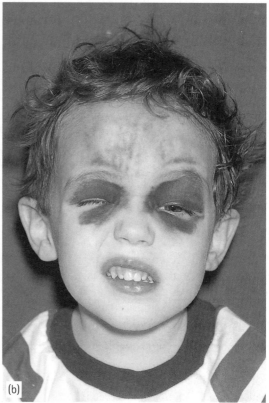

Figure 21.3 (a) Battle's sign; (b) raccoon or panda eyes

PERFORMING THE SECONDARY SURVEY

A "look, feel and listen" technique is used throughout.

Assessment of the head

Look for:

1. lacerations
2. bruising
3. blood and/or cerebrospinal fluid from ears or nose (suggesting basal skull fracture)
4. check pupil size and response
5. battle's sign and "raccoon" or panda eyes (Figure 21.3)
6. pallor and sweating
7. cyanosis.

Battle's sign and raccoon or panda eyes (Figure 21.3) suggest basal skull fracture although they usually only appear some hours after injury.

Feel for:

1. scalp haematomas
2. depressed skull fractures
3. facial tenderness and fractures.

Listen for:

1. airway "noise" suggesting obstruction
2. breathing adequacy and rate.

Assessment of the neck

To assess the neck, the collar may need to be removed while a colleague maintains in-line immobilization of the neck.

Look and feel for:

1. lacerations
2. swelling
3. surgical emphysema – skin "crackling"
4. distension of neck veins
5. spinal deformity, tenderness or haematoma
6. tracheal deviation.
7. largyngeal crepitus.

Assessment of the chest

Look for:

1. wounds and evidence of penetrating injury
2. deformity and abnormal movements

3. breathing distress and pain on inspiration.
4. patterning from clothing or seatbelts.

Feel for:

1. tenderness
2. instability and "clunking" of flail segment
3. surgical emphysema.

Listen for:

1. percussion revealing increased resonance over a pneumothorax or stony dullness over a haemothorax
2. presence of equal breath sounds
3. unilateral absence or reduction of breath sounds suggestive of pneumothorax
4. unilateral, usually basal reduction of breath sounds associated with haemothorax (only if the patient is sitting up).

Assessment of the abdomen

Look for:

1. penetrating wounds and contusions
2. seatbelt contusions and clothing imprints
3. distension.

Feel for:

1. tenderness – either localized or generalized
2. guarding – involuntary muscle spasm on gentle palpation
3. rigidity.

Assessment of the pelvis

Feel for:

1. tenderness and instability from gentle bilateral and anteroposterior compression. If this has already been performed as part of the primary survey, it should not be repeated. Information can be obtained from radiographs after arrival in hospital.

Assessment of lower and upper extremities

Look for:

1. obvious wounds and contusions
2. deformity and swelling associated with fractures
3. voluntary movement.

Feel for:

1. tenderness and deformity
2. distal pulses

3. intact nerve supply – sensation to touch and pain, motor function
4. normal movement in joints.

On completion of the secondary survey, any injuries which are found should be stabilized and any wounds covered.

The patient's condition is monitored frequently during this continued assessment in order to detect any deterioration and if it becomes critical, the survey is abandoned and the patient moved rapidly to an appropriate receiving hospital while undergoing resuscitation.

It cannot be overemphasized that the secondary survey must not be confused with the E of the primary survey. Major or life-threatening peripheral injuries are identified in E while a formal assessment of the totality of the patient's injuries comprises the secondary survey.

CONCLUSION

This process of primary and secondary surveys allows an organized, methodical and rapid assessment of a trauma patient. The patient's condition can be assessed by the findings of the primary survey into critical or non-critical and a decision to go immediately to hospital reached in the first few minutes at the scene.

The secondary survey allows a methodical assessment of the complete range of injuries. In the vast majority of situations the secondary survey should be left until after the patient has arrived in hospital. The key to effective life-saving trauma management is a rapid and organized primary survey. THINK ABCDE! Any deterioration during the primary or secondary survey necessitates a rapid return to airway assessment and rechecking of all the primary survey assessments and interventions in the ABCDE order.

> If the patient deteriorates at any point in the primary or secondary survey, check: Airway, breathing, circulation and disability Reassess these functions and your interventions

These procedures need practice every day and are a good approach to any trauma and many medical emergencies. Unpractised, they will not come readily to hand when they are most needed.

Chapter 22

Shock

CHAPTER CONTENTS

INTRODUCTION

Shock is a clinical syndrome which is defined as *"inadequate tissue perfusion resulting* in *hypoxia and ultimately in cell death"*. Thus the professional's use of the term "shocked" is very different from, and much more specific than, the lay understanding of the term "shocked" which is used to describe the psychological effects of a traumatic experience.

Shock can be classified according to the mechanism by which it occurs.

- *Hypovolaemic shock* due to loss of circulating volume. Causes include: blood loss, burns and diarrhoea and vomiting
- *Cardiogenic shock* due to loss of normal cardiac function ("pump failure"). Causes include: myocardial ischaemia, infarction, contusion, cardiac tamponade, massive pulmonary embolism
- *Septic shock* due to dilation of blood vessels by substances released in overwhelming infection. Causes include: bacterial viral or fungal infection
- *Neurogenic shock* due to dilation of blood vessels caused by spinal injury
- *Anaphylactic shock* due to dilation of blood vessels as part of a severe allergic reaction.

By far the most common cause of shock in the prehospital environment is hypovolaemia (inadequate blood volume), usually related to blood or plasma loss from trauma, ruptured aortic aneurysm, ectopic pregnancy or gastro-intestinal haemorrhage. Less common causes of shock are discussed later in this chapter.

> The most common treatable cause of shock in prehospital care is hypovolaemia

HYPOVOLAEMIC SHOCK

It is important that clinicians are aware of the compensatory mechanisms and pathological responses in hypovolaemia in order to understand the clinical signs and symptoms that occur as shock progresses. The discussion below refers to shock from hypovolaemia because this is the most common clinical scenario in prehospital care.

SHOCK: PATHOLOGY AND COMPENSATORY MECHANISMS

There are many physiological responses which can compensate for blood loss in a healthy individual in order to maintain oxygen delivery and organ perfusion. These mechanisms involve a number of body systems. The pathological processes that occur when the body can no longer compensate for further blood loss are described at organ and cellular level.

Cardiovascular system

The cardiac output is the volume of blood that is pumped around the body every minute. If the total circulating blood volume decreases (because of blood loss), tissue and organ perfusion can only be maintained by the heart working harder to increase the cardiac output. This may be achieved by two mechanisms. First, the quantity of blood ejected by the heart with each cardiac cycle (the stroke volume) can increase. If the amount of blood ejected with each beat falls, the number of beats each minute must increase in order to maintain the same cardiac output. Second, the heart rate can increase in response to sympathetic stimulation, with systemic release of adrenaline and noradrenaline from the adrenal glands and sympathetic nerve endings throughout the vascular system.

> **Cardiac output = Stroke volume × heart rate**

These compensatory mechanisms do have limits. At a critical level the heart muscle reaches the point where each fibre is stretched maximally, further compensation is impossible and the heart begins to fail. Furthermore, the heart rate cannot rise indefinitely. The relaxation or diastolic phase of the cardiac cycle is essential to allow filling of the ventricles and hence "prime" the cardiac pump. With extreme tachycardia the stroke volume is reduced and cardiac output drops. In addition, as the diastolic time decreases, the amount of oxygen reaching the myocardium via the coronary vessels falls, since diastole is the period during which blood enters the coronary circulation. As the heart continues to work in excess of its aerobic ability, anaerobic metabolism develops with the production of a lactic acidosis. This results in a reduction of the strength of myocardial contraction and pump failure.

Finally, if blood loss continues, the decreased venous return to the heart results in distortion of the cardiac chambers and activation of cardiac C-fibres. These cause vagal stimulation and slowing of the heart together with peripheral vasodilation, and a catastrophic (and usually terminal) fall in blood pressure ensues.

The state of the blood vessels into which the heart ejects its contents is also important. There is always a degree of resting tension in the walls of arteries. By increasing this tension under the control of the nervous system, the blood pressure can be maintained in hypovolaemia by effectively reducing the volume of the system. By selective activation of this system, blood can be redirected preferentially to vital organs by vasoconstriction in less important sites such as skin, gut and muscle. This mechanism acts to protect the heart, brain and kidneys, which can control their own blood supplies to a certain extent. The increase in arterial wall tension results from the action of receptors which detect falling blood volume, increasing blood acidity and rising arterial carbon dioxide levels ($PaCO_2$).

Respiratory system

Shock results in tissue hypoxia. The response to shock therefore includes a compensatory increase in the frequency and depth of respiration. This tachypnoeic response is controlled by the respiratory centre in the brain which receives input from peripheral nerves and receptors, which in turn measure blood acidity and carbon dioxide levels.

To improve the uptake of oxygen and excretion of carbon dioxide in the lungs, preferential vasoconstriction diverts pulmonary blood flow to areas of high alveolar oxygen concentration, thus improving the ventilation/perfusion ratio.

The oxygen-carrying capacity of the blood depends upon the haemoglobin concentration and its ability to bind with oxygen. The body has no immediate ability to increase haemoglobin concentration, so the mechanisms regulating oxygen-carrying capacity relate to changes in the affinity of the haemoglobin molecule for oxygen. Increases in acidity, $PaCO_2$ or temperature allow a greater release of oxygen to the cells for a given oxygen saturation.

A number of factors contribute to eventual inadequate ventilation and oxygen uptake by the lungs. A drop in venous return with continued blood loss results in a fall in right heart filling pressures, leading to reduced pulmonary blood flow and oxygen uptake. Anaerobic metabolism producing lactic acid within the respiratory muscles causes muscle fatigue and eventually respiratory failure. Central respiratory depression caused by direct head injury, hypotension or the effects of drugs (such as opioids) will also result in hypoventilation.

Other physiological responses to hypovolaemic shock

Two hormones are released in increased amounts in response to hypovolaemia: aldosterone from the adrenal gland and antidiuretic hormone (ADH) from the pituitary gland. These hormones act to maintain the circulating blood volume by reducing urine output.

The brain's blood supply is protected until late in the pathological process of worsening shock. Eventually, however, autoregulation and preferential supply cannot preserve cerebral perfusion pressure any longer. Once cerebral hypoxia occurs, a downward spiral of events ensues. Vasoconstriction of the reticular formation (that part of the brain concerned with level of consciousness) in some patients leads to marked agitation and apprehension, but as the process continues, central stimulation of the respiratory centre is lost, resulting in hypoventilation and therefore worsening organ oxygenation. Vasomotor and cardiac centres

---

Box 22.1 Compensatory mechanisms in shock

- Tachycardia
- Peripheral vasoconstriction (with diversion of blood to vital organs)
- Increase in frequency and depth of respiration
- Diversion of blood within the lungs to areas of maximal gas exchange
- Increased release of oxygen from haemoglobin
- Reduced urine output (mediated by aldosterone and ADH)

are also depressed, causing slowing of the heart rate and peripheral vasodilation. Accumulation of lactic acid and other waste products of metabolism within cerebral neurones results in depression of the conscious level, and finally coma.

Like the brain, the kidneys are able to regulate their own blood supply during the initial stages of shock. As a consequence renal blood flow is maintained despite falling perfusion. However, as with other organs, a critical period is reached when continued constriction of the renal vessels (increase in vessel wall tension) causes a reduction in renal perfusion and consequently a reduction in function evident by falling urine output.

CLINICAL FEATURES OF HYPOVOLAEMIC SHOCK

The common clinical features of hypovolaemic shock are listed in Box 22.2. It will be seen that they reflect the pathological and compensatory changes discussed above.

In an adult, the normal circulating blood volume is 7% of the *lean* body mass. In an average patient weighing 70–75 kg the total circulating blood volume will be about 5000–5500 ml. In children the blood volume is proportionately greater: 8–9% of body weight or 80–90 ml/kg (see Chapter 35).

Box 22.2 Clinical features of shock

- Tachycardia (arrhythmias may develop)
- Change in blood pressure (initially reduced pulse pressure, later lowered systolic and diastolic pressures)
- Altered mental state
- Tachypnoea
- Cool, clammy skin
- Cyanosis
- Oliguria

Knowledge of the clinical signs and symptoms of shock in a trauma patient is essential to enable resuscitative measures to begin at an appropriate time. The clinical features of hypovolaemia depend upon the magnitude of circulating volume loss. However, these features can act only as general guides and have major limitations, especially in the prehospital setting where advanced monitoring and investigational facilities are unavailable.

CLASSIFICATION OF HAEMORRHAGIC SHOCK

To assist in the assessment of the severity of haemorrhagic shock the symptoms and signs can be subdivided into four grades depending on the extent of circulating volume lost (Table 22.1). This will vary depending on the patient's previous medical and drug history (see below). The extent and severity of soft tissue injury will also affect the degree of interstitial fluid formation and will decrease the accuracy of this classification, as a sizeable part of the soft tissue swelling is fluid that has leaked from the vascular compartment.

The classification in Table 22.1 must be used *only as a guide*; precise estimation of blood loss will never be possible. An easy way to remember the percentage losses is to compare them to the scores in tennis (love-fifteen, fifteen-thirty, thirty-forty, game over).

There are a number of pitfalls in the assessment of the patient with hypovolaemic shock. The following factors must be taken into consideration.

- Age (the elderly are less able to compensate for volume loss)
- Fitness (athletes and fit individuals may compensate and hence have few signs or symptoms even with major losses)
- Medications (drugs such as β-blockers, antihypertensives and antianginals may mask normal responses such as tachycardia)
- Preexisting disease (patients with underlying conditions such as ischaemic heart disease, cerebrovascular disease and pregnancy are less able to cope with the effects of shock).

Table 22.1 Classification of hypovolaemic shock (adult)

Grade	Blood loss	Symptoms	Urine output
Grade I	Up to 750 ml <15%	Minimal Blood pressure unchanged Occasionally tachycardia occurs	Normal
Grade II	750–1500 ml 15–30%	Pallor, tachycardia >100/min, decreased pulse pressure Subtle changes in mood may be seen e.g. anxiety, aggression or fright	Reduced to 20–30 ml/h
Grade III	1500–2000 ml 30–40% This is the minimum volume loss that results in a decrease in blood pressure	Classic signs of inadequate perfusion are usually noticed: pallor, sweating, altered mental state (anxiety, confusion, aggression), tachycardia >120/min, tachypnoea, hypotension	Reduced to 10–20 ml/h
Grade IV	Over 2000 ml Life-threatening and catastrophic	Pulse is weak and thready Tachycardia may deteriorate to bradycardia Systolic blood pressure drops markedly with a very narrow pulse pressure or unobtainable diastolic pressure Drowsiness, lethargy or unconsciousness	Negligible

- Age (the elderly are less able to compensate for volume loss)
- Fitness (athletes and fit individuals may compensate and hence have few signs or symptoms even with major losses)
- Medications (drugs such as beta-blockers, antihypertensives and antianginals may mask normal responses such as tachycardia)
- Pre-existing disease (patients with underlying conditions such as ischaemic heart disease, cerebrovascular disease and pregnancy are less able to cope with the effects of shock)

Figure 22.1 Groups with differing responses to shock

The elderly are less able to compensate for blood loss and may consequently have the signs associated with a higher grade of shock with lower blood loss. Conversely, the very fit may compensate for blood loss, concealing significant haemorrhage until the patient suddenly collapses in grade III or IV shock. A pulse of 95 beats/min may be normal in an elderly patient, but can represent severe vascular compromise in a marathon runner whose resting pulse is 40 beats/min.

It is important that time is not wasted in attempting to decide what grade of shock the patient may be in. All grades of shock will progress if the bleeding is not stopped. The only endpoint of uncontrolled bleeding is death. Every effort must be directed to identifying the presence or possibility of shock and to ensuring that it is controlled either by simple prehospital measures or by urgent surgery.

Medications (especially β-blockers which slow down the pulse) may mask the normal responses to shock, such as tachycardia. The patient's previous medical history should always be considered during the assessment of shock. Patients with ischaemic heart disease, cerebrovascular disease and pregnancy are less able to cope with the effects of shock.

TREATMENT PRINCIPLES

Attention to simple, competently performed procedures executed in the shortest period of time and accompanied by rapid, safe evacuation of the patient to hospital is the key to success in the prehospital management of shock.

The concept that a patient can (or should) be "stabilized" at the scene before transfer to hospital is dangerously wrong. Except where delays are unavoidable because of geographical or environmental problems or entrapment, the delivery of the patient to hospital must never be delayed by interventions such as intravenous access or volume replacement.

Airway and breathing (A + B) on scene

The primary objective in the management of shock is to restore tissue perfusion, with the delivery of adequate oxygen and other metabolites. It should be recognized that only the start of this process will occur before the patient reaches hospital and that this phase of resuscitation is only the beginning of definitive treatment, which may require surgery or other interventions in hospital.

All shocked patients require the highest possible concentration of inspired oxygen delivered to the lungs. Except where a patient is known to have severe chronic obstructive pulmonary disease (COPD), every shocked or potentially shocked patient should be given high-flow oxygen by face mask. Even in cases of COPD and severe trauma the injured tissues require oxygen – a patient who truly has "hypoxic drive" and stops breathing can be ventilated. Clearance and maintenance of a patent upper and lower airway as detailed in Chapters 6 and 7 are mandatory. This may require the patient to be intubated and positive pressure ventilation commenced. Factors impeding ventilation, such as pneumothorax, haemothorax or gastric dilation, will require specific correction.

High-concentration oxygen saves lives

The C of the primary survey has four components.

- Identification of the patient at risk of shock
- Control of compressible haemorrhage
- Circulatory assessment
- Identification of sites of bleeding.

Identification of the patient who is at risk of injury likely to cause shock is the key first stage of the assessment of C. In the early stages, there may be no clinical signs. Unfortunately some of these patients will go on to develop severe shock from which some of them will die. It is essential, therefore, that whenever the severity or mechanism of injury suggests the possibility of severe or life-threatening haemorrhage, the patient is treated as if that bleeding had already been identified and that transfer to definitive care is not delayed.

Where there is an overt source of blood loss, such as an open wound, the affected part should be elevated and direct local pressure applied. Clamping or tying off arterial bleeding points should be avoided and in the majority of cases firm pressure will control external haemorrhage. On very rare occasions, the application of a tourniquet may be the only way to control life-threatening haemorrhage.

Circulatory assessment includes a general assessment of the patient for coldness, clammy skin and sweating as well as an assessment of the mental state. The pulse should be taken, looking for the rate and the quality of the pulse, but a formal measurement of the blood pressure can usually wait until the patient is in transit or has arrived in the resuscitation room. A reasonable idea of the adequacy of the circulation can be gained by checking for the presence of a radial pulse.

Once external bleeding has been identified and controlled, a brief attempt should be made to identify sites of *significant* internal bleeding. Potential sites of bleeding are:

- chest
- abdomen (and retroperitoneum)
- pelvis

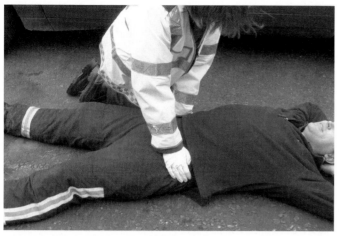

Figure 22.2 Compressing the pelvis to check for fracture

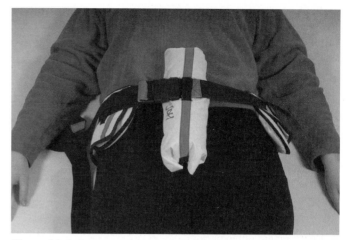

Figure 22.4 A commercial pelvic splint in place

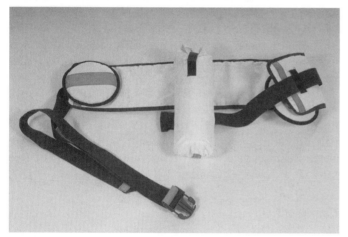

Figure 22.3 A commercial pelvic splint

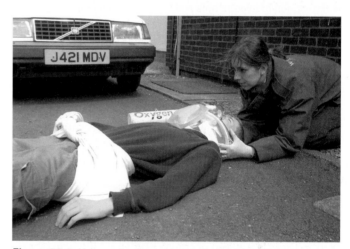

Figure 22.5 Using a sheet as an improvised pelvic splint

- long bones (usually from fractured femurs)
- external.

This is often referred to as "blood on the floor and four more".

Significant bleeding into the chest should have been identified during B of the primary survey. Gentle inspection of the abdomen for swelling and palpation for tenderness as well as a knowledge of the mechanism of injury may suggest intraabdominal bleeding. Retroperitoneal bleeding (into the tissues behind the abdominal cavity) cannot be identified clinically in the prehospital environment and is usually diagnosed by exclusion after arrival in hospital.

In order to identify bleeding from a fractured pelvis, the pelvis should be gently compressed. This involves applying a gentle lateral and then downward force to both anterior iliac spines. An unstable pelvis may be felt on performing this manoeuvre (Figure 22.2). This may exacerbate bleeding and should *never* be performed more than once. It may, however, identify an unstable pelvis associated with life-threatening bleeding and allow immediate treatment. The absence of pelvic instability on compression does not exclude a significant pelvic fracture. In the prehospital environment, the only effective treatment is to attempt to restore the bony continuity of the pelvis. This can be achieved by applying a commercial pelvic splint (Figures 22.3, 22.4) or by the improvised technique of "sheeting" the pelvis (Figure 22.5).

These techniques may be life saving. In partially restoring the continuity of the pelvic ring, they significantly reduce bleeding. They should not, however, be routinely used in the shocked patient but reserved for those patients with an identified unstable pelvis.

The combination of external haemorrhage and bleeding from an unstable pelvis is often known as compressible haemorrhage, as distinct from bleeding in the chest or abdomen which cannot be controlled by the application of pressure (non-compressible haemorrhage). The only way of controlling non-compressible haemorrhage is by urgent surgical intervention.

Major long bone bleeding must also be identified and splinted (see Chapter 27). Splintage not only reduces the pain experienced by the patient but also reduces blood loss from fracture sites by up to 50%. Unless splinted, of course, a leg with significant long bone fractures cannot be elevated!

Intravenous fluid therapy

It will have been noted that vascular access has not yet been discussed. The priorities in the management of shock are:

- identification of the patient at risk of significant bleeding
- identification of shock
- control of compressible haemorrhage
- urgent transfer to hospital for surgical intervention.

There has been a radical change in the use of fluids in shock. Until recently, it has been policy to encourage the vigorous administration of intravenous fluids. There is now increasing evidence that this is actually detrimental to the patient. There are a number of reasons for this.

- Displacement of blood clot
- Dilution of clotting factors
- Promotion of hypothermia and secondary metabolic derangement
- Delay in reaching surgery whilst attempts to gain intravenous access are made.

Equally, it is clearly not acceptable to allow patients to bleed to death! A compromise has to be reached. Therefore, where transfer times are short, the best course of action is immediate transfer to hospital without delay. A maximum of two attempts at intravenous access may be made in the ambulance en route to hospital.

> **Never delay definitive care whilst attempting intravenous access**

If the patient is trapped or transfer times are likely to be prolonged, vascular access should be achieved by the insertion of two intravenous cannulae into accessible peripheral veins (see Chapter 8). In many shocked patients, vascular access is difficult because of the combination of hypovolaemia with collapsed veins, venoconstriction and the problems of performing the technique in adverse conditions where cold, movement and poor lighting render the task difficult. Although, ideally, large-bore cannulae should be used, it is better to insert a small cannula successfully than to suffer repeated failures with large Venflons in small veins.

Once intravenous access has been achieved, intravenous crystalloid should be administered, in sufficient quantity to maintain the presence of a radial pulse. This equates to a blood pressure sufficient to perfuse the vital organs. This blood pressure and the limited amount of fluid which is administered mean that the likelihood of the complications listed above is reduced to a minimum. In the elderly, the presence of a radial pulse is likely to correlate with a higher blood pressure than in a fit young adult. However, a higher blood pressure will also be needed to perfuse the vital organs and as a consequence the radial pulse will still provide an effective monitor for fluid resuscitation.

If the radial pulse is absent, aliquots of 250 ml of crystalloid should be administered until it returns. If the radial

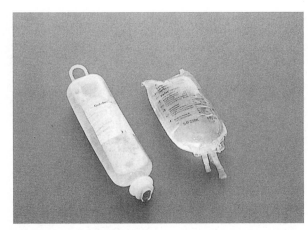

Figure 22.6 Intravenous fluids

pulse is lost, further aliquots should be given until it returns, with a brief pulse check between each. If the presence of a radial pulse cannot be achieved, in the circumstances of prolonged transfer or entrapment, survival is unlikely and vigorous fluid administration pending extrication and transfer to definitive care is the only option available.

Although popular in the 1970s and 1980s in North America, the use of military antishock trousers (MAST) or the pneumatic antishock garment (PASG) for lower limb or pelvic fractures or for hypovolaemic shock has not been shown to improve mortality or morbidity rates. Their use is rarely indicated (see Chapter 26).

Choice of fluid

Although it is the source of much debate, the arguments for choices of intravenous fluid used for volume restoration in shocked patients are based more on dogma than sound clinical evaluation. What is not in doubt is that, if fluids are given, they must contain sodium ions. This apart, a bewildering array of fluids are available, including crystalloids, colloids (Figure 22.6) and both isooncotic and hyperoncotic solutions.

As described above, it is standard practice in the UK to start intravenous volume replacement with isotonic crystalloid solutions such as 0.9% (normal) saline or sodium lactate (Hartmann's or Ringer lactate) solution. Despite the theoretical advantages of Hartmann's solution, no difference has been shown in terms of clinical efficacy. Both are cheap, easy to use, have long shelf-lives and do not cause anaphylactic reactions. Either is therefore suitable for the administration of 250 ml fluid aliquots although a recent expert working party has recommended the use of normal saline.

Colloid solutions available in the UK include gelatin solutions such as Haemaccel or Gelofusine, starch solutions such as hetastarch, dextran solutions such as dextran 70 and human plasma components such as 4.5% albumin and plasma protein fraction (PPF). All of these solutions are significantly more expensive than crystalloids. They all also

Box 22.3 Causes of cardiogenic shock

- Heart muscle (myocardial) dysfunction
  Ischaemia
  Infarction
  Contusion (blunt trauma)
- Cardiac tamponade
  Trauma
  Post infarction
- Pulmonary embolism

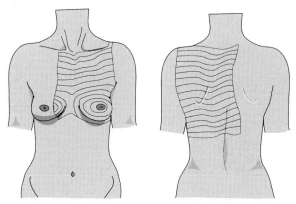

Figure 22.7 Penetrating wounds in the shaded area may be associated with cardiac tamponade

have a small but recognized risk of anaphylactic reaction. In the restoration of hypovolaemic shock, colloids are relatively more efficient volume for volume than crystalloid solutions. For crystalloids, a ratio of 3:1 for volume replacement to blood loss is normally required to reach an appropriate haemodynamic endpoint. For colloid solutions the ratio is nearer to 1:1. In addition, the colloid will stay within the circulation for a longer period. Depending on local protocol, colloid solutions may have a role in fluid therapy during prolonged transfers or in entrapment.

All fluid given should be warmed to 37°C to prevent the adverse effects of rapid infusion of cold fluid into a shocked patient. Boluses of cold fluid reaching the central circulation can cause cardiac arrhythmias, impair myocardial contractility and hence cardiac output, and impede normal blood coagulation.

Blood samples

Except in unusual circumstances, there is no point in taking blood samples from the patient before reaching hospital. The difficulties of patient identification and labelling and the dangers of potential mismatched blood transfusion almost always exceed the potential benefits. An exception to this rule may be where a patient is trapped and full identification of the patient can be made both for the purpose of blood sampling and subsequently if blood or other products are delivered to the scene for on-site management. However, even in this situation it is probably better to use universal donor (O Rh negative) blood rather than relying on the delays involved in blood grouping, crossmatching and then sending type-specific blood to the scene.

CARDIOGENIC SHOCK

Shock is inadequate tissue perfusion: this can also be caused by failure of the pump mechanism (the heart) which is called cardiogenic shock. By analogy, a central heating system can stop working because of a leak (hypovolaemia) or because the pump fails (cardiogenic shock).

Cardiogenic shock may be caused by failure of the heart muscle owing to ischaemia of the myocardium, myocardial infarction or contusion secondary to trauma. Rupture of the

heart following ischaemia or penetrating trauma will also result in cardiogenic shock, exacerbated by compression of the heart caused by blood within the pericardium (*cardiac tamponade*). Management of cardiac tamponade due to trauma is considered in Chapter 25. Massive pulmonary embolism prevents normal cardiac function and will also produce cardiogenic shock.

The most common cause of cardiogenic shock is myocardial infarction producing cardiac muscle or valve rupture. This results in a mortality rate greater than 90%.

Cardiogenic shock due to tamponade may occur as a result of blunt or penetrating trauma. In blunt trauma, the outlook is extremely poor and survival is extremely unlikely whatever interventions are attempted. This is, however, an extremely difficult diagnosis in the prehospital environment, where the only course of action must be immediate transfer to hospital for assessment. The clinical signs of cardiac tamponade are described in Chapter 25.

Cardiac tamponade due to penetrating trauma such as a stab wound may respond to aspiration of blood from the pericardium or thoracotomy, when the chest is opened and the hole in the heart is closed, either by the insertion of a finger, a catheter (with the balloon inflated) or a stitch. The possibility of tamponade should be considered with any penetrating injury in the at-risk area shown in Figure 22.7.

Thoracotomy or pericardiocentesis must be performed by an experienced doctor and is best undertaken in the A&E department rather than delaying departure from the scene whilst waiting for such a person to arrive. Vigorous fluid resuscitation will also be required in hospital; mortality has been shown to be increased where intravenous fluids are given prehospital following penetrating cardiac injury and the guidelines given above should be followed.

If the penetrating object is still in situ (Figure 22.8) it must be left there and carefully protected from dislodgement or movement during a rapid transfer to hospital.

Other causes of cardiogenic shock require only oxygen therapy and immediate evacuation for definitive treatment although symptomatic relief of associated symptoms such as chest pain should be given.

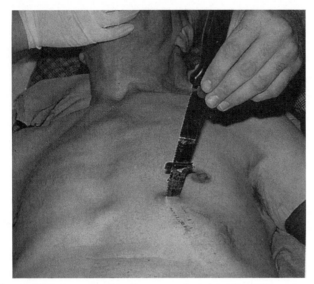

Figure 22.8 A penetrating chest wound resulting in cardiac tamponade

SEPTIC SHOCK

Septic shock results from the action of substances (mediators) released from cells as a consequence of severe infection (usually bacterial). Dilation of blood vessels, leakiness of tissue capillaries and a defect of oxygen utilization by the tissues produce shock. The normal regulation of blood flow to organs breaks down. The appropriate treatment for a patient with septic shock is investigation of the source of infection, intravenous antibiotics and intensive supportive care.

Septic shock usually takes some time to develop following the onset of infection. An exception is shock following suspected meningococcal infection (see Chapter 19) when the patient may progress from health to death within a few hours. In this situation benzylpenicillin should be given intravenously or intramuscularly as soon as the diagnosis is made. All cases of septicaemic shock require oxygen and IV fluids should be started if the transfer is likely to be delayed. No other prehospital treatment is required. Septicaemic shock is rare.

NEUROGENIC SHOCK

Neurogenic shock results from injury to the spinal cord. There is interruption of the nervous mechanism maintaining blood vessel wall tension; as a consequence vessels dilate and peripheral pooling of blood occurs, the effective circulating blood volume is reduced and shock ensues. Neurogenic shock is therefore not associated with cold peripheries, which are instead warm and well perfused. Additionally, the neurological interruption prevents a compensating tachycardia. *The hallmarks of neurogenic shock are hypotension, warm peripheries and bradycardia.*

Head injury never results in hypotension and shock due to spinal injury is rare. Shock in the trauma patient is far more likely to be due to unrecognized haemorrhage. Management priorities should be directed towards identifying and treating hypovolaemia in the shocked patient with a spinal injury. Thus the key to effective management is rapid safe transfer to definitive care.

> **Isolated head injury is not a cause of shock**

ANAPHYLACTIC SHOCK

Anaphylactic shock results from an allergic reaction to a foreign protein such as nuts, bee stings or drugs. The reaction is mediated by immunoglobulins and histamine and results in vasodilation and blood pooling, with reduced effective circulating volume and compensatory tachycardia (compare neurogenic shock). The clinical features and treatment of anaphylactic shock are considered in Chapter 11.

CONCLUSION

Shock is inadequate tissue perfusion. Untreated, it is progressive and leads inexorably to cell death, organ death and death of the patient. The most common cause of shock in prehospital care is bleeding due to trauma. Every effort must be made to identify the bleeding casualty or the casualty who is at risk of severe haemorrhage and, where possible, to arrest the bleeding. If haemorrhage cannot be arrested by compression, the only hope is immediate rapid transfer to hospital for definitive surgical intervention. This must not be delayed whilst attempts are made to gain intravenous access. If the patient is trapped or transfer times are long, fluid infusion must be judicious and calculated not to worsen the patient's condition. Otherwise, intravenous access can be attempted in transit.

Other causes of intravenous shock are less common, but there are likely to be important clinical clues suggesting the diagnosis. In these situations, immediate transfer to hospital with the supportive therapy discussed above is the key to improving patient survival.

FURTHER READING

Greaves I, Porter KM, Ryan JM (eds) 2001 The trauma manual. Arnold, London

Consensus Working Group on Prehospital Fluids 2001 Fluids in prehospital care: a consensus statement. Trauma 3: 4

Chapter 23

Head injuries

CHAPTER CONTENTS

INTRODUCTION

Head injury is a major cause of trauma death and disability. Fortunately, only a small proportion of head-injured patients will require urgent surgical intervention. All patients, however, will benefit from rapid assessment and correction of the abnormalities detected in the primary survey. The key to the optimal management of head-injured patients is the prevention of secondary brain damage by appropriate attention to the airway, breathing and circulation together with expedited transfer to hospital for those who are likely to require surgical intervention, investigation or intensive support.

ANATOMY

The brain is a soft, spongy organ with three main parts (Figure 23.1).

1. The right and left *cerebral hemispheres* forming the cerebrum. The cerebral hemispheres have different lobes. They are concerned with higher functions which include motor and sensory functions such as vision.
2. The *cerebellum* responsible for balance and coordination.
3. The *brainstem* consisting of the midbrain, pons and medulla. The medulla is continuous with the spinal cord. Vital centres controlling cardiac and respiration function are in the lower brainstem.

Various nerves arise from the brain, when they are known as *cranial nerves*, and from the spinal cord as *peripheral nerves*. These nerves supply motor and sensory function to various parts of the body.

Damage to nerve cells is permanent and recovery of central nervous system damage is not possible. Peripheral nerves do have some powers of recovery.

The cerebral hemispheres are responsible for motor and sensory function as well as vision and hearing. They are also responsible for the independent thought processes. The cerebral hemispheres have multiple folds which enlarge the surface area.

The midbrain has many pathways and cross-linkages. It tapers down to the brainstem, becoming continuous with the spinal cord. Because of its shape, swelling and increased intracranial pressure cause compression of the brain and tend to push it through the large hole in the base of skull, known as the *foramen magnum*.

The brain itself has a good blood supply, both internally and externally. However, some arteries are "end arteries" and there is no other blood supply to that area of the brain. Any damage to these arteries, in disease or injury, will lead to ischaemia, infarction and death of that area of the brain.

The coverings of the brain are known as the *meninges* (Figure 23.2). The innermost of these is the *pia mater,* a thin film adherent to the brain surface. Outside this is the *arachnoid* and surrounding the whole brain is the thick, rigid layer of fibrous tissue known as the *dura mater*. Between the pia mater and the arachnoid is a fluid-filled space containing

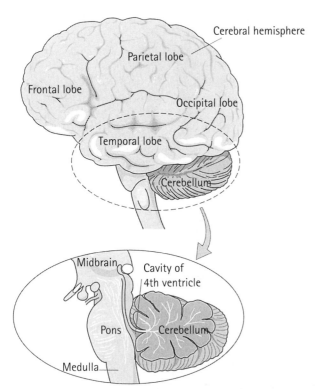

Figure 23.1 The brain

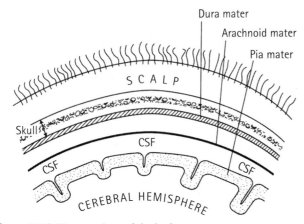

Figure 23.2 The coverings of the brain

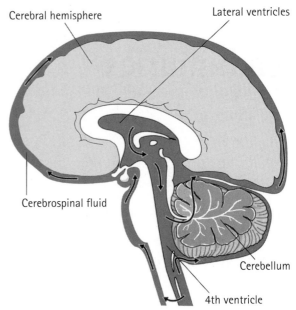

Figure 23.3 Transverse section of the brain showing the flow of cerebrospinal fluid (arrows)

cerebrospinal fluid (CSF). The brain is suspended, or floats, in this fluid, which acts as a shock absorber.

The cerebrospinal fluid is produced inside the brain from the choroid plexuses, mainly in the large lateral ventricles. The ventricular system and various passages (Figure 23.3) can be damaged by natural disease or by injury. This can produce internal swelling of the brain, known as *hydrocephalus*. Hydrocephalus causes a raised intracranial pressure, the treatment of which is CSF decompression through special catheters or shunts. From time to time these become blocked, leading to an altered conscious level. Such patients require emergency treatment.

Reflections of the dura mater form thick, fibrous folds known as *falces* (singular *falx*), which are firmly attached to the skull. Running from front to back is a vertical fold

between the two cerebral hemispheres – the *falx cerebri*. At 90° to this is a transverse horizontal fold separating the cerebral hemispheres and the cerebellum. This partially surrounds the rear of the brain and is called the *tentorium cerebelli*. These fibrous folds act as baffles and hold the brain in position while it is suspended in the cerebrospinal fluid. Large venous sinuses lie between the dural layers and bleed if they are torn.

The skull itself is a rigid box. The cranium is an expanded dome and the wall of the skull is of an uneven thickness. The base or floor of the skull is tiered with numerous ridges and bumps. Any twisting or deceleration injury can cause damage to the undersurface of the brain against these bumps and ridges. Parts of the skeleton of the face and skull have much thinner bone. Above the nasal passages is a thin *cribriform plate*, which communicates with the base of the skull. The middle ear is also close to the base of the skull. With basal skull fractures damage to the cribriform plate and middle ear allows leakage of cerebrospinal fluid and blood from the nose or ears (Figure 23.4).

The skull itself is covered by the scalp, which consists of skin and a fibrous membrane, the *galea*. There is a potential space between the galea and the skull. If bleeding occurs into this space it can produce a large scalp haematoma. The scalp has a good blood supply and bleeds readily, so a large volume of blood can be lost following injury; this is unlikely to cause the symptoms and signs of hypovolaemia, except in children and the elderly (Figure 23.5).

PHYSIOLOGY

One of the important features of the central nervous system is that it has no stores of oxygen, glucose or the other substances required for cell metabolism. If the blood supply is

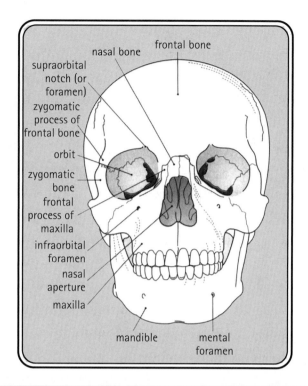

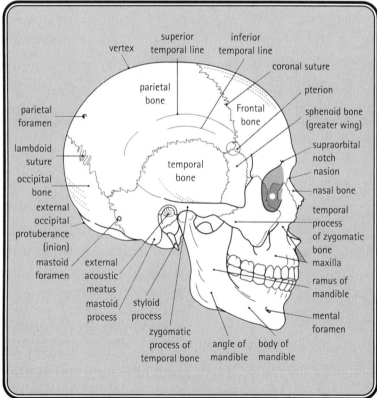

Figure 23.4 Anatomy of the skull

interrupted, depriving the brain of oxygen, consciousness is lost within 15–20 seconds. The brain cells will then die within 3–4 minutes. Any retention of carbon dioxide as a waste product of metabolism will retard brain function and aggravate the effects of *hypoxia* or lack of oxygen. A supply of glucose is also essential for normal brain function.

Because the skull is a rigid box, tissue swelling or bleeding within it will lead to an increase in pressure. As the pressure rises, the brain is pushed down, impacting on rigid structures such as the tentorium and the foramen magnum. The brain is particularly sensitive to increased pressure – nerve cells do not tolerate high pressure well and raised

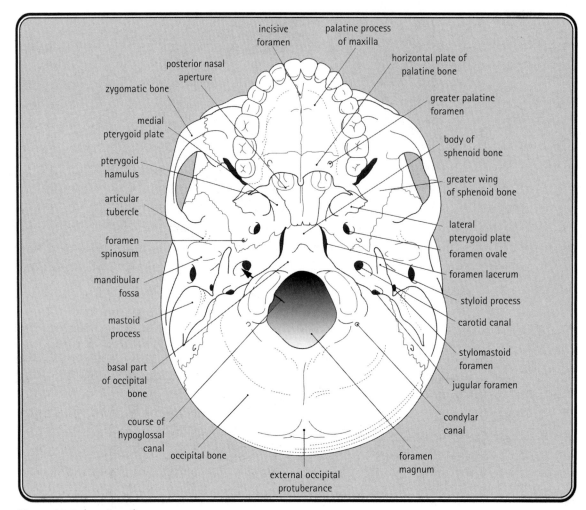

incisive foramen
palatine process of maxilla
horizontal plate of palatine bone
posterior nasal aperture
zygomatic bone
greater palatine foramen
medial pterygoid plate
body of sphenoid bone
pterygoid hamulus
greater wing of sphenoid bone
articular tubercle
lateral pterygoid plate
foramen ovale
foramen spinosum
foramen lacerum
mandibular fossa
styloid process
mastoid process
carotid canal
basal part of occipital bone
stylomastoid foramen
jugular foramen
course of hypoglossal canal
condylar canal
occipital bone
foramen magnum
external occipital protuberance

Figure 23.4 (*continued*)

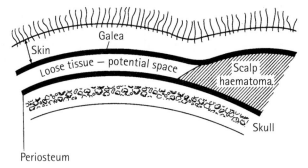

Figure 23.5 Layers of the scalp

Galea
Skin
Loose tissue – potential space
Scalp haematoma
Skull
Periosteum

intracranial pressure will produce a reduction in level of consciousness.

PATHOPHYSIOLOGY

Brain injuries can be classified according to the mechanism of injury:

- blunt brain injury
- penetrating brain injury.

and according to the localization of the injury:

- generalized brain injury
- focal brain injury.

However, for the purposes of optimal management, the most important division is into:

- primary brain injury
- secondary brain injury.

PRIMARY AND SECONDARY BRAIN INJURY

The brain injury sustained at the time of the accident is known as the *primary injury* and it is something that no-one can reduce once it has occurred. What can be minimized is the *secondary brain injury* (Figure 23.6).

> The primary injury is sustained as a result of the original trauma: the management focus is to prevent secondary brain injury

Secondary brain injury is a combination of factors that lead to additional brain injury and cell death in the hours and

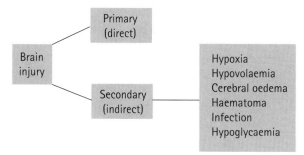

Figure 23.6 Primary and secondary brain injury

days following the primary injury. In the hours immediately after the injury, optimal care of the airway, breathing and circulation is essential to prevent further brain injury from hypoxaemia and hypoperfusion of the brain. Any periods of cerebral hypoxia in the hours after injury significantly add to mortality and morbidity.

The skull is a rigid box and does not expand (although the sutures and fontanelles do allow a little expansion in the infant under 12 months). The development of a haematoma or swelling of the brain within this box causes increases in intracranial pressure. To give an example, if a patient has an extradural haematoma there is bleeding within the skull. Although the initial injury to the brain is liable to have caused concussion, the patient recovers temporarily (a lucid interval) before deteriorating. As the size of the haematoma increases intracranial pressure increases and the conscious level deteriorates. As the pressure increases on one side of the brain, part of the temporal lobe extrudes (herniates) into the small space between the brain stem and the tentorium cerebelli. In this space is the third cranial nerve and as this is compressed, the pupil on the same side dilates. As intracranial pressure continues to rise the herniating temporal lobe forces the brainstem against the opposite fold of tentorium, causing the opposite pupil to dilate and paralysis of the arm and leg of the opposite side of the body to the haematoma. This is a preterminal sign. An alternative site of herniation is the foramen magnum. This is known as "coning" and results in the late development of bradycardia, hypertension and hypoventilation.

Particular factors that affect the brain's blood supply are:

- lack of oxygen (hypoxia)
- carbon dioxide retention.

With hypoxia the brain cells go into an anaerobic metabolism phase. There is damage to the cells, which become swollen. As hypoxia affects the brain as a whole there is generalized swelling – *cerebral oedema* – which results in raised intracranial pressure (ICP). Carbon dioxide retention results in dilation of the intracranial blood vessels which also causes raised intracranial pressure.

The signs of raised intracranial pressure are:

- decreasing level of consciousness
- increasing blood pressure (late)
- falling pulse rate (late)
- decreasing respiratory rate (late)
- pupillary dilation (late).

When the intracranial pressure approaches the arterial pressure, blood cannot flow through the brain and so cells will die. The important blood pressure for the brain is not the mean arterial pressure (MAP) alone, but the *perfusion pressure* (PP). The cerebral perfusion pressure is the mean arterial pressure minus the mean intracranial pressure (MICP).

> Cerebral perfusion pressure is the mean arterial pressure minus the mean intracranial pressure
> PP = MAP − MICP

Both a fall in mean arterial pressure and a rise in intracranial pressure may therefore reduce cerebral perfusion pressure and produce secondary brain injury. In the swollen brain the ICP is also increased if central venous pressure is increased. Treatment should aim to maintain the cerebral perfusion pressure and keep the patient's arterial pressure near normal limits and above 100 mmHg in the adult. Anything that increases central venous pressure, for example a tension pneumothorax, must also be treated.

GENERALIZED AND FOCAL BRAIN INJURY

Generalized brain injury

Generalized or diffuse injuries represent a spectrum of injury from mild concussion with rapid and complete recovery to *diffuse axonal injury* (DAI) which is the principal cause of long-standing coma following head injury. Coma may last days or weeks and may be permanent. It results from microscopic damage to the nerve cells that are sheared and torn. It is not possible to diagnose such injuries outside hospital. These patients should be assumed to have a treatable lesion until the results of a CT scan and a neurosurgical opinion have been obtained.

Focal brain injuries

Localized or focal brain injuries consist of:

- cerebral contusion
- intracranial haemorrhages
- lacerations and penetrating injuries.

Contusion

A contusion is a bruise. It can be small or large, localized or involve a large area of the brain under the site of impact and at the opposite pole of the brain. Most cerebral contusions present with a period of concussion. It is important to realize that patients do not remember the duration of coma; this history is obtained from the observers. For this reason it is essential that all information about loss of consciousness is

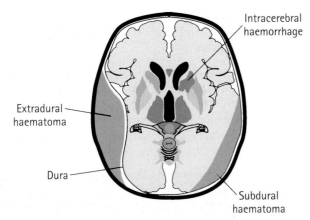

Intracerebral haemorrhage

Extradural haematoma

Dura

Subdural haematoma

Figure 23.7 The anatomy of intracranial bleeding: extradural haematoma, subdural haematoma and intracerebral haemorrhage. A subarachnoid haemorrhage covers the surface of the brain, lying in a thick layer between the arachnoid and the pia mater

documented on the patient's report form. Because of the inflammatory response, there will be a secondary injury around the area of bruising with a collection of fluid causing localized swelling. The secondary oedema around a contusion may cause further deterioration. Modern management of such injuries is non-surgical, but includes monitoring of the intracranial pressure.

Intracranial bleeding

Intracranial haemorrhage may be:

- extradural
- subdural
- intracerebral
- subarachnoid.

Extradural haemorrhage   Intracranial bleeding is usually caused by tearing of veins or arteries. Damage to the middle meningeal artery can cause an *extradural haemorrhage* – bleeding between the skull and the dura mater. It is not a common injury, occurring in less than 1% of head-injured patients, but it can be rapidly fatal. An important feature is that if treated in the optimum time, ideally within 2 hours, the patient may make a complete recovery. Delay beyond 4 hours will significantly alter the degree of recovery (Figure 23.7).

An extradural haematoma characteristically presents as a loss of consciousness (initial concussion), following which the patient may recover, be alert and talkative or have an improved GCS rating. The patient then complains of increasing headache and lapses into unconsciousness as the intracranial pressure increases. For this secondary loss of consciousness treatment has to be surgical and must be prompt. There is often weakness on the opposite side of the body to the head injury, with a dilated and fixed pupil on the same side as the injury. The surgical treatment is to remove the blood clot and seal off the bleeding vessel. If the

pressure on the brain is removed and has not been prolonged, a recovery rate of approaching 100% can be expected.

Subdural haemorrhage   Damage to the vessels in the subdural space (between the dura and the arachnoid) is much more common and accounts for 30% of head injuries. Originally these injuries were thought to have a very poor prognosis. There is increasing evidence that if the patient is operated on within the first 2 hours after injury the survival rate can be as high as 70–80%. Unlike extradural haemorrhages, there is usually a degree of primary brain injury and disability is common in survivors.

Intracerebral haemorrhage   Bleeding may also occur into the tissue of the cerebral hemispheres – *intracerebral haemorrhage*.

Subarachnoid haemorrhage   Bleeding into the subarachnoid space (*subarachnoid haemorrhage*) produces headache and increasing drowsiness. Once the diagnosis has been made there is no immediate surgical treatment.

In prehospital care it is extremely difficult to decide which sort of bleeding is causing unconsciousness. The definitive investigation is a computed tomography (CT) scan. It is therefore important that patients with a significant period of unconsciousness (2–3 minutes or more) are taken to a hospital that has 24-hour CT scanning facilities and appropriate staff to treat the patient once these scans have been obtained. Only after a scan is performed can a long-term prognosis be given.

Lacerations and penetrating injuries

Lacerations are closed brain injuries, often due to shearing forces causing tearing and haemorrhage within the substance of the brain, producing an intracerebral haematoma. This exerts pressure within the substance of the brain, with permanent damage. Specialist neurosurgical centres are able to evacuate such haemorrhages and diminish the effects of the injury. Such injuries can be devastating and have a high mortality rate.

Brain haemorrhage can also be caused by penetrating trauma, inflicted by a low-velocity implement such as a knife, or by impalement in an industrial or traffic accident. The severity of the injury and any long-term disability is determined by the area of the brain which is injured. In gunshot wounds the damage to the brain depends on the size of the bullet and its velocity. In general terms, if the patient is unconscious after the penetrating injury the prognosis is exceedingly poor. Patients who are conscious and talking after such an injury can survive.

SKULL FRACTURES

Blunt injuries can cause fractures of the skull. Such fractures are common and although they are not necessarily serious injuries, they reflect the degree of violence to which the brain

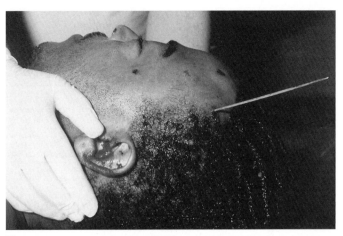

Figure 23.8 Penetrating brain injury

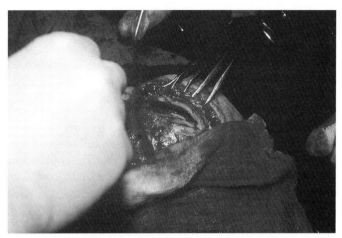

Figure 23.9 A depressed skull fracture

Table 23.1 Risk of intracranial haematoma

Conscious level	Skull X-ray	Risk of intracranial haematoma
Normal	Normal	1 in 5000
Normal	Fracture	1 in 32
Altered	Normal	1 in 120
Altered	Fracture	1 in 4

has been subjected. Damage to the brain is demonstrated by an altered conscious level. The clinical significance of a skull fracture is its potential relation to intracranial bleeding. The combination of a fracture of the skull *and* alteration of consciousness increases the chance of intracranial bleeding from 1 in 5000 to 1 in 4 (Table 23.1).

Linear skull fractures require no specific treatment. The emphasis is on the underlying brain injury. A more severe form of fracture is where the bone is depressed, but surgical treatment will only be required if there is pressure on the brain (Figure 23.9). Unless they are very obvious, skull fractures are extremely difficult to diagnose clinically, especially prehospital, and investigations such as X-rays or CT scanning are necessary.

Leakage of cerebrospinal fluid from the nose or the ears is diagnostic of a basal skull fracture; bleeding from the ears is also highly suggestive although it may result from local trauma. Because there is an open communication with the exterior, there is a clear channel for infection.

Another feature of a basal skull fracture is the presence of black eyes: tracking of blood around both eyes gives the appearance known as "panda" or "raccoon" eyes. Swelling and bruising behind the ear over the mastoid process also indicate leakage of blood from a fractured base of skull. This is known as Battle's sign. These signs may not appear until several hours after the injury and rarely develop before the patient arrives in hospital (see Figure 20.3).

Box 23.1 Signs of basal skull fracture

- CSF leakage from nose (rhinorrhoea)
- CSF leakage from ear (otorrhoea)
- Panda (raccoon) eyes
- Battle's sign
- Bleeding from the ears

Very severe open injuries may expose the brain. Moist non-adherent dressings are needed to cover the area and to stop the brain tissue drying out. Scalp wounds should never be probed with a finger in the prehospital environment. They should be covered and left alone.

> Do not probe scalp wounds – cover them and leave them alone!

PATIENT ASSESSMENT

Patient assessment must follow a systematic approach. Since a patient will lose consciousness within 15–30 seconds because of lack of oxygen, the priorities in management are to:

- protect the airway
- ensure the delivery of oxygen to the brain.

To achieve this there must be an adequate airway (A), uncompromised breathing (B) and adequate cerebral perfusion (C). Faultless assessment and resuscitation during the primary survey are therefore the key to head injury management.

The hallmark of a head injury is an altered conscious level which will vary from drowsiness or irritability to lack of response to verbal commands or to pain and finally to complete unresponsiveness. It should not be forgotten, however, that some patients who appear completely lucid will subsequently undergo deterioration which may be extremely rapid.

Most patients cannot tell you whether they have been knocked out and certainly cannot reliably judge the period of unconsciousness. What they will say is that they lack memory of an event. This lack of memory is known as *amnesia* which can be retrograde or post traumatic.

Retrograde amnesia

Retrograde amnesia is lack of memory or recall of the events before the injury. This can be a period of some minutes or even an hour or so. It suggests a significant brain injury.

Posttraumatic amnesia

Posttraumatic amnesia is loss of memory after the event. The patient may remember up to the time of a fall, a blow or a traffic accident. The next recall is of a specific location, for example the ambulance, the accident and emergency department or the X-ray department. It is important to note the length of time the patient has suffered from posttraumatic amnesia.

"Minor" head injuries, where the patient has been knocked out for 1–2 seconds but then makes a full recovery, are extremely common. The main reason that patients are admitted to hospital after a head injury and loss of consciousness is to make sure they do not have a treatable injury, such as an intracranial haematoma, from which they may subsequently deteriorate and require surgery. As a result, large numbers of patients are admitted to hospital for head injury observation. These patients are suffering from *concussion*.

Any patient who has a witnessed loss of consciousness should be taken to hospital. Patients who have prolonged posttraumatic amnesia of 5 minutes or more should also be observed. Other factors can influence conscious level. These include pre-existing diseases such as epilepsy, where drowsiness is a well-known feature following a grand mal seizure. Alcohol and other drugs will alter the conscious level and because of the risks involved, these patients may need observation, in spite of the fact they have not lost consciousness. Patients who are subject to chronic alcohol abuse can have reduced blood coagulation; they may suffer an insidious intracranial bleed, often without loss of consciousness. These "regular" accident and emergency patients may end up dying because they have an intracranial haematoma that is unrecognized because the patient is labelled as a "drunk". It is dangerous not to take these patients to hospital or to discharge them from the accident and emergency department, in spite of the fact they are regular attenders.

Never accept alcohol as the sole cause of an altered conscious level

Similarly, dementia should never be accepted as the sole cause of an altered conscious level. Serious head injuries are all too often missed in elderly patients who are confused.

Table 23.2 Glasgow Coma Scale – eye opening

Response	Score
Eyes are already open and blinking normally	E = 4
Eyes open in response to speech or specific questions	E = 3
Eyes open in response to pain	E = 2
No response	E = 1

Another high-risk group are those with blood coagulation disorders, whether inherited (for example, haemophilia) or secondary to drugs (such as warfarin).

Assessment of the head-injured patient assumes the primary survey has been carried out, with appropriate management for the airway and protection of the cervical spine in every patient who is concussed or who has an altered conscious level. Cervical spine injury is likely in patients who have had a fall from a height of 3 metres or more or undergone violent deceleration, as in high-speed traffic accidents.

After the airway, breathing and circulation have been assessed and managed appropriately, the neurological status should be assessed. The general neurological state can be observed by assessing whether the patient is alert (A), responds to verbal commands (V), responds to painful stimuli (P) or is completely unresponsive (U). This is known as the AVPU scale.

A > **A**lert **V** > Responds to **v**ocal stimulus **P** > Responds to **p**ainful stimulus **U** > **U**nresponsive

GLASGOW COMA SCALE

A more accurate and detailed examination, which is readily repeated by other observers, is the *Glasgow Coma Scale*. This offers a quantitive score, assessing three functions: eye opening, verbal response and motor response.

Eye opening

Eye opening has four responses (Table 23.2). The painful stimulus should be applied above the neck to ensure that cervical spine injury is not responsible for the lack of response.

Verbal response

If the patient cannot speak it is impossible to carry out this assessment, for example if the patient is intubated. This is relevant and must be documented (Table 23.3).

Table 23.3 Glasgow Coma Scale – verbal response

Response	Score
Fully oriented; for example, patient can state name, address, date of birth and date and time	V = 5
Confused conversation; patient will not volunteer information, disoriented in time, place or person	V = 4
Inappropriate words; patient can produce recognizable words but at random and not in lucid sentences. May also be exclamatory or swearing	V = 3
Incomprehensible sounds (grunts or groans) but no actual words	V = 2
No response to speech	V = 1

Table 23.4 Glasgow Coma Scale – motor response

Response	Score
Spontaneously moves limbs to commands	M = 6
Localizes pain by purpose or motion towards the painful stimuli (this stimulus should be applied to the fingernail bed)	M = 5
Withdraws or pulls away from painful stimuli	M = 4
Abnormal flexion, known as *decorticate* posture	M = 3
Extensor response, known as *decerebrate* posture	M = 2
No movement	M = 1

Motor response

Motor response is assessed as the best response for extremities. It is assessed by the function of the *upper limbs*, assuming no injury to them (Table 23.4). If the response is different on the right and the left, the higher score should be used.

Overall assessment

The E, V and M scores are added up, giving a maximum total for a normal GCS of 15. However, to the specialist a summative score on a GCS has little meaning – it is better to use the scale as a means of documenting the patient's condition on a chart. When messages are passed or when the patient is handed over, the paramedic should state the GCS score for each of the components – for example, opens eyes spontaneously (4), responds only to questions (3) and localizes to pain (5) – which is more meaningful than an overall score of 12 (Table 23.5).

OTHER TESTS

Motor function can be assessed by testing movements of both the right and left upper limbs and the right and left lower limbs. It is important to record that the patient is not

Table 23.5 Examples of different Glasgow Coma Scale assessments with identical total scores

	Example 1	Example 2
Eye opening	3 (speech or questioning)	2 (response to pain)
Verbal response	3 (inappropriate speech)	2 (incomprehensible sounds)
Motor response	3 (abnormal flexion)	5 (localizes pain)
Total score	9	9

moving the lower limbs spontaneously if spontaneous movement of the upper limbs is present. This is highly suggestive of a spinal cord injury. Similarly, assessment of sensation in each of the limbs is important. In certain instances, loss of movement on one side of the body suggests an intracranial bleed – these are known as *lateralizing signs.*

Assessment of pupil function, documenting the size of the pupils and their response to light is an essential part of the primary survey.

The patient's vital signs are of great significance, as they provide direct assessments of brain function. These signs include pulse rate, blood pressure and respiratory rate. In hospital the body temperature which is regulated by the brain will also be recorded.

Knowing the blood glucose level is of value, because hypoglycaemia contributes to secondary brain injury and must be corrected. Recording of blood glucose levels by paramedics should be routine not only in diabetic patients but also in patients with major head injury.

If the victims of head injury are to have the best chance of survival without major neurological deficit, it is essential that such patients are transported to hospital without any unnecessary delay. Therefore paramedics must obtain all this information rapidly and systematically. The assessment of a patient should be completed within 5 minutes, as longer on-scene times will be detrimental. For the purpose of the primary survey, the "mini" neurological examination is adequate: this comprises AVPU and an assessment of the pupillary response to light.

> Primary survey "D" = "mini" neurological examination = AVPU + pupils

MANAGEMENT

Attention must be paid to the normal sequence of resuscitation: airway, breathing and circulation (ABC). Appropriate management of these priorities is the basis of the optimal management of head injuries by prevention of secondary brain injury. Thus airway is the first priority, then breathing, followed by circulation.

AIRWAY

The primary survey requires assessment, establishment and protection of the airway. If simple techniques such as the jaw thrust are inadequate, adjuncts such as the oropharyngeal airway should be used. Even with an adequate airway, the patient may have a problem of hypoventilation (slow or shallow respiratory movements). The effects of hypoventilation can be detected by pulse oximetry and capnography, the first showing low oxygen percentage saturation and the latter low levels of carbon dioxide in expired air. In a patient who is unconscious and comatose (a GCS score of 8 or less, AVPU rating P or U), advanced airway support in the form of intubation will be needed. This can be a straightforward procedure if the patient has no gag reflex.

If the patient is irritable, aggressive and has a gag reflex, adequate airway maintenance can be one of the most difficult prehospital problems. In hospital this situation is resolved by the intervention of a doctor with skills in intubation, using muscle relaxant drugs. If the patient is trapped or cannot be transported to hospital within 15 minutes, the paramedic must consider calling medical help to the scene. A patient airway should be established using the techniques described in Chapters 6 and 7 in sequence. In many cases simple techniques and high flow oxygen will be effective. In others, the only practical course will be to apply oxygen and transfer the patient to hospital urgently.

As well as airway maintenance, the patient must be given oxygen. The best method (if the patient is not intubated) is to use a well-fitting face mask and a high flow of oxygen at 15 litres per minute. To achieve 90% oxygen supply a reservoir bag and mask must be used.

BREATHING

A normal respiratory rate is 10–18 breaths per minute in an adult. A rapid respiratory rate is a sign of hypoxia. Any respiratory rate above 18 breaths per minute should be assumed to be abnormal, indicating that the patient requires oxygen. Slow respiratory rates may be caused by drugs or by significant head injury.

Unequal chest movements can be due to damage of the chest wall, for example pain from rib fractures, or by a flail chest where there is a detached segment of ribs. A major aggravating factor in head injury is a tension pneumothorax. As the pressure builds up in the chest cavity there is an increase of central venous pressure, resulting in a further increase in the intracranial pressure and precipitating further cerebral oedema. Relief of a tension pneumothorax as soon as possible by needle thoracocentesis can have a dramatic effect in reducing high cerebral pressures. It also relieves some of the problems related to the hypoxia secondary to the pneumothorax.

CIRCULATION

Head injuries themselves do not cause low blood pressure, with the possible exception of scalp haemorrhage (see example below). An isolated and closed head injury is likely to have the opposite effect. Significant blood loss into the scalp can be a problem in infants who can lose considerable amounts of blood into their relatively loose scalp, even in closed injuries.

Isolated head injuries do not cause shock

In head injuries patients may lose large volumes of blood from other injuries, such as bleeding into the chest or abdomen, or from multiple fractures. If the patient is hypovolaemic this must be corrected as soon as possible and early evacuation after control of external bleeding is essential. In multiple trauma, if the patient is trapped or in the event of a very long transfer, the blood pressure should not be elevated by infusion sufficiently to precipitate major internal haemorrhage which may be fatal. The policy of maintaining a palpable radial pulse is appropriate. It must be accepted that this is less than ideal physiologically for the brain, as it may reduce cerebral perfusion, and a higher blood pressure endpoint is acceptable if there is definite *isolated* head injury.

TRANSFER TO HOSPITAL

Once the airway and cervical spine and breathing are stabilized, the patient should be rapidly transported to the nearest appropriate hospital. Obtaining IV access is best attempted in transit. At this stage a GCS score can be accurately assessed and can be continually monitored during the journey. An appropriate hospital is one that has a 24-hour accident and emergency department and access to an available and working CT scanner. Serious head injuries need an intensive care unit and surgeons to deal with any complications that develop. For this reason it is best to transfer the patient to a hospital that has trained trauma teams and rapidly available neurosurgeons. It is not efficient to treat patients by transferring them to the nearest hospital where they may be assessed over a period of 1–2 hours and then require a secondary transfer to a neurosurgical unit. The critical time for surgery may have passed, leading to increased mortality and morbidity rates in head-injured patients.

ADVANCES IN TREATMENT

Over the years it has been recognized that it is dangerous to allow patients with head injuries to become hypoxic. With the increased technical skills of paramedics, better airway maintenance has been achieved using basic and advanced life support techniques. In the future there is likely to be increased use of endotracheal intubation with muscle relaxant drugs being given by appropriately trained staff, who will include specially trained medical as well as paramedical personnel. Adequate oxygenation can be monitored noninvasively by pulse oximetry and expired air carbon dioxide levels can also be monitored (capnography or end-tidal CO_2 monitoring) as an indicator of adequate ventilation and gas exchange.

Because of the success of prehospital care by paramedics and immediate-care doctors in maintaining the airway, providing oxygen and maintaining a normal blood pressure, and by careful attention to prehospital times, patients are arriving in hospital in a much better condition. Allied to this are significant advances in the management of head injuries within neurosurgical units. Intracranial pressure monitoring is the norm in the UK and the need of the brain for glucose and other energy sources is now recognized. Brain *function* can be monitored with sophisticated techniques such as the positron emission scan, which identifies the actual levels of glucose being circulated to all parts of the brain. Patients with significant brain injury need to be treated in these specialized centres.

The implication of these developments and their effects on outcome is that paramedics will have the responsibility of transporting a head-injured patient to the most appropriate unit for that patient's injury.

It is of paramount importance that the paramedic pays attention to the basic management of the patient; that is, the provision of a clear airway, good oxygenation, protection of normal breathing and treatment of any complication. Any hypovolaemia will need to be corrected by fluid replacement and continuing assessment of the patient's disability or neurological state is required throughout the transfer to hospital.

The greatest advance for recovery of the injured brain has been attention to detail in the prehospital phase. The sophisticated skills of the modern neurosurgeon will not be effective unless the paramedic adheres to these basic principles.

Chapter 24

Facial injuries

CHAPTER CONTENTS

INTRODUCTION

Facial injuries occur in isolation or in association with multiple trauma. The management of such injuries usually occurs during the secondary survey and forms part of the detailed assessment of the trauma patient. However, severe facial injuries may directly compromise the airway and induce haemorrhage, which may in itself further compromise the airway, and both of these problems should be treated as part of the primary survey.

AIRWAY PROBLEMS

The airway may be directly compromised due to anatomical disruption or obstructed by blood or foreign bodies.

Airway problems arise from:

- inhalation of foreign bodies
- posterior impaction of the fractured maxilla
- loss of tongue control in a fractured mandible
- intraoral tissue swelling
- direct trauma to the larynx
- haemorrhage.

CIRCULATORY PROBLEMS

Haemorrhage from facial fractures may produce:

- airway obstruction
- hypovolaemic shock.

Two percent of facial injuries have associated cervical injuries and the patient's cervical spine should *always* be protected using a semi-rigid collar, spine board and head blocks until adequate radiographs confirm the absence of injury. Severe facial injury may necessitate advanced airway procedures such as cricothyroidotomy (Chapter 7).

Facial injuries can be conveniently divided into soft tissue injuries (including the eye) and hard tissue injuries (teeth and bone).

ANATOMY OF THE FACIAL SKELETON

MANDIBLE (FIGURE 24.1)

The mandible or lower jaw articulates with the rest of the skull at the *condyles*. The thin *neck* of the condyle is connected to the *ramus* of the mandible and this to the *body*. The teeth are held in the bone in the dentoalveolar region.

MAXILLA (FIGURE 24.2)

The upper jaw also supports teeth in the dentoalveolar bone and is closely related to the bones that form the orbit and nose. Lying behind the front wall of the maxilla is the air-filled *maxillary sinus*.

TEETH

In children there are 20 primary (*deciduous*) teeth, divided into four quadrants of the mouth. Visualized from the front

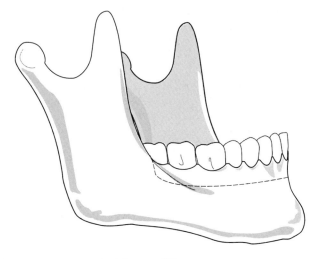

Figure 24.1 Anatomy of the mandible

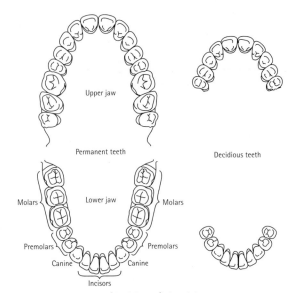

Figure 24.3 The primary (deciduous) dentition

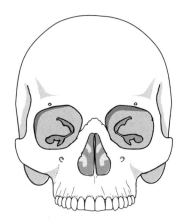

Figure 24.2 Anatomy of the maxilla

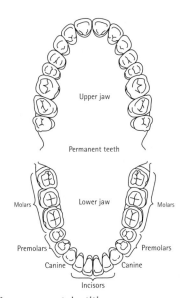

Figure 24.4 The permanent dentition

and starting in the midline, these are situated in the upper left and right jaw and lower left and right jaw and are lettered a to e (Figure 24.3).

In the adult there are 32 permanent teeth, again divided into four quadrants but numbered 1 to 8 (*incisors* 1,2; *canines* 3; *premolars* 4,5; *molars* 6,7,8) as viewed from the front. An upper left canine, for example, may be written as UL3 (Figure 24.4).

ORBIT AND ZYGOMATICOMAXILLARY COMPLEX

The *zygoma* or *malar bone* forms part of the outer margin of the orbital rim and gives the face a cheek prominence. The bone forming the eye socket is very thin and is divided into the floor, the roof and the medial and lateral walls. The lower rim (infraorbital margin) is formed partly by the zygoma and partly by the maxilla. The upper rim (supraorbital margin) is part of the frontal bone of the skull. The eye is contained within the bony orbit and is surrounded by the extraocular muscles and periorbital fat.

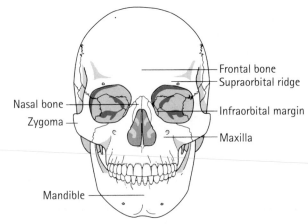

Figure 24.5 The facial skeleton

NASAL COMPLEX

The nose consists of a bony part articulating with the frontal bone and maxilla and a cartilaginous framework. The thin *ethmoid bone* forms the medial aspect of the orbit. The ethmoids contain air-filled sinuses and are closely related to the nose and the frontal region of the brain.

BLOOD SUPPLY TO THE FACE AND SCALP

The blood supply to the face and scalp is excellent and soft tissue wounds may bleed profusely. The *facial artery*, a branch of the external carotid artery, supplies the tissues of the face and there is considerable cross-over from one side to the other. The same applies to the vessels supplying the scalp. In addition, the terminal branches of the *maxillary artery* and the anterior and posterior *ethmoidal arteries* contribute to the midfacial blood supply and can be responsible for life-threatening haemorrhage. Control of massive facial bleeding is discussed below.

NERVE SUPPLY TO THE FACE

The *facial nerve* (VII cranial nerve) is responsible for movement of the muscles of the face. Lacerations to the cheek may damage branches of the nerve, producing a weakness in the muscles on that side. The *trigeminal nerve* (V cranial nerve), which has three divisions (*mandibular, maxillary and ophthalmic*), provides sensation to the mouth and face. A fracture of the mandible may damage a branch of this nerve, resulting in numbness of the lower lip and chin on that side.

CLASSIFICATION AND TREATMENT OF FACIAL INJURIES

Facial injuries can be grouped into soft tissue injuries (including the eye) and hard tissue injuries which may involve teeth or bone.

SOFT TISSUE

Soft tissue injuries may be divided into superficial cuts and grazes, lacerations and penetrating wounds. There may be loss of tissue or degloving injuries, as seen for example in the lower labial sulcus (groove behind the lower lip) when the skin over the chin is forcibly pushed downwards and backwards.

Treatment

Profuse haemorrhage from cuts and lacerations should be stopped during the primary survey. Pressure applied over the wound with a gauze swab held firmly in place may be all that is required. Penetrating injuries should *not* be explored. It is dangerous to explore neck wounds, which should be covered and managed in hospital.

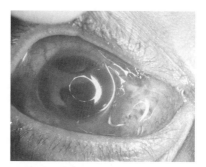

Figure 24.6 A penetrating eye injury

Foreign bodies should be left in place, including those piercing the cheek or penetrating the other intraoral tissues, unless they are causing airway obstruction. A cheek wound may sever the parotid duct, resulting in an escape of saliva onto the cheek.

During the secondary survey a thorough examination of the scalp and face will be carried out in order to identify all the soft tissue injuries.

EYE INJURIES

Eye injuries may be divided into:

- superficial injuries
- penetrating injuries
- foreign bodies
- chemical injury.

The most common superficial injury is a corneal abrasion in which the superficial layers of the cornea are removed. The resulting injury is exactly analogous to an abrasion of the skin and is very painful.

Penetrating injuries of the eye are fortunately rare but can be devastating (Figure 24.6). Such injuries may be immediately apparent, especially given a knowledge of the mechanism of injury. However, the diagnosis is sometimes less obvious; for example, a sudden onset of pain in the eye in a workman who is grinding metal. Foreign bodies on the surface of the eye are remarkably irritant and painful.

Chemical injuries to the eye are extremely common, occurring in both domestic and industrial settings. If not properly treated, the consequences may include loss of vision.

Treatment

No immediate treatment is usually required for corneal abrasions although some patients may gain relief from covering the eye with a pad. Patients with penetrating injuries should be transported to hospital urgently in the supine position. Both eyes should be covered to prevent eye movements but any protruding foreign body must not be forced further into the globe.

Small superficial foreign bodies will require removal in hospital although irrigation with clean water may be

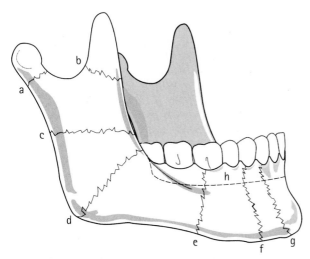

Figure 24.7 Mandibular fractures. (a) Condyle; (b) coronoid; (c) ramus; (d) angle; (e) body; (f) parasymphysis; (g) symphysis; (h) dentoalveolar

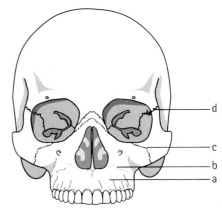

Figure 24.8 Maxillary fractures. (a) Dentoalveolar; (b) Le Fort I (low level); (c) Le Fort II (pyramidal); (d) Le Fort III (high level)

helpful in removing general debris if the injury has occurred in a dirty or contaminated environment.

In the case of chemical injuries, copious irrigation with sterile saline is indicated. Under no circumstances should any attempt be made to "neutralize" an acid with an alkali or vice versa. In general, eye injuries from alkalis have a worse prognosis than those from acids. All such injuries require urgent assessment, including a formal eye examination in the accident and emergency department.

HARD TISSUE

Teeth

Teeth may be loosened, partially extruded or completely avulsed (extracted). They may be fractured at the level of the crown or lower down on the root. Fractures involving segments of tooth-bearing bone may occur and are known as *dentoalveolar fractures.*

Bone

It is convenient to consider the fractures of the facial skeleton according to the anatomical areas described before. Facial fractures can occur on one side (unilateral) or both sides (bilateral) and combinations are frequent.

Fractures of the mandible

A patient with a fractured mandible (Figure 24.7) will give a history of recent trauma to the jaw. For example, a patient who has sustained a blow to the right side of the jaw may have a fracture through the right angle and/or a fracture of the left condylar neck. Alternatively, a patient who has received an injury to the chin may have a midline fracture together with bilateral condylar neck fractures. The patient may complain of pain and swelling over the site of the injury and be unable to open the mouth fully. A number of teeth may have been lost or displaced and the patient may have

difficulty in putting the teeth together properly (abnormal occlusion). Examination of the face may reveal a step deformity along the line of the lower jaw. Intraoral inspection may show lacerated and bleeding gums and loose teeth. Bruising underneath the tongue (*sublingual haematoma*) usually occurs adjacent to the fracture line.

Fractures of the maxilla

A patient with a fractured upper jaw (Figure 24.8) is likely to have sustained high-impact trauma to the face. Gentle manipulation of the maxilla will reveal mobility of the upper jaw and the patient may have a "dish-face" deformity. Marked swelling is a feature of the Le Fort II and Le Fort III fractures and may be accompanied by bruising around the eyes. Again, the patient may complain that the teeth do not meet properly and indeed, the mouth may be gagged open (Figure 24.9).

Orbital and zygomaticomaxillary complex fractures

Fractures in this region are of particular concern because of the potential damage to the eye. Trauma to the cheek can produce marked periorbital swelling and bruising. A step deformity may be felt along the infraorbital margin and there may be flattening of the cheek. Swelling of the eyelids may make examination of the eye more difficult but it is important that any globe injuries are not missed. Gentle pressure on the eyelids for a few minutes will disperse the oedema and allow a full examination of the eye. Subconjunctival haemorrhage can indicate a fracture of the zygoma.

Examination of the pupils should be undertaken to assess size and reactivity. If one pupil is dilated this may suggest an increase in intracranial haemorrhage on the opposite side (Chapter 23). Alternatively a unilateral dilated pupil may be caused by severe concussion to the globe (traumatic mydriasis). Similarly a unilateral constricted pupil may result from blunt trauma to the eyeball (traumatic miosis).

The patient may complain of double vision (diplopia) and examination of the eye movements should be part of the assessment of the eye. Visual acuity can be objectively measured using a Snellen chart in hospital.

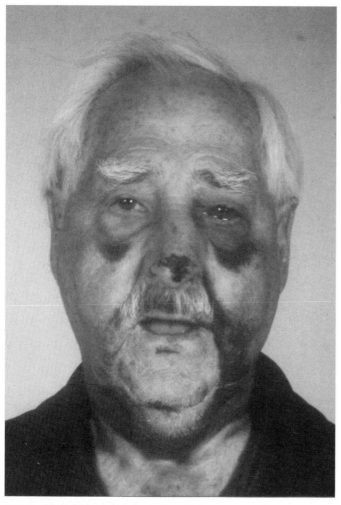

Figure 24.9 A patient with a Le Fort III fracture

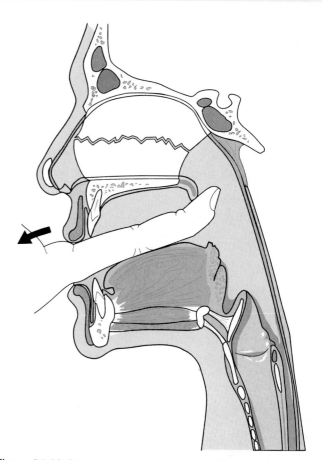

Figure 24.10 Disimpaction of a fractured maxilla

Difficulty in opening the mouth occurs when the zygomatic arch is fractured and restricts the normal movements of the muscles.

Nasal complex fractures

Fractures of the nasal bones occur following trauma from the front and from the side. The subsequent deformity reflects the direction of the injury. Nasal fractures can be accompanied by profuse haemorrhage, the management of which is discussed below. Severe midfacial injury may be sufficient to produce disruption of the thin ethmoidal bones. The patient may have a flattened appearance to the bridge of the nose and widening of the distance between the inner corners (*medial canthi*) of the eyes – known as *hypertelorism*.

Treatment

Teeth

Loose and avulsed teeth may be inhaled and are a cause of airway obstruction. Denture fragments or poorly fitting dentures can also be inhaled, especially in patients with a decreased level of consciousness. Assessment of the patient's airway and inspection of the mouth are mandatory. A finger sweep to remove visible foreign bodies and suction should be part of the primary survey (Chapter 6). Well-fitting dentures may be left in place.

In a patient without a head injury, a completely avulsed tooth (usually a front tooth in a child) can be immediately reinserted. The patient should be asked to hold the tooth in position and the advice of a dentist or maxillofacial surgeon sought. Alternatively, the tooth may be placed in a container of milk and transferred with the patient to hospital. Patients with an associated head injury are at particular risk from inhaling foreign bodies and should not be asked to hold their tooth in the inside of the cheek, as has sometimes been advocated. If the tooth is fractured, where possible, the pieces must be found and taken with the patient to hospital. A chest radiograph may subsequently be necessary if there is any suspicion that a tooth or fragment may have been inhaled.

Posterior impaction of a fractured maxilla

A fractured maxilla may cause obstruction of the nasopharynx by backward and downward displacement along the slope of the base of the skull. Disimpaction of the maxilla can relieve the obstruction and is performed by placing the middle and index fingers behind the soft palate and pulling forwards (Figure 24.10).

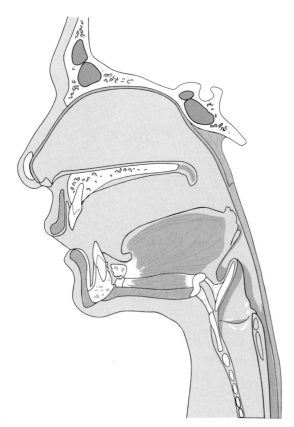

Figure 24.11 Loss of tongue support with a fractured mandible

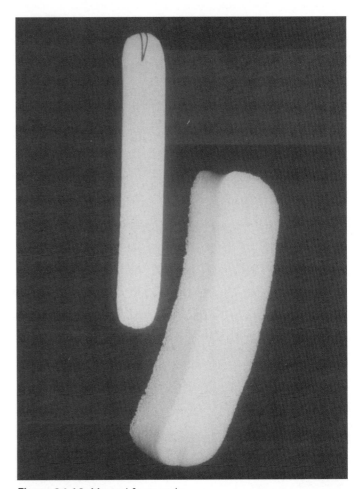

Figure 24.13 Merocel foam packs

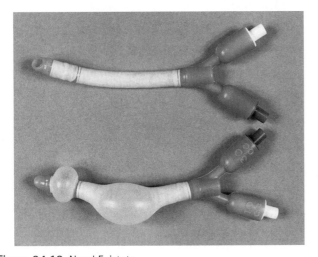

Figure 24.12 Nasal Epistats

Loss of tongue control in a fractured mandible

The fractured mandible may become an immediate airway management problem when there are bilateral symphysial fractures or there is extensive bone loss resulting in loss of tongue support. The musculature of the tongue is attached to the genial tubercles in the midline and if this fragment becomes detached, the tongue may fall backwards to obstruct the oropharynx. Patients at particular risk from this complication are those with a depressed conscious level who are unable to control their tongue (Figure 24.11).

Immediate management involves pulling the tongue forward and holding it in an unobstructed position. This may be achieved manually or a doctor may use a large suture (0 gauge black silk) placed *transversely* through the dorsum of the tongue (a large safety pin may even be used) and the suture taped to the side of the face. A transverse stitch is less likely to cut through the tongue when traction is applied.

Haemorrhage control

Profuse haemorrhage can result from a fractured maxilla after damage to the terminal branches of the maxillary artery and from the anterior and posterior ethmoidal arteries. Bleeding can cause respiratory obstruction or hypovolaemic shock and should be stopped if evident from the mouth and nose. Nasal Epistats (Figure 24.12) will effectively stop most bleeding although if there is a maxillary fracture, they may simply serve to displace the maxilla downwards.

The Epistats are inserted into both nostrils, inflated using normal saline and pulled forward, thus providing a significant compressive force. Nasal bleeding may alternatively be controlled rapidly with expanding foam packs (Merocel – Figure 24.13) inserted into the nostrils.

Chapter 25

Chest injuries

CHAPTER CONTENTS

INTRODUCTION

Deaths following injuries to the thorax usually result from a lack of oxygen (hypoxia) or lack of circulating blood volume (hypovolaemia). To improve the chances of the patient surviving, an ability to recognize and manage these problems and to be aware of conditions that require immediate evacuation is essential. A logical approach to chest trauma is given in this chapter.

In order to better understand the medical management of thoracic trauma, it is helpful to review the anatomy and physiology of the respiratory system described in Chapter 9.

MECHANISMS OF INJURY

Injuries may be blunt or penetrating. These two types can occur separately or in combination, for example following a bomb blast (see Chapter 30). In all cases, however, the severity of the injury is dependent upon the site of the impact and the energy transferred to the tissues from the causative agent.

BLUNT TRAUMA

In blunt trauma the force can be spread over a wide area. This minimizes the energy transfer at any one spot and so reduces local tissue damage. After low-energy impacts, damage is usually localized to the superficial structures. In contrast, following high-energy impacts considerable tissue disruption can be produced with the clinical consequences being dependent upon the organs involved.

PENETRATING TRAUMA

The significance of the local damage following penetrating trauma is dependent on both the site and the depth of penetration. However, the degree of injury is also determined by the amount of energy transferred to surrounding tissues (see Chapter 30). It is important to remember that low-energy transfer can still produce significant clinical problems, depending on the site of penetration; for example, a stab wound to the heart is likely to be rapidly fatal whereas a similar wound involving only the lung is likely to be compatible with longer term survival.

BLAST INJURIES

Following an explosion there is a sudden release of energy which leads to a very rapid rise in pressure in the surrounding air. When this band of high pressure, known as the *shock front* (or *blast wave*), hits the surface of the patient's body, a wave of energy spreads through the thorax causing the tissues to accelerate away from the direction of the impact. This effect is most dramatic at the junctions of areas of different density where the different rates of acceleration of different tissues result in tissue damage (such damage occurs at the air–tissue interface). The extent of tissue damage is directly dependent on both the magnitude and rate of onset of this deformation.

The most serious effects of blast occur in air-containing organs and the lungs and gut are at particular risk, producing damage at the lungs' air–tissue interface and leading to the syndrome known as *blast lung* (see Chapter 30). If it is extensive the patient becomes hypoxic (see below). High blast pressures can also lead to air emboli which may precipitate sudden death if they obstruct the coronary or cerebral arteries.

Behind the shock front comes a movement of air called the *blast wind*. As this spreads out from the epicentre, it carries with it fragments from the bomb or surrounding debris. Close to the explosion, this material will be travelling at high velocity and can produce high-energy transfer wounds.

In addition to these effects, patients may sustain further blunt trauma from surrounding structures damaged by the explosion, (e.g.) falling masonry.

PRIMARY SURVEY AND RESUSCITATION

The initial action plan for patients with chest trauma is the same as that described in Chapter 21. The airway, breathing and circulation must be assessed and stabilized as quickly as possible. This takes the form of a rapid primary survey and resuscitation, followed where appropriate by a more detailed secondary survey. In the vast majority of cases the secondary survey will take place in hospital after any major problems have been identified during the stages of the primary survey (remembering E for exposure).

The aim of the primary survey and resuscitation phase is to detect and correct any immediately life-threatening condition. In chest trauma there are six such conditions which can be remembered using the mnemonic ATOMIC.

- **A**irway obstruction
- **T**ension pneumothorax
- **O**pen chest wound
- **M**assive haemothorax
- **F**lail chest
- **C**ardiac tamponade.

EXAMINATION

To be confident that these conditions have been found or excluded, it is important that the paramedic develops a systematic way of examining the neck and chest. Ideally, all the clothing covering the thorax should be removed so that a full inspection can be carried out. However, if this is impractical the paramedic will have to adapt to the immediate situation.

The neck should always be carefully examined. An initial examination can be carried out just before the cervical collar is applied whilst manual immobilization is maintained. If the mechanism of injury means that a collar is not required, the most appropriate time is immediately after completion of "A".

> The neck is found between the airway and the chest so examine it on the way past!

The neck should be examined for the following.

- Swelling
- Surgical emphysema with crepitus
- Tracheal deviation
- Neck vein distension
- Bruising
- Lacerations.

Lacerations should only be inspected and *never* probed with metal instruments or fingers because catastrophic haemorrhage can be precipitated. In all cases formal surgical exploration will be required.

Once the inspection and palpation have been completed, the chest can then be examined. This involves the following stages.

- Inspection of the chest
- Palpation of the trachea and ribs
- Auscultation of both axillae, top and bottom
- Percussion of both axillae, top and bottom
- Examination of the back: inspection, palpation, auscultation and percussion.

INSPECTION

The respiratory rate, depth and effort of respiration should be checked at frequent intervals. Rapid, shallow breathing and intercostal or supraclavicular indrawing are all sensitive indicators of underlying lung pathology. Both sides of the chest should be inspected and compared for symmetry of movement, bruising, abrasions and penetrating wounds. Paradoxical movement (movement of part of the chest wall in the opposite direction to the rest, inwards on inspiration and outwards on expiration) may be seen and is a sign of a flail segment.

PALPATION

Starting at the top, the clavicles should be carefully palpated for deformity (which may be visible) and the chest wall should be gently felt for tenderness. Instability or crepitus may be noted (Figure 25.1).

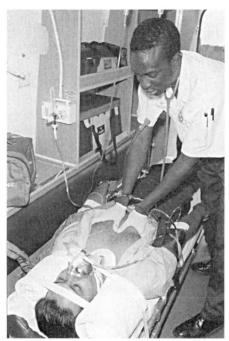

Figure 25.1 Palpation of the chest

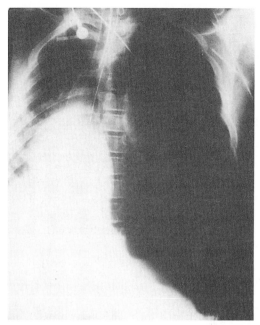

Figure 25.2 Tension pneumothorax

AUSCULTATION

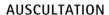

A stethoscope should be used to listen in both axillae in the upper and lower half of the chest to determine if the air entry is equal. Listening over the anterior chest detects air movement in the large airways which can drown out sounds of pulmonary ventilation, particularly if any secretions are present.

PERCUSSION

If there is a difference in auscultation, the findings on percussion of both sides of the chest should be compared. The most likely findings are either hyperresonance (pneumothorax) or dullness (fluid or contusion) on one side compared with the other.

CHECKING THE BACK

It is important to assess the back quickly to determine if there is any evidence of a penetrating injury. If there is time, the examination should include palpation, auscultation and percussion of the posterior aspect of the chest.

All trauma patients have an increased oxygen demand. Therefore, once the airway has been cleared and secured, 100% oxygen should be given at 12–15 litres per minute. The method by which oxygen is administered depends upon resources and the clinical state of the patient (see Chapters 6 and 7).

Patients with chest trauma need high-flow oxygen

LIFE-THREATENING CONDITIONS

Airway obstruction (ATOMIC)

Obstruction of a major airway can occur within the thorax. In many cases, there is little that can be done about this although cardiopulmonary resuscitation or the Heimlich manoeuvre may dislodge the obstruction. Airway obstruction is dealt with in greater detail in Chapters 6 and 7.

Tension pneumothorax (ATOMIC)

If there is a breach in either the lung or chest wall, then air can be sucked into the vacuum of the pleural space and a pneumothorax created. It is important to remember that the pleural cavity and apex of the lung project above the clavicle. Consequently this can occur following penetrating injuries to the lower neck.

Following trauma, a one-way flap valve may be produced on the lung surface. This allows air to be sucked into the pleural cavity during inspiration, but obstructs its escape during expiration. With subsequent respiratory cycles, the volume and pressure of air in the pleural cavity increase. This causes the underlying lung to collapse and profound hypoxia to develop. In the later stages, the mediastinum is displaced towards the opposite hemithorax, impeding venous return and diminishing cardiac output. This condition is known as a *tension pneumothorax* and is fatal if not rapidly relieved (Figures 25.2 and 25.3).

The characteristic signs of a tension pneumothorax are listed below. It is important to remember that this condition can develop rapidly at any stage of the resuscitation. Consequently a high index of suspicion is always required, because

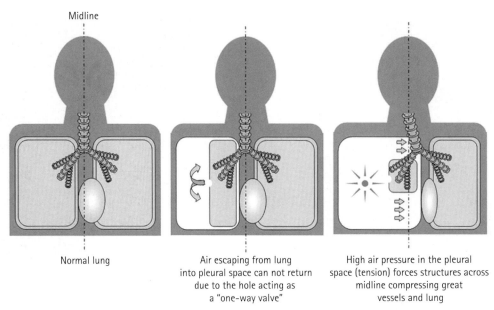

Midline

Normal lung

Air escaping from lung into pleural space can not return due to the hole acting as a "one-way valve"

High air pressure in the pleural space (tension) forces structures across midline compressing great vessels and lung

Figure 25.3 Development of a tension pneumothorax

Box 25.1 Signs of a tension pneumothorax

- Rapid respiratory rate
- Decreased air entry to the hemithorax
- Hyperresonant hemithorax
- Rapid, weak pulse
- Decreasing level of consciousness
- Deviated trachea – away from the affected side
- Raised jugular venous pulse (if no accompanying hypovolaemia)
- Cyanosis (very late)

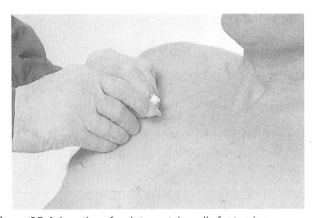

Figure 25.4 Insertion of an intercostal needle for tension pneumothorax (needle thoracocentesis)

patients can die quickly from this condition. Rapid and unexpected deterioration after the establishment of artificial ventilation, associated with the need for increased effort in achieving ventilation, should suggest the possibility of tension pneumothorax as air is transferred to the thoracic space under pressure.

> If the patient deteriorates after artificial ventilation and ventilation becomes progressively more difficult, think: tension pneumothorax

As an emergency measure, a 14 gauge cannula connected to a 10 ml syringe should be inserted into the second intercostal space in the midclavicular line on the affected side aspirating continuously (Figure 25.4). The aim is to decompress the chest by equalizing the pressures on either side of the chest wall. A rapid release of air confirms the diagnosis, following which the cannula is slid over the needle into the pleural cavity and the syringe and needle removed. It should be noted that the cannula can become dislodged

from the pleural space during transfer of the patient. In such circumstances the patient will deteriorate clinically and a further needle thoracocentesis will be required. If a needle is inserted and no tension is demonstrated, the cannula should still be left in place. In this situation, thoracocentesis may result in pneumothorax in a previously normal lung. Insertion of a chest drain will be required when the patient reaches hospital.

Needle thoracocentesis will give enough time to transfer the patient rapidly to hospital. However, if rapid transfer is not possible then a mobile medical team must be summoned so that a chest drain can be inserted. Because the paramedic may well have to assist the doctor in such a situation, it is important to be familiar with this procedure.

Tube thoracocentesis (chest drain) (Figure 25.5)

Prior to the chest drain being inserted, at least one large-bore peripheral venous cannula needs to be in place. Intravenous

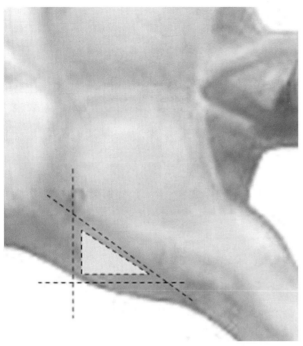

Figure 25.5 Insertion of an intercostal drain

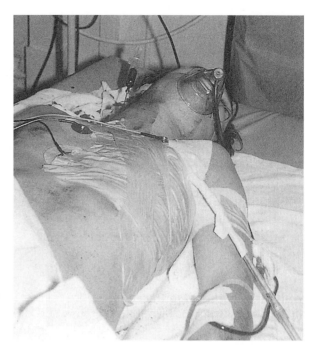

Figure 25.7 An intercostal drain in situ

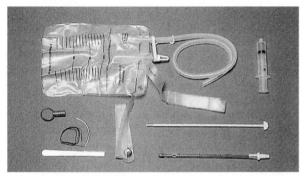

Figure 25.6 Equipment for the insertion of an intercostal drain

access must be available should the patient suddenly develop a significant haemorrhage during this procedure. This is most likely to happen if the chest drain releases a massive haemothorax.

The patient's arm is abducted if possible and the fifth intercostal space palpated, at the level of the nipple in males.

The equipment used for insertion of an intercostal drain is shown in Figure 25.6. Using an aseptic technique, the patient's chest is cleaned. Local anaesthetic solution is injected into the skin and then into deeper structures anterior to the midaxillary line. Finally the needle is directed down onto the sixth rib and local anaesthetic solution is injected onto its periosteum and over its superior surface into the underlying pleura. If the patient is unconscious, local anaesthesia is not necessary. A 3 cm transverse incision is then made down to the sixth rib, through the anaesthetized area.

Using a scalpel, a cut is made down onto the rib, then with a clamp the pleura above the rib is breached and a

track formed perpendicular to the skin. The doctor then inserts a finger through the incision and sweeps around the intrapleural space to detect the presence of intrathoracic bowel, from a ruptured diaphragm, or lung adhesions. If adhesions prevent the passage of a finger, then a fresh incision should be made in the fourth intercostal space, just anterior to the midaxillary line.

The chest drain is inserted into the incision and directed, if necessary, with the curved clamp. It is then connected to an appropriate drainage set and the clamps removed. The chest drain must be secured with both suture and tape. The incision is covered with gauze and tape (Figure 25.7).

Once a chest drain has been inserted, the patient's chest needs to be reexamined to ensure that the lung is now ventilating. Kinking, clogging with blood or displacement of the chest drain may cause a recurrence of the initial symptoms and signs.

The insertion of a chest drain should be done by trained staff because it can give rise to several complications if it is performed incorrectly. The main complications are:

- bleeding
- damage to the intercostal vessels and nerves
- lung and mediastinal injury
- damage to abdominal organs and vessels
- infection
- allergic reactions.

Open chest wound (ATOMIC)

An open chest wound will automatically produce an open pneumothorax on the same side. In addition, if the wound

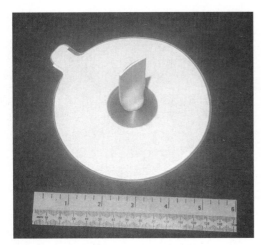

Figure 25.8 An Asherman seal

is greater than two-thirds the diameter of the trachea then air preferentially enters the chest through this hole during inspiration ("sucking" chest wound). This causes failure of ventilation of the lung which eventually collapses. A particularly dangerous situation is when the wound or an inadequately applied dressing acts as a one-way valve. When this occurs air enters the chest via the hole but cannot escape, giving rise to a tension pneumothorax.

The immediate management of an open chest wound is to apply an Asherman seal (Figure 25.8). Air can then escape during expiration, but cannot enter through the wound during inspiration because the valve is sucked closed. The primary survey can then be completed and the patient transferred to hospital where a chest drain is inserted via a freshly created incision. If a tension pneumothorax develops, any occluding dressing must be removed, thereby opening the wound and allowing air to escape. This is more effective than simply inserting a cannula into the chest because the hole will be wider than the cannula and so will produce a more rapid decompression.

If an Asherman seal is not available, a dressing sealed on three sides only can be used. This will allow the escape of air and prevent the development of a tension pneumothorax but not allow air to enter the chest from outside.

Massive haemothorax (ATO*M*IC)

When blood collects in the pleural cavity it is called a haemothorax. Following trauma this is usually caused by tearing of vascular structures. A massive haemothorax is defined as the presence of more than 1.5 litres of blood in the chest cavity; it usually results from laceration of either an intercostal vessel or the internal mammary artery.

The physical signs are listed in Box 25.2. Many of these patients will require early surgery if they are to survive. In the meantime resuscitation following standard protocols should be followed (see Chapter 22). The remainder of the primary survey should be completed and the patient rapidly transferred to hospital.

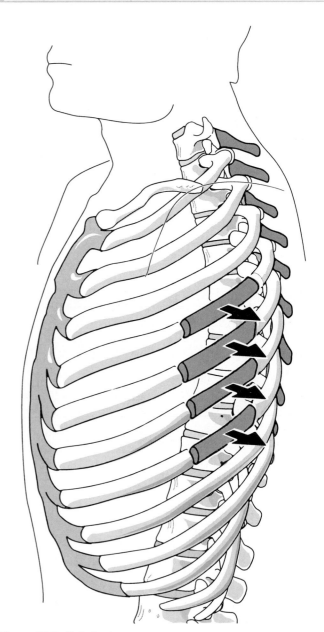

Figure 25.9 Flail chest

Flail chest (ATOM/C)

Flail chest occurs when two or more ribs are fractured in two or more places or when the clavicle and first rib are fractured (Figure 25.9). Normally the chest moves out during inspiration and in with expiration. When a rib is fractured in two places the middle section can move independently from the relatively fixed endpieces and tends to be drawn in during inspiration and pushed out in expiration. This is known as *paradoxical movement.*

Shortly after trauma, this type of movement will only be evident if there is either a large flail chest (over five ribs) or a central flail (multiple bilateral costochondral fractures with a flail sternum). More commonly, the spasm of the chest wall musculature is sufficient to splint the flail segment and mask paradoxical movement. However, this spasm leads to an increased energy expenditure for breathing. Consequently, after a time the intercostal muscles become fatigued and the abnormal chest movement becomes apparent. A flail segment can be a life-threatening condition, mainly because of the underlying pulmonary contusion (see later) which adds greatly to the hypoxia already produced as a result of the impaired breathing.

These patients must be managed in such a way that their hypoxia is corrected. In the majority of cases this will require immediate evacuation so that high-flow, warm, humidified oxygen can be administered. While awaiting this, the patient must be carefully monitored for signs indicating either the development of a tension pneumothorax or that intubation and ventilation are required to prevent further deterioration. These warning signs include:

- exhaustion
- respiratory rate greater than 30/minute
- significant associated injuries of the abdomen and head
- pulse oximeter reading of 85% or less on air
- pulse oximeter reading of 90% or less with supplemental oxygen.

Immediately following injury, and before respiratory failure begins to develop, the condition of the patient can be improved by lying the patient on the injured side (if the other injuries permit), strapping the chest (whilst ensuring that the strapping is not circumferential, which will restrict breathing) or simply stabilizing a flail segment with the clinician's hand.

Cardiac tamponade (ATOMIC)

The heart is covered with a tough, elastic fibrous sac called the *pericardium.* A small collection of blood within the pericardium will constrict the heart, compromising ventricular filling and hence cardiac output. Paradoxically, the jugular venous pulse (JVP) may be raised because of the impaired venous return to the right side of the heart. This condition is known as *cardiac tamponade* and usually follows penetrating chest wound within the anatomical area indicated in Figure 25.10.

Cardiac tamponade may be temporarily relieved by pericardiocentesis. Aspiration of even a few millilitres of blood may be life-saving. However, this is a procedure that requires skill and training and may at best serve only to buy time. It should be performed only by experienced medical personnel.

In all cases an urgent thoracotomy is necessary if the patient is to survive: rapid transfer to hospital is essential.

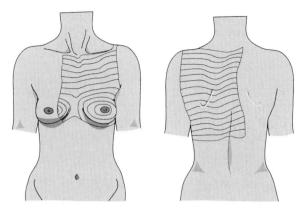

Figure 25.10 Penetrating wounds in the area indicated may result in cardiac tamponade (reproduced with permission from Landon B, Driscoll P, Goodall J 1994 An atlas of trauma management: the first hour. Parthenon Publishing)

MONITORING THE PATIENT

At the end of the primary survey and resuscitation phase it is essential that the life-threatening problems involving the airway, breathing and circulatory systems have been identified and managed appropriately. A policy of continual vigilance is essential in patients with thoracic trauma because serious problems may not only already exist but may develop at any time during resuscitation or transfer. If a patient's condition does deteriorate, then a reassessment must be carried out beginning with the airway in the manner described in Chapter 21 and continuing with assessment of the breathing and circulation.

When available, an automatic blood pressure, pulse oximeter and ECG monitor can be used for frequent measurements of the patient's vital signs. The absence of these devices or their unreliability during transportation will require the person in charge of the patient to record and document the patient's respiratory rate, blood pressure, pulse, skin perfusion and conscious level.

SECONDARY SURVEY

The secondary survey involves a detailed head-to-toe examination as described in Chapter 21. As has been repeatedly emphasized, a secondary survey is rarely appropriate in the prehospital environment; it is best performed in a well-lit resuscitation room or even after the patient has been to theatre. It may occasionally be appropriate in prolonged entrapments or during long transfers. Under no circumstances should it delay transfer to hospital.

There are eight potentially life-threatening conditions.

- Pulmonary contusion
- Cardiac contusion
- Ruptured diaphragm
- Dissecting aorta

- Oesophageal rupture
- Simple pneumothorax
- Haemothorax
- Ruptured bronchi.

Clues to the existence of these injuries may be given by the presence of marks on the chest wall which should lead you to consider particular types of injury. For example, the diagonal seatbelt bruise may overlap a fractured clavicle, a thoracic aortic tear, pulmonary contusion or pancreatic laceration.

Unlike the thoracic problems detected during the primary survey, these conditions cannot be immediately corrected or their presence easily confirmed. This is as true in the emergency department as in the field. Their discovery does indicate the need for urgent evacuation for specialized surgical treatment. Therefore knowledge of the mechanism of the injury and a detailed physical examination are essential for early detection of these conditions.

During the secondary survey, the chest wall must be reinspected for bruising, signs of obstruction, asymmetry of movement and wounds. The sternum and each rib should be palpated. The presence of any crepitus, tenderness or subcutaneous emphysema must be noted. If feasible, auscultation and percussion of the whole chest should be repeated to determine if there is any asymmetry between the right and left sides of the chest.

Examination of the back of the chest is important but it will require sufficient people to enable the patient to be log-rolled safely onto his or her side. It is therefore usually deferred until the end of the secondary survey when the whole of the back (from head to heels) is examined. An indication of bleeding from the back may be obtained by sliding your hands down the back and inspecting your palms for blood. However, if there is evidence of a posterior penetrating injury, for example blood staining on the clothing or floor, then the victim's back *must* be inspected at the earliest opportunity. In doing so, *as much care as possible must be taken in stabilizing the vertebral column*, especially in patients with neurological deficit or pain over the spine or where there is blunt injury anywhere above the level of the clavicles. Considerable care should be exercised in running your hands down a patient's back when there is contamination with broken glass.

LIFE-THREATENING CONDITIONS

Pulmonary contusion

Pulmonary contusion represents one of the most common causes of death following thoracic trauma and usually follows a blunt injury in which energy is transmitted to the underlying lung tissue. It results in an increase in the permeability of the small pulmonary capillaries, leading to fluid collecting both inside the alveoli (alveolar oedema) and in the surrounding connective tissue (interstitial oedema). As a result, the affected lung area becomes more stiff (or less compliant) and less air is drawn into the lungs with each breath. This in turn leads to further hypoxia and additional tissue damage.

As the lungs become "stiff", the effort required by the patient to inflate them increases. The tidal volume decreases and initially the respiratory rate increases in order to maintain alveolar ventilation. As the patient becomes exhausted from the increased effort of breathing, the respiratory rate falls and ventilation is reduced, leading to progressive hypoxia. In addition, infection frequently develops in the contused area at a later stage if the patient survives the initial period.

On examination, respiration is often rapid and shallow and there may be tenderness or marks on the chest wall due to the original injury. Overlying fractured ribs may be present but in children the natural elasticity of the chest wall may prevent this. Auscultation is usually normal in the absence of other pathology such as haemo- or pneumothorax. As the disease process develops the respiratory distress increases and ventilation becomes progressively more difficult. In the majority of cases there are no prehospital signs which can be specifically linked to developing pulmonary contusion other than evidence of significant chest wall injury.

Cardiac contusion

In cardiac contusion there is bleeding into the wall of the heart following blunt trauma to the chest. It can lead to myocardial dysfunction or, occasionally, coronary artery occlusion, giving rise to further myocardial damage.

On examination the patient may have sternal bruising and tenderness due to the force of the impact. There is also an association between cardiac contusions and fractures of the sternum or wedge fractures of the thoracic vertebrae. Should the contusion be significant then the patient may develop arrhythmias, heart failure or hypotension which do not respond to resuscitation. Cardiac contusion cannot be diagnosed in the prehospital environment and there is no specific treatment other than exemplary "ABC" management. The presence of any of the above features is suggestive of the diagnosis which can be confirmed in hospital.

Ruptured diaphragm

Ruptured diaphragm can result from either blunt or penetrating trauma. In the latter case 75% are associated with intraabdominal injury. The reason for this is that during expiration, the diaphragm is elevated and the lower seven ribs overlie the abdominal cavity. Therefore a penetrating wound in this area may enter the peritoneal cavity as well as causing pulmonary injury. Furthermore, a fracture of these ribs can be associated with injury to the underlying liver (10%) and spleen (20%).

> Injuries between the nipple line and the umbilicus should be considered an indicator of potential underlying abdominal damage as well as chest damage

On examination of the patient, suspicion should be raised if a wound is found between the fifth and the 12th ribs. The patient may be breathless and have decreased breath sounds over the lower aspect of the affected side. Occasionally bowel sounds can be heard on auscultation of the chest. This condition requires early surgical treatment and immediate evacuation is required.

Disruption of the thoracic aorta

In patients who have sustained rapid deceleration (for example, a fall from a height or a car crash at speed), movement occurs between the fixed and mobile parts of the thoracic aorta. If only the inner two layers of the aorta are torn, blood escapes but is contained by the third outer layer (10% of cases). If this outer layer is also breached in the injury then the patient rapidly exsanguinates at the scene of the incident (90% of cases).

In the 10% who survive the initial accident, only around 500 ml of blood will be lost from the systemic circulation. Consequently the patient will not demonstrate the characteristic signs of shock (providing there are no other sources of haemorrhage). Variable signs which may be present are hoarseness of the voice (caused by pressure on the recurrent laryngeal nerve from the expanding haematoma), upper limb hypertension and pulse differences between upper and lower limbs. Time should not be wasted searching for these signs, which are rarely present. The diagnosis is usually made after investigation in hospital.

If these patients are to survive then the aorta needs to be surgically repaired before the outer layer ruptures. Time is crucial, because half the immediate survivors will die each day if no operation is performed. Therefore immediate transfer to hospital is essential.

Oesophageal rupture

Following a severe blow to the epigastrium, gastric contents are forced into the lower oesophagus and may tear it. Penetrating trauma can also rupture the oesophagus at any level and is likely to be associated with injuries to neighbouring structures.

On examination, the patient will be shocked and in pain. Surgical emphysema in the neck and upper chest may develop with time. Suspicion should be further raised if there is a left pneumothorax (or pleural effusion) without a history of left chest trauma or fractured ribs on the left side. These patients will require further investigations and in almost all cases a surgical repair.

Simple pneumothorax

Both blunt and penetrating injury may lead to tears of the lung with subsequent air leak into the pleural cavity. This may be detected clinically by the reduction of breath sounds accompanied by increased percussion over the affected side,

but may only be detected on chest X-ray. Hypoxia develops due to local collapse of lung tissue. The treatment is insertion of an intercostal drain as described previously. This may be deferred until arrival at the emergency department.

Haemothorax

Bleeding into the pleural cavity may not be as dramatic as in massive haemothorax. On examination, the patient may have decreased chest wall movement with reduced percussion on the affected side. Again, this may only be detected on chest X-ray. The treatment is insertion of an intercostal drain. Again, this may be deferred until arrival in the emergency department.

Ruptured bronchi

The main bronchi are firmly anchored and so are unable to move when the body is subjected to rapid deceleration forces. A tear can be partial or complete and is associated with a high mortality rate (30%), owing to the other injuries which occur following rapid deceleration.

On examination there may be haemoptysis, surgical emphysema, a pneumothorax and overt signs of a chest injury. If intubation of the trachea is attempted (for another reason), then it may be technically difficult or impossible to perform.

As these patients require the expertise of a thoracic surgeon for their definitive management, immediate evacuation from the scene of the incident is required.

OTHER INJURIES

Chest wall injuries

Fracture of the sternum (see Chapter 27) is common in frontal impacts and may be associated with seatbelt injuries; localized pain and tenderness are characteristic. Fractured ribs (see Chapter 25) are common and may be due to both direct and indirect forces. Although not life threatening, both these conditions are extremely painful and each individual fracture can be associated with the loss of 150 ml of blood. The pain from rib fractures can be improved by adequate analgesia and decreased patient movement. In patients with long-standing chest pathology (for example, the elderly), the reduction in effective ventilation associated with apparently minor chest wall injuries can be enough to precipitate life-threatening respiratory failure.

Surgical emphysema

Surgical emphysema results from leakage of air into the subcutaneous tissues; it may result from either penetrating chest injury or more commonly blunt trauma. Severe surgical emphysema which is impairing ventilation is associated with major airway disruption as well as oesophageal disruption. In the prehospital environment, the presence of surgical emphysema should be assumed to be a sign of significant chest pathology until proven otherwise after investigation in hospital.

TRANSFER

Transfer is a particularly dangerous time for the patient, therefore great care must be taken to anticipate and minimize any potential problems. Where other injuries permit, the patient should be transferred sitting up.

ASSESSMENT

Oxygen should be provided during transfer and all cannulae, tubes and drains must be secured with the knowledge that if they *can* fall out, they *will* fall out!

MONITORING

Monitoring will ensure that ventilation and tissue perfusion are adequate. As a minimum, an ECG monitor, automatic blood pressure recorder and pulse oximeter are essential.

ANALGESIA IN CHEST INJURIES

Nitrous oxide and oxygen inhalation (Entonox) is contraindicated in chest injuries not only because it will reduce the inspired oxygen to 50% but also, and most importantly, because nitrous oxide will diffuse rapidly into a simple or potential pneumothorax to produce a life-threatening tension pneumothorax. The analgesia of choice is therefore intravenous opiates titrated to effect.

> **Entonox is contraindicated in chest injuries**

TRANSFER PERSONNEL

During transit, the patient should be accompanied by a person trained to monitor and intervene should any problems arise. *Where possible, radio contact should be maintained between the ambulance and the receiving hospital.*

SUMMARY

Fatalities in patients with chest trauma commonly result from easily correctable hypoxia or hypovolaemia. The management of these patients therefore follows the standard "ABC" principles. In the majority of cases, immediate transfer to hospital will be required or help from a mobile medical team if the patient cannot be moved.

FURTHER READING

American College of Surgeons Committee on Trauma 1997 Advanced trauma life support course for physicians. American College of Surgeons, Chicago

Driscoll P, Gwinnutt C, Jimmerson C, Goodall O, (eds) 1994 Trauma resuscitation: the team approach. Macmillan, London

Chapter 26

Abdominal and genitourinary trauma

INTRODUCTION

In the UK the incidence of life-threatening abdominal and genitourinary trauma is low, accounting for just over 1% of all trauma admissions to hospital. Nevertheless, serious injury is often overlooked, particularly in the prehospital setting, and this results in an unacceptably high rate of morbidity and mortality. To illustrate this point, in the USA abdominal trauma is the second leading cause of preventable death. This is not due to failure to provide an acceptable standard of care. Physical signs immediately after trauma are often subtle and may even be absent initially. Signs, even when present, may be masked owing to multiple injuries. An associated head injury with alteration in conscious level or intoxication by drugs or alcohol may cause particular difficulty with diagnosis. Also, the presence of an additional painful or easily visible injury may cause further distraction. A high index of suspicion is therefore mandatory, particularly if the mechanism of injury points to the likelihood of abdominal or genitourinary injury. In the UK the majority of injuries are the result of blunt impact following road traffic accidents, and trauma to multiple systems is the rule rather than the exception. Penetrating injury by knife, bullet or fragment is on the increase, particularly in urban areas.

ESSENTIAL ANATOMY

Failure to appreciate the physical extent of the abdominal cavity and the diversity of its contents is an important factor in missed or neglected injury. This is particularly important for prehospital personnel who have to assess patients under arduous conditions and at a time when objective signs may be absent or subtle in presentation. The abdomen has three distinct regions, the true peritoneal cavity, the retroperitoneum and the pelvis. The true peritoneal cavity has two compartments – intrathoracic and abdominal (see Figures 26.1 and 26.2). The intrathoracic abdomen is an extensive area hidden under the lower ribs, comprising the diaphragm, liver, spleen, stomach and transverse colon. The extent of the compartment varies with respiration – in full expiration, the diaphragm may rise to the fourth intercostal space. This is important because vital structures such as the liver are at risk following lower thoracic injury, particularly penetrating injury. In the prehospital setting, if a wound is noted over the lower chest (below the nipple in the male) the paramedic should assume intraabdominal injury and give a high priority to transfer to hospital, even in the absence of physical signs on abdominal examination. Obvious fractures of lower ribs also put abdominal viscera at risk and should heighten suspicion even in the absence of signs. The abdominal compartment contains the soft organs of digestion, the small and large intestines. It is a vulnerable area, protected anteriorly only by the muscles of the abdominal wall. Lying behind the abdominal compartment is the retroperitoneal space containing major blood vessels such as the inferior vena cava and the aorta, genitourinary structures, reproductive organs, pancreas and segments of the intestinal tract including part of the duodenum and colon. This is a notoriously silent area following serious injury – physical

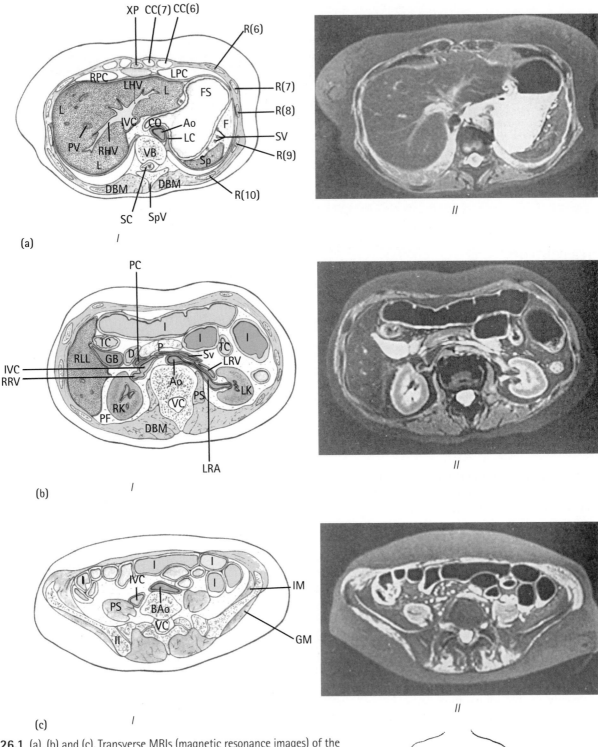

Figure 26.1 (a), (b) and (c), Transverse MRIs (magnetic resonance images) of the abdomen. (Courtesy of Dr. W. Kucharzyck, Clinical Director of Tri-Hospital Resonance Centre, Toronto, Ontario, Canada.) *AO*, indicates aorta: *BAo*, bifurcation of aorta; *CC*, costal cartilage; *CO*, cardiac orifice of stomach; *D*, duodenum; *DBM*, deep back muscles; *DC*, descending colon; *F*, fat; *FS*, fundus of stomach; *GB*, gallbladder; *I*, intestine; *II*, ilium; *IM*, iliacus muscle; *IVC*, inferior vena cava; *L*, liver; *LC*, left crus; *LHV*, left hepatic vein; *LPC*, left pleural cavity; *LK*, left kidney; *LRA*, left renal artery; *P*, pancreas; *PF*, perirenal fat; *PC*, portal confluence; *PS*, psoas major muscle; *PV*, portal vein (traid) *R*, rib; *RHV*, right hepatic vein; *RK*, right kidney; *RLL*, right lobe of liver; *SC*, spinal cord; *RPC*, right pleural cavity; *SP*, spleen; *SpV*, spinous of vertebra; *Sv*, splenic vein; *SV*, splenic vessels; *VB*, vertebral body; *VC*, vertebral canal; *X*, xiphoid process of sternum

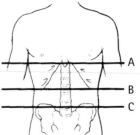

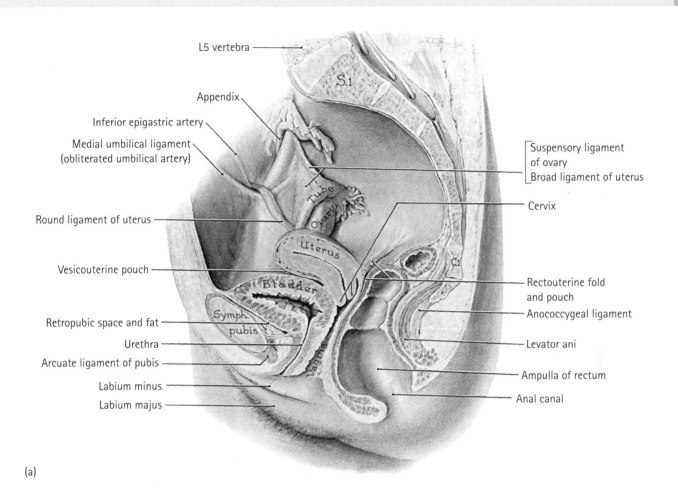

L5 vertebra

Appendix

Inferior epigastric artery

Medial umbilical ligament
(obliterated umbilical artery)

Round ligament of uterus

Vesicouterine pouch

Retropubic space and fat

Urethra

Arcuate ligament of pubis

Labium minus

Labium majus

S.1

Tube

Ovary

Uterus

Bladder

Symph.
pubis

Vagina

Suspensory ligament
of ovary
Broad ligament of uterus

Cervix

Rectouterine fold
and pouch

Anococcygeal ligament

Levator ani

Ampulla of rectum

Anal canal

C.1

(a)

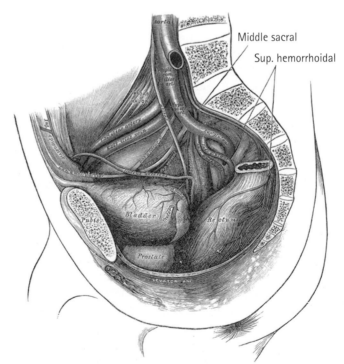

Middle sacral

Sup. hemorrhoidal

Aorta

Pubis

Bladder

Rectum

Prostate

LEVATOR ANI

(b)

Figure 26.2 (a) Median section of a female pelvis. (b) Pelvic vascular tree

signs are masked or may be absent during the "golden hour". The pelvic region contains the bladder, rectum and major vessels in both sexes – in the female the uterus and vagina are present. Although protected by the bony pelvis, intrapelvic structures are prone to injury, particularly in association with pelvic fractures or penetrating injury.

MECHANISMS OF INJURY

Two mechanisms of injury exist – blunt and penetrating. Patients may present with combined injury associated with both mechanisms, a particular feature of injury following terrorist explosions or acts of war. In the majority of instances, injury results from blunt impact following a road traffic accident, sporting accident, fall or industrial accident.

BLUNT INJURIES

Blunt impact results in definable injury patterns, as follows.

Bursting

Sudden, violent compression of the abdominal wall may dramatically raise intraabdominal pressure leading to rupture of a bowel loop. An incorrectly fitted seatbelt is a common factor in these injuries.

Crush

Direct crush injuries occur when a viscus is injured by directly applied pressure. A common event is rupture of the retroperitoneal portion of the duodenum in bicycle accidents – the duodenum is compressed between a handlebar and the lumbar spine. The pancreas, liver and spleen are also readily injured in this way.

Shear

Shear force injuries occur when force is applied tangentially across vascular pedicles; structures at risk include the spleen, liver and small bowel mesentery. These injuries are commonly associated with sudden deceleration.

Collision

Collision injuries result typically from impact of a motor vehicle on a pedestrian. The pattern of injury will depend on the size of the victim – bumper (fender) impact on an adult usually involves the limbs and abdominal injury is relatively uncommon, but in a child the torso takes the brunt of the force and abdominal and chest injury should be assumed in the prehospital setting.

> **Box 26.1 Types of blunt injury**
>
> - Bursting
> - Crush
> - Shear force
> - Collision
> - Ejection

Ejection

Ejection from a vehicle can result in multiple injuries, including damage to the cervical spine, depending on how the casualty lands – the torso is a large target and the likelihood of abdominal injury under these circumstances is high.

Evaluation of blunt injuries

Injury from more than one mechanism is not uncommon and may on occasion be suspected from an inspection of the accident scene, referred to as "reading the wreckage". A head-on collision with a poorly restrained driver may result in compression injury to a bowel loop, if the driver strikes the steering column; direct injury to the abdomen (or chest) may occur and deceleration may result in tearing injury due to shear forces. The paramedic assessing the victim should not be overly concerned with making these deductions; what is important is that an injury has taken place and that the victim has a high priority for transfer to an appropriate hospital. Decision making will be based on a high index of suspicion knowing the mechanism of injury, and supported by physical assessment (discussed later).

PENETRATING INJURIES

Penetrating injury is on the increase throughout the developed world and is already a particular feature of trauma in some UK inner cities.

Intraabdominal penetration may be obvious, for example with a wound clearly visible in the anterior abdominal wall. However, penetrating objects, bullets, fragments, knives or damaged vehicle parts can reach the abdomen from the lower chest, the back, flanks, buttocks and perineum. In the case of bullets and missile fragments, the entry site may be *anywhere*, as they may travel unpredictable distances and readily deflect from their original line of flight. Be particularly wary about discounting torso penetration in any case involving ballistic missiles. Penetration into the abdominal cavity by whatever mechanism is a serious matter – the morbidity and mortality rates are high, particularly if there is a delay in recognition that injury has occurred.

ENERGY TRANSFER FACTORS

It is now conventional to describe penetrating missile injury in terms of injury caused by laceration and crushing in the path of the missile, and in terms of energy transfer to surrounding tissues (see Chapter 30). Penetration by sharp objects in road traffic accidents and stabbings, and wounding by low-velocity (usually handgun) bullets, typically result in *low-energy transfer* with the injury confined to the wound track. The outcome therefore depends on which structures lie in the path of the penetrating object. In contrast, penetration by high-velocity missiles from modern assault rifles and exploding devices is associated with *high-energy transfer,* raising the possibility of injury occurring remote from the track. In practice, this *is* rare in the UK and should not alter prehospital decision making. However, low-velocity missiles may still produce high-energy transfer wounds and vice versa. The initial assessment and resuscitation system for such patients is in no way different from resuscitation in any other trauma situation (see Chapter 30).

RECOGNITION OF INJURY

Serious trauma to abdominal structures is readily missed even in a well-equipped resuscitation room. This is particularly so following blunt impact. As many as 20% of patients with significant intraabdominal bleeding reveal little or nothing in the way of physical signs. How common is it to overlook trauma in the challenging prehospital environment? The attending paramedic may have to rely on an intelligence-gathering exercise, with information gleaned from the mechanism of injury (see above), a history from the patient if possible or from others at the scene and information from an initial clinical assessment or primary survey of the patient, along with a high index of suspicion.

EVENT HISTORY

The event history may be provided by the patient, other victims or bystanders. It is frequently unavailable. A clear history from the patient is the ideal. Ask what happened. Enquire about pain, points of impact or wounds. Ask also if pain is present in the shoulders or back – referred pain from these sites may give clues to the presence of intraabdominal bleeding or faecal spillage. Other questions may yield clues: if the patient was fully conscious and alert after the impact, but now has an altered conscious level or is unresponsive, one of the reasons may be occult intraabdominal bleeding. Remember that head injury, drugs or alcohol, and the absence of witnesses may mean no event history is obtainable (see Chapter 20).

INITIAL CLINICAL ASSESSMENT

Start by being suspicious. Accurate assessment may be difficult because of the environment or because of entrapment. Within the limits imposed the approach should be that described in Chapter 21. There is no point in looking for signs of abdominal trauma if the airway remains in jeopardy.

In the primary survey, the first indication of abdominal trauma typically arises during assessment of "C" (circulation) of the "ABCDE" system, when shock is found and no obvious cause is present – this is known as shock of unexplained aetiology. Another clue may be when the extent of shock is out of proportion to the observed injuries. If shock is not a particular feature and the patient is readily stabilized, the secondary survey may reveal tenderness, rebound tenderness or even rigidity. In particular, the paramedic should:

- expose the abdomen as far as possible
- inspect or look at the abdomen, including flanks, lower chest and pelvic region
- palpate the abdomen, including the flanks and as much of the back as possible.

Wounds, bruises or abrasions should raise the level of suspicion.

> Remember, the paramedic is not concerned with establishing a specific diagnosis and only needs to assess the likelihood of injury being present and arrange expeditious transport to hospital

The secondary survey assessment is only indicated for stable patients. Patients exhibiting shock should be taken immediately to hospital.

PATHOPHYSIOLOGY

It may be helpful to look briefly at the pathophysiological consequences of some intraabdominal injuries. Irrespective of the mechanism of injury, it is safe to assume that solid organs (such as liver and spleen) and vascular structures bleed, while the soft digestive organs will leak bowel contents. Bleeding, if significant, will lead to haemorrhagic shock whose onset may be rapid, dramatic and obvious; while leakage of bowel contents leads to faecal peritonitis and finally septicaemia whose onset may be more gradual and less obvious in the prehospital setting. Of course, both phenomena may be present and this is not unusual. Under these circumstances, signs of haemorrhagic shock present first and may mask evidence of early peritoneal soiling.

GENITOURINARY TRAUMA

Genitourinary trauma is virtually inextricable from abdominal trauma and the two are normally considered together. In general, patients suffering genitourinary trauma are managed as abdominal trauma victims. However, there are a number of points worthy of emphasis. Because the kidneys and ureters lie in the retroperitoneal space (see Figures 26.1 and 26.2), injury is often silent and easily missed. Haematuria is *not* a constant feature. Take particular heed of patients with blunt or penetrating injury to the back and flanks, and regard bruises, contusions or areas of tenderness as significant. Injuries to the lower urinary tract may involve bladder, urethra and external genitalia and are usually more obvious, provided they are looked for. Blood at the external urinary meatus or an inability to pass urine are clear signs of injury. The lower urinary tract is also vulnerable to injury following pelvic trauma. There is little to be done in the prehospital setting apart from injury recognition, understanding the implications and transporting the patient to hospital as a priority.

PELVIC FRACTURES

Pelvic fractures are common components in multisystem injury and they should be particularly looked for. The extent of injury varies from an uncomplicated single bone injury to multiple fractures which disrupt the pelvic ring and render it unstable. The more severe pelvic fractures are usually associated with high-speed impact and should therefore be suspected from the history and mechanism of injury. From a paramedical perspective these are critical injuries to recognize. Unstable, complex pelvic injuries are associated with a very high mortality rate, principally due to uncontrolled haemorrhage.

Physical examination and extrication should be handled with great care. Stabilization of an unstable pelvis is difficult in the prehospital setting and it is reasonable to consider the application of a specialized pelvic splint. More simple techniques include the application of a pelvic binder or drawsheet. In the absence of palpable radial pulses, initial management may require repeated 250 ml aliquots of crystalloid. This should be started en route to hospital if the patient is not trapped. Rapid transportation to hospital is of paramount importance. Large volumes of whole blood are typically needed and some patients will continue to haemorrhage until the pelvis is stabilized by operative fixation.

ABDOMINAL TRAUMA IN PREGNANCY

Trauma in pregnancy is dealt with in Chapter 52 and is not covered here in detail; however, some points specific to abdominal trauma are worth emphasizing. Remember that the pregnant uterus remains inside the protection of the bony pelvis until the 12th week of gestation and pregnancy therefore may not be obvious, particularly in an unconscious patient. After 12 weeks the uterus rises above the pelvic brim and is palpable. *The possibility of pregnancy should always be considered in a woman of childbearing age* and should be actively sought. The best possible care for the fetus is optimal care for the mother and this must be the aim. Trauma to the abdomen in later pregnancy when the uterus is thin-walled may result in uterine rupture or placental abruption associated with significant blood loss. Signs of

shock should be evident in the primary survey and appropriate action taken. Shock management must be prompt and vigorous and the patient quickly transported to hospital. Remember the problem of postural hypotension due to compression of the inferior vena cava by the gravid uterus, which may require manual displacement of the uterus to the left, elevation of the right hip or, if a spine board is available, tipping the spine board and patient towards the left side at a 30° angle during transportation.

> The outcome for the fetus depends on how well the mother is managed

RESUSCITATION IN THE PREHOSPITAL SETTING

The measures appropriate to treat patients with abdominal injuries are outlined in this chapter. It is important again to emphasize the need to transfer patients to the ideal setting of a modern hospital where management can be optimized. However, in certain circumstances, for example entrapment, a prolonged period of prehospital management may be unavoidable. Be guided by the system outlined in Chapter 21 – it provides an approach to trauma life support appropriate for all casualties.

FURTHER READING

Driscoll P, Nancarrow J 1999 Abdominal and genitourinary trauma. In: Greaves I, Porter K (Eds) Prehospital medicine. The principles and practice of intermediate care. Arnold, London

Bickell WH, Pepe PE, Bailey ML, Wyatt CH, Maltox KL 1987 Randomised trial of pneumatic antishock garments in the prehospital management of penetrating abdominal injuries. Annals of Emergency Medicine 16(6): 653–658

Fox MA, Mangiante EC, Fabian TC, Voreller GR, Kudsk KA 1990 Pelvic fractures: an analysis of factors affecting prehospital trials and patient outcome. Southern Medical Journal 83(7): 785–788

Fox MA, Fabian TC, Croce MA, Magiante EC, Carson JP, Kudsk KA 1991 Anatomy of the accident scene: a prospective study of injury and mortality. American Surgery 57(6): 394–397

Vermeulen B, Peter R, Hoffmeyer P, Unger PF 1999 Prehospital stabilisation of pelvic dislocations: a new strap belt to provide temporary haemodynamic stabilisation. Swiss Surgery 5(2): 43–46

Chapter 27

Bone and joint injuries

INTRODUCTION

Bone and joint injuries form a very significant part of the workload of a paramedic. These injuries range from the relatively trivial to the life threatening. The general management of the patient with life-threatening trauma is discussed elsewhere. This chapter will focus on the approach to specific injuries. Serious bony injuries such as open fractures and major dislocations can distract the clinician from paying appropriate attention to the ABC system. It should not be forgotten that however serious a bone or joint injury (Figure 27.1), its true priority is, at best, under C if there is any associated bleeding which might be controlled, for example, by the application of a traction splint.

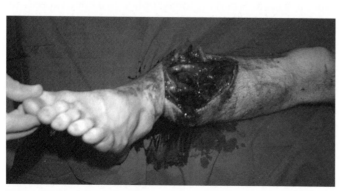

Figure 27.1 Major bony injury

ANATOMY

The human skeleton consists of over 200 bones (Figure 27.2). The functions of this skeleton include:

- support for the organs of the body
- protection for vital organs such as the brain
- forming a frame which allows locomotion in conjunction with the muscular system.

Bones and joints can only rarely be considered in isolation. In the extremities they are intimately related to the muscles, nerves and blood vessels of the limb. The thoracic cage and vertebral column are related to the organs of the thorax, abdomen and pelvis. Injury to the bones and joints invariably results in injury to the soft tissues.

Bones have an outer layer of compact bone called the *cortex*, which is relatively thin. The cortex is surrounded by a layer called the *periosteum*. This has been likened to the "skin" of the bone and contains cells that are able to divide and mature into osteoblasts which in turn form new bone. The inner layer of bone, the *medulla*, has a lattice structure of trabeculae. It contains fat and (in certain bones) the bone marrow.

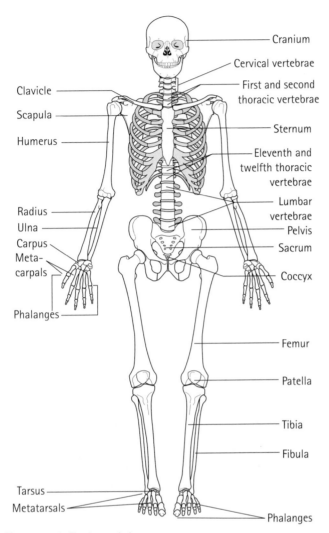

Figure 27.2 The bony skeleton

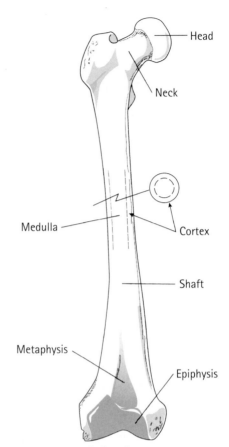

Figure 27.3 The anatomy of a long bone

Bones can be divided into groups, depending on their anatomical structure. *Long bones* include the humerus of the upper arm and the femur of the upper leg. The different parts of a typical long bone are shown in Figure 27.3 *Flat bones* include the mandible and parts of the skull, which are shaped according to their function.

The soft tissues of the limb comprise:

- vascular structures, such as arteries, arterioles, capillaries, venules, veins and lymphatics
- neurological structures, such as nerves (sensory, motor or mixed) and sense organs
- muscular structures, such as muscles, tendons and ligaments
- other soft tissue structures, such as fat, connective tissue and skin.

The bones are connected to each other by articulations or joints which can be of varying type and structure. Joints can be classified as:

- *fibrous* – such as the joints between the individual bones of the skull; there is little or no movement possible at such joints
- *synovial* – movement can occur at these joints which have a capsule lined with a membrane called the synovium; under

normal circumstances these joints contain a small quantity of synovial fluid.

Joints rely on a soft tissue capsule, ligaments and to a lesser extent the tendons and muscles which cross them for their structural stability. Injury to these soft tissues may result in either dislocation or subluxation (partial dislocation with some continuity of the joint surface) of the joint.

MECHANISM OF INJURY

FRACTURES

Fractures occur when the force applied to a bone exceeds its tensile strength. This can be a large force applied to a normal, healthy bone or a moderate or even trivial force applied to a weak bone.

The deceleration forces applied to bone during a road traffic accident or a fall from a significant height can be enormous and will fracture even the healthiest bone. Bones may become weak as a result of a loss of calcium, for example in osteoporosis or perhaps owing to a structural abnormality such as a cyst or a tumour. Such a diseased bone may fracture even after minimal injury, for example a simple fall in the home.

The characteristics of the force applied to the bone lead to different patterns of fractures.

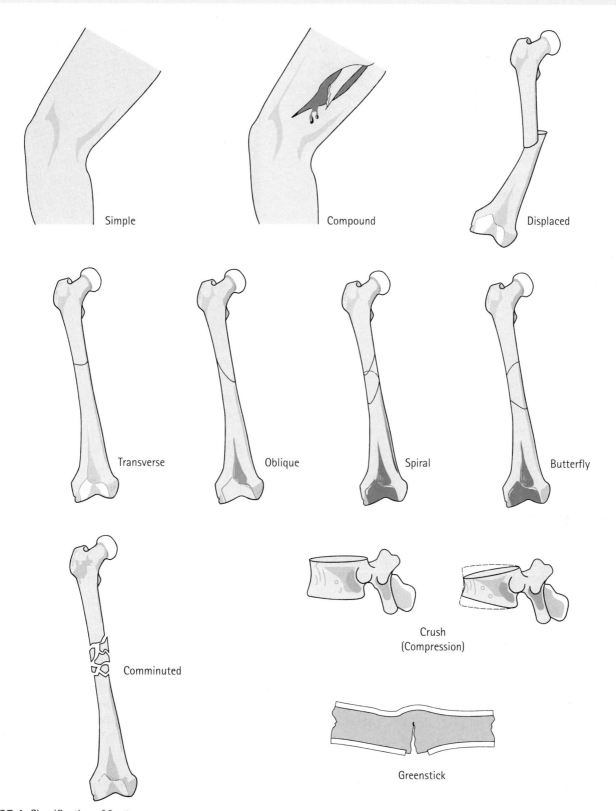

Figure 27.4 Classification of fractures

Fractures may be classified in several ways. Injuries may be *closed* (simple), if the skin and soft tissues overlying the injury are intact, or *open* (compound) if they are not (Figure 27.4). If the fracture is closed then there can be no direct contamination of the fracture site. An open fracture exists where there is a wound overlying the injury. The skin and soft tissues may be breached from the outside, perhaps from abrasion on the road surface or a penetrating object or projectile (*compound from without*). Alternatively, open wounds may be caused directly by the ends of the fractured bone penetrating the skin (*compound from within*). The wound contamination is likely to be greater in the first category. If the fracture is open, then direct contamination may occur from clothes, street debris, bacteria (such as *Staphylococcus aureus*) and spores (such as *Clostridium tetani* which can lead to tetanus). An open fracture of a bone may lose twice as much blood as its closed counterpart.

One of the most important aims in the initial prehospital management of fractures is to prevent the conversion of a closed fracture into an open fracture.

When fractures are treated, wherever possible, the normal anatomical alignment should be reestablished. This reduces pain and bleeding and helps to prevent damage to adjacent structures. It is perfectly acceptable to reduce a bony fragment back into a wound in order to achieve this, as long as the original position of the bone is recorded (preferably by Polaroid photography).

Fracture anatomy

Fractures may also be classified according to the anatomical configuration of the bony injury. After a bone has been fractured, the fragments may remain in their normal anatomical relationship to one another (undisplaced) or their relative positions may change (displaced). The fragments can lie at an angle or the ends of the bone can lose all contact with each other (off-ended). One fragment may rotate with respect to its normal position (malrotation). Muscle spasm may shorten the limb, leading to overlap of the ends of the bone, and may also lead to an increase in blood loss.

The combination of the mechanism and severity of injury, and the strength of the patient's bony skeleton, will lead to the bone breaking in different ways (Figure 27.4). When the shaft (diaphysis) of a long bone such as the tibia or humerus fractures it may do so in a simple *transverse* pattern. If the mechanism of injury includes a rotational force then the fracture may be *oblique* or even *spiral*. If this leads to the separation of a fragment of bone then this is known as a *butterfly fragment*. If the bone shatters into many pieces the fracture is said to be *comminuted*. Falls from a height or rapid vertical deceleration may lead to a *compressed* fracture, typically seen in the vertebral body. This fracture pattern may also be seen in the elderly patient with osteoporotic bone after only minimal injury or it sometimes occurs spontaneously.

Flat bones such as the skull may have simple *linear* fractures. If a complete section of bone becomes detached then it may be pushed inside the skull cavity towards the brain – a *depressed* fracture (Figure 27.5).

Fractures in children

Fractures in children need special consideration. The mechanism and precise type of injury may differ from those of adults. They should, however, be assessed and treated in the same way as similar fractures in adults. Children's bone

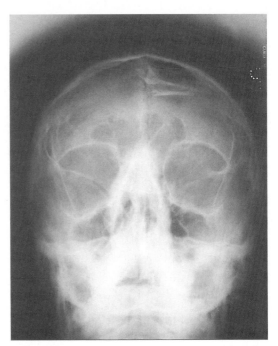

Figure 27.5 Radiograph showing a depressed fracture of the skull

is growing and generally speaking, the younger the patient, the more quickly the bone will heal.

Epiphyseal fractures

The bones of a child have special growth plates or *epiphyses* to enable longitudinal growth. These plates consist of cartilage which divides and is then converted to bone. They are a potentially weak area in the bone and are subject to shear fractures. The fall on the outstretched hand that will produce a fracture of the distal radius in the elderly adult may lead to a fracture of the distal radial epiphysis in a skeletally immature child.

Greenstick fractures

The bone of a child is not as brittle as that of an adult. Forces on that bone may cause an incomplete fracture. If one cortex of the bone is disrupted this is known as a "torus" or buckle fracture. If one cortex and medullary bone are fractured but the other cortex is buckled but intact, the injury is known as a greenstick fracture (Figure 27.6). Anyone who has attempted to snap a wet twig will understand how this name was derived.

DISLOCATIONS

Dislocations may occur when similar forces are placed on joints, but the soft tissue structures fail before the surrounding bone fractures (Figure 27.7).

There are some injuries where fracture and dislocation occur at the same time; for example, posterior dislocation of the hip with a fracture of the posterior lip of the acetabulum (hip socket). In this case, the acetabulum is fractured by the femur as it passes posteriorly, striking the lip.

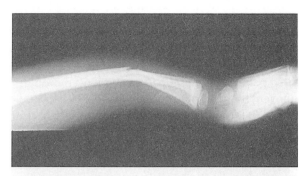

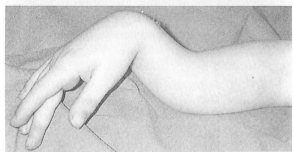

Figure 27.6 A greenstick fracture of the radius

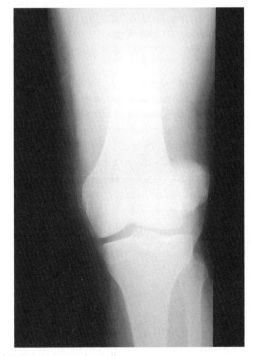

Figure 27.7 A dislocated patella

GENERAL EXAMINATION

The principles of the initial assessment and treatment of life-threatening conditions have been outlined earlier in this book. It is essential that the patient has a primary survey and that immediately life-threatening problems are recognized and treated. The majority of fractures and dislocations are not immediately life-threatening, but exceptions include fractures of the pelvis, multiple closed fractures or compound fractures of long bones, where serious haemorrhage may occur. Fractures of the skull and face may lead to airway obstruction or be associated with life-threatening neurological injuries. Fractures may coexist with injuries to the vital thoracic or abdominal organs.

Limb-threatening injuries are much more common. Many fractures and dislocations can lead to lifelong disability and thus are very important for the individual patient. Correct identification and treatment of such injuries will prevent further damage and reduce long-term disability. Injudicious handling of such injuries may result in increased long-term morbidity.

Fractures, particularly of the limbs, are usually obvious and cause the patient great discomfort. Life-threatening chest, head and abdominal injuries may not be so obvious. It is essential to avoid the temptation to concentrate on the most obvious injuries. Only when life-threatening injuries have been excluded or treated should limb injuries be assessed. The multiply injured patient may require immediate transfer to hospital *without* full assessment or treatment of such injuries. These decisions ("judgement calls") in the field can be difficult, but a common-sense approach based on a proficient primary survey is above criticism.

> **Do not be distracted by bony injuries: REMEMBER ABC**

Examination of bones and joint must be systematic if injuries are to be identified. The system advocated by Apley is simple and easy to master and can be applied in the pre-hospital setting: this is the *look–feel–move* system.

Look The part should be inspected for swelling, deformity and overlying wounds. Are there any preexisting scars? The joint should be compared with the normal side

Feel Is the injured part painful and if so, where? Is there any protective muscle spasm? Are the pulses distal to the injury intact?

Move Can the patient move the injured part?

If there is a fracture then the sensation of grating of the bone ends may be experienced ("crepitus"). This is extremely painful for the patient and deliberate attempts to elicit crepitus should be avoided.

It is essential that all patients who have sustained limb injuries are assessed for vascular injury. The palpation of a distal pulse alone is not sufficient. In the early phase of a compartment syndrome the arterial pressure may be sufficient to produce a pulse, while the tissue pressure is such that there is no effective perfusion of the cells. It is important to assess capillary refill in order to assess tissue perfusion. The nail bed is compressed for 5 seconds. The pressure is released and the time taken for the return of the normal pink colour is measured. If this is greater than 2 seconds (approximately the length of time it takes to say "capillary refill") then tissue perfusion is abnormal.

The capillary refill test is best performed in good light and a warm environment.

A neurological assessment of sensation and muscle power should be made in order to determine whether there is a possibility of any nerve damage.

GENERAL TREATMENT CONSIDERATIONS

PRIORITIES

Life-threatening conditions must be sought and treated where necessary. Perform a primary survey and treat life-threatening injuries before treating any fractures or dislocations. The priorities in fracture management are:

- safety
- airway with cervical spine control
- breathing
- circulation with haemorrhage control
- disability
- exposure.

The patient's history of tetanus immunization must be elicited, along with the features of the AMPLE history (see Chapter 9).

All patients who have sustained a long-bone injury should be given oxygen via a Hudson mask with a non-rebreathe valve and a reservoir bag at a rate of 15 l/min.

> All patients who have a long-bone injury require oxygen

Unnecessary delay at the scene must be avoided. The more serious the injury, the more important this is. If prehospital treatment is contemplated, will it stabilize or improve the patient's condition? If not, then early evacuation to hospital is imperative. If a patient is less than 20 minutes' journey from an appropriate hospital and is not trapped, an intravenous infusion should not be attempted at the scene, but performed en route to hospital.

A succinct history, including the mechanism of injury, and brief but accurate records will ensure efficient transfer of the patient to the care of hospital staff.

ANALGESIA

Pain relief (analgesia) is of prime importance. It can be justified on the grounds of humanity alone, but there is an increasing amount of evidence that adequate pain relief lessens the potential serious complications from major injury.

> Splinting a fracture or dislocation to prevent movement of the injured part is one of the best and simplest forms of pain relief

Most ambulances carry a 50/50 mixture of oxygen and nitrous oxide (Entonox, popularly called "laughing gas"). It is used as the basis for pain relief in most gaseous anaesthetics administered by anaesthetists in hospital. It has excellent pain-relieving properties and if used properly will be sufficient for most situations out of hospital. It should *not* be used if there is any suspicion of significant chest injury. It is best avoided in head injuries. Entonox is excellent for fractures and dislocations sustained as sports injuries.

An increasing number of ambulance services are carrying non-steroidal anti-inflammatory drugs in an injectable form. It is still unclear whether these are an effective adjunct to prehospital treatment. Intravenous opiate analgesia may be required for significant fractures. The types of analgesic agent carried and the indications for their use are variable and beyond the scope of this chapter. Close study of local rules and protocols and adequate practical training are essential before the paramedic administers any analgesia to a patient.

COMPOUND FRACTURES AND SERIOUS WOUNDS

Infection of a fracture is a disaster for the patient. Osteomyelitis can be controlled, but rarely cured. Good wound care starting at the scene of an accident will help reduce the incidence of this complication of compound fractures.

The fracture must be stabilized to avoid further damage to the soft tissues. Some form of manual immobilization or splinting is required. Traction splinting will reduce blood loss, but must not be applied excessively if traction injuries to the nerves are to be avoided.

The wound should be covered in a sterile dressing, soaked in 0.9% saline or aqueous iodine solution. Life-threatening bleeding should be controlled by direct pressure.

SPLINTING

Adequate splintage of a fractured limb (Figure 27.8) will result in:

- pain relief
- reduction of blood loss
- prevention of further soft tissue damage
- a reduced incidence of fat embolism (see below).

There is no substitute for practical experience of splintage techniques, which cannot be learned from a book. Generally splintage can be divided into two categories: simple splintage, and traction splintage.

Simple splintage

Simple splintage of the lower limb may be achieved by securely fastening the injured part to the opposite uninjured leg using triangular bandages or a purpose-built splint. Alternatively, the limb may be placed in a box splint which

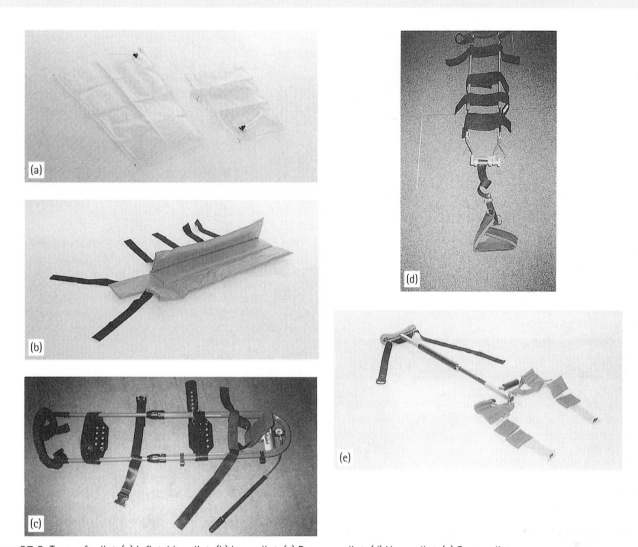

Figure 27.8 Types of splint. (a) Inflatable splint; (b) box splint; (c) Donway splint; (d) Hare splint; (e) Sager splint

should be well padded and should be of the appropriate size for the injured limb. Vacuum splints can also be effective. With the injured upper limb it is often sufficient to immobilize using a simple broad arm sling or allow the patient to support the arm with the uninjured hand.

> Immobilize the joints above and below the fracture

Traction splintage

Traction splintage is generally employed for femoral fractures. The first traction splint, the Thomas splint, was used extensively in the First World War and slashed the mortality rate from open fractured femurs from 80% to 20%. Modern traction splints work on the same principle of traction at the ankle and countertraction via a ring at the ischial tuberosity, except for the Sager splint (a padded T-bar that fits between the legs) which exerts countertraction on the symphysis pubis. The principle is to reduce the fracture and overcome the deforming force of the surrounding muscles which are in spasm. The restoration of the normal length and shape

of the limb also has the advantage of reducing blood loss (by up to 20–30%). Splints that apply traction to one (e.g., the Hare, Donway or Trac-Ill splints) or both lower limbs (e.g., the Sager splint) are effective. The types of splintage are discussed in more detail in Chapter 29. Traction splints can be time-consuming to apply, particularly if used infrequently. Familiarity with the splint used locally is essential.

BONE AND JOINT INJURIES IN SPECIFIC REGIONS

SKULL, FACIAL SKELETON AND CERVICAL SPINE

Head injuries are discussed in Chapter 23. Patients who have sustained a fracture to the skull or facial bones have sustained a serious head injury and must be treated with extreme caution. The airway may be compromised, either directly owing to instability of the facial skeleton (e.g., an unstable fracture of the mandible) or owing to secondary factors such as swelling, bleeding or loss of consciousness.

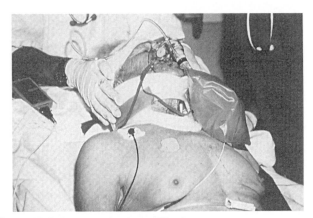

Figure 27.9 Cervical spine immobilization

All patients with a head injury should be assessed for injury to the cervical spine. These are not always symptomatic and an altered level of consciousness may make clinical evaluation unreliable or impossible.

> There is a 5% chance of significant cervical spine injury in the unconscious patient

The airway must take priority, but all reasonable precautions to prevent cervical spine movement must be taken until a radiological and clinical assessment has been made at the hospital. A rigid cervical collar is the minimum requirement. Additional immobilization techniques will be required (Figure 27.9). A blanket placed under the head and rolled at each side, combined with secure tape applied to the stretcher or bed and the patient's forehead, will provide further security. A full spinal immobilization splint such as a Russell Extrication Device or Kendrick Extrication Device combines immobilization of the cervical spine and other areas of the vertebral column during extrication and transport to hospital (see Chapter 29). Neck braces which are combined with immobilization on a spinal board effect the most secure immobilization when properly applied (e.g., the headbox). It must be remembered that pressure necrosis of the skin and soft tissues can be caused by even short periods on a spinal board. This is particularly true in the patient with compromised sensation, which may be a direct result of spinal injury.

Scoop stretchers are invaluable when transferring patients from the floor to a stretcher or bed. They can be adjusted to the correct length and then divided longitudinally to allow the stretcher to be slid under the patient with minimal movement from either side. They can then be reconnected and the patient lifted to safety. It should be noted that they should only be used for short periods and they are designed to transfer the patient from floor to spine board. They should then be removed.

The prevention of pressure sores by good patient care starts with the ambulance crew at the scene and is continued during transport to hospital, in the accident and emergency department, the operating theatre and on the ward. The patient's clothing must be checked for sharp or lumpy objects

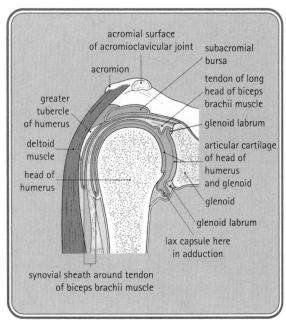

Figure 27.10 Simplified anatomy of the shoulder joint

such as coins or wallets as these will quickly lead to the development of pressure sores in the immobilized patient. This is particularly important in the unconscious patient.

THE UPPER LIMB

The upper limb is suspended from the trunk by the clavicle, scapula and various muscles which include the deltoid (Figure 27.10). Forces from the distal parts of the limb are transmitted to the trunk via these bones and the muscles and ligaments which are attached to them. Following a fall the whole of the upper limb must be examined and this includes the sternoclavicular joint, the clavicle, the acromioclavicular joint and the scapula.

Fractured clavicle

Cause

A fractured clavicle can be caused by a fall on the outstretched hand, when the forces transmitted up the upper limb may indirectly result in a fracture, or by a direct blow. Typically the fall occurs from a bicycle, a horse or a tree in children or from a motorcycle in adults.

Signs and symptoms

Pain occurs at the site of the fracture whenever the upper limb is moved. The patient often supports the injured arm at the elbow in an attempt to reduce movement of the limb. There is usually swelling at the site of the fracture, which typically occurs at the junction of the outer (lateral) third and inner (medial) two-thirds of the bone. There may be a wound associated with the fracture (Figure 27.11).

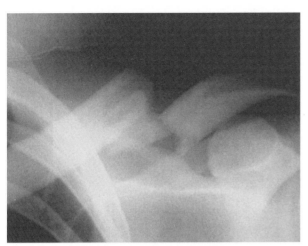

Figure 27.11 Fractured left clavicle. Note the position of the fracture at the junction of the outer third and inner two-thirds of the clavicle

Treatment

The upper limb should be immobilized in a broad arm sling. A collar and cuff should not be used as this will act to separate the bony ends of the fracture due to the weight of the arm.

Potential problems

This is usually a straightforward injury to treat. The sling will often control the pain as it prevents movement at the fracture site. As with all limb injuries, there is a chance of damage to important vascular and neurological structures close to the fracture site. The subclavian artery and vein are in close proximity to the clavicle and although injury is rare, it can be serious. Similarly the nerves that supply the upper limb may be injured, particularly when the fracture has been caused by direct rather than indirect force. Direct injury to this region may also result in chest injury and the assessment must not be confined to the clavicle.

> Always check distal neurovascular function

Fractured scapula

Cause

A fractured scapula is usually due to a direct blow, most commonly after a fall from a motorcycle, from a blunt weapon during an assault or accidentally during a sporting event with a stick or bat (e.g., a hockey stick). The scapula is surrounded by muscle and this is an unusual injury, considerable force being required.

Signs and symptoms

Pain occurs over the site of the fracture and may be made worse with movement of the upper limb.

Treatment

Immobilization of the upper limb in a broad arm sling will reduce the discomfort.

Potential problems

There may be associated injuries to the thoracic cage and ribs and these need careful examination.

Dislocation of the sternoclavicular joint

Cause

Dislocation of the sternoclavicular joint may be caused by a fall on the outstretched hand or by direct injury to the anterior aspect of the shoulder, levering the medial end of the clavicle away from its usual articulation with the manubrium of the sternum.

Signs and symptoms

There is pain localized at the medial end of the clavicle, made worse by movement of the upper limb. There may be swelling and deformity over the sternoclavicular joint.

Treatment

The vast majority of these injuries are subluxations or partial dislocations. They are best treated in a broad arm sling.

Potential problems

Occasionally there is severe displacement. If the medial end of the clavicle has been dislocated posteriorly then the major vessels are in danger of injury. The patient should be examined for signs of chest injury and shock. *If there is evidence of shock, they should be considered to have a severe, potentially life-threatening injury and evacuated to hospital immediately.* Intravenous access can be achieved in transit and any delay in reaching hospital should be avoided. Occasionally posterior dislocation of the sternoclavicular joint may produce airway obstruction: the clavicle should be pulled forwards, as a matter of urgency.

Dislocation of the acromioclavicular joint

Cause

Acromioclavicular joint dislocation occurs with a fall onto the point of the shoulder. It is a common injury in rugby football.

Signs and symptoms

There will be pain situated at the lateral end of the clavicle, made worse by attempting to carry any weight with the affected arm. This injury results from partial or complete disruption of ligaments between the clavicle and the acromion and in severe cases also the ligaments between the clavicle and the underlying coracoid process of the scapula. There will be a variable amount of local swelling and usually a step is visible between the lateral end of the clavicle and the acromion (this is the expanded anterolateral process of the scapula which forms a bony roof over the shoulder joint and muscles and normally articulates with the clavicle).

Treatment

The upper limb should be immobilized in a broad arm sling.

Potential problems

The mechanism of injury should lead to a high level of suspicion of associated injuries to the cervical spine and nerves in the brachial plexus.

Anterior dislocation of the shoulder

Cause

Anterior dislocation (Figure 27.12) is usually caused by forced external rotation of the glenohumeral joint (the joint between the humerus and the glenoid process of the scapula). Typically this results from a fall or a mistimed rugby tackle. If the shoulder has previously been dislocated then less force is required to produce a recurrent injury. Arm wrestling is another cause. Occasionally patients are able to dislocate their shoulder as a "party trick"; they usually have a chronically unstable joint which dislocates without pain.

Symptoms and signs

The acute injury gives rise to severe pain at the site of dislocation and protective spasm of the deltoid muscle. The patient will be supporting the forearm with the elbow flexed. The shoulder will look abnormal (square contour) compared with the other side, with a loss of the usual rounded contour of the upper arm. The lateral edge of the scapula may well appear prominent. It is important to assess the sensory portion of the axillary nerve which provides sensation to the "regimental badge" area of skin on the lateral aspect of the proximal arm. The axillary nerve winds around the neck of the humerus and may be damaged during either the dislocation of the shoulder or its reduction. The motor portion of the axillary nerve is important because it supplies much of the deltoid muscle.

Treatment

Treatment should be directed at immobilizing the upper limb during transfer to hospital for relocation of the joint. An acceptable method is to allow the patient to sit upright and support the arm, perhaps resting it on a pillow. The sooner the joint is relocated the better and at a sporting event there may a doctor present who is able to achieve this at the venue.

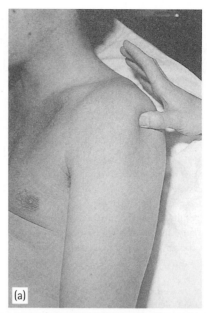

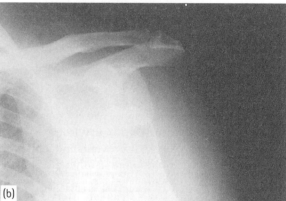

Figure 27.12 Anterior dislocation of the shoulder. (a) Clinical appearance; (b) X-ray

Otherwise the patient requires assessment in the accident and emergency department. In general, it is recommended that the shoulder is X-rayed before reduction, to exclude a fracture dislocation that will require surgical management.

Potential problems

The longer the joint is dislocated, the more permanent damage is done to the articular surface of the bone and to the soft tissues. Damage to the axillary nerve has been mentioned above, but *all* the nerves of the upper limb can be at risk. Damage to the major blood vessels may occur and proper examination and reexamination of the distal limb circulation is essential. Severe fractures and fracture-dislocations of the surgical neck of the humerus may mimic simple anterior dislocation.

Posterior dislocation of the shoulder

Cause

Posterior dislocation may be caused by a fall on the outstretched hand with the arm internally rotated or a direct

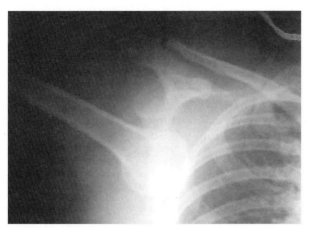

Figure 27.13 Inferior dislocation of the shoulder, clinical appearance

blow to the anterior aspect of the shoulder. An electric shock, epileptic fit or chronic muscle spasticity such as is seen in cerebral palsy can also cause posterior dislocation.

Symptoms and signs

These are similar to those of anterior dislocation, with pain, swelling and local deformity.

Treatment

The arm should be immobilized and the patient transported to hospital.

Potential problems

The nerves in the brachial plexus are particularly susceptible to damage due to pressure from the humeral head. Recognition and early relocation are essential. The X-ray changes are very subtle and this injury can be easily missed in hospital.

Inferior dislocation of the shoulder

Cause

Inferior dislocation (Figure 27.13) is extremely rare but can follow a violent convulsion or an electric shock.

Symptoms and signs

The arm is held extended above the head and the injury is extremely painful. The condition is often bilateral.

Treatment

Analgesia and support during the transfer to the hospital are all that is required.

Potential problems

Fitting the patient onto the stretcher may be difficult.

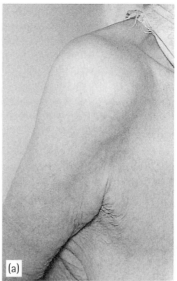

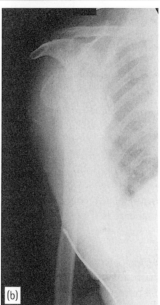

Figure 27.14 Fracture of the humerus. (a) Clinical appearance; (b) X-ray

Fracture of the proximal humerus

Cause

A fracture of the proximal humerus (Figure 27.14) may occur through a fall onto the outstretched hand or a direct fall onto the upper arm, particularly in elderly patients and those with osteoporosis. The fracture can occur in younger patients following violence.

Symptoms and signs

There is pain at the upper end of the arm. The patient will usually be supporting the arm at the elbow with the other hand. There may be obvious deformity. Swelling is almost immediate, but the severe bruising which accompanies this injury may not be apparent for several days and can track distally down the lateral aspect of the arm. In the younger group of patients who have sustained this fracture as a result of extreme violence, care should be taken to assess fully for life-threatening injuries.

Treatment

The arm is supported in a broad arm sling initially. Once the diagnosis has been confirmed in the accident and emergency department, the sling should be changed to a "collar and cuff". This allows the weight of the arm to apply traction to the fracture and tends to reduce the fractured bone into its normal anatomical position.

Potential problems

As with all fractures, the surrounding nerves and blood vessels can be injured directly at the time of the fracture.

Fracture of the shaft of the humerus

Cause

The shaft of the humerus may be fractured through direct injury such as a fall onto the arm or a blow from a blunt weapon. Indirect force can cause these fractures, although the fracture pattern may be different. A fall onto the outstretched hand often results in internal or external rotation at the shoulder – the forearm acts as a long lever and thus the humeral shaft is subjected to significant rotational forces. A spiral fracture is therefore common.

Symptoms and signs

The arm is painful and may be supported at the elbow by the other hand. There may be obvious angular deformity, but rotational malalignment is not always obvious. There may be significant swelling and bruising. It is essential to examine the distal portions of the limb to exclude vascular and neurological injury.

Treatment

The arm should be supported in a broad arm sling.

Potential problems

The radial nerve runs in a groove, closely applied to the humeral shaft posteriorly. It may be damaged directly or secondarily due to swelling (*compartment syndrome*). Loss of radial nerve function may lead to weakness of the muscles that extend the wrist and as a result the patient will demonstrate "wrist drop" (inability to extend the wrist). The arterial blood supply to the upper limb is via just one vessel at this point, the brachial artery. This artery may suffer direct injury or may be constricted owing to a compartment syndrome.

Supracondylar fracture of the humerus

Cause

Supracondylar fractures of the distal portion of the humerus just proximal to the elbow joint are common in childhood. They are typically caused by a fall onto the outstretched hand. The fractures can range from an undisplaced crack to a completely displaced injury with vascular and neurological damage (Figure 27.15).

Symptoms and signs

There is pain at the elbow after a fall. The child will support the elbow with the other hand. There may be obvious swelling and deformity and serious interference with the blood supply to the distal part of the limb.

Treatment

The arm should be immobilized in a broad arm sling in slight extension. Constant evaluation of the distal circulation is essential. If the circulation is compromised the elbow should be extended (straightened).

Potential problems

The brachial artery can be kinked over the bone ends, trapped between the bone ends or directly damaged by the fracture. If the circulation to the distal forearm is not

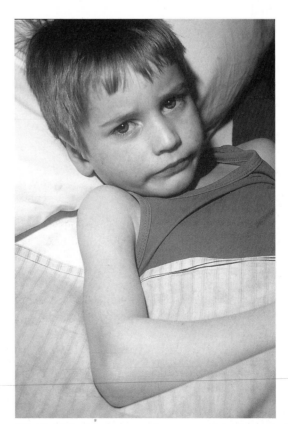

Figure 27.15 Clinical appearance of a supracondylar fracture of the humerus in a child

restored then there is real danger of Volkmann's ischaemic contracture (the death of all the muscle in the forearm), leaving a contracted, painful, useless arm. This can also be the result of compartment syndrome caused by swelling after this injury. Volkmann's contracture is a serious injury which often leads to long-term disability.

Fracture of the radial head

Cause

Fracture of the radial head is caused by a fall on the outstretched hand (Figure 27.16).

Symptoms and signs

There is pain over the lateral aspect of the forearm just distal to the elbow joint. There is often pain on rotation of the forearm (pronation and supination) and the elbow cannot be fully extended.

Treatment

The arm should be placed in a broad arm sling. Once the diagnosis has been confirmed at the accident and emergency department this may be replaced by a collar and cuff.

Potential problems

The distal circulation should be assessed, but this injury rarely leads to complications.

Fracture of the olecranon

Cause

Fracture of the olecranon (Figure 27.17) can result from a fall directly onto the elbow or from violent contraction of the triceps muscle in an attempt to extend the elbow against resistance.

Symptoms and signs

The elbow is very painful and there is considerable swelling. If the triceps tendon is still attached to the distal part of the ulna then it will still be possible to actively extend the elbow, although this will be very painful. If the attachment has been pulled off or is solely to the proximal fragment, then there can be no active extension of the elbow.

Treatment

The arm is immobilized in a broad arm sling. The distal neurological and vascular status is monitored.

Potential problems

The swelling may cause vascular insufficiency and compartment syndrome. There is a potential for damage to the nerves that cross the elbow joint. This is particularly true for the ulnar nerve which is closely applied to the medial side of the joint in the ulnar groove. Damage may lead to altered or lost sensation of the palmar surface of the small and ring fingers of the hand. It may also lead to loss of function of the small muscles of the hand with the exception of those that move the thumb.

Dislocation of the elbow

Cause

Elbow dislocation is caused by a fall on the outstretched hand. This injury may be associated with fractures of the distal humerus and/or the proximal radius and ulna.

Symptoms and signs

There is obvious deformity and gross swelling and the injury is usually very painful. Little movement is possible and attempts to do so are exquisitely painful. There is significant risk of vascular compromise due to swelling and neurological damage due to the stretching of the nerves at the elbow (Figure 27.18).

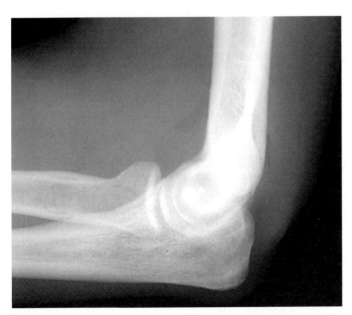

Figure 27.16 Fracture of the radial neck: mechanism of injury

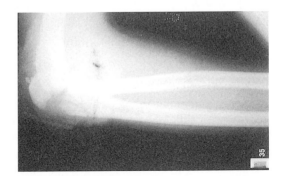

Figure 27.17 Fracture of the olecranon

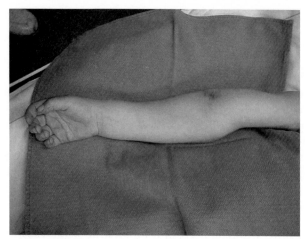

Figure 27.18 Clinical appearance of a dislocated elbow

Treatment

The elbow should be immobilized in a well-padded splint. The distal circulation and neurological status require constant assessment.

Potential problems

The potential for vascular and neurological complications is high and the patient is best served by rapid transfer to hospital to enable early reduction of the dislocation.

Fractures of the shafts of radius and ulna

Cause

Falling on an outstretched hand may cause a fracture of both forearm bones, the radius and ulna (Figure 27.19). Direct injury such as a fall onto the forearm or a direct blow may also fracture both bones, but it is possible to fracture one or the other in isolation. If one bone is fractured there is often an associated dislocation of the proximal or distal joint between the radius and ulna. Children may fracture the radius and ulna in the midshaft region or they may sustain a fracture involving the growth plate of the bones (epiphyseal injuries – see below).

Signs and symptoms

The forearm is painful and is supported by the other hand. There may be an obvious angular deformity.

Treatment

The arm requires immobilization, which is best achieved using some form of splintage. However, if this is difficult to apply because of angulation or discomfort, then a broad arm sling may be appropriate. It is important that the sling prevents movement at the fracture site but that it does not compromise the circulation because it is too tight. It is almost

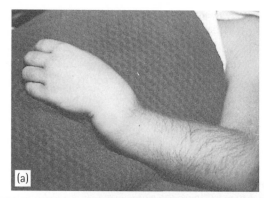

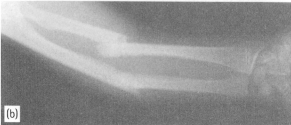

Figure 27.19 Fractures of the radius and ulna. (a) Clinical appearance; (b) X-ray

impossible to apply a splint single-handed and attempts to do so may cause the patient unnecessary discomfort and may even increase the soft tissue damage at the fracture site.

Potential problems

There is the ever-present possibility of circulatory compromise with these fractures and the distal portion of the limb must be regularly assessed. The skin and soft tissues directly overlying the fracture may be placed under tension if there is significant angulation. This may cause local skin ischaemia and necrosis. There is a real danger that closed fractures may become open if the forearm is not immobilized.

Fractures of the distal radius

Cause

Fracture of the distal radius (Colles' fracture, Figure 27.20) is caused by a fall on the outstretched hand. This is particularly common in the elderly with osteoporotic bone. Younger age groups can also sustain fractures of the distal radius. With children the injury is usually through the soft cartilage of the growth plate of the bone or epiphysis. Young adults with mature bone may also sustain a fracture of the distal radius but this is usually due to a highly violent injury such as a road traffic accident or serious fall and should be taken very seriously. This last group will often sustain fractures that extend into the surface of the wrist joint and are often displaced. The wide diversity of injuries illustrates why each distal radius fracture should be treated individually and not just dismissed as a Colles' fracture.

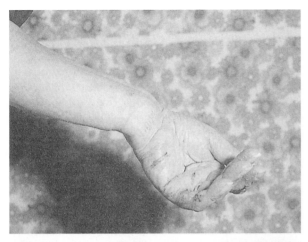

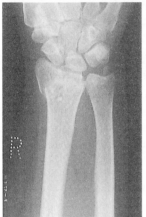
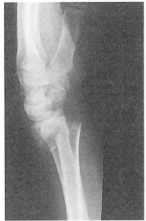

Figure 27.20 Fracture of the distal radius. (a) Clinical appearance; (b) X-ray

If the patient falls onto the back of the wrist with the forearm supinated then the distal fragment of the fracture may be displaced towards the palmar (volar or ventral) surface. This is known as a *Smith's fracture*.

Symptoms and signs

There is pain and swelling at the wrist. If the distal fragment has been displaced dorsally there is said to be a "dinner fork" deformity. If there is volar displacement of the fragment there is said to be a "garden spade" deformity. There may be symptoms of nerve injury in the palm of the hand. The median nerve is situated in the midline of the wrist and enters the hand via the carpal tunnel. It supplies sensation to the palmar surfaces of the thumb, index and middle fingers and supplies the motor branches to the small muscles of the thumb. It may sustain direct damage at the time of fracture or it may be compressed within the carpal tunnel owing to swelling or displacement of the fragments of the bone. The ulnar nerve may also be affected in fractures of the distal radius, but less frequently than the median nerve. The ulnar nerve supplies sensation to the little and ring fingers and motor branches to the remainder of the small muscles of the hand.

Treatment

The distal radius must be immobilized. A broad arm sling may be sufficient in some cases, a short box splint or vacuum splint may be used as alternatives. The sensation and circulation to the hand and fingers must be monitored.

Potential problems

The nerve injuries outlined above may cause symptoms. The hand must be examined to exclude vascular damage. If there is massive swelling then the hand and wrist should be elevated after the fracture has been immobilized.

Fractures of the carpal bones

Cause

Fractures of the carpal bones are caused by a fall on the outstretched hand. Scaphoid fractures (the most common) are caused when the wrist is forced into hyperextension.

Symptoms and signs

The wrist is painful with reduced movements. There may be no significant swelling.

Treatment

The arm should be placed in a broad arm sling.

Potential problems

If fractures of these bones are missed and not immobilized in plaster, the fracture may fail to unite and the patient will be left with a stiff wrist.

Fractures of the metacarpals and fingers

Cause

Injuries to the metacarpals and fingers are usually caused by direct falls or blows.

Symptoms and signs

The injured bone will be painful. There may be considerable swelling on the dorsum (back) of the hand. The palmar skin is firmly attached to the bony skeleton of the hand to allow good grip but the dorsal skin is loose and thus bruising and swelling track dorsally. There may be obvious bony deformity. The fifth metacarpal is most commonly broken, often as a result of a punch.

Treatment

The hand should be elevated in a high arm sling.

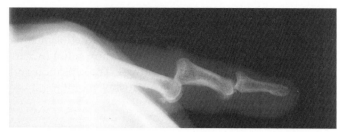

Figure 27.21 Dislocation of an interphalangeal joint

Potential problems

The blood supply to the digits may be compromised, either directly as a result of the injury or secondary to swelling. *It is of paramount importance that rings and jewellery are removed from an injured hand as soon as is practicable. This applies to rings on uninjured digits because they will subsequently swell in any hand injury.* If it is not possible to remove them prehospital then their presence must be communicated to the staff in the accident and emergency department so that arrangements can be made to cut the rings off. Failure to remove rings may lead to swelling, circulatory compromise and even loss of the digit.

Dislocation of the fingers

Cause

Finger dislocation is usually caused by direct injury, for instance by a blow from a cricket ball.

Symptoms and signs

There is obvious deformity of the joint, which is painful (Figure 27.21).

Treatment

It is often said that these dislocations should be reduced quickly, without anaesthesia. This cannot be recommended. Relocation of these joints is not always straightforward and there may be a fracture associated with the dislocation. It is better to transport the patient to the accident and emergency department where a fracture can be excluded by X-ray and reduction can performed painlessly under a ring block or other regional anaesthesia.

THE THORACIC SKELETON

The injuries to organs within the chest have been outlined in Chapter 25. The following section describes the bony injuries that may affect the thoracic cage.

Fractures of the ribs and flail chest

Cause

Rib fractures are usually a result of direct trauma. They may be multiple.

Symptoms and signs

The fractured rib is painful. Clearly it is not possible to stop moving the injured rib without stopping breathing. Thus tenderness is experienced with each inspiratory and expiratory movement. If there have been fractures of more than one rib in more than one place then a segment of the thoracic cage may move independently of the main chest wall. This is referred to as a *flail segment* (flail chest). A flail segment will exhibit paradoxical movement; that is, it will move in the *opposite* direction to the rest of the chest wall. This has significant consequences for the ventilation of the underlying lung (see Chapter 25). Patients with significant chest injuries will have an abnormal respiratory rate (usually high). This is one of the most important factors in the assessment of a severely ill patient. It is also the observation which is most usually omitted by prehospital care professionals, ambulance staff and doctors alike!

> **Record the respiratory rate and monitor changes**

A fractured rib may result in blood loss of up to 150 ml. Multiple rib fractures may therefore be a significant contributory factor in hypovolaemic shock. If facilities for monitoring the percutaneous oxygen saturation (S_pO_2) are available they should be used.

Treatment

The patient must be given high-flow oxygen (15 l/min) through a mask with reservoir bag. Large flail segments may be treated by lying the patient on the injured side (remembering the cervical spine precautions) or by strapping the chest. If strapping is applied it should not be circumferential so as to restrict movement at the uninjured chest wall. In an emergency, stabilizing a flail segment with a hand can be life saving. If the patient is shocked then an intravenous infusion should be started, but this must not delay transfer to hospital.

Fractures of the sternum

Cause

Fractures of the sternum are characteristically caused when the chest strikes the steering wheel in a decelerating vehicle. The correct use of seatbelts, and more recently the deployment of air bags during an accident, will prevent many of these injuries.

Symptoms and signs

There is pain in the anterior aspect of the chest. There may also be symptoms and signs of other significant chest injury (see Chapter 25).

Treatment

It should be assumed that there is also myocardial contusion. The patient should receive oxygen by face mask

(15 l/min through mask with reservoir bag). Monitoring of the pulse, blood pressure, respiratory rate, ECG and oxygen saturation are mandatory. Intravenous access should be obtained following normal protocols. Urgent transfer to hospital is essential

Potential problems

The main problem with these fractures is not the bony injury but contusion or bruising of the heart which lies just posterior to the sternum. This injury requires careful cardiac monitoring and observation in hospital. If cardiac arrhythmias occur they require urgent treatment.

Fractures of the thoracic and lumbar spine

These injuries are described in Chapter 28.

THE PELVIS

Pelvic fractures can be relatively minor or they can be life-threatening. A good history of the mechanism of injury is essential. The anatomy of the pelvis is shown in Figure 27.22.

MINOR PELVIC FRACTURES

Fractures of the pubic ramus

Cause

The cause of a fracture of the pubic ramus is usually a fall, particularly in an elderly patient.

Symptoms and signs

The patient will complain of pain in the hip. Careful elucidation of the site of the pain will reveal that it is in fact groin pain. There is no external rotation or shortening of the leg. The patient is usually unable to walk. The injury is frequently confused with fracture of the femoral neck and correct differentiation of the two may only be possible on X-ray.

Treatment

The patient requires supportive treatment and transfer to hospital.

Avulsion fracture of the pelvis

Cause

Many powerful muscles have attachment to the pelvis (for example, the hamstring muscles). Strong contraction of these, perhaps during sporting activity, may lead to an avulsion fracture (where the muscle inserts onto bone, a small fragment of bone is pulled off).

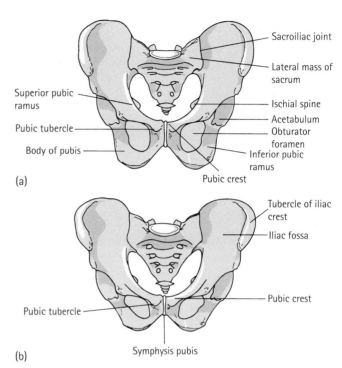

Figure 27.22 Anatomy of the bony pelvis. (a) Male; (b) female

Symptoms and signs

The patient experiences acute pain after a muscular effort and may be unable to stand or walk. The symptoms are similar to those of a severe pulled muscle.

Treatment

The patient will need analgesia and should be transfered to hospital for assessment.

Major pelvic fractures

Cause

Major pelvic fractures are usually caused by severe violence. Falls directly onto the pelvis or force transmitted down the femoral shaft are the usual causes; direct injury by a heavy weight falling on the pelvis can also be responsible. The pelvis can be considered as a ring and usually fails in at least two places. The fracture pattern is dependent on the mechanism of injury.

Symptoms and signs

The patient will be in pain. There may be a leg length discrepancy in pelvic fractures with a vertical shear fracture. Major blood vessels lie on the inner pelvic surface anterior to the sacroiliac joint and pelvic fractures can be complicated by life-threatening haemorrhage. The patient must be examined and assessed for signs of hypovolaemia. The pelvic organs are also at risk of severe injury. The male patient may have blood at the tip of his penis and swelling

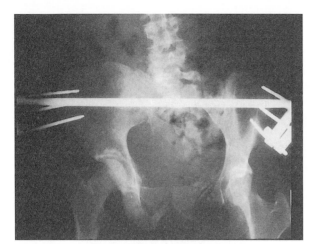

Figure 27.23 Pelvic external fixation and fracture

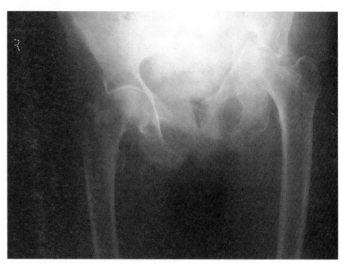

Figure 27.24 A major pelvic fracture

of the scrotum as a result of rupture of the urethra. The pregnant woman will be susceptible to uterine rupture or detachment of the placenta (abruptio placentae). She will also mask the signs of hypovolaemia because she has a proportionately greater blood volume in pregnancy.

Treatment

The diagnosis of a major pelvic fracture may be made when instability is found on pelvic assessment during "C" of the primary survey. The absence of obvious instability does not exclude the diagnosis which may be suspected from the mechanism of injury or in a shocked patient where no other obvious source of bleeding is identified. Under no circumstances should more than one attempt be made to "spring" the pelvis, as this may precipitate or exacerbate haemorrhage. The patient should receive high-flow oxygen (15 l/min through a mask with reservoir). Haemorrhage can be fatal and an external fixator may need to be applied as an emergency at hospital (Figure 27.23). Although ideally intravenous infusion and transfusion should be started prehospital, it is unlikely that the paramedic will be able to keep up with the blood loss and any delay will be detrimental to the patient, who must be transported to hospital quickly. Intravenous access should therefore be obtained during transit or, for short transit times, after arrival in hospital. If it is possible the pelvis should be stabilized during transfer. New pelvic "wrap-around" splints are now available for this purpose and have been proven to improve alignment and reduce bleeding in complex pelvic fractures (Figure 27.24).

Potential problems

Severe hypovolaemic shock may lead to pulseless electrical activity dissociation and death. The patient may also have sustained other life-threatening injuries which must be identified and treated.

Acetabular fractures

Cause

The acetabulum is the bony socket of the hip joint. It is part of the pelvis. Fractures usually occur when force is transmitted indirectly from the femoral shaft. This is a high-violence injury and usually follows a road traffic accident or a fall from a height. The exact injury will depend on the position of the femur. If the hip is flexed or extended then it will usually dislocate, perhaps fracturing the rim of the acetabulum. However, if the hip is in neutral then the force is transmitted directly to the acetabulum which will fracture.

Symptoms and signs

The patient will be in pain which is made worse by any attempt to move the leg. The leg may be short, adducted and internally rotated (see dislocated hip, below). There may be extensive haemorrhage and thus the patient may show signs of shock.

Treatment

The patient should be given high-flow oxygen (15 l/min through a mask with reservoir). An intravenous infusion should be started if this does not delay transporting the patient to hospital. The injured leg should be supported by splinting it to the other leg.

Potential problems

The patient may have sustained other life-threatening injuries which must be identified and treated. If there has been displacement of the femoral head into the pelvis then there may be severe haemorrhage and damage to other pelvic organs.

THE LOWER LIMB

All fractures of the femur and tibia are major injuries and require thoughtful management. The patient requires high-flow oxygen, adequate splintage and analgesia and should be expeditiously transferred to hospital with an intravenous infusion started en route.

Fractured neck of the femur

Cause

Fracture of the neck of the femur occurs in the elderly population. A fall or twisting injury may result in this injury. Some children (often overweight adolescents) have a condition where the upper femoral growth plate slips. Minor trauma in these children may precipitate a complete slipped epiphysis which has similar signs and symptoms to fractured neck of femur.

Symptoms and signs

The hip is painful. There may also be referred pain to the knee of the same side. The leg may be shorter than the normal side and may lie in external rotation (Figure 27.25). All movements of the hip joint cause pain. It is often the case with the elderly person who lives alone that the patient has been lying on the floor for some time since the injury. This increases the possibility of chest infection, pressure necrosis to the skin and hypothermia. The elderly patient may have had some medical event to cause the fall in the first instance (e.g., a myocardial infarction).

Treatment

The leg should be immobilized during transfer to hospital. This is best achieved by using some form of strap or bandage to tie the injured leg to the normal one. The possibility of medical conditions or other injuries should not be forgotten.

Potential problems

Access to and egress from the patient's home may be a problem. The police may be required to effect an entry. There may be difficulty getting the patient out once immobilized on a stretcher. The patient may require airway support and a primary survey is mandatory. Oxygen should be administered and if there is any suspicion of a fall with head injury, however minor, the cervical spine should be immobilized. Precipitating cardiac events may have led to left ventricular failure in which case intravenous infusion may worsen rather than improve the patient's condition; in the vast majority of cases, fluids can safely wait until the patient reaches hospital. Hypothermia may lead to cardiac dysrhythmias. The patient should be kept warm and the pulse, blood pressure, oxygen saturation and ECG monitored.

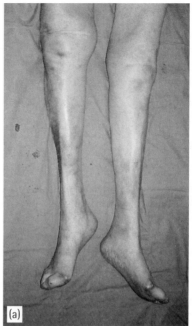

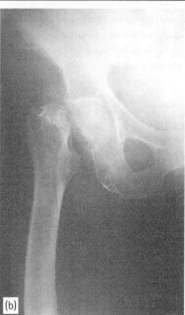

Figure 27.25 Fractured neck of femur. (a) Clinical appearance – note the shortened and externally rotated leg; (b) X-ray

Dislocation of the hip

Cause

Hip dislocation is caused by a high-energy injury. Typically the knee is struck when the hip is flexed, for example on the dashboard of a car in a high-speed road traffic accident. Posterior dislocation is most common and there is often an associated fracture of the lip of the acetabulum (see above). If the hip is in the extended position at the time of injury an acetabular fracture is likely. Hip prostheses are particularly vulnerable to dislocation.

Symptoms and signs

The hip is painful. There may be referred pain down the thigh and in the knee joint. The hip is held flexed and adducted and the leg is internally rotated. There may be associated sciatica. The mechanism of injury is such that other life-threatening injuries are extremely likely and examination should identify these urgently.

Treatment

The patient should be given oxygen (15 l/min through a mask with reservoir). Cervical spine immobilization will be required. The vital signs should be measured and recorded and appropriate treatment for other injuries instituted. An intravenous infusion should be started. It is not possible to place the femur in the normal position until reduction is performed under anaesthesia. Attempts to reduce the dislocation without anaesthesia will be fruitless, extremely painful and delay the patient at the scene. The injured leg should be immobilized by securing it to the uninjured side and the patient transported to hospital as soon as possible. The distal circulation should be monitored. Analgesia will certainly be required. If the patient is trapped then medical assistance should be requested. If the patient is responsive intravenous opiates will probably be required in addition to Entonox.

Potential problems

The mechanism of injury is such that the patient may have multiple injuries. There is considerable disruption to the muscles and soft tissues around the hip joint, leading to haemorrhage. The patient must be monitored and treated for hypovolaemic shock where appropriate but this should not delay transfer to hospital. Good analgesia is essential. The head of the femur will compress the sciatic nerve as it leaves the pelvis which may lead to temporary or permanent damage. If the displacement of the joint is significant then the femoral vessels may become kinked and the distal circulation threatened. It can be difficult to extricate a patient with this injury, even if the vehicle damage is minimal, and good liaison with the fire and rescue services will be essential.

Fracture of the shaft of femur

Fracture of the shaft of the femur is always a major injury (Figure 27.26).

Cause

Fractures of the femoral shaft are usually the result of high-energy injury, such as a road traffic accident or a fall from a height.

Symptoms and signs

The exact symptoms and signs will depend on the level of the fracture. There will be pain and usually swelling at the site of

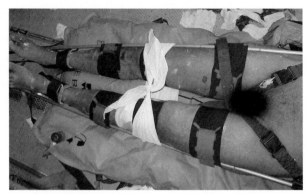

Figure 27.26 Fracture of the shaft of the femur, with kind permission of D. Connell, Ex+Med UK

the injury. There is often some degree of deformity, which may be rotational or angular. The leg may be short. The distal circulation may be compromised. Other coexistent life-threatening injuries should be identified and treated.

Treatment

The patient should receive high-flow oxygen (15 l/min through a mask with reservoir). An intravenous infusion should be started particularly if there is a delay before the patient can be transferred to hospital; otherwise it may be commenced en route. Intravenous opiate analgesia will be required. A regional nerve block (femoral nerve block) administered by an immediate-care doctor are often also indicated. Some form of splintage is required: the best splintage will be afforded by a traction splint (see Chapter 29), but if this is not easily applied or unavailable then a long leg splint (box splint, lollipop splint) or splinting to the other leg will suffice.

Potential problems

Hypoxia must be avoided. Other major injuries must be identified and treated. A femoral fracture may lose up to 1500 ml blood. This may be doubled in a compound injury. The patient should be monitored for the signs of shock and treated with fluids or urgent evacuation. It should be remembered that the infusion volumes achievable in hospital are far greater than those at the roadside. Minimal delay is essential. It may not be possible to immobilize a badly displaced fracture without manipulation. This should be performed with intravenous sedation and analgesia in conjunction with an immediate-care doctor.

Fractures of the patella

Cause

Fracture of the patella (kneecap) may be sustained in a number of ways. The knee may strike the dashboard in a road traffic accident or it may strike the floor in a fall. In both these situations, the association between fractured patella, fracture of the femoral shaft, fracture of the acetabulum of the pelvis and posterior dislocation of the hip should be remembered. Alternatively, a heavy object falling on the knee may cause a patella fracture, as may violent contraction of the quadriceps tendon (which may occur, for instance, when a footballer kicks at the ball, expecting some resistance due to the mass of the ball, but misses, allowing unresisted contraction).

Signs and symptoms

The knee is painful and swollen. There may be a laceration or abrasion over the patella. If the fracture is displaced, it may be possible to feel the gap between the ends of the patella. The extensor mechanism of the knee consists of the quadriceps tendon superiorly, the patella and the patella tendon inferiorly. The latter attaches to the tibia at the tibial tubercle which can be felt 4–5 cm below the patella. If any of these soft tissue or bony structures are disrupted then the knee cannot be extended.

Treatment

The leg should be placed in a well-padded, long leg splint.

Potential problems

A careful history will ensure that potentially serious associated injuries can be identified and treated.

Dislocation of the patella

Cause

The patella may dislocate with minor trauma. The patient will often have experienced this injury previously (see Figure 27.7).

Symptoms and signs

The patella always dislocates laterally. The acute injury is usually painful. The knee appears abnormal with the patella located over the lateral femoral condyle. There may be swelling (effusion) inside the joint. The patient will not be able to move the joint.

Treatment

Analgesia with Entonox may be sufficient to allow relocation of the patella. The important manoeuvre is to extend (straighten) the knee while pressing the kneecap medially. It will be very difficult to reduce while the knee is flexed (bent). If one attempt fails then the leg is placed in a long leg splint and the patient transported to hospital. If the patella is successfully relocated, hospital consultation is still required as the patient will need orthopaedic follow-up.

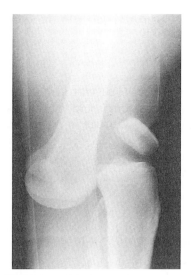

Figure 27.27 Dislocation of the knee

Potential problems

This condition can be extremely painful and the patient may not tolerate a splint.

Dislocation of the knee

Cause

Dislocation of the knee (Figure 27.27) is a serious injury which inevitably means that the majority of the ligaments of the knee have been disrupted. The vessels and nerves to the distal portion of the limb are frequently compromised. Surprisingly, this injury may result from a comparatively trivial event.

Symptoms and signs

The knee will be painful and swollen. There may be significant angular deformity of the joint, although elastic recoil may have returned it to an anatomical position. The disruption of the ligaments and capsule renders the joint unstable. There is a serious possibility of vascular and neurological deficit to all structures below the knee.

Treatment

The vascular status must be assessed and monitored. The leg should be placed in a long leg splint.

Potential problems

The joint is unstable and may have few ligamentous and capsular attachments remaining. Redislocation of the joint may further damage the vascular and neurological structures. When placing the leg in the splint, the limb must be supported above and below the knee.

Soft tissue and ligament injuries to the knee joint (Figure 27.28)

Cause

Injuries to the ligaments of the knee joint are common and are frequently sustained during sporting activities such as football, rugby and skiing. Damage to the menisci of the knee (commonly known as "cartilages") can occur in isolation or in concert with such ligament injuries. A common mechanism of injury is a twisting injury to the knee when the foot is fixed.

Symptoms and signs

The knee will be painful. It may swell immediately (if there is bleeding into the joint, a *haemarthrosis*), or over the next 12–24 hours (an *effusion*). It is important to ascertain the exact mechanism of injury as this will help the medical staff make the diagnosis.

Treatment

The leg should be immobilized in a long leg splint until a fracture has been excluded in hospital. The distal circulation should be assessed and monitored.

Potential problems

The joint may be potentially unstable when severe ligament disruption has occurred and dislocation of the knee may be possible.

Fractures of the tibial plateau

Cause

Fracture of the tibial plateau is caused by a large valgus force (the lower tibia is forced away from the midline) or varus force (the lower tibia is forced towards the midline) (Figure 27.29). This typically occurs when the bumper of a car strikes a pedestrian or when a skier falls but the bindings on the skis fail to release.

Symptoms and signs

There is pain at the knee and often a haemarthrosis (bleeding into the joint). The patient is unable to walk.

Treatment

The limb is immobilized in a well-padded splint.

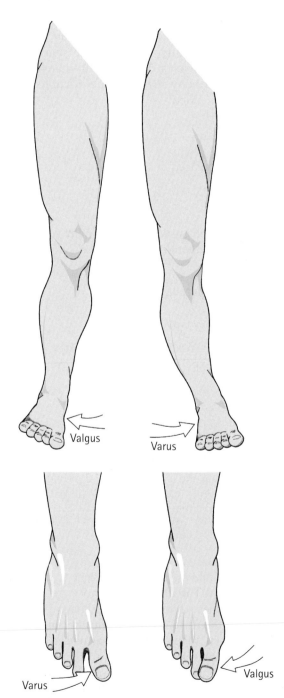

Figure 27.29 Varus and valgus forces

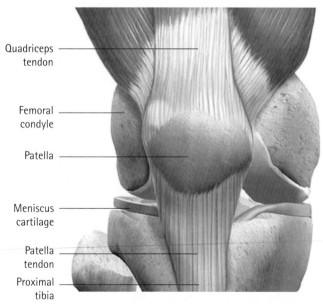

Figure 27.28 Anatomy of the knee

Quadriceps tendon

Femoral condyle

Patella

Meniscus cartilage

Patella tendon

Proximal tibia

Potential problems

The patient should be examined for other major injuries and the distal circulation monitored.

Fractures of the tibial shaft and fibula

Cause

Fractures of the tibial shaft and fibula may be caused by direct injury, such as in road traffic accidents and sporting injuries. In some cases of direct injury either the tibia or fibula may be fractured in isolation. Longitudinal compression as a result of a fall may lead to these fractures and they may also result from indirect torsional forces caused by rotation transmitted from the foot or from the upper body if the foot is fixed. Finally, the tibia may fracture as a result of completion of a preexisting stress fracture.

Symptoms and signs

There is localized pain and swelling. There may be angular or rotational deformity. The distal circulation may be compromised.

Treatment

The patient should be given high-flow oxygen. This is often omitted, particularly in the young athlete. However, these injuries are serious and should be treated with the same respect as a fracture of the femur. Hypoxia is common after tibial fractures and must be avoided. Similarly, there may be considerable haemorrhage. The patient must be examined for circulatory shock and monitored. An intravenous infusion should be started without causing undue delay in transferring the patient to hospital. The injured limb should be immobilized in a long leg splint.

It may be necessary to reduce the fracture before immobilization is possible and therefore opiate analgesia is required. In certain circumstances it may be necessary to ask for medical assistance to allow sedation before this can be achieved and the patient safely immobilized. Only then should the limb be subjected to gentle longitudinal traction to reverse any shortening caused by muscle spasm and overlap of bone. Once the limb is extended to its normal length the fracture is reduced to its anatomical position. Excessive traction must be avoided as this may lead to secondary injury to the vessels and nerves. Accurate fracture reduction will reduce the amount of haemorrhage at the fracture site and from the soft tissues.

Potential problems

The tibia is a subcutaneous bone. It is easy to convert a simple fracture to a compound fracture by careless handling of the limb: this is inexcusable. The vascular supply of the lower parts of the limb may be compromised in several ways. Firstly, the vessels may have been directly injured at the time of the fracture. They may also sustain injury if the sharp bone ends of a displaced fracture are not effectively immobilized. The vessels may be trapped within the fracture site and rough handling during fracture reduction may make this worse.

Compound injuries of the tibia are not uncommon, particularly after motorcycle accidents (Figure 27.30). These are potentially limb-threatening injuries; there is significant soft tissue damage and sometimes loss as a result of the primary injury. Wounds are often seriously contaminated.

There is a significant risk of compartment syndrome following fracture of the tibia. The muscles of the lower legs are enclosed in tough fibrous sheaths. There are four compartments: anterolateral, medial, superficial posterior and deep posterior. If bleeding occurs into these compartments or if there is significant swelling following a soft tissue injury, then the pressure within the compartment will rise. The risk is highest when there is a closed fracture or a soft tissue injury such as a muscle haematoma following a kick. As the pressure rises, perfusion of the tissues and cells decreases and they are starved of oxygen. The pressure in the arteries may be high enough to allow continued flow into the compartment, making the situation worse. *The presence of a palpable distal pulse does not guarantee that the tissues*

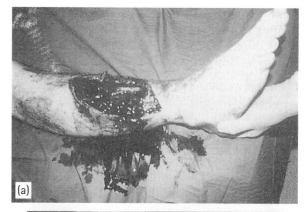

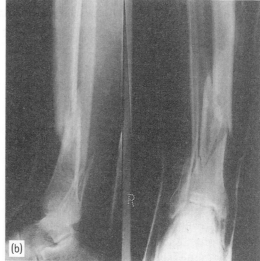

Figure 27.30 A compound fracture of the tibia. (a) Clinical appearance; (b) X-ray

are adequately perfused. The capillary refill test must be performed to allow a more complete assessment of the vascular status of the tissues.

Fractures and dislocations of the ankle

Cause

The anatomy of the ankle joint is shown in Figure 27.31. The exact pattern of fracture depends on the mechanism of injury, but the prehospital treatment is identical regardless of the fracture type. The typical history is of "going over" on or "twisting" the ankle, which may be combined with a fall down a kerbstone or step. These injuries are usually referred to as inversion or eversion injuries and the terms are explained in Figure 27.32. Injuries of this kind are also common on the sports field. The ankle may be trapped by the foot pedals in a motor vehicle or a fall may lead to a fracture or dislocation (Figure 27.33) of the ankle.

Symptoms and signs

The ankle is extremely tender over the fracture site and swelling occurs rapidly. In general, eversion injuries are associated with fractures of the medial malleolus and inversion injuries with fractures of the lateral malleolus. In severe injuries, both may fracture. Any attempt at walking is very painful. There may be associated deformity. Distal nerve or vessel injury may occur.

Treatment

The ankle should be immobilized in a well-padded splint – this will probably require analgesia. The neurological and vascular status of the foot must be carefully monitored. Dislocation of the ankle may occur with obvious deformity (Figure 27.33). This is a limb-threatening emergency requiring rapid reduction. Urgent transfer to hospital (or reduction on scene by a doctor in remote areas) is essential. With an unstable injury, the act of splinting the joint may lead to reduction. However, reduction often requires sedation and intravenous analgesia.

Potential problems

If there is significant deformity following this fracture then the skin overlying the joint can become tightly stretched over the bony fragments. This will quickly lead to pressure necrosis and death of that skin. Penetration of the skin converting a closed to an open injury must be avoided.

At times it can be difficult to distinguish between a fracture and a sprain of the ankle. Typically the pain and swelling of a sprain to the anterior talofibular ligament are distal and anteromedial to the lateral malleolus. Careful examination will show that there is no bony tenderness in

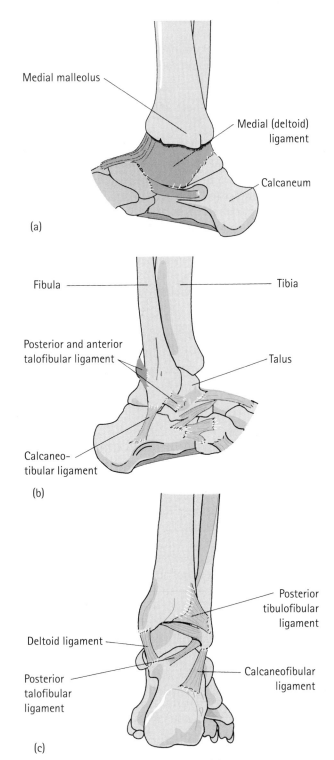

(a)

(b)

(c)

Figure 27.31 Anatomy of the ankle joint. (a) Medial view; (b) lateral view; (c) posterior view

such circumstances. However, the consequences of encouraging weight bearing on a fractured ankle mistakenly believed to be a sprain can be significant and so if there is any doubt in the diagnosis it is best to treat these injuries as fractures until they have been assessed at hospital.

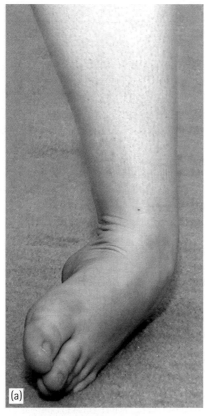
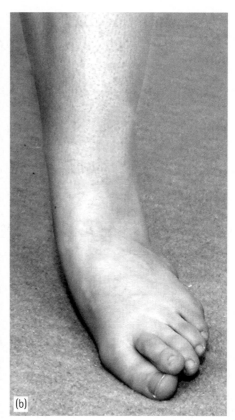

Figure 27.32 (a) Inversion and (b) eversion of the ankle.

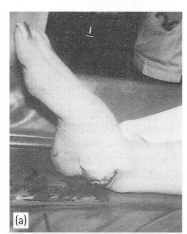

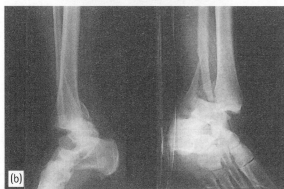

Figure 27.33 Fractures of the ankle. (a) Clinical appearance; (b) X-ray

Fractures of the talus and calcaneum (os calcis)

Cause

The talus is situated between the lower tibia (and forms part of the ankle joint) and the calcaneum or os calcis (heel bone). Both these bones are vulnerable to fracture as a result of falls from a height. They can also fracture when struck or trapped by foot pedals in a motor vehicle.

Symptoms and signs

There is pain on attempts to walk or on direct palpation. There may be significant deformity if these fractures are associated with dislocation of either the ankle or the mid-foot joints.

Treatment

The ankle and foot should be placed in a well-padded splint and elevated. The circulation to the foot should be monitored and the neurological state assessed.

Potential problems

The mechanism of injury usually causes associated injuries. A fall from a height may produce fractures of the calcaneum, talus, femoral neck, acetabulum and vertebrae and a thorough secondary survey is mandatory, although this will usually be deferred until the patient arrives in hospital.

Dislocations of the midfoot

Cause

Midfoot dislocations result from a fall from a height, landing on the foot with the toes pointing downwards (Figure 27.34).

Symptoms and signs

The deformity is usually obvious, although it may be obscured by the footwear, and swelling will occur quickly. There may be associated vascular injury, either directly or indirectly, because of a compartment syndrome.

Treatment

The paramedic should not attempt to relocate the dislocation at the scene. The foot should be placed in a well-padded splint and elevated and the patient evacuated to hospital. The circulation to the distal part of the foot must be assessed and recorded.

Potential problems

The possibility of other associated serious injuries should not be forgotten.

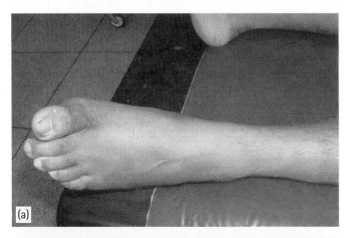

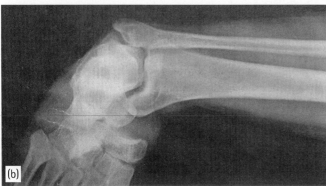

Figure 27.34 A midfoot dislocation

Fractures of the metatarsals and toes

Cause

Fractures of the metatarsals and toes can be caused by direct blows, falls and even by overuse (e.g., the "march fracture" of the second metatarsal seen in army recruits unused to marching in boots). Overuse injuries will rarely present to the ambulance service as an emergency.

Symptoms and signs

There is pain over the fracture which is made worse when attempting to walk. The foot swells dorsally (the top surface), an analogous situation with hand injuries.

Treatment

The foot should be elevated. A splint is not always required, but when used it should be well padded.

Potential problems

The main problem is swelling which may compromise the circulation, particularly of the digits.

TRAUMATIC AMPUTATION

There are many misconceptions about the best way in which to preserve an amputated extremity. Traumatic amputation can range from a relatively minor fingertip injury to a life-threatening avulsion of a limb (Figure 27.35). Recent improvements in microsurgical techniques have increased the likelihood of successful reimplantation of the amputated part.

In order to minimize the damage to the amputated part and thus improve the chances of successful surgery, the following steps should be performed.

1. The time of amputation should be recorded.
2. The amputated part should not be placed in water or directly in ice, as this can cause further cellular damage.

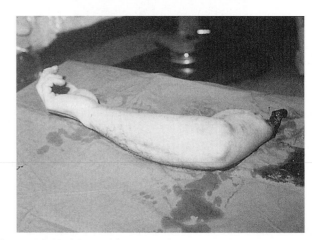

Figure 27.35 A traumatic amputation

3. The amputated part should be securely wrapped up in a sealed plastic bag, which should be placed in a second bag, and the double-wrapped part kept cool. It is safe to place the part in an ice–water mixture after wrapping it in this way as direct contact is avoided.
4. If the patient is still trapped then the part should be clearly labelled and sent to the receiving hospital after discussion with the medical staff who will be receiving and treating the patient.

However damaged the amputated part is, it should always be transported to hospital with the patient. Even if reimplantation is not possible, use of the skin for grafting may be considered.

COMPLICATIONS OF FRACTURES

The complications of any injury can be divided into immediate, early and late. It is not always appreciated that the quality of care given in the immediate period will influence the complication rate at *all* stages of the rehabilitation from injury. For instance, good care of a compound fracture at the scene of injury may, in conjunction with correct treatment in hospital, prevent the long-term sequela of osteomyelitis. Bad immediate care can be life threatening or limb threatening.

IMMEDIATE COMPLICATIONS

A simple fracture may be converted to a compound fracture by injudicious handling of the injured part. This will increase the chance of long-term complications and must be avoided. The deformity that occurs at the time of injury and any subsequent movement at the fracture site may lead to vascular damage. Such damage in the immediate phase is usually due to direct vascular injury, but at later stages indirect compromise such as compartment syndrome may result from swelling.

The direct result of the injury may also lead to neural damage. Nerves can sustain damage due to hypoxia if their blood supply is interrupted. This may be a result of direct or indirect vascular injury or simply prolonged hypotension secondary to hypovalaemic shock.

EARLY COMPLICATIONS

Compartment syndrome has been mentioned earlier. Swelling of an injured limb or digit may lead to a situation where there is no tissue perfusion because no blood flow occurs in the capillaries. In the early stages there may be a palpable peripheral pulse but this alone is not a foolproof guide to the state of a limb's circulation. The consequences of compartment syndrome can be devastating, with the death of or injury to all the muscle groups, leaving a useless, contracted, painful limb.

Infection of a fracture is a similar disaster. Compound fractures are far more likely to become infected. Infection of bone is almost impossible to cure and the patient is committed to lifelong misery with episodic relapse. If a fracture does become infected it is far less likely that it will properly unite. A compound wound must be covered as soon as is practical and preferably with dressings soaked in aqueous iodine solution. *Conversion of a simple to a compound fracture must not be allowed to happen.*

Fat embolism is a rare condition which is still poorly understood. It can occur even after minor fractures, but the incidence seems to be greatest in the case of poorly immobilized long-bone fractures. Fat globules appear in the brain and other tissues. These may be due to a chemical change resultant from factors released due to the injury itself, rather than fat globules transported from the bone marrow direct. The consequences of fat embolism are far worse if there is coexistent hypoxia, so all fractures of long bone *must* be treated with oxygen to minimize hypoxia.

LATE COMPLICATIONS

Infection of the bone, or *osteomyelitis,* is a complication which lasts for the patient's lifetime. Although there may be long periods when infection is dormant and the patient is symptom free, the possibility of recrudescence of the infection will always remain. Steps to reduce the chances of acute infection of a fracture start at the scene of the injury and are of vital importance.

Non-union is the failure of a fracture to heal. There may be no new bone production or there may be massive new bone production, but the functional outcome is the same. If a fracture is slow to unite then the patient must be investigated for infection as this is one of the most common causes of the condition.

Malunion describes a fracture that has united but in the wrong position. The effects of this vary. The mobility of a normal shoulder and elbow may compensate completely for a malunited humeral shaft fracture. Conversely, the forearm bones which rotate around each other during pronation and supination may be adversely affected by only minimal degrees of angular malunion. The accurate positioning of the ends of fractured bones is one of the highest priorities in fracture management.

Arthritis will occur early in a joint that has sustained a displaced fracture of the joint surface. The displacement only needs to be 1 mm before there are massive changes in the stresses placed on the articular cartilage. Point loading occurs and the joint rapidly wears out. This explains the importance of the accurate fixation of fractures involving the joint.

FURTHER READING

Apley AG, Solomon L 1993 *Apley's system of orthopaedics and fractures.* Butterworth, Oxford
McRea R 1989 *Practical fracture treatment,* 2nd edn. Churchill Livingstone, Edinburgh

Chapter 28

Spinal injuries

INTRODUCTION

This chapter is concerned with injuries to the vertebral column that produce (or have the capacity to produce) injuries to the spinal cord. There are around 500 new spinal cord injuries in the UK annually, comprising about 5% of total neck and back injuries. While they are relatively rare (2–3 cases per health district per year), their significance lies in the failure of the central nervous system to regenerate and the consequent disability which results.

Spinal cord injury may be either complete (i.e. with no motor or sensory function below the level of injury) or incomplete (with partial preservation of sensory or motor function, or both). The incomplete cord injury has the capacity to recover in whole or part. Equally, however, it is susceptible to further injury through incorrect management. Complete lesions do not recover.

Since 1980 the proportion of cord injuries that are incomplete has increased from under 50% to over 60%. This is partly a result of seatbelt legislation leading to reduced high-velocity blunt injuries but much of the change is the result of improved standards of patient handling and management. It has been estimated, however, that 75% of spinal cord injuries are incomplete at the moment of primary injury, so there is room for further improvement. The increase in the number of patients with an incomplete cord lesion does mean that many patients will have some partial cord function and the attendant must be capable of recognizing this, rather than regarding incomplete function as evidence of a lack of injury.

In 50% of cases, moreover, there are associated injuries which also may require their own urgent management. Therefore, the responsibilities of those attending are threefold:

- to avoid death or disability from associated injury
- to prevent neurological deterioration or the production of a neurological injury
- to prevent the complications of spinal paralysis.

The first two tasks are interrelated in so far as a secondary injury to the spinal cord is not exclusively due to additional movement of the vertebral column with further mechanical injury during handling. It also arises as a result of an hypoxic injury to the spinal cord through inadequately managed disturbances of ventilation and circulation. Thus, there are two parallel approaches to the stabilization of a patient with a spinal cord injury: the biomechanical stabilization of the vertebral column and the stabilization of the pathophysiological changes to which the damaged spinal cord will be exposed.

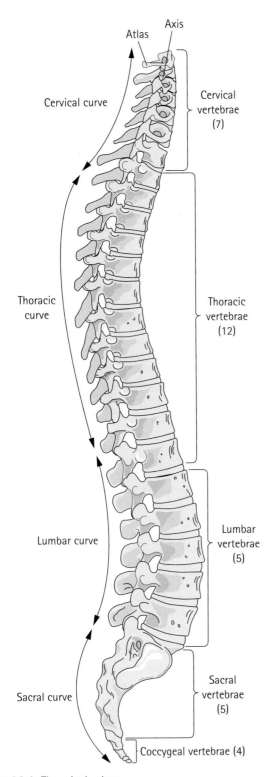

Figure 28.1 The spinal column

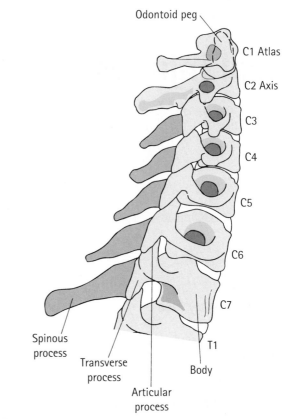

Figure 28.2 The cervical spine

patient as if there were a spinal cord injury even if ultimately no such injury is discovered.

ANATOMY AND PHYSIOLOGY

The spinal column is made up of 33 vertebrae: seven cervical, 12 thoracic, five lumbar and the remainder fused into the sacrum and coccyx (Figure 28.1). The first and second cervical vertebrae are specialized and are known as the *atlas* and the *axis* (Figure 28.2). Movement of the head anteroposteriorly normally occurs at the atlantooccipital joints and rotation of the head takes place between the first and second vertebrae around the odontoid peg. Fractures of these two vertebrae result in a widening of the canal rather than narrowing. However, fracture through the odontoid together with tearing of the ligaments that attach it to the atlas leaves a freely moving body that can cause considerable cord damage. If this occurs then neurogenic respiratory arrest followed by cardiac arrest is possible. Injuries to the first two cervical vertebrae are often associated with severe craniofacial trauma.

The remainder of the cervical vertebrae follow the normal vertebral pattern. Anteriorly lies a large load-bearing mass, the vertebral body, and the body of each vertebra is separated from the next by an intervertebral disc. The spinal canal is formed by backward projections (pedicles) and the posterior part of the arch comprises the two laminae (Figure 28.3).

Acting as anchors for muscle attachments are the three processes, the posterior spinous process and two transverse

The major source of deterioration is a lack of recognition of the potential for a spinal cord injury. In such cases the patient may be either sat up or stood up or is transported sitting or standing, with catastrophic consequences. It is important, therefore, to have a high index of suspicion based on the mechanism of injury and thereafter to manage the

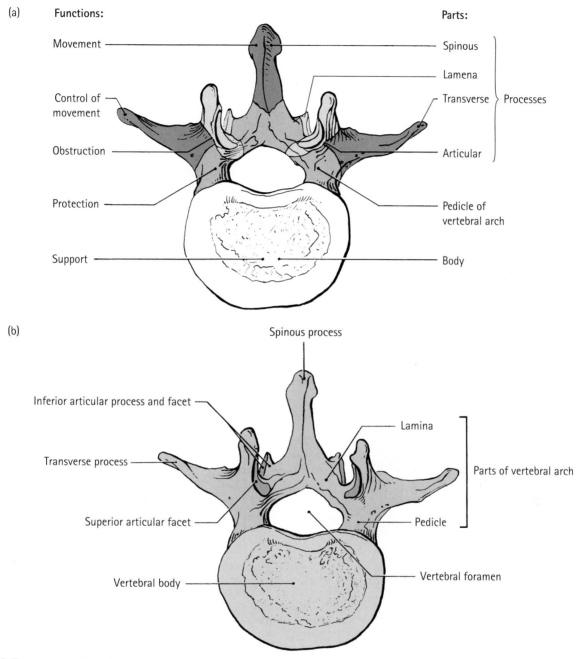

(a) Functions: Parts:

Movement   Spinous

                                                   Lamena
Control of   Transverse } Processes
movement

Obstruction   Articular

Protection   Pedicle of
                                                   vertebral arch

Support   Body

(b)   Spinous process

Inferior articular process and facet

                                                   Lamina

Transverse process   Parts of vertebral arch

Superior articular facet   Pedicle

Vertebral body   Vertebral foramen

Figure 28.3 The anatomy of a vertebra

processes. Each vertebra has two articular processes superiorly which interlock with the inferior articular processes of the vertebra above and likewise that vertebral body's inferior articular processes articulate with the superior processes (facets) of the vertebra below (Figure 28.4).

Injuries to the vertebral column can arise either by a movement of one vertebral body on another, thereby narrowing the canal, or by the vertebral body being sufficiently disrupted to allow fragments to be pushed posteriorly (retropulsion) into the spinal canal, causing compression (Figure 28.5).

The areas substantially at risk are the cervical spine, the thoracolumbar junction and the lumbar spine. This is partly because the natural curve of the spine in these areas is lordotic (concave), partly because the associated muscles are weaker and finally because in the dorsal (thoracic) spine the vertebrae articulate with the ribs (which in turn articulate with the sternum) – if the ribcage and sternum are intact, the chances of a biomechanically unstable vertebral fracture are low. Conversely, the incidence of coincident sternal fracture and vertebral fracture in motor vehicle accidents is high.

> Injuries are more common where mobile parts of the spinal column join more fixed parts

Movement of one vertebral body on another is prevented by strong ligaments anteriorly and posteriorly. If the posterior ligaments are ruptured by forced flexion of the spine it may then be possible for the vertebra above to move anteriorly. Likewise, a forced extension injury tears the anterior ligaments and it is then possible for the superior vertebra to

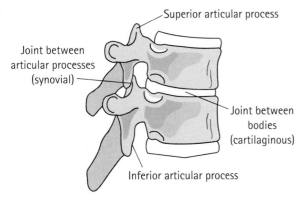

Figure 28.4 Thoracic vertebrae

glide posteriorly upon its inferior neighbour. In the process, damage may occur to the facets or to the anterior part of the vertebral body or to the posterior elements (Figure 28.6).

A combined anterior and posterior ligamentous injury is fortunately rare: with this injury, movement may occur despite the best immobilization techniques. Where there is only one ligamentous tear, it is unlikely that further neurological damage will occur if spinal immobilization procedures are followed.

Compression is the usual mechanism that causes retropulsion of fragments of the vertebral body. Minor degrees of compression may damage the periphery of the body but in the more severe "burst" injury the vertebral body fractures into fragments that can displace backwards into the spinal canal.

In addition to the mechanisms described above, damage to the cord may be caused by rotational forces producing ligamentous and bony damage or by a laterally applied force. A lateral force may occur in "side-swipe" injuries from motor vehicles. In any high-velocity impact where there is

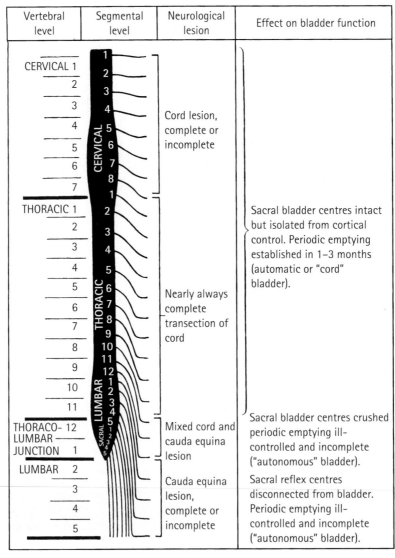

Figure 28.5 Damage to the spinal cord due to displaced bony fragments

flexion and hyperextension, there may also be a rotatory component. The final mechanism is distraction, which occurs either as the result of hanging or by traction on the injured spine by healthcare attendants.

SPINAL CORD ANATOMY

The spinal cord (neuraxis) extends from the foramen magnum to L1 in the adult and to L3 in children. The bottom end of the spinal cord is termed the *conus medullaris* (conus). The nerve roots below L1 hang down inside a sac (*theca*) that surrounds the whole neuraxis and are bathed in cerebrospinal fluid. These nerve roots collectively are known as the *cauda equina*. Injuries to the cauda equina, as to the spinal cord, will cause paralysis and sensory loss and injury to the

autonomic nervous system serving the bladder, bowel and sexual function (Figure 28.7).

The nerves of the spinal cord itself are arranged in a common pattern. Posteriorly lies the point of entry of the sensory roots and anteriorly the exit of the motor roots. There are reflex connections (reflex arcs) (Figure 28.8) between these roots which allow for reflex movements. However, the outflow is regulated by descending bundles of fibres (tracts) coming down the spinal column from the brain and sensory input is transmitted to the brain through ascending tracts. Since the left half of the brain controls the right half of the body and the right half of the brain controls the left side, the ascending and descending fibres have to cross the midline in their journey down the neuraxis. The point of crossover, however, varies between motor tracts and sensory tracts – and

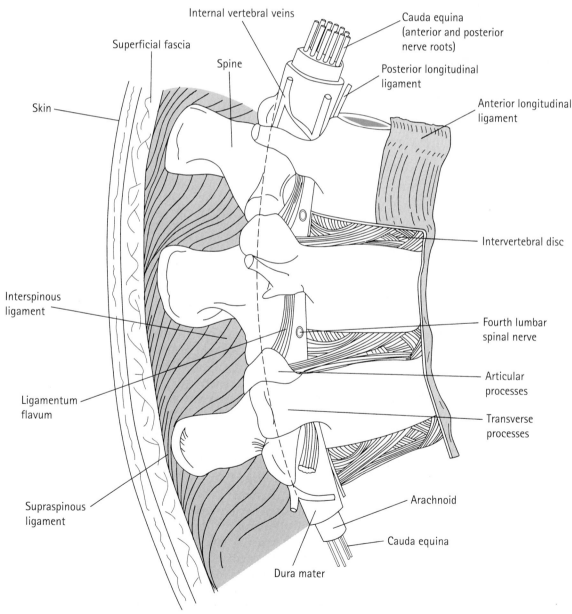

Figure 28.6 Ligaments of the spine

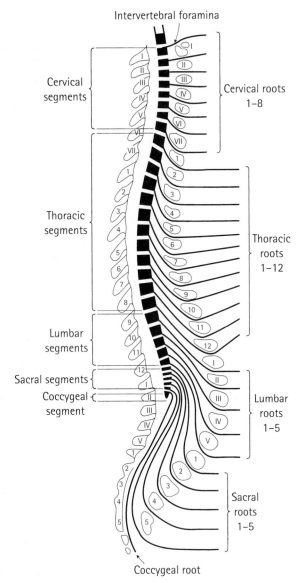

Intervertebral foramina

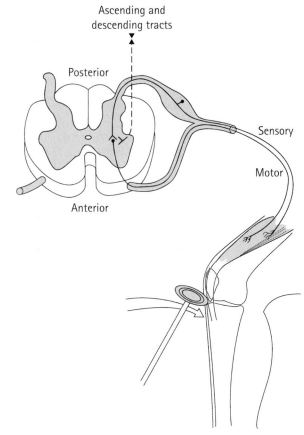

Ascending and descending tracts

Figure 28.8 Nerve roots and reflex arcs

Figure 28.7 The spinal cord. (Reproduced with permission from Lindsay KW 1991 Neurology and neurosurgery illustrated. Churchill Livingstone, Edinburgh)

indeed, within the sensory tracts themselves the point of crossover is different for each type of sensation (vibration, pain, temperature and light touch).

The organization of the ascending and descending tracts shares one similarity – those areas subserving the hands are in the most central part of the cord, with the areas for the arms lying further out and the areas for the legs being the furthest out on the periphery of the spinal cord.

Sensory nerves (touch, pain and temperature) lie in the anterolateral part of the cord, while proprioceptive stimuli (concerned with knowing where a patient's own limbs are in space) are transmitted posteriorly. The significance of this is that discrete anatomical lesions produce specific patterns of sensory and motor change. Unless one is aware of the neuroanatomy these symptoms can occasionally be mistaken for the effects of hysteria or "shock".

PHYSIOLOGY OF THE SPINAL CORD

Anatomic transection of the cord is rare. The majority of mechanical injuries are produced by disruption caused by compression of the cord or the nerve roots of the cauda equina. Whether injury is complete or not will depend, in mechanical terms, upon the severity of the compression force produced.

However, this is not the only factor at work. Damage may be caused (as in head injury) by secondary hypoxic damage to the cord, either by permitting the patient to become hypoxic or as a result of reduced blood flow to the spinal cord.

The blood flow to the spinal cord has two major sources. First, each segment has its own vessel. Additionally, the blood supply of the dorsolumbar (thoracolumbar) cord is provided by a number of vessels collectively known as the *artery of Adamkiewicz*. The blood supply of the cervical spinal cord is derived from the anterior spinal artery, which in turn derives from the two vertebral arteries. There is a zone at the lower limit of the territory of the anterior spinal artery and the upper limit of the territory of the artery of Adamkiewicz where vascular injury is particularly likely. Neglecting to secure the circulation can convert a person who would otherwise be paraplegic into somebody who is tetraplegic. The risk is, however, not solely anatomical. It depends on the microcirculation and the changes that are associated with a spinal cord injury. In cervicothoracic lesions the sympathetic nervous system (which travels in the spinal cord between T1 and L1) is interrupted. This causes a general vasodilation, with a fall in blood pressure even when the patient is lying flat. The hypotension is considerably more pronounced if the patient sits or stands up, because it is the vasomotor tone and the muscle pump in the legs (neither of which is then functioning) that maintain the perfusion pressure. In the uninjured person with an intact nervous system the blood pressure can fall and rise while the blood flow to the brain and spinal cord remains constant. This is known as *autoregulation* and explains why a person who faints is not quadriplegic (all limbs paralysed), paraplegic (lower limbs paralysed) or hemiplegic (limbs on one side paralysed) on recovery. When the neuroaxis is damaged there is a failure of autoregulation and the spinal cord blood flow directly mirrors the blood pressure. Thus, a fall in blood pressure *will* produce a fall in blood flow in the damaged area of the cord and an area of spinal cord already compromised by a compressive force will have a hypoxic insult as well.

Three elements therefore contribute to spinal cord injury:

- biomechanical movement
- hypoxia due to A or B problems
- underperfusion – C problems.

The tendency in treating spinal cord injury has been to dwell on the mechanical factors alone and avoid moving the patient at all, placing the cord at risk of hypoxia, underperfusion or both.

DIAGNOSIS

The symptoms and signs of spinal injury are related to disruption of the spinal column (the bones, ligaments and muscles) and disruption of the spinal cord. Bone injury causes pain, tenderness, swelling, bruising and sometimes an irregularity in the spine on palpation (a "step"). Pain is prominent when there is a dislocation. However, pain from a spinal injury may be masked by more severe pain elsewhere. Superficial bruising is rare and is usually a late sign. When muscles are disrupted and bleeding occurs, an intramuscular haematoma forms which is usually not apparent on the surface. A step, if found, is a useful sign but it is present in only 10% of cases. The feeling of being "severed in two" (agnosognosia) is very rare and occurs in only 4%.

Motor symptoms and signs may be confined to either the proximal or distal muscle groups – the screening test of asking the patient to move fingers and toes is insufficient to exclude motor involvement. Many of the patients who deteriorate do so because their injury is not recognized and they are allowed to sit or stand up during their management. There are two principal reasons for missing the injury. First, the local (spinal column injury) signs traditionally described in textbooks are frequently not present; second, the textbook descriptions of spinal cord injury have often been confined to those of a complete spinal cord injury.

The motor symptoms and signs in the partial cord injury syndromes may be difficult to interpret. In central cord injury the legs may be little affected, the arms more seriously affected and the hands most affected of all. This injury is produced by hyperextension and is a common pattern of injury in the elderly with existing osteoarthritis in the spine. The second pattern of partial cord injury is the *rotational* or *"side-swipe"* injury. This, incidentally, is also produced by stab wounds to the spine. The clinical picture is of a modified hemisection of the cord, where weakness occurs down one side with numbness on the opposite side.

The sensory disturbances are even wider in their spectrum. They include:

- "pins and needles" sensation
- electric shock-like pain at the moment of impact with no other indicator that injury has taken place
- disturbances of proprioception, where the patient feels he or she is still in the same position as at the moment of impact, despite clearly now lying in another
- burning pains throughout both arms or both lower limbs.

Burning pains in the upper limb are seen in motor vehicle deceleration accidents. In the lower limbs burning pains are associated with "hyperpathia" (touch registers as pain), seen most frequently in conus injuries. The result is that touching or moving the patient's legs during extrication produces severe pain and there is a real risk that these patients are misdiagnosed as hysterical or histrionic.

Finally, minor degrees of sensory or motor loss are frequently described by patients either in terms of "clumsiness", "stiffness" or "heaviness" and such complaints must always be treated seriously.

Because of the diversity of symptoms and signs in spinal injury, the management of patients with potential spinal injury requires particular attention to the history and mechanism of injury. Patients who have congenitally abnormal spines or diseases such as ankylosing spondylitis do not require the same degree of force to produce a cord injury as those with a normal spine.

Although the spectrum of sensory and motor neurological abnormalities is wide and complex, it is important not to be deflected from the important management priorities. Time should not be wasted in attempting to make precise neurological diagnoses. The key features of management which take priority are:

- to identify and manage life-threatening injuries elsewhere
- to recognize the presence of a spinal cord injury and to prevent deterioration
- to recognize the potential for spinal injury in a patient without signs or symptoms of established injury and to prevent the progression to established pathology.

CAUSES OF SPINAL CORD INJURY

The principal causes of spinal cord injury are as follows.

- Motor vehicle accidents
- Falls

- Sports:
  - gymnastics and trampolining
  - rugby football
  - horse riding and hunting
  - skiing
  - hang gliding
- Aquatic injuries, for example diving into shallow water
- Weight falling on the back.

Motor vehicle accidents

Fifty percent of all spinal injuries are still produced by motor vehicles and half of these occur to people on motorcycles. The motorcyclist's injury depends on the attitude of the head on falling and characteristically produces compression-flexion or extension with rotation. In motor vehicle accidents the unsecured person can be thrown out of the vehicle either through a door or through the windscreen. A person who is restrained can still have a deceleration injury, particularly to the cervical spine; rollover accidents or underrunning a larger vehicle can produce a compression injury and in vehicles where there are no rear seatbelts the unrestrained backseat passenger can injure the restrained frontseat passenger en passant, as the backseat passenger is thrown through the windscreen (the "flying granny" syndrome). The deceleration injury (whiplash injury) is a combined injury of flexion followed by extension. Vertebral column injury or spinal cord injury can occur in either phase and on some occasions, the vertebral column injury has occurred as the head and neck move in one direction and the cord injury as they move in the other.

Dorsal (thoracic) spine injuries commonly occur in association with injuries to the chest wall (ribs and sternum). Dorsolumbar injuries are more common when a lapstrap only rather than a conventional seatbelt is worn.

Falls

Falls may be from a height onto the feet or a result of jumping (including parachuting). The injuries are usually at the dorsolumbar junction. It should always be remembered that there may have been a medical condition causing the fall in the first place.

Rugby football

Injuries result from either scrum collapse or tackles.

Horse riding

Horse riding is the one cause of spinal cord injury where there is a female preponderance. All the other causes have male preponderance of 5:1.

Aquatic injuries

Aquatic injuries are principally due to diving accidents. There is a compression force and either a flexion or extension force depending on the attitude of the head. There are additional problems: the patient may float to the surface face down and be at risk of inhaling water and drowning and diving accidents are frequently associated with alcohol excess, not only on the part of the victim but also of the victim's companions, and there is therefore a delay in recognition which makes the risk of inhalation much greater. If airway obstruction occurs then the patient will have a predisposition to an anoxic injury over and above the mechanical injury.

A more recent cause of spinal injury associated with aquatic activities is *neurological decompression sickness*. This cause is increasing in importance, not only because diving sport is growing in popularity, with relatively inexperienced people taking part, but also because people ignore the instruction not to dive on the day they fly home from abroad. The combination of a dive to a depth greater than 30 m and then travelling in an aircraft cabin pressurized to only 3000 m will produce decompression symptoms and signs. This injury is the only one which is consistently progressive and also involves the brain and higher function. The result is that the patient arrives home (often inland, where such symptoms are not recognized) with a progressively spastic ataxic gait and a fatuous and elated manner. Unfortunately, the signs are frequently misdiagnosed as intoxication.

Weight falling on the back

Weight falling on the back was the classic mining injury and does still occur in agriculture and industry. Despite the contraction of the coal-mining industry, there has been a relative increase in the number of such injuries in the mines, attributable to the abolition of central direction of mine safety and fragmentation of the industry.

Associated injuries

Gymnastic injuries, rugby football injuries and diving injuries do not generally produce other mechanical trauma in association with spinal injury. However, with the remainder the incidence of associated major injury is of the order of 50%. These injuries will also need rigorous treatment, often with a higher priority than the spinal cord injury.

> The incidence of associated major injury with spinal cord injury is about 50%

ASSESSMENT

Any patient who is unconscious as a result of a head injury (or who could have had a head injury in association with unconsciousness) and any victim of trauma who is unable to give an account of the accident (e.g., through intoxication) must be regarded as having a spinal cord injury until proved otherwise. This also applies to the elderly demented patient and people with learning difficulties, not least as the latter group also harbour abnormalities of the vertebral column.

Also at particular risk are casualties who have signs of degenerative or inflammatory joint disease or those who have other skeletal deformities such as dwarfism.

Finally, the circumstances of the injury must not affect management. A fall is a fall is a fall – it does not matter whether a patient is intoxicated or "high" on a drug of dependence. The fact that thousands of people who get drunk and fall over do not injure their spines is not an excuse for trivializing the incident.

In summary, therefore, it is essential to have a high index of suspicion. If the situation suggests that there could be a spinal cord injury the patient must be treated as if there is.

- Do not let the patient get up.
- Do not allow others to get the patient up.
- Do not get the patient up yourself. *Think spinal cord injury!*

However, when a history is available and clearly excludes the possibility of a spinal injury or when it is apparent from the injury mechanism that a spinal injury has not occurred, immobilization of the spine is not necessary. Universal immobilization of the spine without clinical indication complicates management and may adversely affect outcome.

It is important to be aware that spinal injuries may be overlooked for a number of reasons. The acute stress reaction causes endorphin release which may result in pain masking. Similarly, in the multiply injured patient other injuries elsewhere may distract from the spinal injury. Depression of central sensation may occur from brain injury or intoxication from alcohol or drugs, especially when there is uncooperative or aggressive behaviour. Finally it is tempting to make the diagnosis of "malingering" in the absence of discrete physical signs.

The safe position for the patient is supine with the spine in a neutral position. Patient immobilization and extrication are discussed in detail in Chapter 29.

There are many descriptions of what constitutes an *unstable* or a *stable spinal injury* in orthopaedic terms, often cross-correlated with the radiological features and a retrospective calculation of the mechanism of injury. These analyses are of considerable importance to orthopaedic surgeons and physicians who have to choose between conservative and operative management, but in practical terms such analyses do not affect the immediate handling and management of the patient. It is important on arrival at an accident to identify or predict factors predisposing to any risk and then proceed on the assumption that the injury is biomechanically unstable and that failure to manage the patient properly can and will make the spinal cord injury worse or produce an injury where none existed before.

Neurological examination at the accident site should not be detailed. In motor terms, attendants should be looking at voluntary power, for example bending large joints normally. It is important to observe whether the chest wall moves during breathing or whether it is the diaphragm alone which is responsible for respiratory effort (diaphragmatic breathing, see below). Sensory examination may reveal a "sensory level"

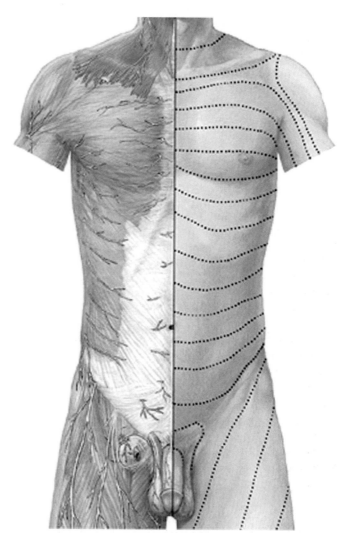

Figure 28.9 Simple sensory levels

below which sensation is altered or lost. The level should be marked on the skin. The following landmarks may be useful: the root of the neck is C4, the nipple line (in the male) is T4, the umbilicus is T10 and the foot (sole) is S1 (Figure 28.9).

IMMEDIATE MANAGEMENT

The causes of deterioration in established or suspected spinal injury are:

- hypoxia from underventilation, airway obstruction or lung damage either as a result of associated injuries or from aspiration of vomit
- underperfusion from reduced cord blood flow which may be due to positioning (e.g. sitting up) or to shock
- mechanical displacement of vertebrae
- displacement of vertebral fragments.

Because of the risk of anoxic damage and damage from underperfusion, airway (A), breathing (B) and circulation (C) must take priority over a cord injury or a potential cord injury.

Initial handling follows these priorities. The problems found in a primary survey are not only life threatening but will inevitably make any spinal injury worse. Careful horizontal movement (e.g., a properly applied "log roll") will not produce further permanent damage. Permanent cord damage is produced by thoughtless, uncontrolled movement of the spine or by applying the force of gravity through the spinal cord.

The patient should be moved as little as possible and there is no place for unnecessary lifts and transfers.

EMERGENCY EXTRICATION

Emergency extrication, that is, without the availability of appropriate extrication devices or the assistance of relevant emergency services, is justifiable only when there is an immediate threat to life. An *isolated* spinal cord injury need not be managed in a hurry. In this situation, depending on whether the patient is indoors or out, and on the weather, it is perfectly permissible to spend an additional 20–40 minutes organizing a safe removal and transfer from the accident site. Where there are multiple injuries these take priority and here the "golden hour" is of crucial importance if life is to be saved.

AIRWAY

Airway obstruction leads to hypoxia and inevitably to cord deterioration. Airway clearance is therefore vital. The technique of jaw thrust (or chin lift if necessary) should be used, whilst the head and neck are simultaneously moved into a neutral position and manual in-line stabilisation is applied. It is appropriate initially to attempt to clear the airway with the patient in the position in which he or she is found, but it may be necessary to move the patient carefully into the supine position.

BREATHING

Ventilation is often impeded in a thoracic or cervical cord injury. This may be because the patient is breathing using only the diaphragm (the intercostal and abdominal muscles being paralysed) or because of chest injuries and associated pain. It should be remembered that pain from chest injuries may mask the pain from the back injury. If ventilation is inadequate ventilatory assistance will be necessary.

> **Always administer high concentration oxygen**

INTUBATION IN POTENTIAL CORD INJURY

There are benefits in intubating the apnoeic and/or unconscious patient in terms of improved airway control, prevention of subsequent bronchial soiling, ease of bronchial toilet and ease of mechanical ventilation.

Against these benefits must be measured the hazards. Neck injury may be associated with laryngeal damage.

> **Box 28.1 Possible indications for intubation**
>
> - Absence of spontaneous ventilation which is not restarted by airway opening
> - Absent or inadequate spontaneous ventilation with evidence of vomiting, reflux or aspiration
> - Adequate supine spontaneous ventilation which is associated with problems in airway control
> - Adequate supine spontaneous ventilation associated with increasing ventilatory difficulty in association with thoracic or abdominal injury
> - The unconscious spinal cord injury patient with isolated head and neck injuries

During intubation the patient may undergo a vagal asystolic arrest. A similar event may occur during endobronchial suction. Both these features are more common if the patient is hypoxic. These complications may be minimized by adequate preoxygenation and the judicious use of atropine (see below). There may, in addition, be movement of the neck with production of a mechanical cord lesion or the induction of vomiting or reflux during intubation.

If there are good grounds for intubating the patient, the possibility of spinal cord injury should not deter the operator. The roadside respiratory arrest is either neurogenic or in the aftermath of aspiration or chest injury. A very high cord lesion, that is C1 to C3 (the *hangman's fracture*), produces diaphragmatic paralysis. The anatomy of the atlas and axis is such that when these vertebrae are damaged the canal is wider, not narrower. If intubation is needed because of chest injury or aspiration the mechanical risks are more than outweighed by the risks of not securing adequate ventilation. At the roadside the patient, even if unconscious, will still have protective muscle spasm of the neck which will not have been ablated by pharmacological paralysing agents or anaesthetic agents. In addition, spinal cord swelling at that stage will be minimal. For these reasons a paramedic should not fight shy of intubating if valid reasons exist.

SPINAL CORD INJURY AND DISORDERED CIRCULATION

Spinal cord injury can be associated with disorders of central circulation, which may cause either a cardiac arrest or an arrhythmia from which a cardiac arrest may develop.

After spinal cord injury, due to loss of function of the sympathetic nervous system, the parasympathetic nervous system can be unopposed. While considerable parasympathetic stimulation is required to induce bradycardia or asystole in non-injured humans, this is not the case in the phase of spinal areflexia with loss of sympathetic function. The stimuli required to trigger adverse parasympathomimetic effects are then considerably less. This phenomenon is aggravated by hypoxia and hypothermia. Hypoxia is particularly significant as it may occur temporarily during upper airway suction, attempts at airway insertion, intubation and endo-bronchial suction through a tracheal tube. The risk rises the further down the airway the stimulus is applied and tends to be more pronounced the higher the cord lesion.

Prehospital management of this bradycardia is the administration of atropine. If the heart rate is below 45 beats per minute, a bolus dose of atropine (500 µg) should be given *before* any of the above interventions are attempted and should be given in any case if the heart rate falls as low as 40 beats/min. If there is no resting bradycardia the pulse should be monitored during the procedure and if it falls below 45 beats/min, a bolus dose of atropine should be given.

The acute signs in the limbs are also derived from the suspension of reflex activity in response to a spinal cord injury. Affected limbs are flaccid and areflexic (so-called spinal shock). The suspension of sympathetic drive produces generalized vasodilation. Thus, even if the circulating blood volume is unchanged there will effectively be underperfusion. This produces the signs of shock and the condition is known as neurogenic shock.

The terms *spinal* shock and *neurogenic* shock often cause some confusion. *Neurogenic* shock is a cardiovascular condition resulting from loss of vascular tone as a result of loss of sympathetic activity and is manifested by a low blood pressure in a well-perfused individual with no evidence of tachycardia. *Spinal* shock is a neurological condition manifested by flaccidity and loss of reflexes.

In an isolated cervical or thoracic cord injury the "normal" systolic arterial blood pressure will be found to be around 90 mmHg. At this level, because the vessels are vasodilated, perfusion should be adequate so long as the patient is kept flat. The heart rate may be either slow or normal. A combination of bradycardia and hypotension should always raise the suspicion of spinal cord injury. Where a patient has a normal pulse and apparent hypotension, both spinal cord injury and covert trauma should be suspected. Shock in the patient with multiple trauma must *never* be assumed to be solely due to spinal cord injury.

In a patient with *multiple injuries* of which the cord injury is one element, the indications for infusion are the same as for any other polytrauma victim. The amount of fluid infused and the rate of infusion should be sufficient to restore perfusion of the vital organs by bringing the systolic blood pressure to a level sufficient to maintain the presence of a radial pulse. In the elderly, hypertensive subject a higher blood pressure may be appropriate. The principle is that whatever infusion is required to establish clinically effective perfusion should be provided subject to the general principle that it should not delay evacuation to hospital.

With the *isolated cord injury*, as may occur in a gymnastic or rugby accident, if given at all, the infusion must be given with extreme care. Because of vasodilation, so long as the patient is kept flat, perfusion should be adequate to maintain a radial pulse. As long as this remains the case, an intravenous infusion is not necessary. Where the radial pulse is lost, an infusion will be necessary to ensure that a palpable radial pulse returns. *Only 500 ml of intravenous fluid should be given prehospital.* This volume is sufficient to compensate for the increased vascular space. Because of the cord damage, however, the circulation is at the limits of vasomotor control. In addition, there is a considerable output of antidiuretic hormone. The result is that it is very easy to overtransfuse a patient – even one who is young – and if a patient is overtransfused it is extremely difficult to correct. Concern about the quantity of fluid infused, however, should not deter the attendant from inserting a cannula or setting up a line while the veins are still easily accessible.

While a head-down tilt can be used temporarily to clear vomit from the airway, continued use of this position on circulatory grounds may cause the abdominal contents to splint the diaphragm and reduce the vital capacity. With associated abdominal injuries and an abdominal cavity filling with gas, blood or both, a secondary ventilatory inadequacy or even arrest may be precipitated.

There are particular problems associated with rescue situations where vertical movement of the casualty may be essential and also in environmental conditions where the cold makes infusion difficult or impossible.

UNCONSCIOUSNESS

There is a strong association of head injury with proven spinal cord injuries. The reverse phenomenon, that is to say the association of spinal cord injury with proven head injury, is, however, only 10–15%.

Reviews of significant deceleration motor vehicle accidents have shown that if the patient is alive when the first rescuer arrives, the incidence of a grossly unstable biomechanical cervical injury is of the order of 1 in 300.

Two maxims derive from this and they are not mutually exclusive. The first is that in the presence of a significant head injury, a spinal cord injury should always be suspected. The overall management picture should presume that a spinal cord injury exists until proved otherwise. Until the patient is adequately stabilized, any *necessary* movement must be carried out carefully, with the best immobilization possible under the circumstances. The second maxim is that because of the relative incidences, any movement which is necessary to save life must take priority and must be carried out in accordance with the priorities of primary survey using the greatest care and best endeavours available. To do otherwise will place at risk the 299 patients with a head injury who do not have a grossly biomechanically unstable neck injury, in favour of the one patient who does.

The major risk of unconsciousness is that of aspiration pneumonia induced by inhalation of vomit or refluxed gastric contents. In spinal cord injury there is a greater risk of silent gastro-oesophageal reflux as some of the muscles forming the sphincter between the oesophagus and stomach are disabled. In addition, there is an immediate ileus coupled to gastric stasis. Third, there are no premonitory signs of vomiting-like reflux, which is silent. Lastly, in many of the associated social circumstances the stomach is full, often with alcohol.

The diagnosis of unconsciousness is definitive, while that of spinal cord injury is presumptive. Unconsciousness takes priority: the airway must be maintained and bronchial soiling avoided. In the absence of advanced airway management, the patient will need to be turned on their side. If there is difficulty in maintaining the airway and there is present or imminent reflux or vomiting an immediate turn onto the side in order to deal with this problem is essential. The mortality of isolated spinal cord injury is under 1%, but this rises to 40% if aspiration pneumonitis supervenes. If the patient is already securely immobilized on a long spine board, they can be effectively turned onto their side without significant risk to the spinal cord, simply by tipping the board.

The normal rules for airway protection apply and must not be compromised because there is inadequate assistance or "packaging" is not yet complete. The attendant must always remember that if a degree of hypoxia is induced which is sufficient to compromise that patient's life then that degree of hypoxia will inevitably render complete an existing incomplete spinal cord lesion.

There are some indicators that a spinal cord injury may coexist in a patient who is unconscious.

- A different level of responsiveness above and below the level of possible cord injury.
- Diaphragmatic ventilation (the cardinal feature of which is that during inspiration the abdominal wall, instead of appearing to recede, balloons out).
- The association of bradycardia, hypotension and a head injury.
- Priapism (sustained erection).

None of these signs is consistently present and it may be that none is present.

The patient with neurogenic shock will appear warm, pink and well perfused, with a low or normal pulse despite a low blood pressure.

In the presence of an isolated spinal cord injury, the patient should be lucid. A patient who subsequently becomes unconscious may have an obstructed airway or be under-ventilating or shocked in association with previously unsuspected associated injuries, or there may be a deteriorating head injury.

BASIC MANAGEMENT SUMMARY

- Always have a high index of suspicion for spinal cord injury.
- Remember the history and mechanism of injury.
- The patient must not stand or sit up.
- Airway, breathing, circulation and unconsciousness require immediate action.
- Slow, careful movement is safe.
- Careful movement in the horizontal axis preserves life and will also preserve residual cord function.

From this list it can be seen that the basic rules are as follows.

- Consider safety.
- Consider the need for resuscitation (primary survey).
- Consider the possibility of a spinal cord injury.
- Control the head and neck position whilst allowing optimal support of the airway, breathing and circulation.
- Organize the team before embarking on complicated extrication and management procedures.

The use of equipment will always require assistance beyond the standard two-person ambulance crew. It may involve summoning ambulance colleagues, making use of fellow emergency service professionals or even seeking help from the general public. Assistants must always be adequately briefed before a task is undertaken.

SPINAL IMMOBILIZATION AND PATIENT HANDLING

CONTROL OF THE HEAD AND NECK

Control of the head and neck must be undertaken as soon as possible. Control is secured by immobilizing the base of the skull without exerting a positive traction force. In the unrecognized spinal injury, traction may induce a secondary distraction injury.

COLLARS

There are many collars on the market, a few of which are effective and safe, many of which are useless and a significant proportion of which are dangerous as well. A semi-rigid collar must be used rather than a soft collar, improvised collar or rehabilitation collar. The only role for an improvised collar is where there are multiple casualties, as a marker to indicate suspicion of a spinal cord injury. The collar should restrict flexion, extension, lateral flexion and rotation of the neck and the resting position of the neck must be in neutral alignment.

The collars must be properly stored and the instructions for application rigorously followed. Another person must always control the head and neck while the collar is applied. If a two-piece collar is applied care must be taken not to obstruct the jugular venous outflow (thereby contributing to raised intracranial pressure) and the front piece and the back piece must be individually sized.

Lastly, any collar is only a restraint and should be supplemented by manual head control or the use of headblocks and tape. A tight collar may interfere with venous return from the cerebral circulation and accordingly raise the intracranial pressure in patients whose cerebral perfusion is already compromised. In cases of head injury with impaired consciousness, a collar can be safely loosened *once a patient has been secured to a board with adequate lateral immobilization* (see below).

MOVEMENT AT THE ACCIDENT SITE

Movement at the scene is usually:

- from prone to supine to maximize ventilation with a conscious patient and place the head in neutral alignment
- from supine to side to protect an otherwise unprotected airway or to assist the clearance of vomit
- from side to supine once vomit has been cleared or to intubate or otherwise maintain ventilation of someone whose ventilation is inadequate on their side.

Traditionally movement is effected by a "log roll". The log roll requires ideally six people and at least five people if it is to be carried out without moving the full length of the spine. Log rolling using three people has been described but this produces a movement of the dorsal and/or lumbar spine. Equally, in hospital, four people can be used but this works only where (a) the conditions are ideal and the patient is at the right height and (b) where the team is highly experienced at the manoeuvre.

Orthopaedic ("Scoop") stretcher

For retrieving casualties from the ground, the scoop stretcher is preferable to the long spinal board which requires a log roll procedure. It is almost exclusively a transfer stretcher, although it can be used to remove people from difficult locations, after which they can be transferred to a conventional stretcher or an evacuation mattress. The disadvantage of the scoop stretcher is that it is composed of rigid metal leaves with sharp edges and can generate pressure sores even in a short journey time, particularly if the patient is underperfused. Once the patient is on the ambulance trolley cot or the evacuation mattress, the scoop stretcher should be removed. It can, however, be positioned under an evacuation mattress to provide greater rigidity for lifting and carrying.

Evacuation (vacuum) mattresses

Whichever type of evacuation mattress is used, the following rules apply. First, it should be tested before the ambulance goes on duty to make sure that there are no leaks. Second, when laid out it needs to be smoothed flat. Third, once the patient is positioned on it manual contouring is required between the legs and around the head, neck and shoulders. As long as it was laid flat in the first instance, it will protect against pressure sores. The scoop stretcher can be placed underneath it with safety and will add to overall rigidity.

Extrication devices

Extrication devices are based around the design of the short spinal board. The designs that are easiest to use have a leading edge which can be applied from either side (and which can be cleared of straps, buckles and other impedimenta so that it can be inserted easily). A minimum of four people are necessary to apply such a device. The ideal device should not "concertina" during insertion behind the patient. It should *not* be applied before a semi-rigid cervical collar is in

place. There should be an effective cushion component to block out the space between the board and the rear of the collar and head. All straps should be applied and tightened, except the leg straps in the presence of a fractured femur. Once secured, the patient can be moved in any suitable direction except the vertical. A vertical lift requires the addition of a vertical movement harness. Some devices have what appears to be a handle at the head end. *This must never be used for lifting the patient.*

Long spinal board

The long spinal board has two uses. The first is aquatic rescue: its use is primarily a lifeguard skill, although ambulance service personnel may be required to assist the lifeguards. The second is as part of vehicular extrication. The technique of choice is to bring the device in behind the patient from the rear of the wreckage and to move the patient up the long axis of the spinal board. However, this requires removal of the roof of the vehicle. If a rapid extrication is mandated by the presence of a time-critical injury, the patient may be rotated onto a spine board through the adjacent doorway of the vehicle. The spinal board should therefore be rigid, thin, have contoured edges and have a low coefficient of friction for both the undersurface and the top surface. The spinal board is used with head immobilizers attached to it which prevent lateral movement.

Helmet removal

It is recognized that the removal of motorcycle helmets is essential even in the presence of a spinal cord injury. Opening the visor is not sufficient to manage the airway. Ideally every motorcyclist would wear a *BMW pattern* helmet where the front elements canbe hinged away and the helmet removed with relative safety, as with the old-style "coal-scuttle" helmets before the development of full-face helmets. However, the occipital portion of all helmets will move the head into flexion, reducing the diameter of the spinal canal. Helmet removal is, therefore, essential to obtaining neutral alignment of the cervical spine. Helmet removal is not an emergency if the airway is clear and protected.

Helmet removal should, wherever possible, be undertaken by two people. A common error is failure to undo the chin strap. One person supports the neck from the front and gradually moves their hands up the back of the neck and head while the helmet is tipped backwards and forwards in the vertical plane to clear the occiput and then the nose. Whilst the helmet is being removed, it should be carefully expanded laterally. At every stage, the person holding the neck must have complete control and should ask his colleague to stop if problems arise (Figure 28.10).

If circumstances demand that a helmet is removed by a single rescuer, the procedure in Figure 28.11 should be followed. The rescuer kneels above the patient's head, the chin

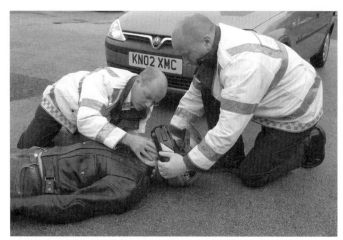

Figure 28.10 Safe helmet removal with two rescuers

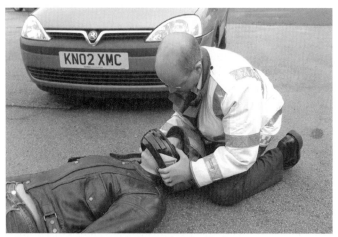

Figure 28.11 Safe helmet removal with one rescuer

strap is undone and the helmet is expanded laterally and gently tilted forwards until it is clear of the occiput. Once this has been achieved, the helmet can then be tilted backwards in order to release the chin from the chin bar. Having done this, the rescuer maintains in-line stabilization by placing his hands along the sides of the patient's head whilst using his forearms to complete the helmet removal.

GENERAL RULES FOR EQUIPMENT

The equipment used today for the management of spinal cord injury is effective, but equally has the capacity to cause mischief in unskilled, unpractised hands. Therefore, not only should personnel be trained, but they should also be practised. None of the equipment can be applied as effectively by a single person as by two or more. Even applying a cervical collar or removing a helmet (by whatever means) requires two people. The use of a scoop stretcher requires a minimum of two trained ambulance personnel, with other people assisting by lifting the sides to prevent it bending. The use of the long spinal board, short spinal board and

evacuation mattress all require a minimum of four people – six people is optimal. These people need not necessarily be fully trained ambulance personnel – help from other emergency service workers, first-aiders or members of the public may be appropriate. Neurological deterioration is never due to equipment failure, it is due to errors on the part of the people using it.

PRESSURE SORES

Paralysed patients are at risk from pressure sores because they cannot feel and cannot move. Pressure sores can start to develop within an hour of a spinal cord injury occurring. These sores usually occur in the usual pressure sites – the bony prominences where only a small amount of tissue interposes between the bone and the hard surface of the stretcher. In the supine position these are the heels, the buttocks, the scapulae and the back of the head. Primary journeys are usually short and pressure sores are produced at this stage largely by the misapplication of splinting systems, by hard objects in the pockets of the patient, such as bunches of keys, and by certain extrication devices. Therefore, clothing should be loosened, including the shoelaces. Hard objects should be removed from pockets where they are next to the skin. Padding should be placed between the legs. Any additional splintage should be padded. The spinal board should be perceived as a rescue board and patients should be splinted on it for only a short period of time, ideally no more than 30 minutes. At the receiving hospital, the patient should be released from the board as soon as possible.

The scoop stretcher, too, because of its sharp-edged leaves, can produce pressure sores even on a short journey. It should only be used as a transfer stretcher and patients should *not* be left lying directly on it. Ideally the evacuation of spinal injury patients should be carried out on a vacuum mattress. This device is essential for long journeys or secondary transfers or for aeromedical flights.

HYPOTHERMIA

A paralysed person cannot sweat or shiver. Temperature perception is impeded because of sensory impairment and the control mechanism, stripped of its input and output, also becomes erratic. Patients with spinal injuries must be protected from the cold; they must be warmed passively by being wrapped up well. During the primary journey this is not usually a problem, but because of the large distances between spinal units, it can be a problem on a secondary journey from the receiving hospital to the spinal unit, for which the ambulance service is also responsible. The problem is likely to arise if, mistakenly, it is thought appropriate to drive an ambulance at 5 miles per hour for the entire distance. Clear directions have now been issued by the Spinal Injuries Consultants in the UK as to how it is possible to move patients at normal road speeds, together with protocols favouring the use of helicopters under certain conditions.

In the UK the major problem is hypothermia. However, in hot weather the reverse problem – heat stroke – can also occur. It is also a major problem during aeromedical evacuation of people who may well have been lying out in the sun on the tarmac at a foreign airfield for a long period.

SUMMARY

Spinal cord injury management aims to avoid neurological deterioration, prevent death from acute effects or associated injury and prevent long-term complications.

It depends first on a high index of suspicion and an ability to make a diagnosis, particularly where the cord injury is incomplete. Deterioration may be produced by either biomechanical, anoxic or vascular mechanisms.

The overall rule is to move patients as little as possible, but correct positioning to protect or maintain the airway, provide adequate ventilation and maintain the circulation is essential and takes precedence. Intubation should be undertaken where clear indications exist. An intravenous cannula should be inserted and conventional fluid protocols should be followed. Cardiac arrest may be induced through parasympathetic stimulation and can be prevented with the use of prophylactic atropine. Manual control of the head is crucial and should be instituted at the earliest possible opportunity. The only safe position for the spine is lying supine in neutral alignment.

In addition, patients should be protected against development of pressure sores and hypothermia. Mishandling is not merely mechanical, it also compromises the spinal cord on a pathophysiological basis. Serial mishandling produces cumulative effects greater than that produced by each individual element.

Chapter 29

Patient immobilization and extrication

INTRODUCTION

Following an accident it is accepted clinical practice that casualties should be transported to hospital for definitive care as rapidly as possible. The need to differentiate time-critical from non-time critical conditions early in any rescue is imperative. This management decision will significantly alter the way patients are handled and "packaged" in preparation for transport to hospital. However, not only should we have the patients' interests and care at heart, but it is also essential to remember the needs and safety of the rescuers and to be alert to any risks posed by environmental factors.

It is therefore crucial that decisions about stabilization, extrication and subsequent evacuation are taken early on in the rescue. The techniques used for stabilization must not be viewed in isolation, but should be part of the total rescue activity and should complement the other treatments used to provide care and comfort to the patient. Whichever technique is used, the method of transport must first be determined, to make sure the equipment needed will fit the vehicle to be used.

In choosing a method of stabilization for the known or suspected injuries, the paramedic must remember the two underlying principles of prehospital care. First, to do no harm while ensuring the patient's comfort and second, to ensure there is no delay in the provision of rapid definitive care.

PRINCIPLES OF IMMOBILIZATION

In the prehospital setting, the principles of skeletal management are to prevent further injury, ensure neurovascular supply and to make the patient comfortable. Immobilization also helps to reduce further blood loss and reduces the risk of fat embolism.

The overriding importance of managing the airway with cervical spine protection, breathing and circulation (ABC) is fundamental to the treatment of any injury. With the exception of cervical spine care, fracture management and extrication follow the primary survey unless a "snatch rescue" is necessary.

The principles of definitive fracture management are *reduction, immobilization* and *preservation of function*. How these principles are applied or modified in the prehospital setting, and the equipment available, are considered below.

Reduction
Immobilization
Preservation of function

Since nearly every piece of equipment will cover or hide the patient to a greater or lesser extent, it is essential that any immediate local treatment and observations are carried out before the immobilization device is applied. Examination should be as complete as the situation allows and the injuries dictate. Wounds should wherever possible be photographed using an instant-print camera, and appropriately dressed before immobilization.

BENEFITS TO THE PATIENT

The benefits of immobilization are:

- pain relief
- reduction of blood loss
- prevention of neurovascular damage
- prevention of fat embolism.

Any prehospital treatment should always be considered from the standpoint of the patient. Remembering the ABC principles, splinting or extrication devices should never produce any airway, breathing or circulation compromise.

The patient should always feel more comfortable after the splint or device has been applied, so that handling becomes easier. This will help to reduce the patient's fear and, as a consequence, reduce circulating catecholamines and their potentially harmful effects (peripheral vasoconstriction with reduced peripheral tissue oxygenation). By correct splinting, bleeding into the tissues may be reduced, thereby lowering the life-threatening risk of hypovolaemia. Fat emboli resulting from fractured long bones will also be reduced by early and correct splinting, particularly if it is combined with oxygen therapy.

FORMS OF SPLINTAGE

Most of the forms of splintage considered in this chapter relate to spinal immobilization, but limb splintage and the pneumatic antishock garment (PASG), also known as military antishock trousers (MAST), are also considered.

BOX SPLINTS

Box splints are simple in design and are often overlooked. They are useful for some arm, lower leg and ankle injuries and are carried by every front-line ambulance (Figure 29.1).

The splint forms an oblong box, open along one side with the other three sides able to be folded in such a way as to form a gutter. There may be a foot support at one end. Box splints are available in adult and child sizes.

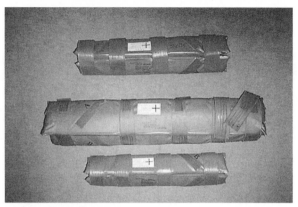

Figure 29.1 Box splints

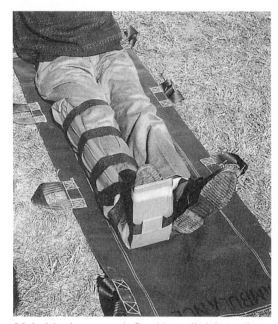

Figure 29.2 A leg in a correctly fitted lower limb box splint

Application

The injured leg should be exposed and the footwear removed (if possible). Appropriate dressings should be applied to any wounds and the ankle straightened. The peripheral pulses should be checked.

There may be rare occasions when only available boots or footwear provide a splint for ankle injuries and in these situations they may be left on. Otherwise they should be removed to allow assessment of neurovascular function and to avoid compression arising from swelling.

The leg should be raised and the splint passed underneath the leg. The two sides of the splint are then folded so they fit closely against the leg. The ankle support should hold the foot at right angles or in a position of comfort if there is significant deformity, bearing in mind that this may be a limb-threatening problem requiring urgent reduction. The Velcro straps are passed over the top of the leg and around the front of the ankle. This arrangement forms a firm support and immobilizes the lower leg effectively (Figure 29.2).

If any strap passes near to an injury, care should be taken that it does not cause pain; if it does, it should be left loose. Once the splint is applied, the patient should be rechecked – specifically, the pulses in the limb and the distal sensation must be noted and recorded.

Always check the pulses distal to an injury

Some box splints have a side pocket and a long wooden splint can be inserted to form a long leg splint. This, together with fracture straps or broad-fold triangular bandages and padding, can be used to immobilize a fractured femur.

Care should be taken when a box splint has been applied in case there has been any bleeding since this may not be obvious and the box splint may retain a considerable volume of blood within it.

TRACTION SPLINTS

The primary function of a traction splint is to immobilize the fracture (of a lower limb) in a reduced position. This will greatly aid patient comfort but, more importantly, will prevent further neurovascular damage and reduce the severity of shock by reducing blood loss and pain from the fracture site.

Following a fracture of the shaft of the femur, if the muscles of the thigh are left without traction they will shorten the leg, causing the bone ends to override, which not only presents a serious potential for neurovascular damage and entrapment but also increases the radius of the thigh so that it becomes more spherical: this shape has a larger internal volume than a cylinder and so presents a larger space into which blood can escape. Application of traction will restore the cylindrical shape of the thigh, reducing its volume and reducing the overall blood loss. Traction splinting in association with early surgical intervention reduces the incidence of fat embolus.

Three types of traction splint are found in prehospital care: the Hare or Trac-3 splint, the Sager splint and the Donway splint. The Sager splint is the most effective and convenient for prehospital use.

Hare or Trac-3 traction splint

The Hare traction splint (Figure 29.3) and the Trac-3 traction splint are useful pieces of equipment. Not only can they be used with traction to maintain a reduced fracture of the lower limb, but they can also be used without traction simply for support.

Indications

There is some debate about the indications for use of this type of splint and it is wise to check with the local receiving hospital for their views.

Indications with traction
- Closed (simple) fractures of the femoral shaft
- Closed (simple) fractures of the proximal two-thirds of the tibia and fibula

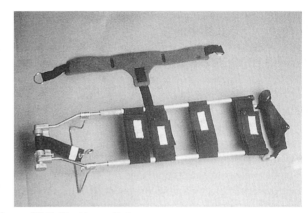

Figure 29.3 The Hare splint

- Compound fractures of the femur, and the proximal two-thirds of the tibia and fibula (this is open to debate and local guidance must be sought).

All compound fractures must be surgically explored and cleaned. Therefore the receiving hospital must know that a fracture was compound. If the fracture was reduced at the scene then it is mandatory to ensure that the receiving doctor is completely aware that the fracture was compound (if possible a photograph should be taken using an instant-print camera).

It is worth emphasizing that compound fractures should be reduced into an anatomical position before splinting, even if this means reducing exposed bone ends back into the wound. The important thing is to tell the hospital that the fracture was compound.

Contraindications to traction

- Fractures around the knee
- Dislocation of the hip
- Fracture dislocation of the knee
- Ankle injuries
- Simple undisplaced fracture of the lower third of the tibia and fibula (better immobilized with a box splint)
- Fractures of the pelvis
- Fractures of the neck of femur (Sager type *not* contraindicated).

Application

Application must be practised regularly. It requires two people to apply the splint correctly. It should be remembered that just because a patient has a fracture that can be dealt with by traction splinting, it does not follow that it is in that person's interests always to have a splint put on. There may be other more life-threatening injuries which must take priority. Patients are far less likely to die from a fracture of the lower limb than they are from a blocked airway. In time-critical patients, the traction splint may be applied en route to hospital.

The splint should be set up as follows.

1. The patient is given analgesia as required.
2. The fracture site is exposed (clothes should be cut if necessary). Motorcycle leathers should not be removed as these can be dramatically effective in the control of lower limb and pelvic fracture bleeding (see below).
3. The limb should be examined thoroughly and the footwear removed. The pulses distal to the fracture together with the colour and warmth of the limb and sensation and motor function distal to the fracture should also be assessed (the neurovascular examination). An oximeter can be helpful if the probe is applied to a toe and both limbs compared.
4. Wounds are dressed if required.
5. The splint is prepared.
   - The appropriate ankle hitch is selected.
   - The splint is placed by the good leg, measured for length and adjusted accordingly, then laid by the injured leg.
   - All the straps are checked; these should be open and placed at the correct intervals down the splint.
   - Some of the traction strap should be unwound.
   - The splint is rechecked from top to bottom immediately prior to application.
6. The ankle hitch is placed under the ankle. The foot is straightened and the hitch placed well under the ankle. The side straps are then tightly folded over the ankle (not around the foot) and the rings brought together below the foot. Finally the strap at the bottom of the foot is firmly grasped (Figure 29.4). Traction *must* be applied along the longitudinal axis of the femur, *not* over the dorsum of the foot, which can cause permanent damage to the limb. Poor application of the ankle hitch is the cause of misaligned traction.
7. Manual traction is started with one hand while the other hand supports the leg.
8. The splint is then put in the correct position. Circumstances will dictate to an extent how this is done, but the best method is to roll the patient away from the splint while a colleague slides the splint under the leg. The top padded ring *must* fit under the ischial tuberosity. The patient is then rolled back onto the splint. If the position is still not correct then the patient can be moved down slightly so that he is sitting on the padded ring. *Manual traction MUST be maintained THROUGHOUT this procedure.*
9. The top strap is done up and padding applied if required. The external genitalia should be avoided in males. If correctly positioned, this strap will lie parallel to the crease of the groin.
10. The traction hook is then put through the "D" rings and traction taken up, ensuring that manual traction is not released before the splint's mechanical traction is tightened.
11. Traction is applied until the limb is comfortable (to a maximum of 7 kg in adults).
12. The neurovascular examination is repeated and the oximeter reading rechecked.
13. The leg is elevated by raising the foot stand.
14. The Velcro straps are positioned and tightened to support the site of the fracture.
15. The leg is covered to keep it warm.

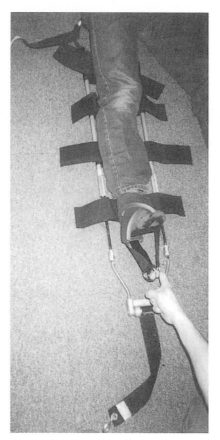

Figure 29.4 Manual traction using a Hare splint

En route to hospital

1. The neurovascular examination should be repeated every 5–10 minutes.
2. The straps should be checked and loosened if required – the leg may swell.
3. The tension of traction should be checked; as a result of reduced spasm in the muscles, tension can be lost.

To release traction

The two splints (Hare and Trac-3) have slightly different release mechanisms. Manual traction is taken up and then the mechanical traction is released after all the supporting Velcro straps have been removed. The Hare splint has a pull ring which releases the traction suddenly, whereas the Trac-3 has a knob which has to be unwound to release the traction (which is less likely to be accidentally released).

Complications

The only real complication that can occur is damage to the neurovascular supply to the leg. This can be prevented by careful examination of the distal limb function. Absence or change in distal function must be reported to the A&E department. If it is found that the distal pulses diminish or are absent after traction has been applied, the tightness of

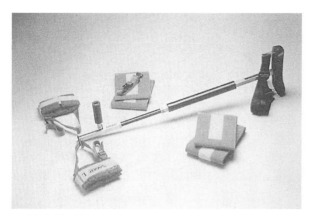

Figure 29.5 The Sager splint

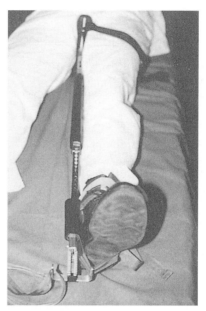

Figure 29.6 Applying the ankle harness

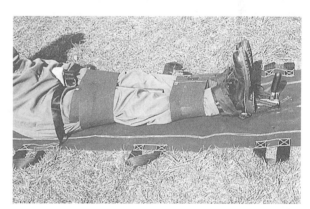

Figure 29.7 Leg in a Sager splint

the straps should be assessed in case circumferential occlusion has occurred and if so, under manual control the traction must be gently reduced until the pulse returns.

The pulse oximeter can be used to detect alterations in the blood flow if the probe is placed on one of the toes of the fractured leg. However, this can be unreliable.

One problem with a traction splint of this type is that it will extend well beyond the patient's body and therefore handling on a trolley or in a vehicle may be difficult (it may be impossible in some helicopters). When treating bilateral fractures, two splints are required and this can make handling very difficult. These problems are not encountered with the Sager splint (see below).

Sager traction splint

The Sager traction splint weighs less than 2 kg and can be used to treat single or bilateral fractures of the lower limb, especially of the femur (Figure 29.5).

It is claimed that the Sager splint can be applied with the patient in any position so long as the leg can be straightened. A great advantage of the Sager splint is that it does not extend far beyond the end of the leg following application, which makes handling and transport easier.

Application

1. The shoe and sock are removed and the leg exposed as necessary.
2. The distal pulses and sensation in the injured leg are assessed.
3. The cushioned end of the splint is applied between the patient's legs, against the perineum and symphysis pubis (avoiding the external genitalia in males).
4. The bridle "S" strap is applied around the top of the thigh.
5. The splint is extended so that the ankle hitch lies between the patient's heels or at the level of the normal heel if the fractured leg has been shortened.
6. The ankle harness is applied beneath the heel and wrapped around just above the malleoli, adjusting the cushions on the strap to fit the size of the leg (Figure 29.6).
7. Traction is applied (recommended at 10% of the body weight) until the patient is comfortable.
8. The leg cravats are applied.
9. The bridle around the thigh is tightened if necessary.
10. The cravats are secured.
11. The foot-binding strap is placed around the feet and ankles in a figure-of-eight.
12. The foot pulses must be checked following application.

The splinted leg is shown in Figure 29.7.

It is vital that the ABC priorities have been dealt with before the splint is applied. Additional pain relief may be required.

A report form should be completed, including photographs if taken.

To release traction

Manual traction is taken up. The cravats and ankle hitch are removed. Along the shaft of the splint there is a small sprung piece of metal, which should be lifted to release the tension.

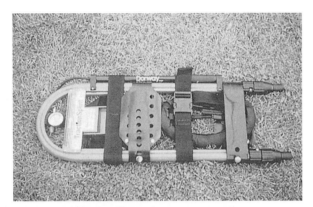

Figure 29.8 The Donway splint

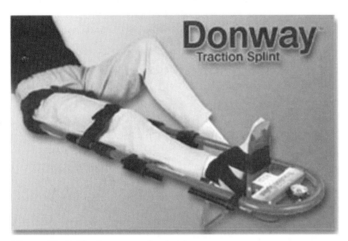

Figure 29.9 The Donway splint in place

Donway splint

The Donway splint (Figure 29.8) employs a different method to achieve traction. The fractured leg is cradled by the splint with the foot firmly fixed to the ankle support. The top strapping is put around the thigh and then, using the pump provided, the two halves of the splint (lower and upper) are pushed apart by increased pressure (like the slide on a trombone). Once the patient is comfortable the securing screws are tightened; the pressure in the splint is then released through a valve. The leg straps are applied and (as with other forms of traction splint) the pulses and sensation in the limb must be checked. As with the Hare and Trac3 splints, particular care must be taken to ensure the ankle hitch is applied in a manner that avoids traction over the dorsum of the foot.

PNEUMATIC ANTISHOCK GARMENT

The pneumatic antishock garment (PASG), also known as the military antishock trousers (MAST), is an inflatable garment that surrounds the legs and abdomen and can be inflated to a pressure of 100 mmHg (Figure 29.10).

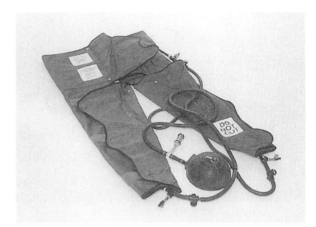

Figure 29.10 Pneumatic antishock garment

Indications

Indications for use of the PASG are:

- splinting of pelvic and lower limb fractures
- intraabdominal trauma – tamponade of bleeding vessels.

The PASG is no longer recommended for hypovolaemic shock except in exceptional circumstances (see below) and there are better alternatives for lower limb fracture splintage. A description of its use is included because it may occasionally be seen in use by immediate care doctors in remote situations.

Method of action

The PASG acts by applying direct pressure to bleeding vessels and splinting fractures. Investigations have shown that it reduces intraabdominal haemorrhage. It was originally thought to act by physically squeezing blood from the lower limbs into the central circulation, but later evidence suggests this is not the case. The mechanism is now thought to be that the PASG increases the peripheral vascular resistance.

The net effect is equivalent to giving a 2–3 unit blood transfusion in an adult. Blood pressure rises, as does cardiac output, stroke volume and mean arterial pressure (see Chapter 22).

Contraindications

Absolute contraindications:

- cardiac failure
- pulmonary oedema
- ruptured diaphragm (to use of the abdominal compartment only)
- second and third trimester of pregnancy (to use of the abdominal compartment only)
- uncontrolled bleeding above garment (particularly in the thorax).

Relative contraindications:

- head injury
- application lasting more than 6 hours.

Dangers

The use of a PASG is associated with a number of problems. Visual examination of covered areas is prevented (injuries should be photographed first with an instant-print camera). Respiratory embarrassment may occur and it is vital that the PASG is not seen as a reason for failing to monitor vital signs.

Application

As will be seen, the application of a PASG is a complex and relatively prolonged procedure, especially in inexperienced hands. As a consequence, its use is NOT RECOMMENDED when reasonably rapid transfer to definitive care is possible. The PASG may have a role in remote areas associated with long transfer times and in these circumstances, local protocols should be carefully followed.

If the use of a PASG is indicated, the garment should be applied as follows, after the patient's vital signs have been recorded.

1. The PASG is unpacked and laid on an ambulance cot spineboard, or a flat, hard surface.
2. Although it is possible to place the PASG under the patient by rolling, it is much easier to lay the patient onto a prepared PASG. The top of the PASG should be just below the lower border of the costal margin.
3. Any potentially harmful objects must be removed from the patient's pockets.
4. The left leg of the PASG is wrapped around the patient's left leg and secured with the Velcro straps.
5. The right leg of the PASG is wrapped around the patient's right leg and secured with the Velcro straps.
6. The abdominal compartment (if it is to be used) is fitted and secured with the Velcro straps.
7. The air tubes are connected and the stopcocks appropriately set ("open").

The fitted PASG is shown in Figure 29.11.

Inflation

Before inflating the PASG, the patient's vital signs must be checked. The leg compartments are inflated first – if possible, equality of pressure is maintained in each compartment.

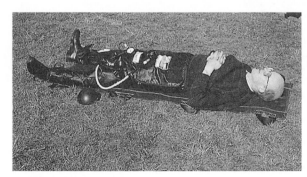

Figure 29.11 Patient in a PASG

Inflation should stop when the patient's radial pulses have returned (see Chapter 22); at this point the stopcocks are closed. It is important to remember that the PASG is inflated according to the presence of radial pulses, *not* according to the pressure reading of the garment.

The patient's vital signs should be continuously monitored and the pressure adjusted accordingly. Safety pressure valves are incorporated in the compartments of the garment. Finally, the peripheral pulses are checked.

Deflation

Deflation must not be attempted by inexperienced staff

Deflation of the PASG must only take place when definitive surgical facilities for the control of haemorrhage are available; this is most likely to be in the operating theatre although it may be in the A&E department.

1. Before deflation is attempted, one or two large-bore intravenous cannulae must be in place and adequate venous access established.
2. The vital signs must be continuously monitored.
3. The abdominal segment is deflated first; only when it is completely deflated can the deflation of the leg compartments begin.
4. The pressure must be reduced slowly and monitored continually. If the patient's blood pressure falls by 5–10 mmHg, deflation must be stopped and fluid given whilst being prepared to reinflate the PASG.
5. It is essential to be prepared for rapid surgical intervention.
6. Deflation may take 20 minutes at least.

Complications

Complications of PASG use are:

- extreme hypotension, possibly irreversible, if the garment is inappropriately removed
- a possible association with ischaemic compartment syndrome, tissue damage, metabolic acidosis and respiratory embarrassment
- exacerbation of:
  cardiac/thoracic vascular bleeding
  pulmonary oedema
  congestive cardiac failure.

In most cases, prehospital personnel do not have the necessary experience for its safe use, and the complexity of its application, as well as the problems associated with its removal, mean that its use is contraindicated. Inflation of the abdominal compartment alone has been used successfully in the reduction of bleeding from unstable pelvic fractures.

CERVICAL SPINE IMMOBILIZATION

Cervical spine immobilization may be achieved manually with or without the additional use of a cervical collar. For full immobilization the patient should be firmly strapped with neck blocks to a long board or similar device.

MANUAL METHODS

Whenever the accident scene or the nature of the injuries suggests the potential for cervical spine damage, as the airway is opened or protected, the cervical spine should be immobilized manually. This can be achieved from behind, from the side or from in front of the patient.

Behind the patient

From behind the patient, the rescuer's palms are placed behind the patient's ears. The little fingers should lie just under the angle of the jaw and the thumbs should be extended upwards behind the posterior aspect of the skull. The rescuer's hands should be adjusted so that the patient's ears lie between the fingers. It is important not to cover the ears: the last thing an anxious patient needs is to be rendered deaf as well!

If the head is not in a neutral position, it should be moved slowly and gently into a neutral position. If resistance is felt during this procedure the patient should be managed in the position in which he has been found.

Having reached a supported neutral position, the neck is held until the patient is secured to a short or long spine board (Figure 29.12). Traction is *not* applied. The rescuer should move into a comfortable braced position in order to support his own arms to prevent them from becoming tired.

> **Never apply traction to a cervical spine**

Side

One hand should be placed behind the patient's head so the occiput lies in its palm. The other hand should support the jaw between the thumb and second finger. The two hands now hold the neck in a similar way to a cervical collar. The head can be moved into a neutral position. The anterior arm should be braced against the patient's sternum (Figure 29.13).

Front

The rescuer's hands are placed over the patient's cheeks so that the fingers pass around the neck and the extended thumbs lie just in front of the ears over the temporomandibular joint. The head may be moved into a neutral position. The anterior arm should be braced against the patient's sternum (Figure 29.14).

CERVICAL COLLARS

A number of different types of cervical collar are available. Some are "one piece" and require a range of sizes to be carried

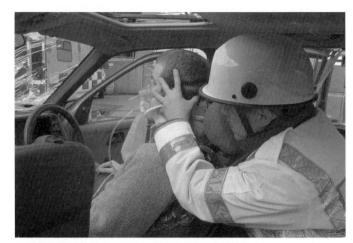

Figure 29.12 Manual immobilization from behind

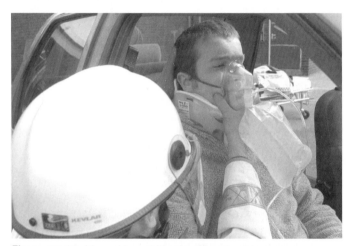

Figure 29.13 Manual immobilization from the side

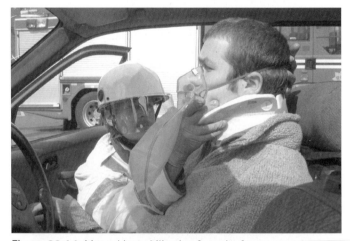

Figure 29.14 Manual immobilization from the front

(for example, the Stiffneck collar; Figure 29.15); others come in one piece but are adjustable (Figure 29.16). Occasionally, although increasingly rarely, two-piece collars are seen (Figure 29.17).

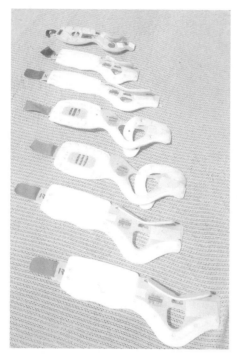

Figure 29.15 A range of Stiffneck© semi-rigid collars

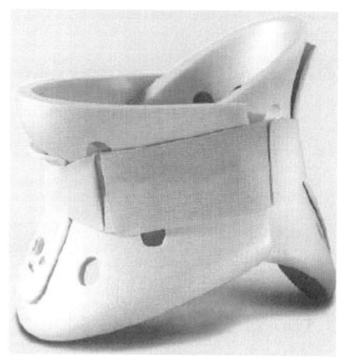

Figure 29.17 A two-piece cervical collar

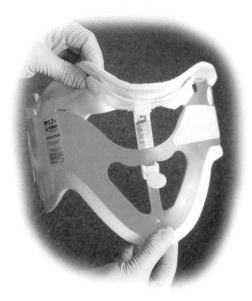

Figure 29.16 An adjustable one-piece collar

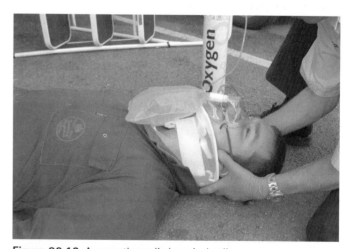

Figure 29.18 A correctly applied cervical collar

The collars have to be sized according to the manufacturer's instructions and then applied correctly while maintaining manual immobilization. *Collars do not completely immobilize the cervical spine* and it is essential to continue manual immobilization until this is replaced by a short spine board or long spine board and head immobilizer. It is of little use merely to hold on to the collar: the hands have to support the head and should be placed *above* the collar. A correctly applied collar is shown in Figure 29.18.

A correctly sized collar will reduce flexion and extension and to lesser extent sideways movement, but will not stop rotation – it is rotation that the rescuer's hands or headblock and tape will prevent. Access to the airway and trachea is available at all times through the gap in the front of the collar.

There is research evidence to suggest that the application of a cervical collar, even when correctly sized, will cause a rise in intracranial pressure (through venous compression), but from a practical viewpoint it is accepted that a correctly fitting cervical collar should be used in the prehospital setting when the situation suggests a cervical spine injury.

There has recently been a position statement from the Royal College of Surgeons which sets out the management of the cervical spine as well as the thoracic and lumbar spine.

Patients who are unconscious should have their cervical spine protected and be fully immobilized. However, patients who are conscious should be carefully assessed to include:

- consideration of the mechanism of injury
- the presence of drugs or alcohol
- a long bone injury or other distracting injury
- the presence of midline cervical spine tenderness.

The presence of any of these features following an accident with possible cervical spine injury should mandate full immobilization.

Similarly patients who complain of pain and are reluctant to move their neck of their own volition should receive full immobilization. A large study in Quebec has attempted to develop a protocol for the application of cervical spine immobilization. If followed carefully, these protocols will ensure that those patients at risk will receive cervical spine immobilization whilst those patients who do not require any form of cervical spine immobilization will be spared the potential dangers of raised intracranial pressure and transportation on a long board with its associated hazards.

Correct scene and patient assessment will ensure the correct management of the cervical spine.

LOG ROLL TECHNIQUE

Log rolling is a method of turning patients either to inspect their backs or to help put them on to a long spinal board. To log roll a patient, there should be a minimum of four people but more can be utilized if available. The patient should lie with his arms by his sides and the palms placed against the legs. Alternatively the patient can place his arms in a crossed position on his chest (Figure 29.19).

The object is to keep the whole spine in alignment and to achieve this, the cervical spine is stabilized and the patient moved with the neck, shoulders and pelvis kept in the same plane.

One person takes the head and this person controls the manoeuvre. The next person grips the patient's shoulder on the opposite side and also the further arm. The third person grips the pelvis, and the fourth person controls the legs. The person at the head calls the instructions and the whole body is rolled over, keeping the spine from twisting. The roll should be only as far as is needed to inspect the back or insert a long board underneath the patient (Figure 29.20).

A fifth person should examine the patient's back and perform any necessary treatment (for example, dressing a bleeding wound).

The patient is then rolled back into the supine position, again controlled by the person controlling the head and neck. The person at the head should inform his colleagues what command will be given before the manoeuvre begins: *"I will say one, two, three, move. Everybody ready? Good. One, two …"*.

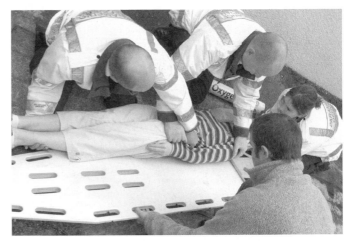

Figure 29.19 Initial position for the log roll

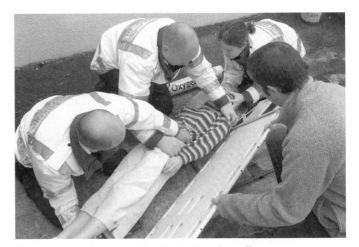

Figure 29.20 Patient on his side during a log roll

SCOOP STRETCHER

The scoop stretcher provides a means of lifting a patient onto a trolley or ambulance cot with minimal movement. The scoop stretcher can be split in half longitudinally and may have a head cushion. The bottom half can be extended to fit the patient (Figure 29.21).

The scoop should be laid beside the patient and extended to the required length. The patient should be told what is about to happen. The halves are then slid underneath the patient's body from the sides, taking care not to pinch the body as the halves are brought together. The patient may have to be rolled slightly to allow each half stretcher to be slid underneath.

Once the stretcher is in place and the halves are locked together, the head cushion is secured and the patient is lifted onto the trolley or cot. The distance that the stretcher has to be carried should be kept to a minimum and if rough ground or stairs have to be negotiated, restraining straps can be used to increase the patient's security (Figure 29.22).

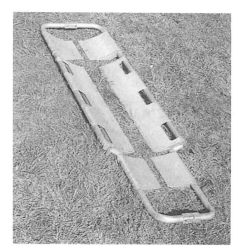

Figure 29.21 The scoop stretcher

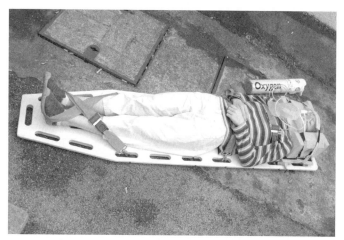

Figure 29.23 A long spinal board with headblocks

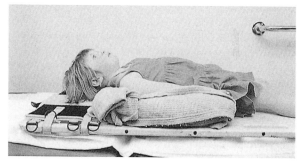

Figure 29.24 Padding under a child's shoulders on a long spinal board

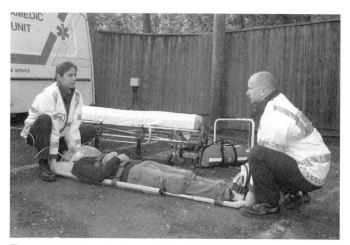

Figure 29.22 A patient secured to a scoop stretcher

A spinal board is a much better device for carrying a patient downstairs.

Once the patient is on the trolley, the scoop stretcher should be removed to prevent pressure sores developing, unless the transfer time is short and the removal of the stretcher would delay definitive treatment.

Recently a new design of a scoop stretcher has evolved. Known as a "Combi-board", this has attempted to combine the scoop and long board. The new board splits diagonally. It is shorter than a long board and, unlike a scoop, cannot be extended. Its place in prehospital care has yet to be determined.

SPINAL BOARDS

Spinal boards are used to assist in the movement (extrication) of casualties from an accident scene (Figure 29.23). They provide a secure and stable base onto which a patient may be strapped, so providing full spinal immobilization.

Despite the recent concern that patients may develop pressure sores from prolonged use of a spinal board, such boards are still the best form of protection in prehospital care. The vacuum mattress (perhaps used in conjunction with a spinal board) provides an alternative.

A spinal board may be used to secure and move a person who is on the ground, to assist in controlled extrication or, if time is a critical factor, to rapidly extricate a patient from a vehicle.

The use of a long board requires many hands and everyone must be aware of his role because teamwork is all-important. Before using a long board, the method of log rolling a patient must be understood (see above).

LONG BOARD

A patient may be rolled onto a long board or lifted onto a board using a scoop stretcher. Depending on the situation of the patient, a cervical collar may be applied before or after placing the patient on the board. Either way, manual in-line cervical stabilization will be required until the patient is secured to the board.

The head should be supported in a head immobilizer ("headbox"). The straps on the board are applied according to the manufacturer's instructions (Figure 29.23).

If a child is placed on a long board, because of the relatively larger size of the child's head, a pad may be required below the shoulders to prevent any forward flexion of the neck (Figure 29.24). Some paediatric boards are formed so as to accommodate the larger occiput of the child.

However, it is perfectly possible to use an adult board in the prehospital environment to prevent the ambulance having to carry a further piece of equipment. In this situation several blanket rolls will be required to secure the child comfortably on the board.

Extrication

Access to a patient in a vehicle is obtained either by springing the front door or by removing the roof of the vehicle.

If the roof of the car has been removed, the long board can be slid behind the patient. If the patient is in a front seat, the seat can be reclined as the patient is slid onto the long board and lifted clear. If it is impossible to remove the roof, the front door must be forced open. One person maintains in-line cervical stabilization from the back seat; a second person will apply a cervical collar from the side, while the third brings the long board, which is placed on the seat under the patient (Figure 29.25). When room is limited, the long board should not be put under the patient until later in the procedure. Unless a "snatch" rescue is necessary, a brief assessment should be performed.

The patient's feet and legs are then freed. The first rescuer maintains manual in-line cervical stabilization, while the third rescuer should be beside the patient in the front of the car, ready to lift the patient's legs across the unoccupied front seat. The second rescuer assumes the command of all movements, placing one hand on the patient's midthoracic spine and the other hand on the sternum.

The second rescuer uses both hands to sense any twisting of the patient's spine, and directs the movement of the patient. The legs are swung onto the seat so that the patient's back faces the open door; this movement should be done in short steps. Depending on the position of the first rescuer, another may have to control the patient's neck while the first rescuer negotiates the doorpost.

Once the patient is sitting across the front seat, the long board (if not already in place) is pushed onto the seat, and then elevated to meet the patient's back. The patient and the board should then be lowered together, ideally onto a waiting ambulance trolley. The patient is then slid in small movements up the board.

As the patient is slid up the board, rescuer 1 maintains in-line cervical stabilization, rescuer 2's hands are placed in the

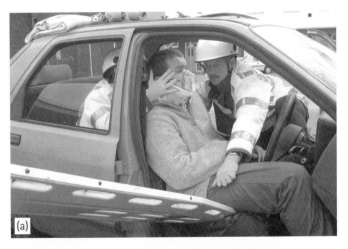

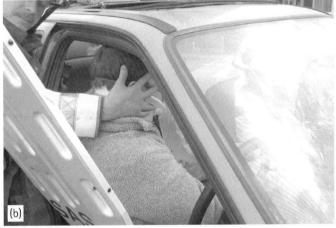

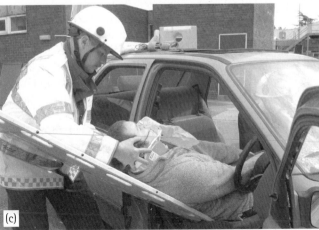

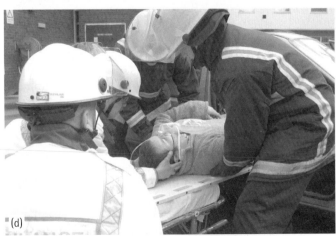

Figure 29.25 Extrication using a long spinal board

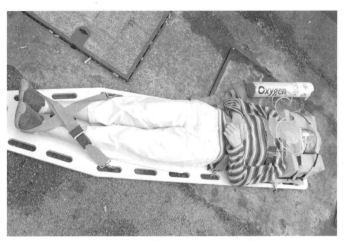

Figure 29.26 A patient secured to a long spinal board

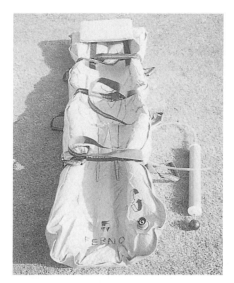

Figure 29.27 A vacuum mattress

patient's armpits and the third rescuer steadies the hips, pelvis and legs. Once the patient is on the long board he can be carried away from any danger and appropriate resuscitation started, during which time the patient will be properly stabilized on the long board.

All straps should be applied *before* the head immobilizer is fitted to avoid a moving patient "hinging" at the neck. Apply two straps across the thorax, extending over the clavicles and crossing to the opposite pelvic crest. Ensure strap buckles do not rest on the clavicles. Attach a third strap across the pelvis, and a fourth in a figure of eight from the proximal tibia and around the ankles. Ensure a close fit when applying head blocks, and apply the forehead strap first, tightening both sides together to limit rotational forces. The chin strap should be applied over the point of the chin and collar, never under the chin, to avoid obstructing the airway (Figure 29.26).

VACUUM SPLINTS

Vacuum splints provide rigid support to the body and can be very comfortable. They are bags of polystyrene beads enclosed in tough plastic. The injured limb or the whole patient can be placed onto the splint, which is actively moulded around the injured part. Suction is then applied to the bag, creating a vacuum: the contents take up a rigid form, supporting and splinting the injury.

Vacuum splints can be used to immobilize:

- limbs (upper or lower)
- the cervical spine, in conjugation with a semi-rigid collar
- other spinal injuries.

The whole-body splint (or vacuum mattress; Figure 29.27) should be laid onto the trolley and the patient is laid onto the mattress, which is secured around the patient's body using Velcro straps or a continuous webbing strap. The mattress is actively moulded around the patient. Care must be taken to ensure the vacuum mattress is smooth and flat

before positioning the patient, and then to support the head as the mattress is moulded around the neck and side of the head. A vacuum is then created inside the mattress using the suction pump provided. The mattress will conform to the patient's shape and provide whole-body support. Finally, the valve mechanism is secured and the pump removed. The splint can be removed by opening the valve and allowing air back into the mattress.

A vacuum mattress is a good immobilization device but a poor lifting device. It is important therefore to place a long spinal board or scoop stretcher under the vacuum mattress if the patient is to be lifted or carried any distance.

STRETCHERS

The scoop or orthopaedic stretcher has already been described.

Sometimes it is appropriate to use a canvas that can be slipped under the patient's body. The canvas can then be lifted in hospital using poles and spreader bars.

Other forms of stretchers which can be used in rescue situations are the Neil Robertson and Paraguard stretchers.

NEIL ROBERTSON STRETCHER

The Neil Robertson stretcher is constructed in canvas with wood slats sewn into the canvas (Figures 29.28, 29.29). It has side straps to fasten the stretcher around the patient's body and rope handles at the head, bottom and sides to help lower or raise the stretcher. The person is placed on the stretcher which is then fastened round the body, securing the feet and head to the stretcher. The stretcher can either be carried using the side handles or poles can be passed through the handles so it can be carried end-to-end.

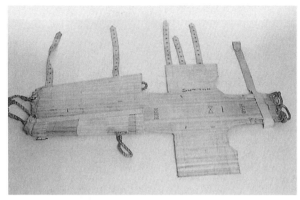

Figure 29.28 The Neil Robertson stretcher

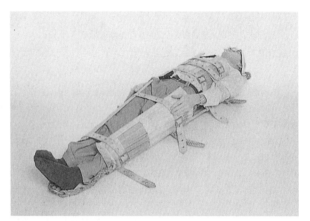

Figure 29.29 Patient in a Neil Robertson stretcher

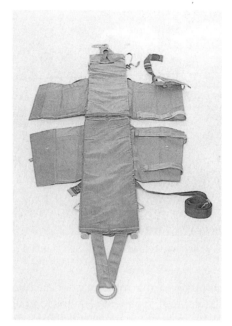

Figure 29.30 The Paraguard stretcher

PARAGUARD STRETCHER

Although the Paraguard stretcher is similar to the Neil Robertson stretcher, there are some significant differences. The Paraguard has a hinge in the middle and can, even with a patient fixed on the stretcher, be bent around obstacles. It has approved lifting points and can be used for helicopter rescue (Figures 29.30, 29.31).

When unpacked, the Paraguard stretcher should be folded straight and the hinge secured with the metal sleeves. The patient is laid on the stretcher and the corset fitted and secured with the straps. The ankle hitch and head restraints are secured.

Once the patient is firmly strapped onto the stretcher it may be moved horizontally or vertically.

EXTRICATION DEVICES

There are a number of different types of extrication device available. In current use are the Kendrick Extrication Device (KED) (Figure 29.32), the Russell Extrication Device (RED) (Figure 29.33) and the ED2000. These have replaced the short wooden board, which was always difficult to use and became increasingly so as car seats became shaped.

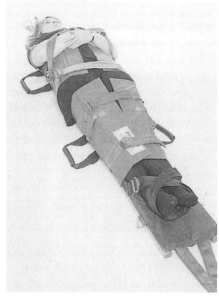

Figure 29.31 A patient in a Paraguard stretcher

These devices have a similar method of application, but each has its own characteristics. It is important for the practitioner to be familiar with the model which he will be using.

The devices are to an extent flexible and can therefore be slipped between the patient and the car seat. Once applied, they offer some protection to the spine and allow the patient to be lifted from the vehicle onto a trolley or other device.

The patient must first be assessed, and the cervical spine immobilized manually and with a cervical collar. The extrication device can then be slipped down behind the patient, making sure the various straps do not become caught on any object. While this is being done the cervical

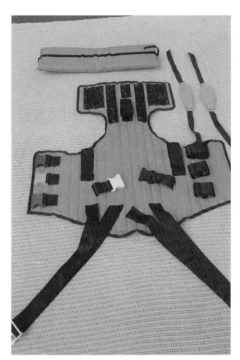

Figure 29.32 The Kendrick Extrication Device (KED)

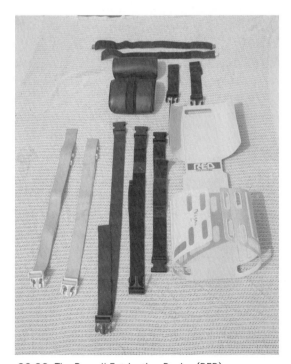

Figure 29.33 The Russell Extrication Device (RED)

spine is immobilized both with a collar and manually. The device is then positioned correctly in relation to the patient's head and shoulders (Figure 29.34).

The wings of the device forming the chest sides are drawn together with the chest straps, which are then tightened, in the sequence upper, bottom, middle, ensuring that this produces no respiratory embarrassment or pain. The leg straps are passed under the patient's legs and then fitted back onto the device. These straps are tightened.

The shoulder straps are placed across the body and fixed to the opposite side of the device; they must not overlap the cervical collar (Figure 29.35). The head straps are applied after making sure that any space behind the head is filled in with the padding supplied. These straps will hold the head and cervical spine firmly and the person who has been immobilizing the cervical spine can now let go. All straps are checked for tightness and adjusted so they are even (Figure 29.36).

The patient can now be lifted out of the vehicle using a long spine board and placed on a trolley. The leg straps must be loosened to allow the legs to extend.

PRINCIPLES OF EXTRICATION

Entrapment is relatively common in high-speed road traffic accidents, but can also be encountered in industrial, recreational, aircraft, train, farming or domestic incidents. In dealing with the trapped patient, the prehospital worker's role is vital. The time-specific response cannot be applied when casualties are trapped but the concept of the "golden hour" is still important. Therefore the medical priorities must be sorted out at a very early stage.

It is important that early consultation takes place between all the emergency services working at the scene in order to establish the priorities. It must be appreciated that this involvement should include the hospital staff – first to alert them of the prehospital problem, so that they may be prepared, and second to seek their help if extra equipment or skills are required. If a patient is not trapped and the environment is hazardous then a snatch rescue may be needed, with minimal intervention under ABC. Life-threatening airway, cervical spine and breathing problems must be managed before transfer to the ambulance along with control of significant external haemorrhage. All other interventions should be carried out en route to hospital.

Patients with time-critical problems who are not trapped should be in the ambulance within 10 minutes of the paramedic's arrival. However, life-saving interventions (for example oxygen administration, needle thoracocentesis) should be performed prior to extrication where indicated. Whilst extrication for these patients must be rapid, manual in-line stabilization of the cervical spine must be maintained and a cervical collar fitted. Since the requirement for speed mandates against the fire service cutting off the roof of the car, the patient should be extricated using a long spine board through the adjacent vehicle doorway. Similarly, time does not permit the use of an extrication device (for example the KED) for these time-critical patients.

It must be recognized that if casualties are trapped and have time-critical injuries they may die before being rescued,

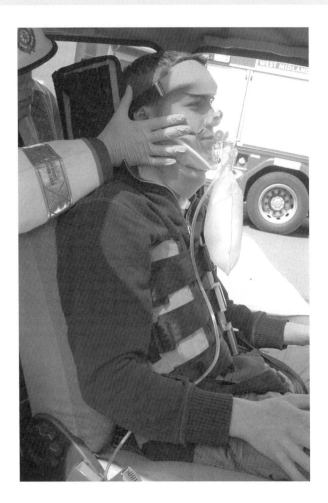

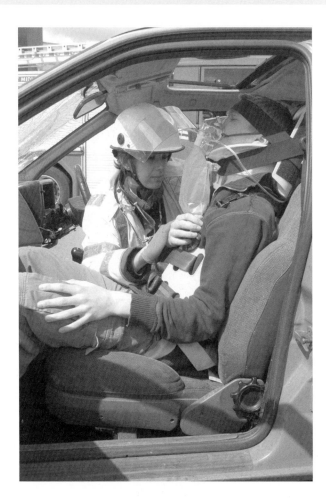

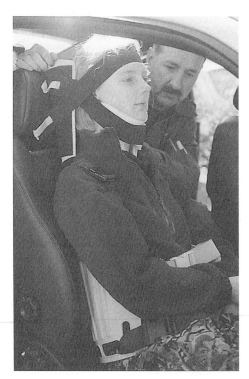

Figure 29.34 An extrication device being used

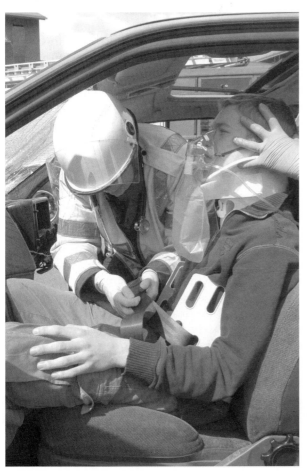

Figure 29.35 Fastening the shoulder straps

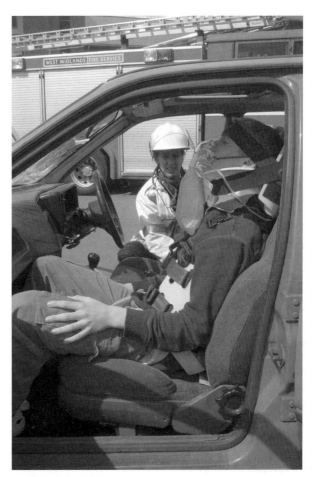

Figure 29.36 Adjusting the straps

simply because of the technical difficulties involved in the extrication.

DEFINITIONS

Entrapment itself may be:

- actual
- relative.

Actual entrapment

Actual entrapment occurs when the victim is physically enclosed or held in a vehicle or area by the structure impinging on his body – for example, a deformed vehicle following an RTA, a roof fall following a mining or caving accident or building collapse following an explosion or bomb blast where rocks or masonry may be lying on the patient.

Relative entrapment

Relative entrapment occurs when the victim needs help because of his location, the environment or physical injury.

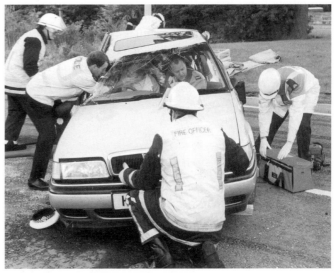

Figure 29.37 Rescue of an entrapped patient

For example, a traffic accident victim may have a fractured humerus. It is the pain that immobilizes the patient as well as the fracture. If a few minutes are spent on relatively simple splinting to immobilize the fracture or the provision of appropriate analgesia, then the patient may be able to escape from the vehicle with minimal assistance.

In other examples injuries, such as a broken ankle, may prevent accident victims climbing out of a cave or up a cliff. The rescue team may have to use devices such as coastguard equipment or helicopters as an aerial crane or elevator, rather than sophisticated medical equipment. Once the rescue has been achieved it may be necessary to release the helicopter for other work and use road ambulances for the hospital transfer. A non-time-critical patient in an RTA with a suspected spine injury is relatively entrapped, since removal of the roof of the vehicle is mandatory to application of an extrication device and for longitudinal movement of the victim onto a long spine board placed behind them.

MANAGEMENT

The basic prehospital approach of primary survey, resuscitation and stabilization is even more important when dealing with the trapped patient. The ABC principles apply and continuing reassessments will be required during the rescue. With a trapped patient, problems created by a missed critical injury cannot always be retrieved by early evacuation to hospital.

Preparation

Preparation includes training and a knowledge of the rescue teams and other services. It is essential to know the equipment they carry and their potential skills and benefits.

The paramedic's own equipment must be checked and kept up to date. The function of all equipment needs to be known. There is nothing worse than having equipment that one does not know how to use or finding that equipment is incomplete or faulty after struggling to reach the accident scene.

Teamwork

Each professional group must recognize their own limitations. The ambulance crew or the immediate care doctor will have some basic rescue equipment. If power-operated tools are required then this part of the rescue should be left to the specialists (the fire service). Equally, these specialists should have a clear understanding of what the medical priorities are. That may mean giving early access to the paramedic to allow stabilization of the casualty. The paramedics can then concentrate on controlling the cervical spine during the rescue and monitoring the patient including ECG, pulse oximetry and non-invasive blood pressure monitoring, as well as directing the movement of the patient onto a spine board.

Clothing

Entrapments can be dangerous to the rescue worker and therefore proper clothing should be worn. This should include a helmet and robust footwear that gives protection from sharp metal and glass. Latex rubber or plastic gloves may be easily breached at the scene of the accident because of the many sharp objects and edges found there and once breached, will no longer protect the rescuer or the casualty from disease. Despite the difficulties, hand and eye protection are needed to prevent the potential spread of disease.

Safety

Any entrapment scenario will have its associated dangers. Road traffic accidents, for example, are associated with the dangers of moving vehicles whose drivers are not concentrating on their driving owing to a morbid interest in the accident scene. Industrial accidents may well involve unfamiliar machinery or chemicals. In domestic entrapments risks from falling debris, electricity or gas may be present. The movement and actions of fellow rescue personnel and their associated equipment must not be ignored as a potential cause of additional injury.

> **Always think safety**

Assessment

Assessment begins by looking at the scene and looking at the forces of violence and understanding the energy exchange which took place. At the same time the number of casualties involved can be identified. Each casualty's priority should be assessed according to ABC criteria. This may be facilitated by asking other rescue workers with first aid training to help check that every casualty is breathing. Usually the fire service has plenty of personnel at the scene who can see that each casualty has an open airway and is breathing (see Chapter 6). This frees the medical workers to perform practical procedures and helps to identify the critical problems.

The assessment of the individual casualty involves talking to the person, examining him for injuries and assessing the wreckage. At this stage the identification of actual or relative entrapment can be made. The casualty must be protected not only from the dangers found within the accident scene but also from the effects of the environment, for example from broken glass, fire or noxious fumes. It should be remembered that casualties will not be able to escape if they are still entrapped (whether relatively or actually). The stability of the vehicle or structures such as a building roof is also assessed at this stage. The specialist services should help in stabilizing or gaining access to the area.

Once these early stages of assessment have been completed the patient's ABC can be assessed, followed by D and then E. Significant fractures are often identified under E. Team discussions can take place on how best to tackle the extrication, allowing for the additional hazards that the environment may pose.

Monitoring

Continual monitoring is essential and must be performed by the ambulance crew who will be close to the patient. The use of monitoring equipment with electronic readouts must not encourage patient monitoring at a distance whilst other aspects of the rescue continue. Electronic blood pressure monitoring, electrocardiography and pulse oximetry are useful, but none of these replaces clinical observation.

Entrapment scenes are often noisy and electronic equipment can be used without requiring shutdown of the rescue field. Chest auscultation or assessment is almost impossible, so rescue field shutdown is required to enable this procedure to be completed. When there is relative silence, it is important to take the opportunity to check the whole patient. The fire service will always help but they should not be expected to stop the rescue unnecessarily or more frequently than is needed.

In a hostile environment a rapid extrication may be necessary. There is little point in unprotected paramedics entering smoky or fume-filled environments such as a coal mine or ship's cargo hold. Their own survival would be put at risk and it would not be possible to treat the casualties. Rescue should be left to specialist crews in protective clothing. In the first instance rapid extrication from a hostile environment is all that can be achieved.

Planning

Dealing with an entrapped patient may take several hours. Early decisions should be made about the method of transportation. If the casualty is going to be trapped for 1–2 hours then the "golden hour" will be exceeded by the time hospital is reached. If road transport is likely to take some time, air evacuation by helicopter or other means should be considered and requested early.

SNATCH RESCUE

Snatch rescue is the retrieval of the casualty from a difficult environment with minimal stabilization and resuscitation until a place of safety is reached. An example is a person who is drowning in the sea. The coastguard or lifeboat service will have to rescue the person before they can protect the airway. Fires and chemical accidents are further examples.

Similar problems occur in mountain and cave rescue and other situations where access is difficult. Because of the location only a minimum of first aid equipment can be carried to the scene of the rescue.

In civil disturbance or terrorist situations the rescue workers may be under hostile fire. Both rescuers and casualties are at risk. In these situations the airway and cervical spine protection, breathing and circulation management must be restricted to the basics, safety of all personnel being paramount. Once the casualty is retrieved to a safer area then the primary survey can be repeated and more advanced ABC techniques used if necessary.

Working with a trapped casualty is one of the most challenging and difficult areas for prehospital personnel: it is noisy, dangerous and difficult and is not without risk to the rescue worker. Strong team bonds are formed in such rescue situations.

RESOURCES

Ambulance service

The ambulance service has a full range of prehospital clinical care equipment, communications systems, including telemetry, and paramedic staff. Their vehicles include single stretcher ambulances, four wheel drive vehicles, sitting ambulances and in some parts of the country helicopter support.

Recently the responsibility for the decontamination of injured casualties has passed to the ambulance service.

Police

The police are experienced in scene management, traffic control, escorting ambulances from the scene and sometimes escorting special equipment or staff to the scene. They have special responsibility for victims who have been pronounced dead. They also have a responsibility to investigate any criminal activity associated with the incident. They have a duty to protect property.

Fire service

The fire service are experienced in scene management, heavy and light rescue and are able to supply large numbers of staff, often for long periods if required. They have a special responsibility for chemical and radiation incidents and the safety of such scenes. Each fire service has special rescue units including rock rescue, RTA rescue and radiation and chemical decontamination units. A selection of fire service rescue equipment is shown in Figure 29.38.

Medical immediate care schemes

Immediate care doctors are experienced in trauma and medical care and can provide rapid assistance to the ambulance technician or paramedic. In entrapments, this is most likely to take the form of the provision of additional analgesia or anaesthesia prior to extrication, although on rare occasions amputation may be necessary.

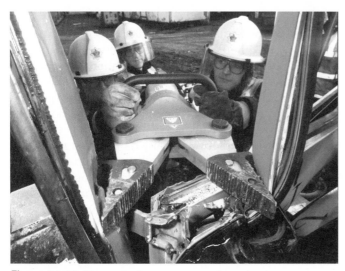 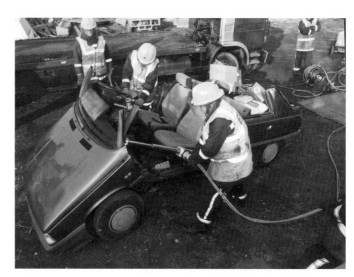

Figure 29.38 Fire service heavy rescue equipment

CONCLUSION

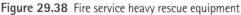

"Casualty packaging" is an art that requires an understanding of injury patterns, a knowledge of equipment and, above all, teamwork. The removal of the injured person from the accident scene is an often unplanned and almost forgotten part of the rescue.

There can be no argument about the necessity to perform a rapid primary survey before attempting immobilization and the removal of the patient from the scene. Only if a snatch rescue is needed should this principle be altered.

Some methods of immobilization may appear cumbersome and in retrospect (when the casualty's injuries are known) may be regarded as unnecessary, but the paramedic has a duty to prevent *potential* injuries. This does not mean that the paramedic must be obsessive about techniques and manoeuvres to the extent of losing sight of the patient's needs and the necessity to reach hospital quickly.

Prehospital care is a rapidly changing, specialist area and each new technique must be evaluated carefully. All too often techniques may be introduced which have not been fully assessed and for which there may be little objective evidence of resulting improvement in the welfare of patients.

Chapter 30

Blast and gunshot injuries

INTRODUCTION

Trauma caused by bomb blast and gunshot is an increasing problem in all developed societies (Figure 30.1) Paramedics, particularly those working in large urban areas, can expect to manage such patients from time to time. However, it is important to place the injuries caused in context and to re-assure medical attendants. Perhaps the most important state-ment to be made is that victims should be medically managed in the same way as other trauma patients – that is a period of initial assessment and resuscitation and then transport to hospital. The general approach of primary sur-vey, resuscitation, limited secondary survey and transport to hospital is not altered because of the nature of injury. However, there are other aspects of shootings and bomb blasts which must be noted. The first is the element of dan-ger for paramedic personnel, particularly following a bomb blast. These incidents are controlled by the security services and approach by medical personnel to victims will be restricted and may be delayed until the area is secure.

There are a number of basic rules governing behaviour which must be followed.

- Do not become a casualty yourself. Do not approach the scene until it has been declared safe – risks of secondary explosions, fire and building collapse are high.
- Do not disturb or remove objects found in the environment – they may have forensic or other non-medical implications.

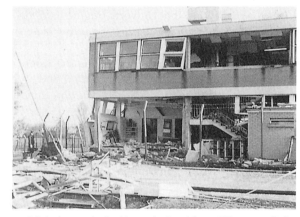

Figure 30.1 A terrorist incident: the bombing of Musgrave Park Hospital, Belfast, in 1991

- Do not disturb obviously dead victims or move body parts.
- If there are multiple victims, triage will be necessary so that those most in need are identified, assessed and resuscitated first. This will normally be coordinated by an ambulance incident officer (in liaison with a medical incident officer) (see Chapter 58).
- Care for multiple victims involves teamwork and it may be necessary to summon medical teams to the site – particularly if entrapment of victims is a feature.

Blast and gunshot injuries are discussed separately in this chapter, although the victims have much in common, both in the nature of their injuries and in their management needs.

PHYSICAL EFFECTS OF BLAST

Explosives when detonated produce large quantities of gas at very high pressure. At the moment of detonation the explosive substance undergoes compression and chemical decomposition into gaseous products at very high temperature and pressure. A resulting front of high pressure or *shock wave* is formed which is characterized by an instantaneous rise to a peak level. The shock wave then travels through the surrounding environment with a velocity greater than the speed of sound in air. It is the instantaneous rise to peak pressure and the supersonic velocity that distinguish a shock wave from an ordinary sound wave. As the shock wave or front moves away it declines in velocity (or decays) to ambient levels and then falls below ambient level for a short time, forming a negative pressure component which has little or no biological significance (Figure 30.2).

Behind the shock front is an area of turbulence defined as the dynamic pressure or *blast wind*. The forces generated by the blast wind can be considerable and have notable biological consequences. The effects of the two phenomena can be simply illustrated. If a shock wave passes through a building with glass windows, the glass will be broken by the shock wave; however, the dangerous showering of glass fragments is caused by the blast wind. Equally, when the shock front causes the collapse or disintegration of buildings, it is the blast wind that converts fragments of the collapsed structures into lethal missiles of varying size, shape and velocity.

The magnitude of an explosion, that is the extent and duration of overpressure and the pressure exerted by blast wind, is determined to a large degree by the type and quantity of explosive used. Another influencing factor is the environment – whether the explosion occurs in an open space or is confined inside a building. Other features of medical significance are the flash from the explosion, the risk of fires developing and the collapse of buildings.

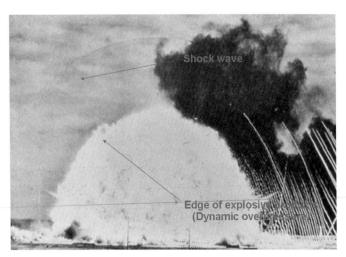

Figure 30.2 Pressure changes in a shock wave

BIOLOGICAL EFFECTS OF BLAST

PRIMARY EFFECTS

Primary effects result from exposure of the body to the overpressure associated with the shock wave. The most notable effects are in areas of the body where there are air–fluid interfaces. These include the ears, the lungs and the bowel.

The tympanic membrane or eardrum is very susceptible and injury is common. The extent varies from mild vascular congestion of the membrane to rupture with possible disruption of the ossicular chain leading to severe hearing loss. Ear injury is curiously unpredictable following an explosion – the victim's ear must be correctly oriented to the shock wave for significant blast loading to occur.

Injury to abdominal structures is uncommon in air blasts but is a particular feature of exposure to blast in water. Injuries range from mild contusion of bowel wall to areas of frank perforation with faecal spillage and subsequent peritonitis. It is possible that blast injury to bowel is more common than is realized and experimental work supports this view. However, injury appears to be mild in most cases of air exposure and is therefore of limited significance to the prehospital assessment and management.

The most significant clinical primary effect is contusion injury to the lungs, which may progress in some cases to "blast lung". The problem results from widespread pulmonary bruising with haemorrhage into the alveolar spaces – the "haemorrhagic contamination of lung" as described by some blast research scientists. The clinical consequence of this contusion injury is ineffective gas exchange with resultant hypoxia. In addition, the damaged lung continues to accumulate fluid for a period of upto 24–48 hours, leading to a progressive deterioration if appropriate treatment is not instituted. The clinical presentation in the prehospital setting is one of breathlessness; the victim may be in acute distress, refusing to lie down and using accessory muscles of respiration. There may be associated pneumothorax or haemothorax compounding the respiratory distress.

Blast lung is not common in survivors of terrorist explosions: the overall incidence is under 5% as severe blast lung in isolation is usually rapidly fatal at the scene and the proximity to the device is often associated with multiple fragmentation injuries that also result in death. The reason for

---

Box 30.1 Mechanisms of bomb injury

- Blast shock wave
- Blast wind
- Fragmentation
- Crush
- Burn
- Psychological

such a low incidence is clear – casualties close enough to an exploding terrorist device to develop blast lung will usually die from multiple hits by fragments.

An even rarer but striking feature of exposure to blast over-pressure is sudden death in individuals with no external signs of injury. This was noted and reported during the blitz on London in World War II. Possible explanations include coronary artery air embolization or cardiac arrhythmias.

SECONDARY EFFECTS

The most common serious clinical problems facing para-medics after an explosion are the penetrating and non-penetrating injuries caused by fragments. These may arise from the casing of the exploding device, or from the environment, such as pieces of glass, masonry and wood propelled by the blast wind. Size, shape, type of material, velocity and terminal effectiveness vary enormously. Following a car bombing, vehicle parts are generated as fragments and typically produce severe and often lethal injury.

Unlike fragmentation injury in war, which is somewhat predictable, injury after a terrorist explosion is very variable. At one end of the spectrum, there are superficial injuries to exposed parts; at the other, multiple, irregular wounds across more than one body system. Widespread contamination by foreign bodies and mixed bacterial species is common to all.

The nature and extent of injuries will depend on many factors; the size of the charge, proximity to the device, the environment and its propensity to generate fragments all play a part. Ballistic aspects of penetrating injury are discussed in the section on gunshot wounds.

TERTIARY EFFECTS

Tertiary effects result from gross displacement of the body by the blast wind. The clinical consequences include trau-matic amputation and even complete body disintegration. Injury may also be caused by a body being thrown onto a hard or irregular surface. Finally, tertiary injury may result from building collapse caused by the blast winds.

BURN INJURY

Burns are common and may be caused by flash, flame or both. Flash burns occur at the moment of detonation and particularly affect exposed parts such as face, arms and legs. Although dramatic in appearance, injury tends to be superficial. However, frontal exposure to flash may lead to airway burn with critical consequences – early intubation must be considered in all these patients (see Chapter 6 and 7). Flame burn occurs if the surrounding environment ignites – patterns of injury, immediate man-agement and outlook are as for flame burns under normal circumstances.

PSYCHOLOGICAL INJURY

Over 40% of those involved in incidents such as terrorist explosions may expect to suffer some form of psychological distress in the aftermath period. For the majority of trained personnel, the outlook is very good, particularly if their efforts were successful in reducing morbidity and mortality. Debriefing and stress counselling may be helpful and is now mandatory for many emergency personnel after expos-ure to a stressful incident such as a bomb explosion.

WOUND BALLISTICS AND MECHANISMS OF INJURY

Before discussing gunshot wounds it is worth considering ballistic injury in general. The field is fraught with contro-versy, mainly because of disagreement among ballistic sci-entists, which need not concern paramedic personnel.

Wound ballistics is the study of injury caused by pene-trating ballistic missiles. The list of potential wounding agents is prodigious: Box 30.2 is far from complete.

Wounding missiles, irrespective of type, cause injury by penetrating the body and transferring energy to the tissue. Therefore the wounding capacity of a particular missile wound may be defined by:

- the degree of penetration into the body, resulting in laceration and crushing of tissues and structures in its path – the severity or

---

Box 30.2 Wounding missiles

Bullets
  Police handgun (many varieties)
  Military handgun
  Military assault rifle (5.56mm, 7.62mm)
  Hunting rifle (many varieties)
  Machine gun

Fragments
Primary:
  Natural (fragments from bomb casing, shells and mortars)
  Preformed (claymore mine, etched wire from hand grenades)
  Flechettes (individual darts preloaded into a cargo-carrying munition)

Secondary:
  Masonry
  Glass
  Wood
  Metal

Intrinsic:
Body parts – typically fragments of bone

clinical outcome will be determined by the nature of structures in its path: for example, laceration of soft tissue in a forearm will differ in outcome from the same degree of penetration and laceration in the liver or myocardium

- the capacity of the missile to cause injury to structures surrounding and remote from the missile track.

The degree of penetration of the missile will be determined by the mass, presenting area of the missile (fragments will usually be large, bullets small), impact velocity and the density of the tissues penetrated.

The capacity to produce remote injury will be determined initially by the efficiency of the missile in imparting kinetic energy (KE) to the tissue. The available KE can be calculated from the formula:

$$KE = 1/2\ MV^2$$

where M is the mass of the missile and V its velocity. There is a critical difference between the *available* KE and the *actual* amount imparted during the wounding. It is important to grasp this principle, as a high-velocity missile with considerable available KE may actually impart very little to the tissue during wounding. The factors that ultimately determine energy disposition or transfer include the impact velocity, tissue characteristics, wound track length and missile characteristics.

What should now be obvious is that it is foolhardy to approach any victim of missile injury with preconceived notions concerning wound severity. In particular, the older system of classifying wounds according to known or presumed missile velocity is now considered unsafe. Thus, it must not be assumed that high-velocity or low-velocity missiles produce high-velocity or low-velocity wounds – the terms are misleading and are best abandoned. Most clinicians and ballistic experts now use the terms "high-energy transfer" and "low-energy transfer" wounds (Figure 30.3) – the distinction can only be made by surgeons at surgical exploration. This means that medical personnel involved in assessment and resuscitation should be unconcerned by the niceties of wound ballistics – patients with missile wounds are managed in the same way as any other trauma victim: primary survey, resuscitation, limited secondary survey and transport to hospital. There is nothing magical or mystical about missile velocity or ballistic injury.

GUNSHOT INJURIES

In the UK, gunshot wounds are mainly caused by handguns and shotguns. Although patients are now being seen with wounds caused by bullets from military assault rifles and other military automatic weapons, these are still fortunately rare.

HANDGUNS

If there is no event history a gunshot wound may be missed and indeed, this has happened in the resuscitation area of

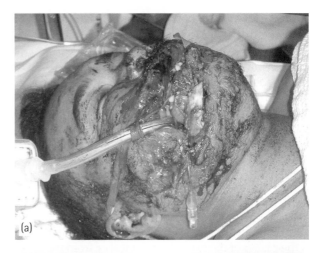

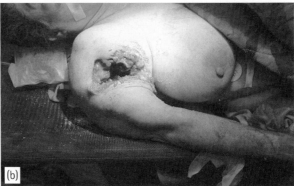

Figure 30.3 A high-energy transfer wounds from handguns (a) facial, (b) to right shoulder. (From Lt Col Hodgetts)

a large London hospital. The approach to assessment, resuscitation and decision making is as directed in earlier chapters. There are no special rules! Do not come to any decision concerning wound severity based on knowledge, actual or assumed, of the wounding missile or wound appearance. In general, bullet wound entry and exit wounds give very little information on the patient's condition. Assume serious injury in all cases and arrange rapid transfer to hospital.

Remember that bullets may travel an erratic and unpredictable path and may enter several body cavities. A careful primary survey should detect evidence of intrathoracic or abdominal penetration, which is a particularly ominous feature. Deal with thoracic and abdominal problems as directed in Chapters 25 and 26.

SHOTGUNS

Shotguns have a smooth bore and are designed to fire multiple pellets or shot; some fire large, solid lead or plastic slugs. Pellet size varies from large buckshot to small birdshot.

Wound severity varies enormously and depends on range, body region and size of shot. In general wounds tend to be extensive, with heavy foreign body contamination which may include the wadding from the shotgun cartridge. Assess and manage as for any form of trauma – external haemorrhage control may necessitate firm pressure over a large wounded area. The risk of local and systemic sepsis is particularly high. In the longer term, lead levels may need monitoring.

MILITARY WEAPONS

Assault rifles and automatic weapons are now readily available to criminals and terrorists. This need not unduly trouble prehospital personnel. Treat victims as described earlier. It would be sensible to presume anyone wounded by bullets from military weapons to have serious injury until proved otherwise.

FURTHER READING

Knight B 1991 Simpson's Forensic Medicine, 10th edn. Edward Arnold, London

Ryan JM 2000 Warfare injuries. In: Russell, Williams, Bulstrode (eds) Bailey and Love's short practice of surgery, 23rd edn. Arnold, London

Ryan JM, Rich NM, Dale RF, Morgans BT, Cooper GJ 1997 Ballistic trauma – clinical relevance in peace and war. Arnold, London

Chapter 31

Burns

INTRODUCTION

Burns are the third highest cause of deaths due to accidents. In 1988 in England and Wales 900 people died from fire and serious burns resulted in 15 000 admissions to hospital. Almost 150 000 patients present to accident and emergency departments in the UK with burns each year. Half of these patients will be children and two-thirds of these will be under 5, with scalds being more common in this age group.

ANATOMY OF THE SKIN

The cells of the epidermis come from the germinal layer; they gradually migrate upwards and the outer layer is shed continuously. The epidermis acts as a barrier against water, bacteria and external injurious substances as well as protecting against wear and tear. The dermis consists of strong connective tissue containing numerous nerve endings to provide sensation and the skin adnexa which include sweat glands, hair follicles and sebaceous glands. The functions of the skin are:

- protection from injury
- temperature control
- prevention of excess water loss
- detection of the nature of the immediate environment.

DEPTH OF BURNS

The anatomy of burn depth is shown in Figure 31.1.

Simple erythema

Simple erythema is a superficial burn with no skin loss, for example sunburn. The skin is red and tender; this heals in 5–10 days with no scarring.

Superficial partial-thickness burn

Blisters are thin walled and the burn is extremely painful. The skin is red and moist with a granular appearance and the germinal layer is not penetrated; an example is a scald from boiling water. Healing takes 10–20 days and there is minimal scarring.

Deep partial-thickness burn

A deep partial-thickness burn can be produced, for example, by boiling fat; it is deeper than the superficial partial-thickness

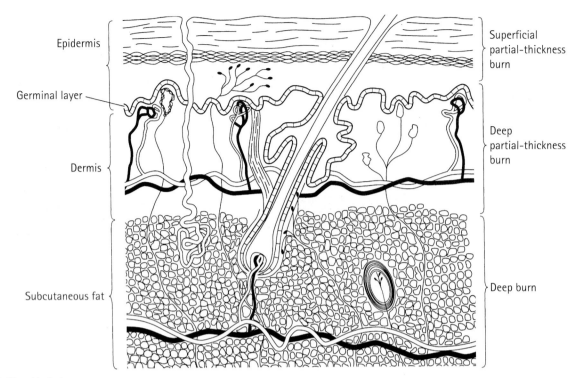

Figure 31.1 The skin in burns

burn and the blisters are thick walled. The underlying skin is granular and white in appearance, with pinpoint red mottling; sensation may be dulled. Healing is by migration of epithelial cells from the edge of the wound or skin adnexa, which takes 25–60 days.

Deep full-thickness burn

Full-thickness burns are caused by prolonged contact with the burning agent or dry heat. The appearance is white, leathery or charred. Although the areas of full-thickness burn are painless, the depth of the burn is usually shallower around its margins and these areas will be painful. This burn affects the full thickness of the skin and may extend further into fat, muscle or bone; it does not heal. Treatment includes tangential excision and either skin graft or free flap repair, depending on the depth.

FACTORS AFFECTING THE DEPTH OF THE BURN

TYPE OF BURNING AGENT

Wet heat

Wet heat is the most common burning agent, for example boiling water from a kettle; this produces a scald which is a superficial partial-thickness burn. Superheated steam may produce deep partial-thickness burns as the temperature is greater and large amounts of energy are released as the steam condenses.

Dry heat

Dry heat may be a flame burn or a contact burn, for example from hot tar. These are direct burns and are often deep. Flame burns are also often associated with inhalation and other injuries.

Flash burns

Flash burns are associated with explosions where the patient is subject to intense heat for a few seconds. These are usually partial-thickness burns and the patients commonly have other associated injuries.

Chemical burns

The severity of chemical burns depends upon the agent, the time of contact and the concentration. Some alkaline substances, such as wet cement, are highly corrosive and will continue to burn until completely removed. Acid burns usually produce less damage but will continue to burn if left on the skin. An exception to this is hydrofluoric acid which penetrates deeply and produces extensive tissue destruction and pain; these burns require treatment with calcium gluconate applied topically.

Electrical burns

See Chapter 43 on electrocution.

Radiation burns

The most common radiation burn is sunburn. Radiation burns may, very rarely, result from exposure to ionizing radiation.

DURATION OF EXPOSURE TO THE BURNING AGENT

As the time of exposure to the burning agent is increased, the severity of the burn increases.

PATHOPHYSIOLOGY OF BURNS

In a burn wound there are three zones:

- the zone of coagulation
- the zone of stasis
- the zone of hyperaemia.

The *zone of coagulation* is the central zone where cells have been destroyed by the thermal injury, producing an avascular area.

In the *zone of stasis* cells have been injured by the heat and should survive; however, they may die during the first 48 hours owing to associated vasoconstriction and microthrombus formation which reduce the blood supply.

In the *zone of hyperaemia* there is minimal thermal damage but marked vasodilation and an acute inflammatory response. Owing to vasodilation and changes in the blood vessel walls, large amounts of fluid leak from the surface of the burn. The amount of fluid loss is dependent on the extent of the burn. This fluid loss tends to occur over the first 36 hours after the burn injury and if the burn is large enough, this can result in hypovolaemia. Thus fluid replacement is vital in burn management and the type and the amount of fluid to be given are discussed below.

The pain from a burn is produced by the exposure of nerve endings in burnt skin as well as by inflammatory mediators.

Thermal damage to cells allows sodium to enter the injured cells, producing a serum sodium deficit. Dead red blood cells release haemoglobin and damaged muscle releases myoglobin. This, combined with hypovolaemia, can lead to renal impairment. If the burn injury is severe, cardiac output can drop owing to the metabolic effects of the burn on the myocardium. Cardiac output also decreases if the burn injury is extensive and there is a large fluid loss with no replacement. This leads to an increase in heart rate and peripheral vascular resistance to maintain blood pressure and coronary and cerebral blood flow. As a result there is a reduction in blood flow to peripheral tissues and the gut, which leads to bacterial transfer from the gut into the bloodstream, producing burn sepsis.

The patient's immune system is depressed following a burn, leading to an increased susceptibility to infection. Bacterial infection delays healing and can convert a partial-thickness burn into a full-thickness burn. Thus it is important to wear gloves when treating or moving a burns patient.

If a burn is extensive it is important to remember that the patient will lose heat rapidly and become hypothermic.

FACTORS AFFECTING THE OUTCOME OF BURNS

Factors affecting the outcome of burn injuries include the source and the depth of the burn – see above. Other factors are discussed below.

EXTENT OF BURN

It is important to assess the extent of the burn accurately. In most accident and emergency departments the Lund and Browder chart is used for the estimation of percentage burn (Figure 31.2). This chart takes into account the differences in body surface area between adults and children when assessing the extent of the burn, so that the volume of fluid lost can be calculated correctly when estimating fluid replacement. Other methods are the Wallace *rule of nines* for adults and the *rule of fives* for children and infants (Figure 31.3), and using the approximation that the patient's hand (flat with the fingers together) is equal to 1% of the patient's body surface area. This method is useful in assessing patchy burns present all over the body (Figure 31.4). The preferred method in the prehospital setting is serial halving. Ask "Does the patient have 100% burns?" If not, "Does the patient have 50% burns?" and so on until an estimation is reached that reflects total body surface area burnt (excluding erythema).

BURN SITE

Burns in certain areas of the body have a worse prognosis than others. Burn sites with a poor prognosis are:

- face
- hands and feet
- eyes
- ears
- perineum.

Burns to the hands and feet, especially deep or deep partial-thickness burns, can produce extensive scarring and disability. Any facial burns can produce scarring and are often associated with an inhalation injury. Burns to the ears and eyes can produce long-term problems. A burn to an eye can cause blindness, eyelid deformities or corneal scarring. Ear burns can lead to deformity and infection. Burns to the perineum are difficult to dress and are susceptible to infection.

CIRCUMFERENTIAL BURNS

If there is a circumferential burn to the neck this can cause airway obstruction. Circumferential burns to the limbs produce constriction, causing oedema and distal ischaemia.

NAME _____ WARD _____ NUMBER _____ DATE _____

AGE _____ ADMISSION WEIGHT _____

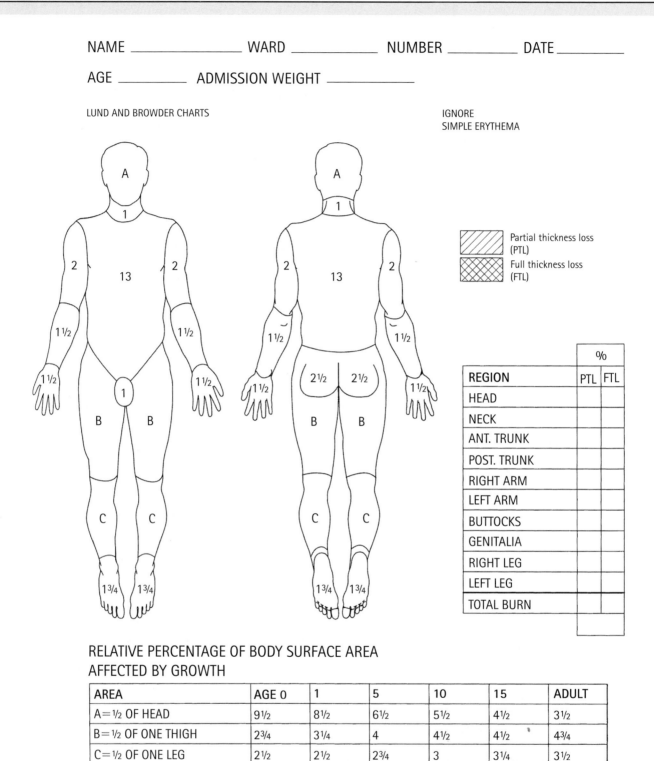

LUND AND BROWDER CHARTS

IGNORE
SIMPLE ERYTHEMA

Partial thickness loss (PTL)

Full thickness loss (FTL)

REGION	%	
	PTL	FTL
HEAD		
NECK		
ANT. TRUNK		
POST. TRUNK		
RIGHT ARM		
LEFT ARM		
BUTTOCKS		
GENITALIA		
RIGHT LEG		
LEFT LEG		
TOTAL BURN		

RELATIVE PERCENTAGE OF BODY SURFACE AREA
AFFECTED BY GROWTH

AREA	AGE 0	1	5	10	15	ADULT
A = ½ OF HEAD	9½	8½	6½	5½	4½	3½
B = ½ OF ONE THIGH	2¾	3¼	4	4½	4½	4¾
C = ½ OF ONE LEG	2½	2½	2¾	3	3¼	3½

Figure 31.2 Lund and Browder chart. (Reproduced with permission from Settle J 1986 Burns: the first five days. Smith and Nephew)

A circumferential burn to the chest can lead to respiratory failure.

INHALATION INJURY

Inhalation injury is now the major cause of death in burns and occurs in 15% of burn patients who are admitted to hospital. It results in three different pathological processes:

- direct thermal injury
- inhalation of smoke containing harmful chemicals
- systemic poisoning.

WALLACE'S RULE OF NINES

RULE OF FIVES FOR CHILDREN AND INFANTS

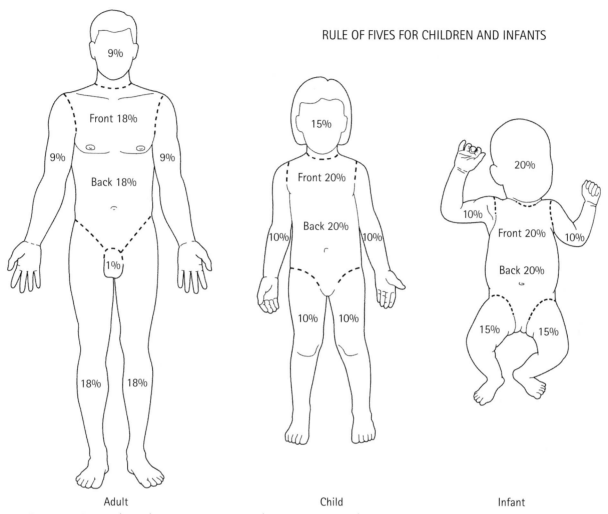

Adult

Child

Infant

Figure 31.3 The "rule of nines" (adults) and the "rule of fives" (children and infants)

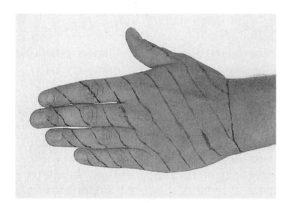

Figure 31.4 One percent of the body area

Direct thermal injury results from inhalation of flames, steam or hot gases. Inhaled smoke contains water-soluble substances which react to form alkalis or acids, for example hydrogen chloride, ammonia or phosgene (produced by burning polyvinyl chloride), and lipid-soluble substances such as acrolein which can be attached to inhaled carbon particles. The third mechanism of injury is systemic poisoning (e.g., carbon monoxide or cyanide).

The upper airway is damaged by either direct thermal injury or smoke inhalation. This leads to oedema and sometimes obstruction of the upper airway which can have a rapid onset. The lower airway is damaged by smoke; in addition, superheated steam can produce thermal damage to the alveoli and this has a poor prognosis. Smoke inhalation can cause sloughing of the airway lining, producing obstruction and inflammation. The latter leads to the loss of protein-rich fluid into the lungs, causing pulmonary oedema and hypoxia.

Systemic toxicity is caused by the inhalation of chemicals, for example cyanide from burning polyurethane foam, which cause cell death. Another common inhaled gas is carbon monoxide, which binds to haemoglobin to produce carboxyhaemoglobin, making the haemoglobin unavailable for oxygen carriage. Inhalation injury should be rapidly assessed and treated promptly.

ELECTRICAL INJURY

Electrical injuries are discussed in Chapter 43.

AGE OF THE PATIENT

There is a greater mortality rate in children under 5 years old, as a child's surface area is greater in relation to their total body size and they will thus lose proportionally more fluid from the same percentage burn compared with an adult. In the elderly the mortality rate is also greater, first because ageing tissue does not heal as well as younger tissue and second, because patients often have associated medical conditions which affect morbidity and mortality, as well as a reduced physiological reserve.

ASSOCIATED INJURY

Associated injuries are common in patients suffering from burns who may have jumped to escape the fire or have been involved in an explosion or a road traffic accident where petrol has ignited. In all these cases associated injuries should be looked for in the primary and secondary surveys.

ASSOCIATED MEDICAL CONDITIONS

If a patient has a respiratory disorder the mortality from an inhalation injury will increase. A burn may cause further problems for patients with heart conditions through either emotional or physical stress. Patients with diabetes mellitus, on steroid therapy or with peripheral vascular disease will have delayed healing.

CRITICAL BURNS

The burns listed in Box 31.1 should be regarded as critical and will normally require specialist management in a burns centre following assessment in the accident and emergency department. Consideration should be given to direct transfer from the scene of the accident to a regional burns centre. Such transfers can only be considered if there is no significant associated injury or the receiving hospital has the facilities to deal with a full range of other injuries.

ASSESSMENT AND MANAGEMENT

SAFETY AT THE SCENE

The approach to the scene is described in Chapter 1. It is essential to ensure that the environment is safe. It may be necessary to wait for the fire service to put the fire out or to rescue the burned patient. It should be remembered that simply opening a door or window enhances the oxygen supply to the fire, increasing its intensity or possibly causing a flash-over and thus endangering the lives of both rescuer and patient.

STOPPING THE BURN PROCESS

Dry and wet heat

Once the patient is safe it is necessary to prevent further harm. If the patient's clothes are smouldering or in flames, they should be placed on the floor and wrapped up in a blanket in order to put the flames out. If the clothes are smouldering or have hot liquid on them, they must be removed quickly; if the clothing is stuck or burnt onto the skin the clothes must be cut around the adhesive area and soaked with clean cold water to minimize the burn process. Burns that are extensive from either dry or wet heat (e.g., flame or scald) can be soaked with clean cold water but cold water must not be left on the burn for more than 10 minutes unless it is less than 5% of body surface area, as this will increase heat loss from the body surface and the patient may become hypothermic. It is vital to wrap patients with extensive burns in blankets to minimize the risk of hypothermia.

> **Cool the burn, warm the patient**

Tar burns

The tar should not be removed but immersed in cold water to cool the area and to stop the burning process.

Chemical burns

All clothing should be removed from the affected area and any dry powdered chemical brushed off. The burn should be copiously washed with large quantities of water for up to 10 minutes at the scene. The patient may then be transferred to hospital. If there is associated life-threatening trauma, irrigation should take place during transit.

PRIMARY SURVEY

Assessing the airway

The airway should be assessed as explained in Chapters 2, 6 and 7.

Assessment of breathing

The breathing should be assessed as explained in Chapter 2.

Specific signs and symptoms of inhalation must be looked for, including certain aspects of the history. These include:

- history of being confined with the fire in a closed space
- history of unconsciousness at the time of the incident
- exposure to smoke or gas during the incident
- evidence of burns to the face
- singed nasal hair
- cough or carbonaceous sputum
- blistering or redness in the mouth
- evidence of laryngeal oedema, e.g. hoarseness, stridor
- wheezing
- signs of airway obstruction or respiratory distress
- full-thickness burns to the nasolabial area of the face or posterior pharyngeal swelling
- signs of respiratory failure: the patient who is unable to speak owing to shortness of breath or exhaustion or who is unconscious.

If the patient is unconscious and unresponsive then oxygen should be given via a bag and mask and only in extreme circumstances (respiratory or cardiac arrest) should intubation be considered in the field. A smaller tube than normal must be available because the airway will often be narrowed owing to oedema. It is best to transfer the patient to the nearest accident and emergency department for definitive airway management.

If there is marked wheezing, nebulized salbutamol at the scene may help.

> If there is any evidence of an inhalation injury or a critical burn the patient should be given the highest concentration of oxygen available (100%)

Assessment and treatment of carbon monoxide poisoning

Most burns patients from a fire in an enclosed environment will have inhaled carbon monoxide. Carbon monoxide is a byproduct of incomplete combustion of carbon and has a higher affinity for haemoglobin than oxygen (approximately 200 times greater). If large amounts of carbon monoxide are present, oxygen is displaced from haemoglobin and large quantities of carboxyhaemoglobin are produced. Because the binding of carbon monoxide to haemoglobin is much stronger than that of oxygen it also makes it difficult for the haemoglobin to release oxygen at the tissues, which further aggravates tissue hypoxia. The half-life of carboxyhaemoglobin in room air is 320 minutes; on 100% oxygen it is 80 minutes and on 100% oxygen at 3 atmospheres (hyperbaric oxygen) it is 23 minutes. The signs and symptoms of carbon monoxide poisoning include lethargy, muscle weakness, headache, nausea and vomiting. When carbon monoxide poisoning is more severe the patient will have dilated pupils,

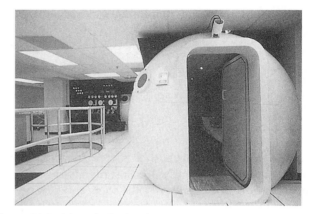

Figure 31.5 A hyperbaric chamber

cyanosis and pulmonary oedema. However, the cherry-red colour which is classically described is rarely seen.

The signs and symptoms of mild carbon monoxide poisoning are:

- lethargy
- muscle weakness
- headache
- nausea
- vomiting.

The signs and symptoms of severe carbon monoxide poisoning are:

- cyanosis
- coma
- pulmonary oedema
- dilated pupils.

Any person with carbon monoxide poisoning should be given 100% oxygen and transferred to the accident and emergency department immediately. Pulse oximetry, which measures oxygen saturation, does not alter in carbon monoxide poisoning as it will not detect the difference between carboxyhaemoglobin and oxyhaemoglobin. Pulse oximetry may therefore appear falsely reassuring. The levels of carboxyhaemoglobin can only be measured from an arterial blood sample. After arrival at hospital, the patient is considered for hyperbaric oxygen (Figure 31.5) if:

- the patient is unconscious at any time
- the carboxyhaemoglobin concentration exceeds 20%
- neurological signs and symptoms are present
- the patient is pregnant.

Patients with carboxyhaemoglobin levels of 50–60% are comatose and require ventilatory support.

The diagnosis of carbon monoxide poisoning may be straightforward if the patient is found in a fume-filled car with the exhaust connected to the interior. However, the symptoms are unfortunately vague and non-specific and a high index of suspicion must be maintained, especially in chronic carbon monoxide poisoning, which may occur in poorly ventilated accommodation.

Assessment of circulation

It is important to assess pulse, blood pressure and capillary refill in any burn, but especially in a critical burn (>15% in an adult; >10% in a child). An intravenous infusion must be started in a patient with a burn greater than 25% of body surface area or if the transfer time is greater than one hour, as vast quantities of plasma will be lost from the burn. There should, however, be no delay at the scene and intravenous access can usually be obtained during transit.

It is important to realize that a patient suffering from burns alone is unlikely to be hypovolaemic at the scene. If the burns patient is in hypovolaemic shock immediately after the burn it is advisable to give the locally recommended fluid for hypovolaemic shock due to trauma and the cause of the hypovolaemia should be assumed *not* to be the burn.

Intravenous access is usually inserted into the antecubital fossa. If this area is burnt it is preferable to site the intravenous line somewhere else in the upper limb; if this is not practicable the lower limb should be considered. If there is no alternative, vascular access can be obtained through burnt skin but this is technically difficult. If vascular access is problematical, the most appropriate action is rapid evacuation to hospital where a wider range of techniques and better conditions are available.

In burns units, human albumin solutions have been recommended as the ideal replacement fluid for burns as it closely resembles the fluid lost and maintains body functions as close to normal as possible. This is not practical outside hospital. It is also suggested that plasma substitutes are of value if there has been a delay of 1 hour or more in giving a patient fluid after a burn; this is because of their plasma-expanding properties. There is less controversy over which fluid to give in the prehospital environment. The recommended initial fluid is Hartmann's solution. If this is unavailable normal saline is a suitable alternative.

Fluid requirement

In the prehospital setting patients with burns greater than 25% of body surface area or more than one hour from hosptial should receive Hartmann's or normal saline infusions. Adults should be given 1000 ml, and children under 15 years 10 ml/kg.

A number of formulae for fluid replacement following a burn are available. These formulae are not relevant to prehospital care and are given here for information only.

The *Muir and Barclay formula* is commonly used in burns units and in accident and emergency departments in the UK. This gives the amount of colloid required in the first 4 hours:

Fluid (ml) = 0.5 × (weight in kg × percentage surface area burnt)

The *Parkland formula* is commonly used in North America to calculate crystalloid requirements, which are greater than the volume of colloid which would be required. The amount of fluid (Hartmann's solution) required in the first 8 hours is:

Fluid (ml) = 2 × (weight in kg × percentage surface area burnt)

ANALGESIA

The ideal analgesic agent is morphine at 0.1 mg/kg body weight, given intravenously with an appropriate antiemetic. Partial-thickness burns are extremely painful and either Entonox can be self-administered by the patient or the patient can be given intravenous morphine. Morphine is given as small intravenous aliquots of 2 mg (in adults), titrated according to effect. No analgesic drug should be given intramuscularly or subcutaneously in severe or moderate burns, as it will remain unabsorbed owing to poor circulation. Non-steroidal antiinflammatory drugs are contraindicated due to the risk of gastrointestinal problems or ulcer formation. Entonox should only be considered as a second-line analgesic due to its variable efficacy and 50% oxygen concentration.

> It is essential that hospital medical staff are made aware that opiate analgesia has been given

SECONDARY SURVEY

A formal secondary survey is rarely performed prehospital. At the scene and during transit, the following details should be ascertained.

- Time of the burn
- Burning agent
- Is the patient complaining of pain?
- Has the patient jumped or been involved in an explosion?
- Was the patient in a confined space?
- Has the patient lost consciousness at any time?
- A brief medical history, drug and allergy history (AMPLE)
- Tetanus status of the patient.

During the secondary survey in hospital a head-to-toe examination is performed to see if any other injuries have been sustained by the patient.

INITIAL DRESSINGS FOR BURNS

The burned area should be wrapped in clingfilm or sterile towels to reduce pain. If the burn is less than 5% of body surface area, sterile cold water or saline soaks are placed on top of the clingfilm to reduce contact with the air, reduce pain and cool the burn. If clingfilm is unavailable, clean sterile towels can be placed on the burn prior to rapid transfer to hospital. Circumferential clingfilm should never be applied to the thorax or limbs. Individual sheets of cling film should be gently laid on the burned area.

> Under no circumstances should any cream (antibiotic or otherwise) be applied to a burn before hospital assessment

DISPOSAL

All burn patients should be transferred to hospital and there a decision can be taken as to whether the patient needs to be transferred to a burns unit, admitted to the hospital from the accident and emergency department or treated as an outpatient. Patients should not be taken to isolated burns units without prior assessment. Critical burns should be sent, wherever possible, to a hospital with a burns unit as long as general resuscitative and treatment facilities are available:

- partial-thickness burns over 10% in a child or an adult over 60 and over 15% in an adult
- full-thickness burn at any age
- any flexure burn, particularly neck and axilla
- any circumferential dermal/full-thickness burn to limb, torso or neck
- extensive burns to the hands, feet, genitalia, perineum or face
- severe electrical burn

- severe chemical burn $\geq 5\%$ total body surface area
- hydrofluoric acid burn $>1\%$ total body surface area
- inhalation injuries.

FURTHER READING

Allison K, Porter K 2004 *Consensus on the pre-hospital approach to burns management*. Injury, Int. J Care Injured, 35:734–738.

Crawford ME, Rask H 1996 *Prehospital care of the burned patient*. European Journal of Emergency Medicine 3:247–251

Lawrence JC 1996 *First-aid measures for the treatment of burns and scalds*. Journal of Wound Care 5:319–322

Pre-Hospital Trauma Life Support Committee of the National Association of Emergency Medicine Technicians 1990 *Pre-hospital trauma life support*, 2nd edn. Committee on Trauma of the American College of Surgeons, Washington DC

Shaw A, Anderson J, Hayward A, Parkhouse N 1995 *The early management of large burns*. British Journal of Hospital Medicine 53:247–250

Skinner D, Driscoll P, Irlam R 1991 *ABC of major trauma*. BMJ Books, London

Wardrope J, Smith JAR *Management of wounds and burns*. Oxford Handbooks in Emergency Medicine. Oxford University Press, Oxford

Chapter 32

Wound management

INTRODUCTION

According to the 1987 mortality statistics of the Office of Population Censuses and Surveys, 432 deaths (2.5% of deaths from accidents) in the UK were due to wounding. Throughout the country 3 million wounds are treated annually in accident and emergency departments; 1.4 million children attend accident and emergency departments in the UK each year because of injury and a large proportion of these children will have suffered a wound of one form or another. Apparently minor wounds can have devastating consequences if they are not properly managed. Attention to the basic principles of wound management will significantly reduce the adverse consequences of these common injuries.

ANATOMY OF THE SKIN

See Chapter 31.

DEFINITIONS

Wound   Any interruption by violence or surgery of the continuity of the external surface of the body or the surface of an internal organ. Legally this used to mean the whole thickness of the skin must be broken and an internal injury alone would not qualify as a "wound". However, this part of the definition is no longer used.

Strictly, *a wound is a disruption of the continuity of tissue*.

Cut (incised wound)   A breach of the skin caused by a sharp edge.

Laceration   A breach of the skin caused by a blunt force; it is usually irregular in shape.

Contused wound   Loss of continuity of the tissue with surrounding bruising.

Contusion   An area of bruising due to the effect of a blunt force.

Haematoma   An accumulation of blood due to bleeding beneath the skin as a result of a blunt direct force.

Abrasion   Removal of part of the surface of the skin. It is usually the outer layers of the skin that are damaged and there is often oozing from the capillaries on the surface of the dermis. Conventionally referred to as a "graze".

Puncture wound   A wound with a narrow path made by, for example, a nail.

Avulsion   The forced separation of two parts; with wounding, this is when a flap of skin and associated tissue has been partially or completely removed.

Amputation   Removal of a portion of a limb or the complete limb.

Closed wound   An internal injury caused by a blunt direct force to the surface of the body. The skin itself is intact but there is injury to the underlying tissues.

PATHOPHYSIOLOGY

Wound healing can be divided into two types. Healing by *primary intention* occurs when the edges of the wound are already adjacent or can be brought together (e.g. with sutures or Steristrips). Healing by *secondary intention* occurs when there is significant tissue loss from the wound and regrowth of skin cover is required. The phases of wound healing are the same in primary and secondary intention.

PHASES OF HEALING

Inflammation

Blood vessels that are torn during wounding initially contract in order to reduce blood loss from the open end of the vessel. Nevertheless, blood is released into the wound which triggers the activation of platelets and initiates the coagulation cascade which ultimately leads to the production of fibrin from fibrinogen and produces a clot in the wound. A complex sequence of events gives rise to the activation of other biological compounds, including vasodilators, which increase the capillary permeability in the area, producing swelling and oedema; other compounds are released which attract cells to the wound. These cells include polymorphonuclear cells, granulocytes and macrophages which remove tissue debris and bacteria. The macrophages initiate the healing of the wound by stimulating the production of blood vessels and attracting fibroblasts, cells that produce the extracellular matrix which contains collagen. The inflammation process occurs over a period of up to 4 days, with a maximum response at 24 hours. The wound at this stage will have a clot on the surface and the surrounding tissue will be red and oedematous.

Cell proliferation and matrix deposition

During the next stage, which lasts up to 30 days, there is an increase in cell proliferation, especially in fibroblasts which produce collagen. Collagen is laid down haphazardly in the scar tissue. At the same time epithelial cells at the wound margins start to move in to cover the wound. New capillaries are formed, giving the base of the wound a granulated appearance (*granulation tissue*) and the epithelial cells grow over the granulation tissue beneath the clot. The epithelium over the granulation tissue is extremely delicate and can often be damaged with either removal of the clot or repeated dressings. At this stage the wound space becomes organized and it is very vascular. The scar and surrounding tissue are red owing to the increase in blood flow to the area. During this phase the contraction of the wound is initiated. This is caused by two components: first by certain types of cells and second by the maturation of collagen which occurs in the third phase.

Matrix remodelling

This third phase overlaps with the first two phases and occurs between days 1 and 300. However, the wound is regarded as "healed" at 30 days. During phase three the matrix of collagen is remodelled, there are changes in orientation of the collagen fibres and the collagen becomes cross-linked biochemically, producing an increase in its tensile strength. This, together with the mechanisms described above, produces further contraction of the scar tissue. The scar becomes less vascular, less cellular and paler.

With primary intention healing the two edges of the wound are opposed and there is healing with minimal scarring. With secondary intention healing there is a defect in the wound and the vascular granulation tissue matures in the base of the defect, initially producing a red, very vascular area which converts into a dense mass of fibrotic tissue which is white and avascular. With secondary intention healing wound contraction is more prominent. This can lead to significant deformity or contractures if the defect has been large.

FACTORS AFFECTING WOUND HEALING

Age

As tissue ages, the healing process slows.

Nutrition

Any decrease in protein intake causes a reduction in the essential amino acids available for tissue repair. A decrease in vitamin C intake causes poor tissue healing and produces the characteristic picture of scurvy. Zinc is also vitally important for the synthesis of collagen.

Diseases

Disease processes, specifically diabetes mellitus and haematological problems such as anaemia, will decrease the efficacy of wound healing.

Drugs

Steroids dampen the inflammatory response and over long periods can cause the skin to thin, making it more susceptible to damage.

Infection

If there are more than 100 000 bacteria per gram of tissue at the time the wound is repaired, infection is likely to occur.

Foreign body

Any foreign material in a wound which is not removed at the time of repair can give rise to further inflammation and infection and prevent wound healing.

Poor blood supply

Pretibial wounds, especially in the elderly, have a reduced blood supply. This reduces the influx of inflammatory cells and the supply of oxygen and nutrients required for healing.

Adhesions, movement and drying

All these affect the degree of wound healing. "Adhesions" occur when dressings stick to a wound: every time the dressing is replaced the reepithelialization is disrupted and the granulation tissue bleeds. This also occurs if there is movement of the dressing around the wound. Drying of a wound, although once thought to be ideal for healing, reduces the amount of reepithelialization and thus reduces the rate of healing.

Ionizing radiation

Ionizing radiation causes a reduction in the rate of healing.

Hypoxia

Hypoxia is associated with poor blood supply. If a patient is severely wounded with a reduction in oxygenation of the tissue and a reduction in the blood supply due to hypovolaemia, both of these will be detrimental to the establishment of the initial phase of wound healing. Thus it is vitally important to maintain the airway, breathing and circulation during wound management.

Psychological stress

Recent research has shown that stress, anxiety, sleep deprivation and emotional disturbances can disrupt the inflammatory response, leading to delayed healing in adults of all ages.

IMMEDIATE MANAGEMENT OF WOUNDS

First, it must be remembered that the primary survey comes before dealing with any soft tissue injury.

AIRWAY

The airway must be secured using the procedure described in Chapters 6 and 7. Any severe facial injury can produce major bleeding. This may be external from obvious lacerations or internal from facial fractures (see Chapter 24).

BREATHING

Appropriate attention must be paid to the diagnosis and treatment of immediately life-threatening breathing problems. If there is a penetrating wound to the chest the object must be left in situ (if it has not already been removed). If there is an open pneumothorax, an Asherman chest seal or a dressing sealed on three sides must be placed over the wound, thus preventing a sucking chest wound (see Chapter 25).

CIRCULATION

Circulation must be assessed (see Chapters 2 and 22). Intravenous access must be obtained and intravenous fluids commenced subject to the guidelines given in Chapter 22.

Control of external haemorrhage

There are three different kinds of bleeding:

- arterial
- venous
- capillary.

Arterial bleeding is bright red in colour and may be seen spurting from the wound. If a large artery has been severed (e.g., the femoral artery) a large volume of blood may be lost. Venous bleeding is dark red in colour and tends to be slower than arterial. However, the veins are capacitance vessels and a large amount of blood can still be lost. Capillary bleeding or oozing typically occurs with an abrasion. If capillary bleeding is caused by a blow to the skin with no break, this will produce damage to the capillaries beneath the skin and cause a bruise or haematoma.

When treating a wound, adequate personal protection (gloves, glasses or face guard and overalls) must be worn. If a wound is bleeding, clothing should be cut away from the wounded area, thus exposing the wound. At this time it is useful to make a mental note of the size and depth of the wound and the sort of bleeding occurring. The majority of wounds show a mixture of both arterial and venous bleeding. It is important to note if it is a major arterial bleed.

Control of bleeding from an open wound

Direct pressure is applied to the wound with a clean, large gauze pad (dry or moist). The gauze pad can be moistened with sterile water or saline if it is available. The direct pressure must be constant. If a gauze pad is not immediately available a gloved hand can be used initially, provided that it can be confirmed that there are no sharp objects in the base of the wound. Several layers of gauze can then be placed on the wound and a bandage placed over these layers of gauze to secure them in position. The entire wound should be covered and the bandage secured. It is important to elevate the injured area above the heart if possible to reduce blood flow to the area.

If direct pressure to the wound is not sufficient and the wound is still bleeding, the dressing should not be removed but may be reinforced with further dressings. If the wound continues to bleed through the dressings indirect pressure may be applied to specific pressure points. These are areas where the arteries providing blood to specific areas can be pressed against bone, thereby reducing the flow of blood to the wound. Five important pressure points are:

- the femoral artery in the groin, which can be compressed against the pelvis

- the brachial artery approximately 2 cm in from the medial epicondyle of the elbow, which can be compressed against the lower end of the humerus
- the superficial temporal artery, which can be palpated just anterior to the tragus of the ear and can be compressed against the temporal bone to reduce bleeding from scalp lacerations on that side
- the supraorbital and supratrochlear arteries supplying the forehead, which can be compressed against the supraorbital margin to reduce bleeding from lacerations of the forehead
- the facial artery, which can be compressed against the mandible approximately halfway from the angle of the mandible to the tip of the chin to reduce bleeding from the lower half of the face.

Direct pressure to the pressure point should only be applied for 10 minutes at a time with release of the pressure and review to see if the bleeding has stopped. If it has not stopped then the pressure can be reapplied. The key to successful management of these patients is rapid evacuation to hospital.

Splinting is also effective in reducing movement of the limb, thereby reducing the amount of bleeding. Splinting is also an advantage in patients who have an open fracture (see Chapter 29).

> **Tourniquets are only used as a last resort**

Tourniquets are used as a last resort where the patient is exsanguinating, for example from a traumatic amputation, or in a severe crush injury when the application of a tourniquet may protect the patient from toxins arising from the crushed part. If a tourniquet is to be applied it should be tight enough to prevent both arterial and venous flow. If the tourniquet is too loose it allows arterial flow and leads to venous engorgement in the limb and further bleeding. It is important to use wide, flat material and apply a rolled pad to the artery underneath. The tourniquet must be tightened until no further bleeding occurs. The time of application of the tourniquet, the name of the person applying it and its position must be recorded. The tourniquet must never be covered. It should be released when an adequate external compression bandage has been applied to the area. It is advisable to mark on the patient that a tourniquet has been applied so that it is not forgotten once the patient has been transferred to hospital.

An alternative method of haemorrhage control is the windlass technique applied directly over the wound. Gauze and a bandage are applied to the wound and a triangular bandage, folded to produce a broad strip, is tied tightly round the limb with the knot directly over the wound. A pencil or similar object is then inserted under the bandage and twisted to apply pressure, then secured in place (Figure 32.1). A blood pressure cuff applied over or preferably proximal to the wound and inflated to 5 to 10 mmHg above the systolic blood pressure is a highly effective method of haemorrhage control. However, this procedure carries the same risks as those of tourniquets. Consequently similar cautions must be used in applying this technique.

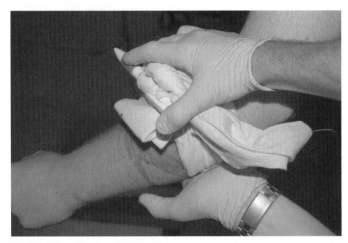

Figure 32.1 The windlass technique

Control of external haemorrhage of an open wound with a sharp object protruding

When a sharp object is protruding from a wound it must not be removed. Pads or thick dressings are placed around the protruding object to support it and reduce unwanted movement. The dressings are then secured firmly in place.

SPECIFIC WOUND MANAGEMENT

WOUND ASSESSMENT

During the history relevant details regarding the patient should be obtained (see Chapter 20). The mechanism of injury should be clearly established.

Blunt injury

Blunt injury may occur, for example, in a road traffic accident. The severity of the blunt injury depends on the speed and direction of impact; in road traffic accidents, the greater the speed of the vehicle, the greater the severity of the injury to the occupant and injury patterns can be predicted. For example, a frontal collision is more likely to result in injury to the front of the head, the neck, the front of the chest, abdomen, pelvis and the femur. However, a side impact will cause rotational injury to the head and neck and injure the side of the chest and abdomen as well as the hip (see Chapter 20).

Blunt injuries are also caused by being hit with a blunt object (e.g., a baseball bat). The skin may not always be broken, even in the presence of severe underlying injury.

Another type of blunt injury is the crush injury; this typically occurs when fingers are trapped, for instance in machinery, a car door or underneath someone's foot in a contact sport. In this instance the skin may not be damaged, although there often is a split laceration due to pressure. There is marked contusion and eventually gross swelling of the part crushed, owing to the tissue damage which occurs underneath the skin. There may be no bony injury, but there is often long-term swelling and damage to the soft tissue which takes time to heal.

Penetrating wounds

The damage produced by a *stab wound* depends on the area of the body involved and the velocity and force with which the stab has been inflicted. It is important to remember in a stab wound that only structures lying in the path of the stabbing implement are damaged. Thus if there is a stab wound to the leg muscle, nerve or vessel damage may also occur. However, if there is a stab wound to the abdomen, any of the viscera underlying that area of the stab wound can be damaged.

The damage caused by a *bullet wound* depends on the shape of the bullet, the velocity, the angle at which it was fired, the distance of the person from the weapon and the position of the victim at the time of impact. When a bullet penetrates the skin, the energy is dissipated from the bullet to the tissue and the cells of the tissue are moved directly away from the site of impact by the energy exchange. This causes damage to the tissue on either side of the pathway of the bullet as well as along the direct wound track. In addition, the path of the bullet may be erratic and cannot always be predicted from the apparent wounds. Attempts to match "entry" and "exit" wounds are unnecessary and will only lead to confusion. It is also important to note that there is a great deal of contamination from a bullet wound due to clothing and foreign material being drawn in with the bullet.

Bites

The most significant risk in the management of bites is the development of infection, especially in human bites, the most common of which is a laceration over the knuckle from a punch to the face which has struck the opponent's teeth. Bites that produce lacerations can damage underlying tissue and bites from large animals (including powerful dogs) may be associated with underlying fractures.

Puncture wounds

These wounds are caused by a sharp point and since the wound closes over, they are prone to infection, especially with anaerobic bacteria. These patients need antibiotic cover. With a puncture wound, only structures in the path of the puncturing object are damaged. This usually involves muscle and occasionally nerves and tendons.

Environment in which the injury occurred

It is important to establish the circumstances in which the wound occurred, for example indoors or outside, and also if the area outside was tetanus prone.

Wounds which are tetanus prone include wounds more than 6 hours old which have not been thoroughly cleaned, those with a large amount of necrotic tissue present and wounds that have been in contact with soil or manure

Table 32.1 Tetanus treatment and prophylaxis (reproduced with permission from the Chorley and Royal Preston NHS Trust handbook)

	Clean wound	Tetanus–prone wound
Five doses of tetanus toxoid in lifetime (course + 2 boosters)	Nil	Consider tetanus immunoglobulin if particularly high risk (e.g. manure contamination)
Complete course or booster within last 10 years (<5 doses in life)	Nil	Consider tetanus immunoglobulin if particularly high risk (e.g. manure contamination)
Complete course or booster over 10 years ago (<5 doses in life)	Tetanus toxoid booster (Td)	Tetanus toxoid booster (Td) + tetanus immunoglobulin
Not immunized	Tetanus toxoid course	Tetanus toxoid course + tetanus immunoglobulin
Immune status unknown	Patient to check with GP within 72 hours (? Needs booster/course or check antibody levels)	Tetanus immunoglobulin and patient to check with GP within 72 hours (? Needs booster/course)

Due to the increasing incidence of diphtheria all adults who need a tetanus toxoid booster should be given the tetanus/diphtheria combined booster (**Td**).

The dose of tetanus immunoglobulin is 250 iu which must be **doubled** if the wound is more than 12 hours old or the patient weighs over 90 kg.

(Table 32.1). The temperature of the environment is also important; frostbite will reduce wound healing.

Time of injury

The longer a wound is left without appropriate cleaning and dressing, the more likely it is to be infected. An untreated wound more than 3 hours old will have more than one million bacteria per gram of tissue. In all traumatic wounds there is an infection rate of approximately 15%. The chances of wound infection are reduced by clearing debris from the wound, applying a clean sterile dressing or gauze and transferring the patient to an emergency department so that the wound can be cleaned and treated. Older wounds are more likely to be contaminated and are usually cleaned and allowed to remain open with an appropriate dressing.

Examination

Prehospital examination of the wound includes observation of the size, shape and depth of the wound and of any underlying structures that have been exposed or are protruding from the wound (e.g. bone, tendons, vessels, nerves or subcutaneous tissue). At the scene it is important to note movement and sensation distal to the wound so the examining hospital doctor can assess if distal function has deteriorated.

WOUNDS AT SPECIFIC SITES

Scalp wounds

For scalp wounds it is important to replace any skin flaps and to provide direct pressure on the site of the wound with a sterile gauze and secured with a bandage. In the absence of other injuries, these patients are best transferred sitting up.

Neck wounds

Neck wounds may be associated with airway compromise due to pressure from external bleeding or bleeding into the airway, pneumothorax (simple or tension), shock or severe damage to underlying structures. Foreign bodies should be left in situ and a simple dressing applied. If there is an air leak, an occlusive dressing must be applied to prevent air embolism. Direct pressure may be necessary to control bleeding, but simultaneous pressure on both carotids must be avoided.

Wounds of the palm of the hand

A sterile pad should be placed over the wound, with the patient's fingers over the gauze to apply pressure over the injury. The fingers can then be bandaged down. The same principles apply for wounds in joint creases; for example, at the elbow the pad can be placed in the crease of the elbow and the elbow flexed to exert pressure over the pad to reduce the bleeding. The limb should be elevated. The pressure can be released every 10 minutes to see if the bleeding has stopped.

Bleeding from the ear, nose or facial injuries

See Chapter 24.

Chest wounds

See Chapter 25.

Abdominal injuries

See Chapter 26.

Eye wounds

Any contusion, laceration or penetrating wound to the eye should be covered by a sterile dressing and the sterile dressing bandaged in situ. The bandage should ideally cover both eyes as this prevents any consensual movement of the eye which could cause further damage. The patient should be kept supine.

Varicose vein injuries in the lower leg

Direct pressure should be applied to the wound with gauze, the patient should be laid down and the leg elevated during transfer.

MANAGEMENT OF SPECIFIC TYPES OF WOUNDS

Flap wounds

It is important to make sure that the flaps are replaced and that a sterile gauze dressing, dry or moist, is placed over the top.

Foreign body wounds

If there is a large impaled object then this should not be removed and a dressing should be applied around the area. If there is a small foreign body, either glass or grit, on the surface which is not embedded, it can be removed. If small particles of glass or grit are embedded these will be more difficult to remove and a sterile dressing, dry or moist, should be placed over the wound and the personnel at the hospital notified on arrival.

Crush injuries

Crush injuries can range from a fingertip crushed in a car door to a crushed chest in a major road traffic accident. Fingertip crush injuries are common and cause local tissue damage, often with an underlying fracture and marked swelling. The injured digit should be covered with either a dry dressing or a moist saline soak, elevated and the patient taken to hospital. With extensive crush injuries to the limbs it must always be borne in mind that toxins may be released once the crush has been released. Before the patient is released (or en route to hospital if this is not possible) fluid resuscitation should be commenced. If life-threatening thoraco-abdominal bleeding is present, give 250 ml aliquots of normal saline to maintain the presence of a radial pulse. In the absence of thoraco-abdominal bleeding, give a fluid bolus of 2 litres of normal saline, followed by 1 to 1.5 litres of normal saline per hour. Children should receive a fluid bolus of 20 ml/kg. Intravenous opiate analgesia is likely to be required to control pain. Once the object crushing the limb has been removed it is important to cover the external wound, splint the limb and transfer the patient to hospital as soon as possible.

High-pressure injection injuries

Injuries may occur from a high-pressure oil or grease gun and initially very little injury may be evident. However, these injuries must be seen in hospital as there may be severe damage and necrosis to the tissue underlying the skin. These injuries can lead to extensive loss of soft tissue.

Puncture wounds

See above.

Bites

See above.

Amputation

When either a limb or a digit has been completely severed there can be massive bleeding, but bleeding is usually limited as the vessels go into spasm and retract into the wound. The area should be covered with a sterile saline soak or sterile gauze, direct pressure applied and the stump elevated. The amputated part should be wrapped in a polythene bag. The bag can then be placed in a second bag which can then be placed in iced water. It is important not to place the amputated part directly in contact with either cotton wool, gauze or ice as this will cause tissue damage or contamination.

Abrasions

Abrasions are superficial wounds which are usually caused by shearing or friction and usually contain grit or debris. It is important not to try to clean them at the scene, as this can be extremely painful. The abrasion should be covered with a sterile dressing, preferably moist, and the patient transferred to hospital so that the abrasion can be cleaned adequately under local anaesthesia.

Contusions

Where there are severe contusions to a limb, hand or digit, the injured part should be immobilized in a splint, elevated and, where possible, ice or a cold compress used to alleviate the pain and swelling.

BASIC DRESSINGS

It was originally thought that wounds should be kept dry to prevent infection and aid healing. However, it has been shown that it is important to keep the wound environment moist and a specific level of moisture is required for ideal healing. Reepithelialization of wounds occurs 40% faster in a moist environment; this is because a wound deprived completely of any exudate actually heals more slowly, as the exudate contains growth factors required to encourage new vessel formation and reepithelialization.

The ideal wound dressing should promote gaseous exchange, maintaining the correct oxygen tension and pH of the wound surface. There should be high humidity in the wound and an equilibrium between exudate absorption and the amount of moisture at the wound surface. The temperature of the wound should be maintained near to core temperature which enables the cells to function maximally for regeneration and removal of debris. The dressing should aid the removal of dead tissue, bacteria and any unwanted chemicals and should provide a barrier to the outside environment, preventing bacteria entering the wound as well as protecting against environmental changes in temperature. It should preferably be non-adherent, non-allergenic and have good mechanical properties to protect the wound from external forces.

Currently there is no one particular dressing that provides all of these features. However, there are numerous micro-environment dressings available which include thin films, hydrocolloids, hydrogels, foams and alginates. All of these may be used at different times with different wounds and all are utilized in the long-term treatment of wounds.

In prehospital wound treatment where the wound needs to be covered quickly with the cleanest possible material, the most useful dressings should be sterile, usually gauze pads or larger bulky dressings if it is necessary to stop excessive bleeding. Sterile water or saline may be used to moisten the dressing and reduce adherence of the dressing to the wound surface. The dressing can be secured in place using a bandage. Occlusive dressings can be used for wounds of the abdomen or chest, particularly of the abdomen where bowel has been exposed, as this prevents loss of moisture. Clingfilm has already been mentioned as a dressing for burns.

FURTHER READING

Greaves J, Porter K Consensus statement on crush injury and crush syndrome. Accid Emerg Nurs, 2004;12(1):47–52.

Wardrope J, Smith JAR The management of wounds and burns. Oxford University Press, Oxford

Chapter **33**

Overview of trauma resuscitation

INTRODUCTION

This chapter provides an overview of the management of the trauma patient. It is designed to emphasize the integration of material from the preceding chapters into a logical and systematic approach to the injured casualty. For details of the management of specific systems or injuries, the reader should refer to the relevant chapter.

SAFETY

The first priority at all times is to be safe: are you safe, is the scene safe, is the casualty safe?

> **Safety – self, scene, casualty**

It is important to remember that the fire service have overall responsibility for the safety of an accident scene.

ASSESSMENT

The first role of the paramedic, particularly if the ambulance service is the first emergency responder to arrive, is a brief assessment of the scene. What is the nature of the incident? Are there any specific hazards? What emergency response is present and what will be required? Is the necessary equipment available? How many casualties are

> **Box 33.1 Assess**
>
> - Safety
> - Hazards
> - Casualties – numbers
> - Mechanisms of injury
> - Emergency services – present and required

involved and what are the mechanisms and nature of their injuries?

On arriving at the scene of an accident, one should always identify oneself to the senior representatives of the other emergency services.

An important early priority must be to assess the casualties for priority of treatment and evacuation: this is *triage* (see Chapter 59).

> **On arrival at an accident, identify yourself to the other emergency services**

PATIENT MANAGEMENT

The first and most important part of the management of any trauma victim is the *primary survey*. This must be performed rapidly, carefully and in a standard manner; it is the basis of all good trauma care. During the primary survey, life-threatening problems are identified and dealt with; other problems can wait.

> The role of the primary survey is to identify and treat life-threatening problems

The primary survey not only identifies but treats life-threatening problems.

> Primary survey = identification of problems + treatment

THE PRIMARY SURVEY

Obstruction of the airway causes death more rapidly than disruption of breathing, which in turn is more rapidly fatal than circulatory compromise. For this reason, the primary survey must rigidly follow the "ABC" sequence – airway, breathing and circulation – to which are added control of the cervical spine to prevent progression of neurological deficit (potential or actual) due to neck injury and control of overt haemorrhage as an adjunct to management of the circulation, thus:

- airway with cervical spine control
- breathing
- circulation with control of overt haemorrhage.

The primary survey is completed by "disability" and "exposure". In the primary survey, the assessment of disability is AVPU (see below) and pupillary response to light. The degree of exposure must be judged according to the patient's injuries (severity and location), environment, sex and age. Although due regard must always be given to the patient's modesty, exposure must be sufficient for the proper management of the patient's injuries.

Approaching the patient

On approaching the patient, an introduction is essential (and good manners), as is an explanation of what is about to happen. It should be remembered that casualties can often hear what is said to them although they give no sign of this at the time. If the patient can speak, however incoherently, it means that the airway is clear and the patient is breathing; otherwise the first step is to assess the airway.

Airway with cervical spine control

If the patient is breathing quietly and comfortably, no other action may be necessary other than to apply oxygen at 12–15 litres per minute via a face mask with reservoir. If, however,

> **Box 33.2 The full primary survey**
>
> - Airway with cervical spine control
> - Breathing with oxygen
> - Circulation with control of overt haemorrhage
> - Disability
> - Exposure

the airway is at risk, either the insertion of an airway (nasopharyngeal or oropharyngeal) or putting the patient in the recovery position should be considered (remembering the possibility of a cervical spine injury). If the airway appears obstructed or partially obstructed, any obvious removable obstruction should be removed digitally or by suction and simple airway manoeuvres should applied (see Chapter 6). These are *chin lift* and *jaw thrust*.

> All trauma victims require high-flow oxygen

Both the head tilt and chin lift, as well as the recovery position, are best avoided if there is any possibility of cervical spine injury and immobilization of the cervical spine should be maintained manually at first, then by semi-rigid collar, head blocks and tape throughout resuscitation. It must be remembered, however, that the airway takes precedence over the cervical spine and if it is absolutely necessary to compromise the cervical spine (e.g., by performing a head tilt) in order to achieve a patent protected airway, then this must be done.

> Airway takes precedence over cervical spine

The jaw thrust manoeuvre is safe in cervical spine injury. If simple airway manoeuvres are successful in clearing the airway, an oral or nasopharyngeal airway can be inserted, if the patient will tolerate it, and oxygen applied. Otherwise it will be necessary to proceed with *stepped airway care* as follows.

1. Airway clearance – manual and aspiration
2. Manual airway opening manoeuvres:
   – chin lift
   – jaw thrust
3. Oropharyngeal airway
4. Nasopharyngeal airway
5. Oral tracheal intubation
6. Cricothyroid ventilation

Nasopharyngeal airways are often better tolerated than oral ones but are a last resort if there is any possibility of basal skull fracture (they should be considered, for example, in the patient with a partial obstruction and clenched teeth).

When – and *only* when – the airway is patent and protected, it is possible to move on to the assessment of breathing. However complex the airway manoeuvre that is required, it must be completed before the breathing is considered.

Breathing

Assessment of breathing begins with the *neck*:

- tracheal shift
- wounds
- emphysema (surgical)
- laryngeal crepitus

- vein distension
- swelling.

Penetrating neck wounds should be sealed with an occlusive dressing to reduce the risk of air embolism.
Then the *chest*.

- LOOK for movement, instability, flail segments, wounds
- PALPATE for surgical emphysema, tenderness, wounds, paradoxical movement
- PERCUSSION for resonance or dullness
- LISTEN with a stethoscope for breath sounds

Hyperresonance with reduced breath sounds suggests a tension pneumothorax; dullness with reduced breath sounds is indicative of a haemothorax. Remember, the role of the primary survey is the identification and treatment of life-threatening injuries.

If the clinical signs suggest a tension pneumothorax, an intercostal needle thoracocentesis should be performed (Chapter 25). Penetrating chest wounds should be covered with an Asherman seal or a dressing sealed on three sides.

Remember to examine the back of the chest

When – and *only* when – life-threatening breathing problems have been identified and treated, where possible, is it appropriate to move on to the circulation.

Circulation with control of external haemorrhage

The patient must be assessed for signs of shock; at the same time obvious external haemorrhage should be controlled by external pressure. In the trauma patient the causes of shock are:

- hypovolaemia
- cardiogenic
- neurogenic.

Septic shock is unlikely to be a problem in the trauma victim unless rescue is particularly prolonged (e.g., following a natural disaster such as an earthquake). *Hypovolaemic shock* is by far the most likely cause for shock in the trauma victim and may be classified as in Table 33.1.

Haemorrhage may be divided into:

- external
- internal.

Box 33.3 Life-threatening chest injuries (ATOMIC)

- Airway obstruction
- Tension pneumothorax
- Open pneumothorax
- Massive haemothorax
- Flail chest
- Cardiac tamponade

Significant external haemorrhage is likely to be obvious but this is not always the case and an appropriate search should be made. The location of internal (concealed) haemorrhage may be:

- chest
- abdomen
- pelvis
- thigh.

Brief palpation of the abdomen and pelvis (springing the pelvis, Figure 33.2) will aid the location of bleeding. Springing the pelvis should only be performed once (see below).

Box 33.4 Overview of examination findings in chest trauma

- Chest wall contusion
- Surgical emphysema
- Penetrating object
- Pneumothorax
- Tension pneumothorax
- Rib fractures
- Flail chest
  1. Small rib panel
  2. Complete anterior flail
  3. Hemi flail
- Open chest wound (Sucking)
- Open chest wound (Bleeding)
- Fractures of the clavicle/shoulder/scapula
- Ruptured diaphragm (bowel sounds in chest cavity [difficult to detect])

Table 33.1 Classification of hypovolaemic shock (adult)

	Class I	Class II	Class III	Class IV
Blood loss (ml)	Up to 750	750–1500	1500–2000	>2000
Blood loss (%BV)	Up to 15%	15–30%	30–40%	>40%
Pulse rate	<100	>100	>120	>40
Blood pressure	Normal	Normal	Decreased	Decreased
Pulse pressure (mmHg)	Normal or increased	Decreased	Decreased	Decreased
Respiratory rate	14–20	20–30	30–40	>35
Urine output (ml/hr)	>30	20–30	5–15	Negligible
CNS/mental status	Slightly anxious	Mildly anxious	Anxious and confused	Confused and lethargic
Fluid replacement (3:1 rule)	Crystalloid	Crystalloid	Crystalloid and blood	Crystalloid and blood

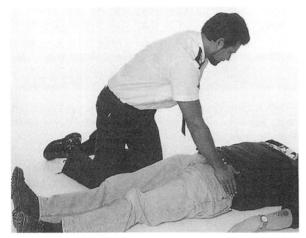

Figure 33.1 Springing the pelvis

Significant haemorrhage into the chest should already have been identified during the assessment of breathing. Severe shock may result from bleeding into the thighs from femoral fractures, although this is uncommon.

Cardiogenic shock may result from tension pneumothorax or cardiac tamponade, usually secondary to penetrating injury.

Neurogenic shock is rare. It should never be assumed that shock is neurogenic since any accident severe enough to cause spinal injury is also likely to be capable of producing haemorrhage from other associated injuries. Isolated head injury is not a cause of shock in adults (shock occasionally occurs in babies due to bleeding into the layers of the scalp).

> Isolated head injuries do not cause shock

All patients with significant trauma should have an intravenous cannula inserted and should receive fluid replacement in order to maintain the presence of a radial pulse. In the presence of a significant head injury the same protocol should be followed. However, even moderate hypotension is detrimental in head injuries and it is imperative therefore that the patient is evacuated as rapidly as possible to hospital. The patient will need urgent definitive haemorrhage control.

> In uncontrolled haemorrhage, time is of the essence

Unless the patient is trapped, intravenous access (using the largest possible cannula, usually 16 or 14 gauge) should be obtained in transit. If the transfer times are very short (only a few minutes) this may legitimately be left until arrival in the accident and emergency department. Under no circumstances should achieving intravenous access be allowed to delay transfer to hospital.

> Intravenous access must never delay patient transfer

Disability

Disability is assessed during the primary survey using the AVPU system and pupillary assessment to light (PERL – "pupils equal and reactive to light").

The pupillary reactions are examined and the patient's response is classified as follows.

> **A** > Alert
> **V** > Patient responds to voice
> **P** > Patient responds to pain
> **U** > Patient unresponsive

Exposure

In the primary survey, E is for exposure. The degree of exposure that is appropriate depends on the clinical situation. Exposure of the chest is always necessary for assessment of B and other exposure must be performed as necessary to ensure that *no significant injury is missed*. For reasons of privacy, warmth and good lighting, this part of the primary survey is often best performed in the ambulance. Motorcycle leather trousers should only be removed after very careful consideration, as they may act to tamponade significant lower limb bleeding from pelvic or long-bone fractures by acting like a pneumatic antishock garment.

Once the primary survey is complete, it may be appropriate to move on to the secondary survey. Short transfer times and the identification of significant problems during the primary survey usually mean that the secondary survey is delayed until arrival at hospital and after the primary survey has been repeated.

> Performing a secondary survey must never delay patient transfer to hospital

If there is any suggestion of a change in the patient's condition during either the primary or secondary surveys, the same routine should always be followed: go back to airway (A). If the change in the patient's condition is an increase in respiratory rate it is essential not to be distracted into returning to breathing (B) or, if bleeding, into returning to circulation (C): always return (however briefly) to A. The same principle applies if one becomes distracted during the examination.

> If in doubt, go back to A (airway)

The *golden hour* is defined as the time from injury to definitive surgical treatment. It is an artificial concept designed to emphasize the importance of achieving rapid definitive care. It should never be used as an excuse for delay: "It's only

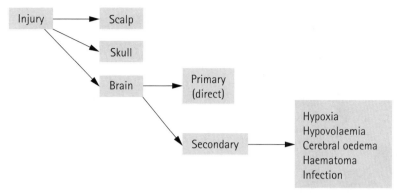

Figure 33.2 Classification of head injuries

half an hour since the injury, we've got plenty of time to get this guy to hospital before the golden hour is up!".

THE SECONDARY SURVEY

The secondary survey is a "head-to-toe" assessment of the patient with assessment of vital signs (including the Glasgow Coma Scale), during which all the patient's injuries will be identified.

It is vital to remember that the secondary survey was originally described for use in the accident and emergency department and included appropriate X-rays. The clinical examination itself, if it is to be appropriately thorough, will take time. The following description of a detailed survey, therefore, will rarely be appropriate in the pre-hospital environment which is often cold, uncomfortable and poorly lit. Furthermore, there is no point in delaying transfer to definitive treatment to perform an examination which will be repeated in hospital: the life-threatening problems will have been identified during the primary survey.

The secondary survey should follow a logical order, starting at the head and working towards the feet. In principle a "log roll" examination of the cervical spine should be included, but practical considerations suggest that this is best performed in hospital.

Head

The most important role of head injury management is to prevent secondary brain injury. Head injuries are classified in Figure 33.2. The scalp should be examined for lacerations, paying particular attention to the possibility of compound skull fractures.

> Do not insert your fingers into deep scalp lacerations!

The face, scalp and behind the ears should be checked for bruising and swelling and any alteration in facial contour should be identified and recorded. Leakage of blood or possible cerebrospinal fluid from the nose or ears should also be recorded.

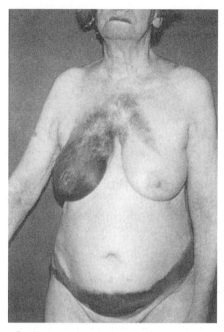

Figure 33.3 Secondary survey chest injuries

Chest

Life-threatening problems should already have been identified during the primary survey. This sequence should be repeated in the secondary survey.

- Trachea
- Neck veins
- Visual inspection
- Auscultation
- Percussion
- Palpation.

In addition, the presence of bony injury to the chest (ribs, clavicles, scapulae, sternum), bruising, pattern bruising, lacerations and abrasions should be noted and recorded. Particular attention should be paid to seatbelt bruising (or its absence) in road traffic accidents (Figure 33.3).

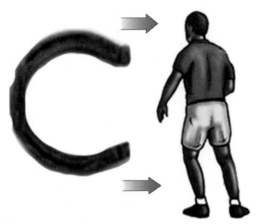

Figure 33.4 The "giant horseshoe". Unless the victim has been hit by a giant horseshoe, injury to the legs and chest is unlikely to occur in the absence of abdominal injury

Box 33.5 Limb examination	
Superficial	Lacerations
	Bruises
	Abrasions
	Swelling
Bones	Simple fractures
	Compound fractures
Joints	Swelling
	Deformity
	Abnormal movements:
	fracture
	dislocation
Nerves	Neurological damage
Arteries	Vascular compromise

Upper limbs

The first clue to an upper limb injury may be an abnormal position of the arm: assessment should include checking for this as well for swelling, bruising, lacerations and abrasions. Compound fractures should be noted. It is mandatory to record that a fracture was compound before it was reduced. Each joint should be examined in turn for swelling, deformity and range of movement (normal and abnormal). Evidence of vascular or neurological compromise must also be sought.

Abdomen

The abdomen should be observed for swelling, bruising, abrasions or lacerations and their presence recorded. The abdomen should be gently examined for tenderness or rebound (see Chapter 26). Intraabdominal pathology may be associated with tenderness, rebound and swelling, but it is vital to remember that in the early stages abdominal injuries may be concealed ("silent"). Patients who have blunt chest and leg injuries probably have abdominal injuries as well, since the mechanism of injury is unlikely to have missed the unprotected part of the body that lies between (Figure 33.5).

> Chest injury + leg injury = abdominal injury

There is no role for the measurement of pelvic girth or for auscultation of the abdomen in the prehospital environment.

Pelvis

Bleeding into the pelvis is a common cause of concealed haemorrhage and should not be forgotten if there is shock without external bleeding or evidence of intrathoracic or intraabdominal haemorrhage. Springing the pelvis (see Figure 33.2) may give some indication of pelvic injury, but is not particularly reliable and may exacerbate or precipitate

haemorrhage. A single attempt under C of the primary survey is useful in identifying potential sources of bleeding. This procedure should not be repeated in the secondary survey – a pelvic radiograph should be performed after arrival in hospital. Suspicion of the possibility of pelvic injury should arise from a knowledge of the mechanism of injury.

Lower limb

The lower limbs are examined for abnormal position, deformity, swelling, bruising, lacerations and abrasions. Compound fractures may be noted. The knee and ankle should be examined for evidence of fracture, dislocation, deformity or swelling and movement (normal or abnormal) as well as the superficial injuries listed above. As with the arms, neurological and vascular damage must be confirmed or excluded (Box 33.5).

Having completed the secondary survey, all the findings (positive and negative) must be recorded.

> If it isn't written down, it wasn't done

PREPARATION FOR TRANSPORT

More often than not, transfer of the patient will begin before the secondary survey, at a time when only ABCDE have been completed and major injuries have been identified. Major fractures, dislocations and soft tissue injuries should be identified during E of the primary survey and not during the secondary survey. Whenever preparations for transport are made the principles remain the same.

Airway

The patient's airway must be safe and secure during handling. The patient should continue to receive high-concentration oxygen and should be moved in such a way that the risk of spinal injury is minimized.

Breathing

The patient must be breathing or, if not, supported respiration must be in progress and maintainable during transfer. Cannulae or chest drains must be fastened securely.

Circulation

During transit, it is essential that the patient's condition can be observed and that a central pulse is easily to hand. During short periods of transfer (e.g., into an ambulance) drips should be switched off and the fluid bags placed against the patient; alternatively, if enough pairs of hands are available, infusion bags may be carried at shoulder height and handed into the vehicle. Always tape a loop of the IV giving set to the patients arm to reduce the risk of the cannula being inadvertently pulled out.

Disability

Assessment of AVPU and pupillary reactions should be repeated as soon as the patient is in the back of the ambulance.

Exposure

The patient should be reasonably covered during transfer. It may be appropriate to remove clothes or blankets during transport to facilitate observations. When positioning the patient in the ambulance, if the patient has severe unilateral injuries (or more significant injuries on one side), they should be placed with the injured side against the gangway. This will aid access for both observation and practical intervention if it is required.

IN HOSPITAL

The role of the paramedic in the hospital management of trauma is vital. Only the paramedic can give details of the accident and, most importantly, of the mechanism of injury. The ambulance service report form should be given (ideally) to a doctor or to the senior nurse involved with the case. A brief verbal handover is essential and hospital staff should have the courtesy to remain silent and listen. The MIST system can be used as a basis for the handover:

Mechanism
Injuries
Symptoms and signs
Treatment given

Section 5

PAEDIATRICS

Chapter 34

Obtaining a paediatric history

INTRODUCTION

A paediatric history is made up of two elements:

- the account of what has happened
- background information about the child which might affect the current or future situation.

Even in the early stages of treating a patient, there are essential facts which provide vital help in deciding what to do. In addition, a considerable amount of information is available in the prehospital situation which is difficult or even impossible to obtain later. Conversely, the past medical records are usually obtainable by hospital staff whereas out of hospital only verbal information is available.

Immediate assessment: a few brief details are AMPLE

THE AMPLE FORMAT

Immediate assessment and appropriate action take precedence over the history at all times. However, even in the first few seconds some relevant information can be vital. This should take the form of a few short, structured questions. The AMPLE format is widely used and is easy to remember:

A > Allergies
M > Medicines
P > Past medical history
L > Last food and drink
E > Events leading up to the current problem

ALLERGIES

It is especially important to know about allergies if any drugs may be given. Occasionally, an allergic reaction to medicines or foods is the *cause* of the illness.

MEDICINES

Any medicines that the child may have already taken will influence his treatment. Regular medication gives much information about known medical problems and the current state of health. For instance, a child with asthma who is taking regular steroids has an illness which has been difficult to control.

PAST MEDICAL HISTORY

The medical history has a major bearing on the current problem. At this stage just a list of important past illnesses is required. Even in young children the past history can be surprisingly complicated! Children with congenital problems frequently present with urgent problems such as fits and chest infections. Certain illnesses such as asthma also lead to recurrent problems.

LAST FOOD AND DRINK

The presence of food and drink in the stomach is a major risk factor for regurgitation. This may lead to airway and breathing problems. To be forewarned is to be in a position to take action if necessary. This knowledge is particularly important in the child with a reduced level of consciousness or in whom narcotic analgesic drugs may be given. Children often vomit after minor injuries and during the course of many illnesses.

EVENTS LEADING UP TO THE CURRENT PROBLEM

Brief details of the course of an illness or the mechanism of an injury together with the nature of the present complaints are extremely helpful.

THE STORY FROM THE SCENE

Every police officer knows how much information can be gathered from the scene of an incident. The prehospital worker has a unique insight into this source of information. At a child's home, the normal living environment reveals much about the child's daily life. The family's social circumstances and habits may give useful clues as to the current problems. The apparent health and well-being of the other children in the household is also important.

When attending an accident, the circumstances leading up to the event can be a valuable guide as to the nature and severity of any injuries. The environmental conditions, the position of casualties and the proximity of other objects such as vehicles all give useful clues as to the mechanism of injury.

THE CARER'S TALE

Children are unique in often having someone in close proximity who is looking after them. This person, who is usually a parent but may be a relative, friend or teacher, can usually give a good account of what has happened. Depending on their relationship to the child, they may also know about other parts of the history. Teachers, for instance, often know about illnesses and medication.

WHAT THE BYSTANDER SAW

People at the scene of an incident often give valuable information. Such people may include passers-by, neighbours or professionals such as police officers and fire-fighters. Sometimes the accounts may differ, but usually the essential details are consistent. After the incident, all these people disperse and this part of the history may be lost for ever.

THE CHILD'S OWN ACCOUNT

It goes without saying that children vary widely in their ability to communicate. A neonate may make signals that are only understood by its mother whereas teenagers use the same level of communication as adults. The type and level of language used is also influenced by the child's intelligence and environment. Consequently, communicating with a child is a difficult art which comes more naturally to some than to others.

The person trying to elicit a medical history from a child must pitch the questions at the right level and continually reassess the responses of the child. It is obviously a mistake to phrase a question in language that a small child cannot understand. However, it is equally ineffective to address older children with questions in "baby language" that leave them feeling patronized. Children often respond very well to appropriate questions. Their account of events can be extremely accurate. It should not be assumed that an adult's story of events is any more credible than an older child's.

WHAT OTHER HEALTH PROFESSIONALS ASK

Doctors and nurses all take histories; they use slightly different structures according to differing professional needs. The AMPLE format described above is probably the best one in the immediate-care situation, but it is important to understand other methods. Doctors divide the information into:

- presenting complaint and history of presenting complaint – what has been happening to prompt the current need for help
- past medical history – past illnesses and operations
- social history – the environment that the child lives in and the people that they live with

- family history – medical problems of other family members
- drugs and allergies – the child's current and past medication and known allergies
- review of systems – a checklist of the different body systems involving inquiry into possible problems with each.

Nurses use a variety of structures which focus on the environment needed to care for the child during the illness.

> Never delay urgent treatment to collect unnecessary data

RELEVANT IMMEDIATE QUESTIONS

The AMPLE structure describes most relevant details; the depth of inquiry should vary with the immediacy of the situation. Once again it should be emphasized that immediate assessment and corrective interventions take precedence over almost all questioning. The questions below should be addressed to the most appropriate person, be that the carer or the child.

Breathing problems, fits, pain, injury and general symptoms of infection are responsible for the majority of paediatric emergencies. A systemic consideration of some useful urgent questions is helpful. These questions make up the E (events) and some of the P (past medical history) of AMPLE. The list below is by no means exhaustive, but it serves to illustrate the technique of direct questioning to ascertain the need for urgent action. The form of the question must be tailored to the situation and the people.

AIRWAY

Diagnosis of the problem

- When did the problem start?
- Is there reason to suspect an inhaled foreign body?

Severity of the problem

- Has the child been distressed?
- Has the child been drooling?
- Can the child eat and drink?

BREATHING

Diagnosis of the problem

- When did it start?
- Has it ever happened before?

Severity of the problem

- Has the child been responding normally?
- Has the child been distressed?
- Has the child ever needed steroids?

- Has the child ever been admitted to hospital with breathing problems before?
- If admitted, has the child ever been on an intensive care unit?

CIRCULATION

Diagnosis of the problem

- When did it start?
- Has the child any heart problems?
- Does the child have a rash? Meningococcal septicaemia causes purpura (bruises)
- Has the child had any diarrhoea or vomiting?

Severity of the problem

- Has the child been responding normally?

DISABILITY

- When did it start?
- Has the child been responding normally?
- Does the child have a rash?
- Has the mother (or other carer) noticed any agitation or an odd cry or affect?

ENVIRONMENT

- In what position is the child most comfortable?
- Is the child too hot or too cold?

FITS

Diagnosis of the problem

- Has the child ever had fits before?
- Has the child been generally unwell in any way before the fit?
- Has the child had a raised temperature?
- Have the child's eyes rolled up at the time of the attack? (Mothers often notice this)
- Was the child playing when he or she went limp and collapsed? Febrile convulsions often occur with minimal tonic/clonic activity.

Severity of the problem

- How long did the fit last?

GLUCOSE

Diagnosis of the problem

- Does the child have diabetes?
- Has the child had his or her normal insulin dose?
- Has the child been eating and drinking normally?

Young children have limited stores of glucose. Always check blood sugar in seriously ill children and correct if evidence exists of hypoglycaemia, regardless of whether or not the child is diabetic.

> **Hypoglycaemia in any child is a life-threatening emergency**

Severity of the problem

- Has the child been behaving and responding normally?

IMMEDIATE NEEDS

- Where does it hurt?
- How bad is it?

SUMMARY

- Airway
- Breathing
- Circulation
- Disability
- Environment
- Fits
- Glucose
- Immediate needs.

It is important to note the differences (and similarities) between this system and the ABCDE of trauma resuscitation.

FURTHER BACKGROUND QUESTIONS

In the situation of immediate care, extensive consideration of the child's background is often irrelevant and may be counterproductive. However, it is useful to have some appreciation of the special features of a child's history.

MATERNAL HEALTH AND PREGNANCY

The health of the mother may affect the development of the fetus. Maternal infections such as rubella may lead to a damaged baby.

BIRTH PROBLEMS

A difficult birth (caesarean section or forceps delivery) may later manifest itself as developmental problems or fits. Was the child on the special care baby unit (SCBU)? If so, then the perinatal period was not as smooth as it might have been.

DEVELOPMENT

The continuing rapid development of a child distinguishes it from the adult. Questions should be asked about relationships, behaviour, play, school, sports and activities.

IMMUNIZATIONS

Children in the UK benefit from a planned programme of immunizations. The immunizations received by the child should be ascertained.

SIBLINGS

The health of brothers and sisters may give useful information concerning a child's illness.

EXPLORATION OF THE CURRENT PROBLEM

It is important to listen to the story told by the child or the carer. Direct questions will involve expanding on the AMPLE format and the systematic A–I approach above. The particular complaints that are common in children may also involve:

- raised temperature or shivering
- lethargy or drowsiness
- headache and neck stiffness
- aches and pains
- cough, cold, sore throat and earache
- feeding problems
- diarrhoea and vomiting
- reduced or increased urine output (? normal wet nappies in a small child)
- difficulty sleeping.

Sometimes the worries of the parents and other carers predominate over the symptoms of the child and these problems must be explored also.

LANGUAGE PROBLEMS

The UK is a multicultural society and children reflect this in the languages that they speak. Most children speak excellent English, but in a crisis they may revert to the language that they speak at home. Gentle rephrasing of the questions may be successful, but sometimes another person is needed to act as a translator.

EARLY SUSPICIONS OF CHILD ABUSE

Several different types of child abuse are now recognized.

- Physical abuse (non-accidental injury)
- Emotional abuse
- Neglect
- Sexual abuse
- Organized or ritual abuse.

There are patterns of physical signs for some types of abuse, but the history and the context in which the events occurred are the most important first indicators to alert the health worker. The following features of a history of injury might point to abuse.

- Inappropriate delay in seeking help and advice after a significant injury
- Previous history of frequent accidents
- The history of the accident is not a likely mechanism for that injury
- Vague or absent history of an accident
- Different carers give different explanations for the same injury
- The child gives a different history
- The injury is supposed to have been sustained in a way that is inconsistent with the child's development, for example, a fall before the child has started walking
- The adults with the child are either unconcerned or hostile during questioning.

The prehospital worker is in a unique position to note two particular factors.

1. The *home* – the environment from which a child comes is often seen by prehospital workers. This environment may have changed by the time others (such as social workers) can visit it.
2. The *initial story* – one of the best pointers to physical abuse is inconsistency in the history, both between those telling it and in respect of the likely mechanism of injury. Such inconsistencies may well have been "ironed out" by the time the tale is told to hospital staff.

> Suspicions of child abuse, in whatever form, should not be voiced in the prehospital environment. Such concerns should be brought to the attention of the senior doctor after arrival in hospital. It is also the individual responsibility of paramedics to ensure any concerns are reported to the relevant social services department. All ambulance trusts should have a child welfare policy in place that details the correct procedure.

RECORD–KEEPING

Good, legible records are of vital importance, although "good" should not be taken as meaning "long". Accurate details help medical and nursing staff to deliver appropriate care while giving due consideration to the prehospital situation and treatment. The history given (and recorded) often makes sense of what later seem to be inexplicable events and actions. In addition, paramedics are often judged by the quality of their written information.

Sometimes, many months or years later, the prehospital records provide important information. Cases involving children may be the subject of social investigation and legal actions may be delayed until the child reaches maturity. At such a time, the paramedic may be called to give evidence in court. Failure to make sense of one's own records is acutely embarrassing, to say the least! In cases of litigation where a health worker is involved, the court may sometimes take the view that the quality of the records may reflect the quality of the care given. In any case, actions omitted from the records will be taken as omissions from the actions of the worker involved.

Derogatory comments or criticisms are best not recorded in the notes. Children can be very difficult to manage – but they learn their strange behaviour from adults! However, a record of the paramedic's opinion on such episodes is often hard to justify at a later date. Any concerns are best communicated directly to hospital staff.

HOW TO HAND OVER THE HISTORY TO THE HOSPITAL

Good communication is vital at the point where the care of the patient is transferred from the prehospital workers to the hospital. It should include both handing over the written records of the history and some direct discussion. What happened after the ambulance arrived and during the journey to the hospital is now part of the history!

FURTHER READING

Advanced Life Support Group 1997 Advanced paediatric life support, 2nd edn. BMJ Publications, London

Advanced Life Support Group 2005 Pre-hospital paediatric life support, 2nd edn. Blackwell Publishing, Oxford

American Heart Association & American Academy of Pediatrics 1997 Pediatric advanced life support. American Heart Association, Dallas

Morton RJ, Phillips BM 1992 Accidents and emergencies in children. Oxford University Press, Oxford

Moulton C, Yates DW 1999 Lecture notes on emergency medicine. Blackwell Science, Oxford

Chapter 35

Assessment of the ill or injured child

INTRODUCTION

Assessment should be carried out in a structured fashion, correcting problems as they are identified. The aim of the prehospital assessment is management of the child's condition rather than specific diagnosis.

DIFFERENCES BETWEEN ASSESSING ADULTS AND CHILDREN

The principles of paediatric assessment are identical to those applicable for an adult. Problems arise because the range of ages – and hence sizes – of children affects physiological measurements, drug doses and equipment sizes. An expected adult weight range is 45–90 kg; that is, a two-fold difference. Children's weights may easily vary from 3 kg to 60 kg; a 20-fold range. A factor of two is often disregarded – most adults are given a standard dose of drugs and assumed to have similar physiological parameters. A 20-fold difference is impossible to ignore; treatment must be tailored to the size of the child.

The age of a child is usually known but the weight is more difficult to ascertain. Because of this it is important to be able to estimate a child's weight from a knowledge of the age. A method of doing this is shown in Table 35.1.

The weight of a child in kilograms can be approximately calculated by the formula:

Weight in kg = (age in years + 4) × 2

This works well between the ages of 1 year and 10 years.

Table 35.1 Estimating a child's weight

Age	Weight (kg)
2 months	5
6 months	7.5
1 year	10
3.5 years	15
6 years	20
10 years	30
13 years	40
14 years	50

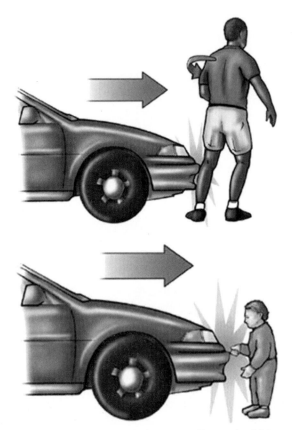

Figure 35.1 A different pattern of injuries will occur in children and adults even if the mechanism is the same

The average birthweight of a full-term infant is 3.5 kg; this has usually doubled by 5 months of age and tripled by 12 months.

Surface area is needed to assess the area of a burn. It is best to use a Lund and Browder chart but a quick estimate can be made on the basis that the palm of the patient's hand and adducted fingers are approximately equivalent to 1% of the body surface area. Serial halving is also a useful technique (see Chapter 37).

The conditions with which children present are different. They do not generally suffer from the degenerative diseases of adult life, but have problems with infective conditions. Their fast metabolism and low reserves mean that they become ill (and cold) very quickly, but their general health and high capacity for repair make for a speedy recovery.

Children usually die from *hypoxia* (secondary to respiratory distress or depression) or from *hypovolaemia* (fluid loss or maldistribution). These lead to cardiac asystole which has a very poor prognosis. Therefore, it is vital to recognize and reverse these conditions before terminal bradycardia supervenes. Coronary artery disease and thus ventricular fibrillation is uncommon in children.

Children differ in their body proportions from adults. They also have a more elastic skeleton. These facts make for a different pattern of injury and for an airway that can be more difficult to manage.

The interaction with the assessor is as variable as the age of the child. Only practice can teach the subtle parts of this relationship, but those with children of their own have a distinct advantage.

IMMEDIATE ASSESSMENT

The SAFE approach should be used. Children are usually easy to move to a safer place.

For paediatric cardiac arrest protocols see Chapter 37.

AIRWAY

First, *check for responsiveness.* A response is usually immediately obvious. If it is not, then gentle shaking may establish verbal communication with an older child. The young child will respond by eye movement, cry or body posture – the mother will know. Failure to respond indicates a significantly lowered level of consciousness and therefore an airway at risk. There may be a need for airway opening manoeuvres and action to protect the airway.

Partial upper airway obstruction is suggested by:

- snoring – the familiar sound of obstruction caused by the soft tissues of the mouth and pharynx ("the tongue falling back" is the usual oversimplified but easily understood explanation); it often accompanies the reduced muscle tone of a lowered level of consciousness
- rattling or gurgling – the sound of fluids in the upper airway.

For airway opening manoeuvres, recovery position and suction clearance of the airway, see Chapter 6.

Stridor is a harsh, "crowing" noise which is heard best in inspiration – this differentiates it from wheezing, which is usually loudest in expiration. Stridor suggests obstruction at the level of the larynx and upper trachea. General illness and raised temperature usually indicate an infection causing swelling. Obstruction by a foreign body is the other main cause.

> Do not examine the throat with any instrument in children with stridor or suspected partial airway obstruction – doing so may convert the problem to complete obstruction

Drooling, the inability to swallow saliva, suggests blockage at the back of the throat.

> Cyanosis and reduced haemoglobin saturation readings on a pulse oximeter are very late signs of airway obstruction

For management of laryngotracheal obstruction see Chapter 6. For choking protocols see Chapter 6.

Ask yourself if this child needs:

- the recovery position?
- a sitting-up position?
- suctioning?

Box 35.1 Airway and endotracheal tube sizes

Oropharyngeal airway size = approximately the distance from the centre of the lips to the angle of the jaw
Nasopharyngeal airway size = approximately the distance from the tip of the nose to the tragus of the ear
Endotracheal tube size:

Internal diameter (mm) $= \dfrac{\text{age in years}}{4} + 4$ (neonate 3–3.5 mm tube)

Oral tube length (cm) $= \dfrac{\text{age in years}}{2} + 12$

Nasal tube length (cm) $= \dfrac{\text{age in years}}{2} + 15$

- manual maintenance of the airway?
- an airway adjunct?
- intubation?
- oxygen?

All children with the problems identified below will benefit from high-concentration oxygen therapy. There is no need to assess "risk" as in adults with chronic lung disease. Only a small group of infants with congenital heart disease need controlled oxygen therapy.

> It is not worth struggling to make an unwilling child wear an oxygen mask

The need for aids to maintain the airway is assessed on the same criteria in the child as in the adult. However, if a child's airway can be maintained by simple manoeuvres, an oropharyngeal (Guedel) airway is best avoided. This is because retching is easily induced in children and may be followed by laryngospasm or aspiration. For assessment of artificial airway and endotracheal tube sizes, see Box 35.1

> Assess the need for cervical spine protection before any airway intervention

The presence or absence of the gag reflex gives no useful information. Testing for it in children may easily induce retching or laryngospasm and create an airway problem.

BREATHING

Look, listen and feel for breathing. The absence of breath sounds indicates the need to follow procedures for cardiorespiratory arrest (Chapter 37).
Look for:

1. difficulty in talking – a child who is unable to speak because of laboured breathing is very unwell
2. an abnormal respiratory rate – usually fast, laboured breathing (Table 35.2). Very slow respiratory rates may occur just before

Table 35.2 Respiratory and pulse rates in children

Age (years)	Respiratory rate (breaths/minute)	Pulse rate (beats/minute)
Under 1	30–40	110–160
1–5	25–30	95–140
6–12	20–25	80–120

respiratory arrest or in children poisoned with narcotic drugs, e.g. methadone
3. recession of the chest wall – the indrawing of the elastic tissues of a child caused by increased respiratory effort
4. wheezing and rattling, grunting and panting
5. nasal flaring and use of the shoulder and neck muscles during breathing
6. unequal or diminished breath sounds.

> Absence of breath sounds means that the movement of air in the lungs is so diminished that it cannot be heard

All the above suggest that the child is struggling to achieve normal respiration. Failure to adequately oxygenate the blood and hence the tissues is shown by:

- tachycardia – the hypoxic nervous system is stimulating the heart (for normal values see Table 35.2)
- cyanosis – a late sign
- irritability, confusion or reduced responsiveness mean that the brain is short of oxygen – this is an extremely worrying sign.

> The oxygen saturation shown by the pulse oximeter should be close to 100% in a normal, healthy child

Ask yourself if this child needs:

- oxygen?
- a bronchodilator, e.g. salbutamol?
- intubation and ventilation?

All wheezy children will benefit from nebulized bronchodilators, whether they are known to be asthmatic or not. Ask the parents how much of this type of drug the child has already had and look for agitation, tachycardia and tremor – the signs of overdosage. Remember, however, that these may also be signs of hypoxia.

Ventilation is indicated as an emergency procedure for respiratory insufficiency in a child in the same way as in an adult. Suggested ventilator settings for children are:

- tidal volume 10 ml per kg
- minute volume 100 ml per kg.

The assessment of chest injury uses the same techniques in children as in adults. Because of the elastic chest wall, children are far less likely to have rib fractures than adults, although they may have severe underlying lung damage (see Chapter 25).

Breathing: what to look for.

- Difficulty talking
- Abnormal respiratory rate
- Chest wall recession
- Wheezing and rattling, grunting and panting
- Nasal flaring and accessory muscles
- Unequal or diminished breath sounds
- Tachycardia
- Cyanosis
- Irritability, confusion, drowsiness.

CIRCULATION

Check for a central pulse (over 10 seconds). The brachial or femoral pulses should be used in infants rather than the carotid pulse, as their necks make carotid palpation difficult. The absence of a central pulse (or a rate of less than 60 beats per minute in infants) indicates the need to follow procedures for cardiorespiratory arrest (see Chapter 37).

> In a child with ventricular fibrillation and no obvious precipitating factors, the cause could be poisoning with tricyclic antidepressants

Look for the following.

1. A fast or slow heart rate (for normal values see Table 35.2). Fast heart rates usually mean that either (a) there is a cardiac arrhythmia or, more commonly (b) the nervous system has detected a problem with the body (such as hypoxia, hypoglycaemia, pain or fear) and is "instructing" the heart to beat faster. A slow heart rate usually means that something is wrong with the heart itself. The worst cause of this is severe hypoxia (or hypovolaemia) and, in this case, terminal bradycardia and asystole are only seconds away. This is the mechanism of most cardiac arrests in children. Occasionally, bradycardia is seen with poisoning and severe head injury; it may also occur in syncopal attacks.

2. Abnormal systolic blood pressure – this varies with age. A useful formula to calculate the expected systolic blood pressure is:

$$\text{systolic blood pressure (mmHg)} = 80 + (\text{age in years} \times 2)$$

Blood pressure can be difficult to measure in young, restless children and requires a cuff of the correct size. It will not fall until very late in shock. It may be raised with intracerebral and renal problems.

3. A raised capillary refill time – it should be less than 2 seconds if the circulation is satisfactory. However, peripheral shut down in a cold, wet child can easily produce a prolonged refill time.

4. Pallor and coolness of the skin – the body diverts blood away from the skin when there are circulatory problems and these signs are thus very useful.

5. Active bleeding.

> A child's blood volume is approximately 80 ml/kg

Inadequate circulation will reduce tissue oxygenation and thus may also cause:

- a raised respiratory rate
- altered mental status as detailed above.

Circulation: what to look for.

- Fast or slow heart rate
- Abnormal systolic blood pressure
- Increased capillary refill time
- Pallor and coolness of the skin
- Active bleeding
- Raised respiratory rate
- Instability, confusion, drowsiness.

The ECG is rarely as helpful in making a diagnosis in children as it is in adults, except for arrhythmias. A cardiac monitor does, however, provide constant information about the heart rate.

Ask yourself if this child needs:

- oxygen?
- pressure haemostasis?
- intravenous fluids?
- vagal manoeuvres (tachyarrhythmia)?
- sitting up (pulmonary oedema)?
- urgent penicillin therapy (meningococcal septicaemia)?

The need for venous access and the site should be assessed carefully. There is nothing worse than looking for veins on a screaming child who is covered with bruises from previous attempts by someone else. Remember the possibility of intraosseous infusion.

> Bolus fluid therapy should be calculated at 20ml/kg and after further assessment repeated as necessary

DISABILITY

Look for the following.

1. A reduced level of consciousness. This is the most important sign of any problem which is affecting the brain. Even sleepy

children should be fairly easy to rouse. The AVPU scoring system is as useful for children as for adults:

A > Alert
V > Voice elicits a response
P > Pain elicits a response
U > Unresponsive

Note: the parents of an ill child are usually in a highly distressed state, so be careful how you elicit the pain response; pressure on a fingernail is probably the most subtle way.

> Consider hypoglycaemia as a cause for a reduced level of consciousness

2. Abnormal pupils – look for size, equality and reactivity. These features can be affected by both drugs and brain disease. Dilated, fixed or unequal pupils are worrying signs in children as they are in adults.
3. Abnormal posture and limb movements – children may be flaccid or show abnormal posturing. Limb movements may be unequal; sometimes this is congenital but it is best never to assume so.

Severe intracerebral problems may also cause:

- airway obstruction
- respiratory depression (respiration, unlike the heart beat, requires an intact brainstem)
- bradycardia and hypertension.

Signs of an intracerebral problem

- Reduced level of consciousness
- Abnormal pupils
- Abnormal posture and limbs movement
- Airway obstruction
- Respiratory depression
- Bradycardia and hypertension

Ask yourself if this child needs:

- the recovery position?
- other airway care?
- oxygen?
- ventilation?
- intravenous access?
- glucose?
- urgent penicillin therapy?

EXPOSURE AND ENVIRONMENT

Look for:

1. cold extremities
2. shivering
3. wet clothing
4. pyrexia and clamminess
5. the position in which the child is most comfortable
6. the proximity of the mother or other carer.

> In a child, cold limbs usually indicate a cold trunk and head

Attention to these details early on can radically change the well-being (and demeanour) of a child.

A child may well need clothing removed to facilitate assessment. However, children easily become cold and embarrassed.

Ask yourself if this child needs:

- wet clothing removed?
- warmth?
- cooling measures?
- repositioning or support of a limb?
- his or her mother?
- covering up (embarrassment)?

FITS

Look for:

1. frank tonic or clonic activity
2. spasmodic twitching
3. postictal drowsiness
4. gurgling, rattling or other signs of airway obstruction
5. cyanosis – during a fit there is a very high demand for oxygen, coupled with respiratory inadequacy
6. signs of head injury
7. signs of other injury caused by a convulsion (e.g. a bitten tongue and intraoral bleeding)
8. reasons to consider hypoglycaemia.

It is very difficult to assess or manage a fitting child. Hence termination of the convulsion must be an immediate aim.

Ask yourself if this child needs:

- the recovery position?
- other airway care?
- oxygen?
- intravenous access?
- anticonvulsant therapy, for example rectal diazepam?
- glucose?
- urgent penicillin therapy?

GLUCOSE

Children are like fast-burning little engines and become short of oxygen and fuel very quickly. Their fuel is glucose and they have relatively low glycogen reserves. Glucagon will therefore be less consistently effective than in adults.

Look for:

1. restlessness, agitation or other mental change ("jitteriness" in a neonate)

2. a reduced level of consciousness
3. signs of insulin usage. (All diabetic children will be on insulin – oral hypoglycaemic drugs are generally only used in adults. This does not mean, of course, that a child cannot take someone else's drugs and become hypoglycaemic!)
4. a low blood glucose level on testing with a reagent strip
5. convulsions – can be caused by hypoglycaemia.

Ask yourself if this child needs:

- the recovery position?
- other airway care?
- oxygen?
- intravenous access?
- glucose therapy?

Glucose: 5 mls per kg of 10% dextrose solution (ie. 0.5 mg per kg of glucose)

HISTORY

After immediate problems have been assessed and appropriate action has been initiated, further information may be sought. The AMPLE structure is recommended as providing adequate historical detail in the prehospital situation. Appropriate immediate questions are discussed in Chapter 34. Some of the answers will give enormous help in the assessment of both the type of problem and the likely severity.

Ask yourself:

- are the answers to these questions going to affect the immediate management of this child?

IMMEDIATE NEEDS OF THE CHILD

Some immediate needs will have been assessed, under "environment". These needs include the provision of warmth, the removal of wet clothing and the need to ensure psychological support from the mother or other carer. A position of comfort is also mandatory; it may be life-saving in conditions such as epiglottitis.

The relief of suffering is as usual of paramount importance. This may entail assessing the following.

1. *The need for analgesia* – this can be very difficult to assess in a distressed child. Exact localization of pain is difficult in very young children, but careful observation and discussion with the mother often helps. If analgesic drugs are available, they can turn an unmanageable situation into a calm one. They also reassure the carers. It is far better to give analgesia freely to children who may be in pain than to withhold it on the spurious grounds that it alters conscious level or masks pupillary or abdominal signs. Gaseous analgesia (Entonox) may be inappropriate for younger children as they find it frightening and do not have enough inspiratory force to open the demand valve.
2. *The need for limb splintage* – simple limb support with troughs and pillows can be very helpful in children with limb injuries.

Distal circulation should be assessed before and after positioning limbs in the same way in children as in adults.

3. *The tolerance of cervical and spinal splintage* – conscious children often do not tolerate this sort of device very well. If a collar is distressing a child significantly, it is better to remove it. The mother's hands and pillows can be more acceptable substitutes. A child who is struggling to remove a collar is actually moving the neck more than a child with no splint who is lying still. This is also true for immobilization on a spine board. The indications for spinal immobilization are the same in children as in adults, although young children are less accurate in localizing the pain of spinal injury.

Ask yourself if this child needs:

- drugs to relieve pain
- splintage
- freedom from splintage.

FURTHER ASSESSMENT

For further information concerning the recognition of the seriously ill child, see Chapter 36.

For further assessment of injuries see Chapter 38.

THE NEEDS OF THE PARENTS

The needs of the carers cannot be ignored. These may vary from simple reassurance to medical treatment. The satisfactory treatment of children depends on the support of those closest to them. The mental state of a child may be inseparable from that of the mother. Parental anxiety or difficulty coping is a good reason for admitting a child to hospital.

FLUID LOSS AND DEHYDRATION

Look for the following.

1. Purpura – these small bruises may be the first sign of meningococcal septicaemia.
2. Abdominal pain, tenderness or rigidity following trauma or illness. Large amounts of fluid or blood can be "lost" into the abdomen. The elastic ribs and low liver and spleen increase the possibility of intraabdominal damage.
3. Dehydration, shown by a dry, non-elastic skin or sunken eyes. In infants a floppy anterior fontanelle is a useful, if late, sign of severe fluid loss. Diarrhoea and vomiting can quickly dehydrate a small child.
4. Wet nappies confirm urine output in young children. The child's carer will know their normal state.

LEVEL OF CONSCIOUSNESS

Although the AVPU method is quick and convenient, the Glasgow Coma Scale (GCS) is the standard method of scoring a reduced level of consciousness from any cause. The

Box 35.2 The Glasgow Coma Scale in children

Response elicited	Score
BEST EYE OPENING RESPONSE	
Open spontaneously	4
React to speech	3
React to pain	2
No response	1
BEST MOTOR RESPONSE	
Moves normally and spontaneously or obeys commands	6
Localizes pain	5
Withdraws in response to pain	4
Flexes abnormally to pain (decorticate movements)	3
Extends abnormally to pain (decerebrate movements)	2
No response	1
BEST "VERBAL" RESPONSE	
Smiles, follows sounds and objects, interacts	5
Cries consolably or interacts inappropriately	4
Cries with inconsistent relief or moans	3
Cries inconsolably or is irritable	2
No response	1

standard (adult) GCS is suitable for children of school age, but a special variant of the GCS is more appropriate in children under 4 years old. Box 35.2 gives the children's coma scale.

Even in experienced hands, the children's coma scale is difficult to apply and even more difficult to remember. Do not delay a transfer to perform a coma scale assessment; use "AVPU and pupils".

POISONING

Bizarre symptoms and signs and unexplained combinations of findings suggest poisoning. Younger children may ingest substances accidentally; older children may experiment with drugs. Look for the most common signs:

- confusion, agitation and drowsiness
- tachycardia
- dilated pupils
- evidence at the scene (which is of enormous help to hospital staff).

OTHER IMPORTANT FINDINGS

1. Raised temperature – a hand on the abdomen may reveal an obvious pyrexia. This often accompanies a fit: febrile convulsions are common between 5 months and 5 years of age. Children with epilepsy are more likely to have a fit during a pyrexia.
2. Neck stiffness indicates inflammation of the meninges, i.e. meningitis. This is often accompanied by pyrexia, headache and drowsiness; however, the diagnosis can be difficult.

3. Rashes usually indicate systemic infection, allergy or specific skin disease. Purpura is the most worrying skin sign (suggesting possible meningococcal septicaemia or other cause of vasculitis).
4. Drawing up of the knees suggests pain in the abdomen.
5. Signs of congenital abnormality – children with congenital problems are often prone to fits and chest infections.
6. The relationship and interaction with the parents and the other family members is always important.

UPPER RESPIRATORY TRACT INFECTION

Young children may have upper respiratory problems up to 10 times a year. Such infections may precipitate asthma attacks or lead to more serious chest infections.

Look for the following.

1. A cough and/or a runny nose – the most common signs of infection. The barking cough of croup is important to recognize as it may accompany stridor. Whooping cough is very distressing (Severe coughing empties the lungs and is followed by an inspiratory "whoop".) Children with upper respiratory infections often have a sore throat. There may be enlarged lymph nodes in the neck or even in the abdomen (mesenteric adenitis) which can mimic appendicitis. Asthma may cause nocturnal coughing.
2. Pulling at the ears – young children may pull at their ears if they have earache. Otitis media (infection of the middle ear) is a frequent accompaniment of upper respiratory infection in children.

SIGNS OF CHILD ABUSE

See Chapter 34 for elements of a history which lead to suspicions of abuse.

Signs suggestive of non-accidental injury

- Unexplained head, facial, chest or limb injuries – especially in children who are not able to walk and thus fall (few children walk before the age of 11 months)
- Multiple bruising
- Injuries of different ages
- Unusual burns (e.g. those of a "glove" or "stocking" distribution)
- Unusual cuts and bruises – imprints of hands, sticks, cords, shoes, belts and teeth may be present.

CONTINUING ASSESSMENT

Assessment should continue during initial treatment and transportation. Children may change their physiological status very rapidly. It is particularly important to assess the effect of any interventions.

Monitoring needs to be appropriate to the child's condition and should not replace careful observation. It needs to be considered in terms of usefulness of information obtained and acceptability to the child. In a conscious child, this probably means *pulse oximetry* is better than *ECG monitoring* which is better than *blood pressure monitoring*.

CONSIDERATION OF OTHER CHILDREN IN THE VICINITY

In many situations, such as severe infections, fires, poisoning and abuse, other children may have been exposed to the same agents as the patient. In such cases it is appropriate to assess the risk to these children also. Sometimes, full assessment (and the need for speed) may necessitate bringing other children into hospital along with the primary patient.

FURTHER READING

Advanced Life Support Group 1997 Advanced paediatric life support 2nd edn. BMJ Publications, London

Advanced Life Support Group 2005 Pre-hospital paediatric life support 2nd edn. Blackwell Publishing

American Heart Association and the American Academy of Pediatrics 1997 Pediatric advanced life support. American Heart Association, Dallas

Morton RJ, Phillips BM 1992 Accidents and emergencies in children. Oxford University Press, Oxford

Moulton C, Yates DW 1999 Lecture notes on emergency medicine. Blackwell science, Oxford

Chapter 36

The sick child

CHAPTER CONTENTS

INTRODUCTION

Children tend to be treated with a greater sense of urgency than adults. This reflects both the instinct that most adults have to protect the young and the generally held view that children can "go off" quickly. This sense of urgency is useful in that it focuses care on the child. It must not, however, be allowed to deteriorate into a sense of panic. If carers are happy about their diagnostic and treatment abilities then they will be able to care for children with confidence. Gaining this confidence requires both training and practice.

It may seem obvious to state that recognizing that a child is ill is the key to ensuring that the best outcome is obtained. In fact, there is a definite skill to this and this skill has to be studied and practised like any other. The importance of the ability to recognize the severity of childhood illness cannot be overemphasized – a decision to rapidly transport a child to hospital may mean the difference between life and death. A considerable proportion of this chapter is devoted to this skill.

Once the seriousness of their condition has been established some children may need interventions prior to and during transport. Some appropriate treatments are discussed at the end of this chapter. Specific conditions are not dealt with in detail since the priority for seriously ill children is rapid, safe transportation to an advanced facility, rather than diagnosis and treatment at the scene.

RECOGNITION OF SERIOUS ILLNESS

Health workers with a great deal of paediatric experience will intuitively recognize a very sick child. Those with less experience should approach the assessment of each child systematically in order to decide whether they are seriously ill or not. This systematic approach should follow the familiar ABC pattern.

AIRWAY

The airway may be patent or obstructed, protected or unprotected. Obstruction may be partial or complete and protection may be secure or insecure. Any child who has anything other than an open and securely protected airway is seriously ill.

Airway patency

If the child is conscious then a simple question such as *"How are you?"* or *"What's wrong?"* should start the assessment. Even the examination of babies begins with quiet gentle reassuring speech, which should be maintained throughout the examination. If the child answers then this confirms that the airway is patent and implies that pharyngeal and laryngeal function are such that it is protected. It is important to remember that there are many reasons why a child fails to answer such questions (fear of strangers and inability to talk being two obvious ones), and silence does not therefore imply that the airway is obstructed.

In an unconscious child an appropriate airway-opening manoeuvre should be performed and breathing should be assessed as described below.

Airway protection

An airway may be insecure either because the protective pharyngeal and laryngeal reflexes are absent (usually because conscious level is decreased for whatever reason) or because there is a developing pathological condition which places the airway at risk. A child with a significantly reduced conscious level (responding to pain or verbal stimuli only or unresponsive) should be considered to be seriously ill since the airway is at risk.

> The airway is at risk in any child who is not fully conscious

BREATHING

An apnoeic child is fairly easy to spot and is clearly seriously ill. It is much more difficult to recognize children with inadequate breathing, but these children are potentially as ill as those who are apnoeic and the earlier they are picked out, the better their prognosis. Adequacy of breathing should be examined as follows.

Effort of breathing

As breathing becomes more difficult, more effort is required to maintain it. This fact can be used to try and spot children with breathing difficulty. The respiratory rate will increase from normal. Normal ranges vary depending on the age of the child (Table 36.1).

The respiratory rate should be counted by exposing the chest. Exposure will also enable another major sign of increased respiratory rate to be seen – *recession*. Recession is the appearance of indrawing of the chest wall that occurs while it is expanding during inspiration. It can be seen in a number of areas: intercostal (between the ribs), subcostal (below the ribs) and sternal. The last is usually only apparent in younger children (<2 years old) who have very elastic chests.

Extra noises may be heard during the breathing cycle. Wheezes (during both inspiration and expiration) indicate

Age (years)	Respiratory rate (breaths/min)
<1	30–40
1–5	25–30
6–12	20–25

Table 36.1 Normal respiratory rates in children

that respiratory work is raised because of the increased pressure associated with narrowing of the airways. Severe upper airway obstruction (such as that caused by a foreign body) can result in stridor. It is important to note that the loudness does not correspond to the severity of the problem. In fact, silence in a previously noisy chest can be one of the most worrying signs of all, in that it may indicate either exhaustion or total obstruction.

Effectiveness of efforts to breathe

Initially, as the work of breathing increases, effectiveness will be maintained but eventually the body will not be able to keep up the effort and signs of inadequate breathing will appear. Depth of breathing (or in infants abdominal movement) can be a useful indicator, as can a falling respiratory rate.

If breathing is inadequate, the effects do not only manifest themselves in the chest. Hypoxia (reduction in oxygenation) initially causes the heart rate to rise as the body attempts to deliver more blood to the tissues to make up for the lower concentration of oxygen. Eventually, however, the heart rate falls to below normal levels: this is a very serious sign and usually indicates imminent death. Hypoxia will also affect conscious level. First of all the child becomes agitated but as the low oxygen delivery continues, drowsiness and then unconsciousness will ensue.

> Bradycardia in a sick child or infant is a critical sign

The advent of pulse oximetry has been a great advance in non-invasive monitoring. It allows oxygen saturation to be measured in any situation and is an invaluable tool in assessing the adequacy of breathing. Saturation may be normal if breathing is adequate, may be low (less than 95% on air) if there is some impairment or very low (less than 90% on air or less than 95% on oxygen) if breathing is seriously impaired. The great advantage of using pulse oximetry is that continuous objective assessment of breathing can be undertaken.

CIRCULATION

Circulation may be present or absent and, if present, may be adequate or inadequate. It is fairly easy to decide that circulation is absent by palpating a large artery (carotid or femoral in a child or brachial in an infant) for 5 seconds to see whether any pulse is present. As with breathing, however, it is not the ability to spot the child who has already died that is important but rather the recognition of the child who is critically ill and whose life is threatened. In order to achieve this, the state of the child's circulation must be systematically examined.

Decreased capillary refill time and increasing peripheral pallor and coolness are early signs of a failing circulation in children. The capillary refill is measured by applying gentle pressure (enough to squeeze out the blood) over the forehead or sternum for 5 seconds, then releasing the pressure and counting the time in seconds that it takes for the blood to return. The normal time is less than 2 seconds.

Both pulse rate and blood pressure can be measured, but the assessment and interpretation of these figures are fraught with difficulty, especially in the very young. The normal values vary with age and, in the case of blood pressure, the equipment needed for accurate measurement is also age specific. Furthermore, significant interpretable changes occur later rather than earlier. For those who do manage to measure these parameters accurately, normal values are shown in Table 36.2.

A raised respiratory rate and a decreased level of consciousness may both result from circulatory inadequacy.

DISABILITY

Disability assessment involves a rapid evaluation of conscious level. Children with a reduced conscious level for whatever reason should be classed as seriously ill and

treated accordingly. The simple AVPU system shown below is recommended.

A	**A**lert
V	Responds to **V**oice
P	Responds to **P**ain
U	**U**nresponsive

Any voice prompt can be used but calling the child's name is recommended. It must be remembered that very young children may not recognize words but all should recognize the sound of a voice. The painful stimulus should only be applied if there is no response to voice. Initially a peripheral stimulus such as fingernail bed pressure should be used; if there is no reaction this should be followed by a central stimulus such as supraorbital ridge pressure.

An examination of the pupils for size and reactivity should be carried out at this stage, although there are no pupillary signs of serious illness which are present when conscious level is normal.

ASSESSMENT SUMMARY

The recommended approach to assessing whether a child is seriously ill is summarized in Figure 36.1. It is worth noting that there are three possible outcomes. First, the child may be found to be in respiratory or cardiorespiratory arrest; in such a case the appropriate resuscitation should be started and rapid transport to an advanced facility should be arranged (Chapter 37). Second, the child may be assessed as seriously ill; in these cases appropriate levels of resuscitation should be commenced (see below) and again rapid

Table 36.2 Normal pulse rate and systolic blood pressure in children

Age (years)	Pulse rate (beats/min)	Systolic blood pressure (mmHg)
Newborn	160	60–80
<1	110–160	70–90
1–5	95–140	80–100
6–12	80–120	90–110
13+	60–100	100–120

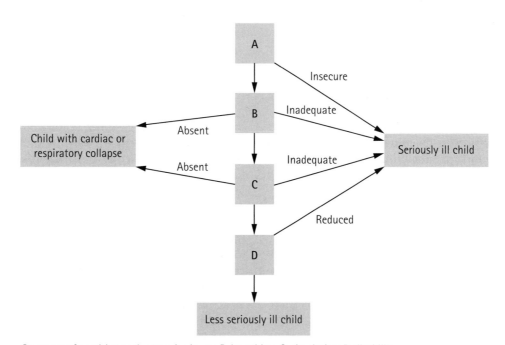

Summary of regnition pathways; A, airway; B, breathing; C, circulation; D, disability

Figure 36.1 Assessment of whether a child is seriously ill

transport should be arranged. Finally, the child may be found to be less seriously ill. In such cases transport to another facility where further evaluation can be carried out will usually be appropriate; speed is less important in these latter cases but this does not imply that time should be spent attempting procedures at the scene that could be done as well or better in hospital.

APPROPRIATE TREATMENT

Even in the best of circumstances, performing procedures on children can be practically difficult and emotionally draining for the professional involved. The difficulties encountered are worsened by adverse conditions and by inexperience in the operator. Since the circumstances of most prehospital care are not ideal, and because very few paramedics will attend seriously ill children often enough to keep a high level of proficiency in practical procedures, resuscitative procedures should be limited to those necessary for safe transportation.

AIRWAY

Opening and maintenance of the airway are both essential. Simple opening manoeuvres should be performed first – head tilt, chin lift and jaw thrust can be used in children. The head should be kept in the neutral position in infants (<1 year old), since overextension may cause deformation of the soft trachea with consequent airway obstruction.

Oropharyngeal airways can be used as simple adjuncts to airway opening. The appropriate size should be found by placing the airway vertically at the side of the face and selecting the one that reaches from the angle of the jaw to the level of the incisor teeth. The selected airway should be inserted the "right way up" by depressing the tongue (using a tongue depressor or a laryngoscope blade) and slipping the airway into the mouth until the flange lies at the lips. Attempts to insert an airway using the adult twisting technique may cause considerable damage to the soft palate and may compromise the airway as bleeding occurs. Nasopharyngeal airways are not routinely used in children.

It is important to beware of interfering with a child who has severe stridor and is managing to maintain a critically threatened airway. These children often wish to sit up during transport and should be allowed to do so. Attempts to make things better by lying the child down and opening the airway may prove to be the last straw and can precipitate respiratory arrest. Once this has occurred it can be extremely difficult to reestablish ventilation. The sensible approach to such a situation is to provide high-flow oxygen (but not to force a mask on the child) and to transport the child calmly to an advanced facility (preferably warning that facility of one's imminent arrival so that appropriate preparations can be made).

BREATHING

All children with inadequate breathing should be given oxygen in the highest possible concentration. Worries about potential oxygen toxicity are totally misplaced in such situations. Paediatric oxygen masks with rebreathing bags are available and can achieve an inspired concentration of 85% with high gas flow rates.

If respiratory support is required it can be given either by using a bag–valve–mask system or by intubating the child and using a self-inflating bag or mechanical ventilator for ventilation. The bag–valve–mask option is technically simple and can be initiated quickly when necessary. A child need not be apnoeic or unresponsive before support is given in this way. An appropriately sized mask can be quickly selected by considering the size of the child's face; the mask should cover both the mouth and nose but the choice between round and shaped masks is largely a matter of operator preference. Three sizes of self-inflating bag are available – infant, child and adult. If there is any doubt, the larger bag should be used since it is always worse to underventilate than to overventilate. Adequacy of ventilation can be judged by looking for chest excursion.

Attempts at intubation are only indicated in apnoeic children and then only once other avenues have been exhausted. Paramedics are unlikely to be skilled or practised in these techniques in children and critical time should not be lost to failed attempts. However, if the decision to intubate has been made then the correct equipment must be selected and the correct technique used; these will depend on the age of the child.

A correctly sized tube can be selected by looking at the size of the child's little finger or by using the formula below.

$$\text{Internal diameter (mm)} = \frac{\text{age in years}}{4} + 4$$

Infants and very young children (below the age of 2 years) have a long, floppy epiglottis and this cannot be elevated sufficiently to allow the cords to be seen if the standard intubation technique is used (Figure 36.2). Consequently it is necessary to directly lift the epiglottis with the laryngoscope. This is achieved by passing the laryngoscope almost to the oesophagus and slowly withdrawing it in the midline. As the laryngoscope is withdrawn the epiglottis will remain elevated and the cords will come into view. A tube can then be passed through the cords and ventilation commenced. It is said that a straight paediatric blade is necessary to allow this technique to be performed, and it is certainly true that having one can make things easier. However, a standard or even a long adult blade can be used with success, since in a small mouth the curve of an adult blade is almost indiscernible.

In children over 2 years old the standard technique of passing the laryngoscope blade into the vallecula and lifting the epiglottis upwards and forwards to reveal the cords

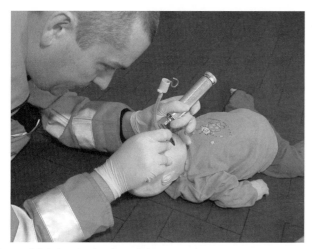

Figure 36.2 Intubation in an infant

can be used. As discussed above, adult-sized blades can be used if necessary.

Once the child is intubated, ventilation should be started and the position of the tube checked by listening with a stethoscope and observing chest movements. Adequacy of ventilation is judged by looking for a reasonable rise and fall of the chest.

CIRCULATION

If circulation is present then circulatory resuscitation is rarely necessary in the prehospital phase of care. Gaining intravenous access can be extremely difficult in children and time should not be wasted unless access is essential.

If vascular access is required (usually because of progression or imminent progression to cardiorespiratory arrest) then strict time-limiting protocols should be adopted. A vein should be identified and the area prepared as usual; if standard techniques do not work within *90 seconds* then the procedure should be abandoned and an intraosseous line should be inserted. This is usually achieved in the medial surface of the upper tibia using a specially designed intraosseous needle. Both drugs and fluid can be introduced through this route.

TREATMENT SUMMARY

Once the seriousness of a child's condition has been recognized it is important that treatment is limited to that necessary for rapid, safe transportation. This will include attention to the airway and to breathing, but will rarely involve circulatory management. Sticking to these appropriate levels of paramedical intervention is essential if the benefits of prehospital care are to be maximized. A diagnosis can be made and specific treatments administered in the receiving unit on arrival.

CONCLUSION

Dealing with a seriously ill child is a rare experience for most paramedics and a highly stressful one with considerable emotional overlay. The stress of the situation and an awareness of the consequences of failure, together with lack of experience, only make an already difficult situation worse. For all these reasons, it is essential to have a system. This chapter has described a system which allows recognition of the acutely ill child. Once such a situation has been recognized, immediate evacuation to hospital must be the priority. Unnecessary procedures, during which the child will continue to deteriorate, must be avoided. If a simple and logical approach is combined with an appropriate sense of urgency, many young lives will be saved.

Chapter 37

Paediatric cardiac arrest*

INTRODUCTION

Cardiorespiratory arrest in children is a much rarer event than in adults. Unfortunately, the outcome for children is much poorer. In adults cardiac arrest is usually secondary to a primary cardiac event such as myocardial infarction.

Primary cardiac event (e.g. myocardial infarction)

↓

Cardiac arrest (ventricular fibrillation, asystole, pulseless electrical activity)

↓

Respiratory arrest

This is not true for children, in whom the underlying event is usually hypoxia followed by respiratory arrest.

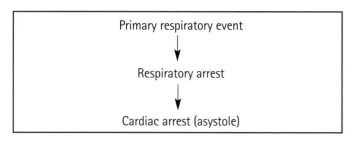

Primary respiratory event

↓

Respiratory arrest

↓

Cardiac arrest (asystole)

*The authors are aware of impending changes in resuscitation guidelines (late 2005). Refer to www.resus.org.uk for further information

The outcome of paediatric cardiac arrest is worse because the arrest takes place late in a sequence of deteriorating illness. In addition, because of the sequence of events leading to cardiac arrest, asystole is by far the most common arrest rhythm. It is easier to prevent paediatric respiratory arrest than to treat it.

For the youngest children (i.e. infants) the most common clinical cause is sudden infant death syndrome. For older children, the underlying cause is hypoxia which is secondary to severe sepsis, drowning, poisoning, aspiration and trauma, amongst other things.

Paediatric cardiac arrest guidelines are now well established. The latest were issued in 2000 and are internationally accepted. They include guidance on the delivery of both basic and advanced life support in children. Paramedics have a clear role to play in the institution of both basic and advanced life support for paediatric cardiac arrests occurring out of hospital.

BASIC LIFE SUPPORT

Because there are considerable variations in size within the paediatric population, the basic life support procedures are artificially divided into those for infants (aged under 1 year) and for children (aged 1 year to 15 years).

INFANTS

For infants, basic life support starts with checking for responsiveness by shaking whilst shouting for help. The next step

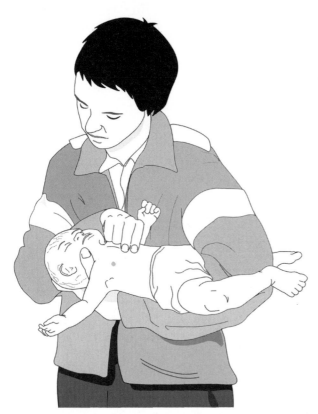

Figure 37.1 Correct hand position for cardiopulmonary resuscitation in infants

is to open the airway by the chin-lift manoeuvre. When this is achieved, the presence of breathing is assessed by looking, listening and feeling for any signs of respiration. If breathing is found to be absent it is necessary to deliver two effective breaths, taking no more than 10 seconds to achieve this. When this has been performed, the next step is to check for a brachial pulse – it is very difficult to feel a carotid pulse in infants because of their short necks over 10 seconds.

In infants check the brachial pulse

If the pulse is absent or the infant is found to be significantly bradycardic (i.e. the pulse rate is less than 60 per minute) then chest compressions should begin. To achieve this two fingers are placed on the lower sternum, a finger's breadth beneath the nipple line (Figure 37.1). The chest is compressed by approximately one-third of its depth and five rapid compressions are administered. This should be followed by further cycles of one breath to five compressions.

If the pulse is below 60/min commence basic life support

The paramedic crew attending such a call should continue basic life support measures whilst more advanced life support techniques are considered. The crew will have adjuncts to aid this cardiopulmonary resuscitation (CPR).

CHILDREN

For children over 1 year old the following sequence is used.

- Check responsiveness
- Open airway
- Check breathing
- Check (carotid) pulse
- Commence respiratory support or CPR as appropriate.

Chest compressions are given using the heel of one hand for children aged 1–8 years and a two-handed technique for children aged 9 and above. In both instances the heel of one hand is placed on the lower sternum, one finger's breadth above the xiphisternum, and the chest compressed to a depth of 3 cm. Five chest compressions are given and then a cycle of one breath to each five compressions is maintained.

The approach to paediatric cardiac arrest is summarized in Figure 37.2.

ADVANCED LIFE SUPPORT

The trained paramedic should be able to institute more advanced life support measures to augment cerebral and coronary circulation during basic life support and to attempt to terminate the cardiac arrest and restart the cardiovascular and respiratory systems.

The paramedic needs training in the use of all the above equipment. Training will be required to connect the child to a cardiac monitor and to determine correctly what cardiac rhythm underlies the cardiorespiratory arrest. Training is also required in intubation and securing an airway. The paramedic needs to be familiar with the methods of intravenous and intraosseous access to the circulatory system (see Chapter 8). Finally, the paramedic needs training in the use of drugs useful in treating cardiac arrest.

The size of the endotracheal tube used for intubation and the dosage of the drugs used in arrest depend on the age and size of the child. Two important formulae will assist the paramedic to choose correctly. To estimate the weight of the child, 4 is added to the child's age in years and the result doubled. For instance, a 4-year-old child will weigh approximately 16 kg.

Weight in kg = (age in years + 4) × 2

To estimate the endotracheal tube size (internal diameter in mm), the age is divided by 4 and 4 added:

Endotracheal tube size = $\dfrac{\text{age in years}}{4}$ + 4

For example, a 6-year-old child would require an endotracheal tube of 5.5 mm.

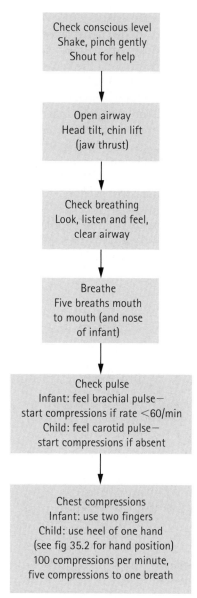

Figure 37.2 An approach to cardiac arrest in infants (less than 1 year old) and children (over 1 year old)

ARREST ALGORITHMS

When the child is placed on a cardiac monitor, the first decision, as in adult practice, is to determine which arrest rhythm the child is suffering from.

Asystole

The algorithm for the management of paediatric asystole is given in Figure 37.3. Asystole is by far the most common rhythm found in paediatric cardiac arrest, particularly arrest occurring outside hospital. The treatment is intubation and ventilation with supplemental oxygen to try to give an inspired oxygen content of 100%. Circulatory access should then be gained as rapidly as possible.

With skill it is possible in some cases to gain intravenous access. For younger children this may involve using a vein on

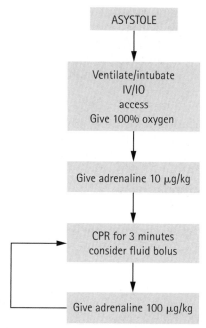

Figure 37.3 Management of asystole in children

the back of the hand or the dorsum of the foot, as large antecubital veins are not as readily found as in adults. If intravenous access is not successful, intraosseous access should be obtained (Chapter 8). Research shows that with a minimum of training it is easy to gain intraosseous access. Fluids or drugs given by this route are rapidly diffused into the venous system and therefore gain access to the central circulation as effectively as by peripheral cannulation.

Once access is achieved, adrenaline in a dose of $10\,\mu g/kg$ ($0.1\,ml/kg$ of 1:10000 solution) is administered. Thus, for a child aged 1 year the weight will be 10 kg and the first dose of adrenaline will be $100\,\mu g$, and the paramedic would give 1 ml of adrenaline 1:10000 solution as the first dose.

> The initial dose of adrenaline is $10\,\mu g/kg$

Cardiopulmonary resuscitation is then continued for 3 minutes, by which time there is a need for a further dose of adrenaline. The dose of adrenaline for the second and successive doses is up to $100\,\mu g/kg$ ($0.1\,ml$ of 1:1000 solution). Therefore, the second dose for a 10 kg child would be a maximum of $1000\,\mu g$, which is 1 ml of 1:1000 adrenaline. Cardiopulmonary resuscitation is then continued for a further 3 minutes, after which a further dose of adrenaline of $10–100\,\mu g/kg$ is necessary. The higher dose of adrenaline is used in cases of circulatory collapse (anaphylaxis or septicaemia).

> The subsequent doses of adrenaline are $10–100\,\mu g/kg$

While this cycle continues, the next step is to consider whether to augment the resuscitation by giving the child a fluid bolus, normally $20\,ml/kg$ of normal saline, particularly if the history suggests hypovolaemia.

If intravenous or intraosseous access is not possible, adrenaline may be delivered at a dose of 100 μg/kg via the endotracheal tube. However, if 1:10 000 adrenaline is used for this, large volumes would be required, so for this method of administration more concentrated adrenaline (typically 1:1000) is recommended.

The use of vagolytic drugs such as atropine is controversial and is not included in the European Resuscitation Council guidelines for asystole. However, the drugs do have a role in treating bradycardia before asystole ensues.

Pulseless electrical activity

Electromechanical dissociation (EMD) can be found in paediatric practice. The treatment is as follows.

- Intubation
- Ventilation with 100% oxygen
- Intravenous or intraosseous access
- Adrenaline 10 μg/kg
- IV fluid bolus 20 ml/kg
- CPR for 3 minutes
- Consideration of underlying cause of EMD
- High-dose adrenaline 100 μg/kg
- Continue CPR.

This is shown as an algorithm in Figure 37.4.

Electromechanical dissociation is usually secondary to some known cause, such as profound hypovolaemia, tension pneumothorax, cardiac tamponade, drug overdose or hypothermia. It is therefore necessary for the paramedic to consider whether any of these problems are present. Since hypovolaemia is common, it is reasonable to administer a challenge of 20 ml/kg of fluid such as normal saline for this particular arrest rhythm unless it is specifically contraindicated.

Ventricular fibrillation

Ventricular fibrillation in paediatric cardiac arrest occurring out of hospital is rare, but may occur typically with some poisons, such as with tricyclic antidepressant drugs, and also with drowning in cold water and hypothermia.

A first shock of 2 joules per kg should be given. If there is no response a further shock of 2 J/kg is delivered and if again there is no response, the shock is increased to 4 J/kg. If after these three shocks the child is still in ventricular fibrillation, the next step is intubation and ventilation with supplementary oxygen. This is followed by gaining circulatory access through an intravenous or intraosseous route and giving a dose of adrenaline (10 μg/kg). Cardiopulmonary resuscitation is continued for 1 minute only before the rhythm is checked on the monitor and if the child remains in ventricular fibrillation, three further shocks all at 4 J/kg are delivered, with pauses in between to check for any return of pulse. If this second set of shocks is unsuccessful then further adrenaline (10–100 μg/kg) is used and CPR continued again in a cycle for 1 minute.

Thereafter treatment consists of a cycle of CPR resuscitation for 1 minute followed by three shocks of 4 J/kg, followed by high-dose adrenaline with continuation of CPR, and so on. If the cause of the ventricular fibrillation is known to be secondary to imbalance of electrolytes (particularly potassium) or hypothermia, then measures to correct the underlying situation should be taken. If these measures are unsuccessful after three cycles, the use of specific antiarrhythmic drugs such as amiodarone, in a dose of 5 mg/kg, can be considered. The management is summarized in Figure 37.5.

In order to give a safe defibrillatory shock to a young child or infant, it may be necessary to use special paediatric paddles which are smaller than adult paddles (Figure 37.6). It is also necessary to use some form of electrogel or electrode pad between the child's skin and the defibrillator paddles.

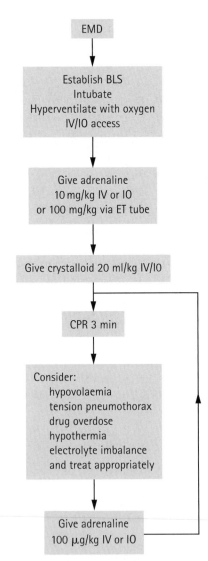

Figure 37.4 Management of electromechanical dissociation (EMD) in children. BLS, basic life support; CPR, cardiopulmonary resuscitation; ET, endotracheal, IO, intraosseous; IV, intravenous

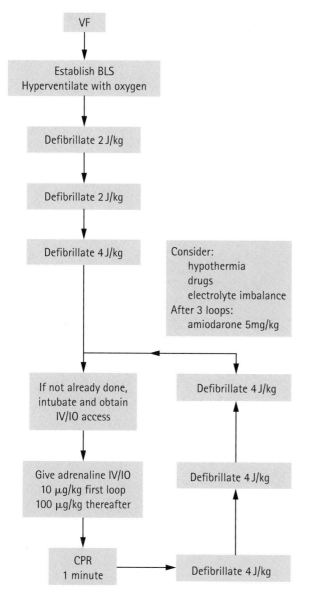

Figure 37.5 Management of ventricular fibrillation (VF) in children. BLS, basic life support; CPR, cardiopulmonary resuscitation; IO, intraosseous; IV, intravenous

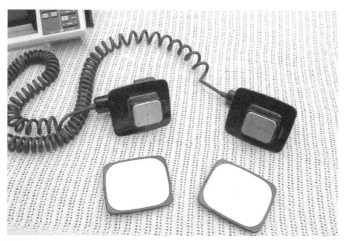

Figure 37.6 Adult and paediatric defibrillator paddles

AUTOMATIC EXTERNAL DEFIBRILLATORS

The energy delivery from most automatic defibrillators (AEDs) is fixed at that which is appropriate for adults. It is therefore too high for most young children (less than 8 years old). Whilst the use of an AED in young children cannot be recommended, if it is the only means of defibrillation available, then it should be used.

CONTINUATION OF CARE

The paramedic team, having instituted or continued basic life support and started the advanced life support appropriate to the child's clinical situation, next need to consider transporting the child to hospital. This should be achieved without any break in CPR.

In addition, adequate warning should be given to the receiving hospital who may have a specific team for paediatric cardiac arrest that can be present to receive the child on arrival at the emergency department. At the very least, additional and more senior paediatric and emergency department staff can be summoned.

It is hoped that the improvement in first aid skills by members of the public, the use of skilled paramedics to take over resuscitation in prehospital care and the establishment of specialized paediatric arrest teams will improve the outcome for children who suffer such an unfortunate event.

CONCLUSION

Paediatric cardiac arrest is a desperately distressing and stressful situation. Knowledge of, and adherence to, the protocols described in this chapter will ensure the best possible outcome for the child and, in addition, go some way to avoiding those feelings of *"Is there anything else I could have done?"* which are almost universal when these events sadly all too often have an adverse outcome.

FURTHER READING

Advanced Life Support Group 2000 *Advanced paediatric life support*, 2nd edn BMJ Books, London

Advanced Life Support Group 2005 Pre-hospital paediatric life support 2nd edn. Blackwell Publishing, Oxford

American Heart Association & American Academy of Pediatrics 1990 *Pediatric advanced life support manual*. American Heart Association, Dallas

Paediatric Life Support Working Party 2000 *Guidelines for paediatric life support*. European Resuscitation Council, Antwerp

Chapter 38

The injured child

INTRODUCTION

Major injury in childhood poses special difficulties for healthcare professionals. The greatest of these is that although injury in childhood is very common (one in three children are injured each year), true multisystem trauma occurs relatively infrequently and any one practitioner is likely to have only limited experience of it. It is therefore of vital importance that certain rules are followed so that assessment and resuscitation can be approached methodically, efficiently and thoroughly. These rules are:

- the ABC priorities are the same as for adults
- the practicalities are different.

DIFFERENCES BETWEEN CHILDREN AND ADULTS

Children differ from adults in the following ways.

SIZE

Smaller size means that a child sustains more injuries than an adult would sustain from the same force and that multisystem injury is more likely (Figure 38.1).

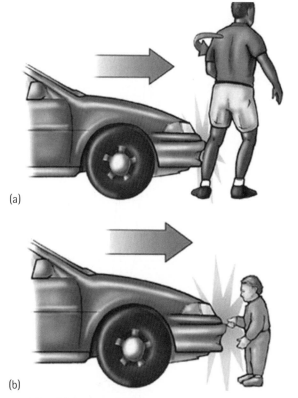

(a)

(b)

Figure 38.1 (a) An adult hit by the front of a car; (b) a child involved in the same impact. Note the much greater distribution of injuries sustained by the child

SHAPE

The child's relatively large head means that more forces may be applied through the neck during deceleration. A falling child tends to land head first. Formulae for calculating the area of a burn are also different as the percentage body surface area varies with age (Figure 38.2; see Chapter 31).

SKELETON

The skeleton in children is very elastic. The child may sustain internal organ damage without overlying fracture; for example, spinal cord damage may occur without radiological evidence of any fracture or dislocation of the spine. More importantly, lung contusion may occur without overlying rib fracture because the ribs are more pliable. Fracture of one or more ribs in childhood is extremely uncommon and is very serious since it indicates that enormous force has been applied and internal damage is likely to be severe.

SURFACE AREA

The larger surface area relative to body size in children means more rapid heat loss can occur and the child easily loses heat.

SEQUELAE

The physical results of the injury may remain with the child for a long time. Damage to the growing plates of long bones can affect later stature or cause asymmetrical growth which can impact on associated skeletal and muscle development.

PSYCHOLOGICAL PROBLEMS

A careful and gentle approach is needed to the assessment and treatment of a frightened child who is in pain. Children almost invariably find the presence of a parent calming and

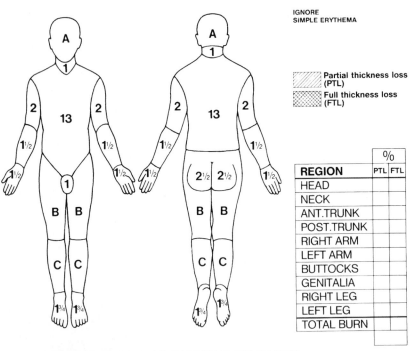

Figure 38.2 Burns and body surface area in children

although they may not understand what is said, continuous quiet speech is also reassuring. The psychological impact on the carer of having to deal with a distressed child may also significantly alter performance. Under stressful circumstances, the child may regress to a younger age and may not behave as might be expected for his chronological age. In addition, the psychological effects of trauma may be very prolonged. There is no substitute for a knowledge of "normal" uninjured children in setting "alarm bells" ringing.

EQUIPMENT

Appropriately sized and designed equipment must be available in order to allow appropriate treatment.

SPECIFIC DIFFERENCES IN TREATMENT

Specific differences exist between the anatomy and physiology of the child which have an immediate practical bearing on what injuries may have been sustained and on how the child is treated. These differences are listed below under the ABCD headings.

> **A** Airway with cervical spine control
> **B** Breathing with oxygen
> **C** Circulation with haemorrhage control
> **D** Disability

Airway

The differences in a child's airway when compared with an adult are (Figure 38.3):

- relatively large tongue and easily damaged soft palate
- relatively large epiglottis
- relatively short trachea
- the narrowest part of the upper airway is below the level of the cords at the level of the cricoid
- the larynx is more difficult to visualize.

The practical consequences of these differences are as follows.

1. The best way to insert an oral airway is by depressing the tongue with a tongue depressor or the blade of a laryngoscope. The oral

airway is then inserted directly (the right way up) rather than rotated through 180° as in an adult.

2. Nasopharyngeal airways are more difficult to insert in the very small child.

3. Orotracheal intubation requires a different technique. The large, floppy epiglottis may be picked up directly by the laryngoscope blade and lifted out of the way to allow better visualization of the cords (Figure 38.4).

4. In children under 6 years old an uncuffed tube should be used. A useful way of remembering the right size of tube is that it should be the size of the child's small finger. Alternatively, the following formula may be used:

$$\text{Internal diameter (mm)} = \frac{\text{Age in years}}{4} + 4$$

When inserted, the black vocal cord marker near the tip of the endotracheal tube should be placed at the level of the cords. After placement it is essential to ensure that both lungs are expanding normally in order to be certain that intubation of

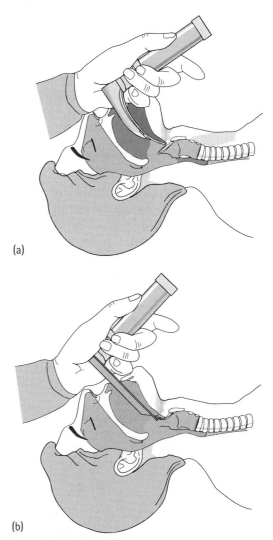

(a)

(b)

Figure 38.4 (a) Endotracheal intubation in an adult; (b) endotracheal intubation in a child. Note the position of the tip of the laryngoscope

> - Large head (Occiput)
> - Short fat neck
> - Small mandible
> - Obligate nasal breathers
> - Short and soft trachea
> - Large tongue

Figure 38.3 The child's airway highlighting the differences from the airway of an adult

the right main bronchus has been excluded. In addition, it is important to listen for air entry high in the axillae to confirm equal air entry.

5. Surgical cricothyroidotomy should not be performed in children; only needle cricothyroidotomy is appropriate.

Breathing

Children breathe rapidly. They have low oxygen reserves and their metabolism uses oxygen very quickly; if ventilation is impaired, cyanosis rapidly ensues. If ventilatory support is needed then the rate of ventilation should be around 20 breaths per minute for a child and 40 breaths per minute for an infant. The volume of the ventilation is best judged by watching the child's chest move.

Children do not tolerate tension pneumothorax well. This is because the mediastinum is very mobile and it can be pushed across to compress the other lung by the increased pressure within the injured hemithorax. Repeated assessment of air entry in the ventilated child and early needle cricothyrotomy are therefore of paramount importance.

Circulation

The heart rate in children is faster than in adults (Table 38.1). The blood pressure also varies with age. In children under 1 year old the minimum acceptable normal systolic pressure is 70 mmHg. In children older than 1 year the expected systolic pressure can be worked out by the formula:

Systolic pressure (mmHg) = 80 + (age in years × 2)

The circulating blood volume of a child is approximately 80 ml per kilogram, which means that the total blood volume of a neonate is likely to be around 240 ml. A child's first response to a decrease in blood volume is a tachycardia. The next response is usually cool skin at the peripheries, with a drop in blood pressure as a late sign. The practical implication of this is that assessment of a child's circulatory status can be very difficult.

There are a number of important pitfalls. Tachycardia, the first sign of blood loss, is also affected by fear and pain, peripheral skin temperature will be affected by ambient conditions (just as it is in adults) and low blood pressure is a late feature and its absence does not exclude the diagnosis of shock.

Repeated and frequent assessments are therefore necessary so that changes can be detected early and intervention can take place as soon as possible.

If there is a suspicion of circulatory compromise or if injuries are apparent which would indicate significant blood loss then fluid therapy will be required. In the majority of cases immediate evacuation to hospital for fluid therapy and possible surgical intervention is the most appropriate course of action. In cases of prolonged transfer or entrapment, however, prehospital fluid administration may be required. The best route of access to the circulation is through the antecubital fossa, as in an adult, or in the dorsum of the hand or foot in a child under 1 year old. Venous access can be extremely difficult due to a combination of small veins, an uncooperative unrestrained patient and suboptimal ambient conditions. For all these reasons, access is more easily achievable in hospital. Intraosseous access is an effective alternative if two attempts at intravenous access fail in a child or as a first resort in an infant.

Once access has been achieved, the fluid bolus that should be administered is 20 ml/kg of crystalloid solution (preferably warmed). Under no circumstances should intravenous access delay transfer to definitive care, and should be performed en route to hospital if the child is not trapped.

Disability (neurological status)

Children frequently sustain head injuries because of the relatively large size of their head. Vomiting after head injury is common and does not necessarily imply increased intracranial pressure. Many children will vomit once or twice without any sinister significance. Persistent vomiting is more worrying, however, and such children will require admission for observation and possible investigation. Children sustain fewer intracranial haematomas after head injury but are more liable to develop cerebral oedema than adults. It is therefore especially important that episodes of hypotension or hypoxia are avoided wherever possible. Adequate ventilation with a high concentration of oxygen is therefore mandatory and correction of hypotension is a high priority.

Seizures after head injury are more common in children than in adults but are usually self-limiting. Infants can lose a large proportion of their circulating volume from scalp lacerations or into haematomas within the scalp. Head injuries do not otherwise cause hypotension.

Assessment using the Glasgow Coma Scale is likely to be more difficult than in an adult because of the child's inability to cooperate. However, the key to optimum management is the prevention of secondary brain injury by paying attention to the airway, breathing and circulation. This, combined with rapid evacuation to definitive care, is far more important than attempts at neurological assessment. The AVPU assessment can be used in children but the Glasgow Coma Scale has to be modified for children younger than 4 years of age. The assessment of the verbal component of the score is as outlined in Table 38.2.

Table 38.1 Mean heart rate in children	
Age	**Mean heart rate (beats/min)**
Newborn–3 months	140
3 months–2 years	130
2 years–10 years	80
More than 10 years	75

Table 38.2 Glasgow Coma Scale for children under 4 years old

Verbal Response	Score
Smiles, follows sound and objects, interacts	5
Cries consolably or interacts inappropriately	4
Cries with inconsistent relief or moans	3
Cries inconsolably or is irritable	2
No response	1

NON-ACCIDENTAL INJURY

Healthcare professionals have a responsibility for the protection of children. It is important that a child who is being deliberately abused is identified and protected from further injury. All healthcare professionals need to be aware of the features of non-accidental injury. Suspicion should be aroused by:

- a history that does not fit the apparent injuries
- a delay in seeking help
- an inappropriate response from the child or carers
- inconsistent history of the injury.

Injuries that are especially associated with a non-accidental cause include:

- injuries around the mouth
- injuries around the genital area
- long-bone fractures in children under 3 years old
- bizarre injuries such as cigarette burns or rope burns.

It is important that prehospital personnel pass on any suspicions to the healthcare professionals to whom the case is handed on at the hospital.

SUMMARY

Multiple system injury in childhood is relatively uncommon and is distressing for healthcare professionals. The principles and priorities of assessment and management are the same as for the adult population. There are some differences in resuscitation techniques and equipment but the key is, as in adults, scrupulous attention to the primary survey.

FURTHER READING

Advanced Life Support Group 2000 *Advanced paediatric life support*, 2nd edn. BMJ Books, London

American College of Surgeons 1993 *Advanced trauma life support programme for physicians*. American College of Surgeons, Chicago

American Heart Association and American Academy of Pediatrics 1990 *Pediatric advanced life support*. American Heart Association, Dallas

Morton R, Barbara P 1996 *Accidents and emergencies in children*. Oxford University Press, Oxford

Section 6

CARE OF THE ELDERLY

Chapter 39

Care of the elderly

INTRODUCTION: THE ELDERLY PATIENT

Throughout the 20th century in the UK there have been improvements in public health, nutrition and housing and medical advances, especially the discovery of antibiotics. These have led to a steady increase in the numbers of people reaching not only the statutory retirement age but their 80s and 90s and older; for example, the number of centenarians in the UK rose from around 200 in 1951 to 4000 in 1989. In the second half of the 20th century the number of pensioners was estimated to have increased from 5.25 million in 1951 to a projected 10 million at the millennium. Furthermore, the greatest increase is in the numbers of the very old, with a rise in those aged over 80 years from 0.75 million to 2.5 million, accompanied by no change in the overall population. We see therefore a relative reduction in numbers of younger people who may be called upon to support their elders both financially and physically. The burgeoning cost of caring for our oldest citizens is the subject of vigorous political debate as we look to the year 2020, with a further projected increase in people aged over 75 years of over 30%. The decrease in the proportion of those able and willing to care for the old highlights the ever more precarious support systems for our most frail citizens.

Why do old women outnumber men by 2 or 3 to 1? The ravages of two world wars and other factors (such as the capacity for young and middle-aged men to "self-destruct" with industrial accidents, smoking and excess alcohol consumption) have left many widows now in their 80s and 90s. Thus, nearly half of women over 75 will live alone. Old age may also bring with it an accumulation of illnesses which result in a reduced capacity to function independently: half of those old people over 85 will be housebound or unable to leave their homes without assistance.

In summary, old age may bring a combination of factors rendering the old person especially vulnerable to an acute breakdown in their capacity to cope:

- social isolation
- poor housing
- low income
- precarious functional capacity
- dependency on others.

Moreover, many old people are fiercely proud and independent and may fail to recognize or acknowledge their increasing vulnerability. This is the backdrop to emergencies occurring in vulnerable old people and the factors described here are essential for an understanding of the emergency situations

Table 39.1 Physiological changes in the elderly

Change	Clinical consequences
Brain	
Shrinkage and loss of neurones (cerebral atrophy)	Increasing forgetfulness. Dementia. Vulnerability to toxic confusional states
Peripheral and autonomic nervous system	
Reduced awareness of touch, temperature, pain. Impaired proprioception. Impaired control of posture and balance	Hypothermia. Postural hypotension. Falls, urinary incontinence, constipation
Eye	
Cataracts. Macular degeneration. Stiffening of lens	Impaired eyesight. Presbyopia (failure to accommodate to near and distant vision)
Ear	Deafness
Bones, joints and muscles	
Thinning of bones (osteoporosis) Osteoarthritis Loss of muscle, strength and bulk capacity to respond to displacement	Fractures of femoral neck, wrist and vertebrae. Increased curvature of spine (kyphosis) Stiffening of knees, hips and fingers Immobility, falls

involving old people to which the paramedic may be called.

THE AGEING PROCESS

PHYSICAL AGEING

Scientists have great difficulty in distinguishing the "pure" effects of ageing from abnormal or pathological ageing. Strictly speaking, for a process to be due entirely to ageing, it should be present in everyone and should be progressive and deleterious. In practical terms, most clinicians will include conditions which have a strong association with growing older. Table 39.1 describes some important physiological changes associated with growing older and the common clinical consequences of these changes. What is remarkable is the extraordinary variability in individuals' susceptibility to the ravages of ageing. Thus, while the changes described in muscle are true for most old people, a marathon runner aged 80 will have muscle which is virtually indistinguishable structurally and physiologically from that of a fit 20-year-old. Inspection of the major clinical consequences of ageing highlights some of the major problems of old age which will be described later.

AGEING OF THE PSYCHE

Popular stereotypes need to be judged with caution. Many behaviours described as being associated with ageing may well be the habits of middle age carried into late life:

- rigidity of personality
- reduced sexual drive
- decreased repertoire of activities
- hypochondriasis
- bowel obsession.

Successful ageing embodies maintenance of interests, hobbies and work, adapting to changing capability, maximizing current abilities and avoiding negative attitudes to old age (ageism).

THE NATURE OF ACUTE ILLNESS IN OLD AGE

Some generalizations can be made. First, acute illnesses in old people often fail to present with convenient and characteristic symptoms or physical signs.

- A myocardial infarct may not present with crushing central chest pain but rather with a fall, acute onset of mental confusion or simply breathlessness.
- Acute infections may fail to mount the response of an immune reaction (raised white cell count) or a raised body temperature.

Acute illnesses in old people arise in the context of a general background of failing health such as:

- memory loss and impairment of intellect. The elderly brain is especially susceptible to the toxic effects of any acute illness, so that acute onset of mental confusion may be a presenting symptom which resolves provided that the underlying cause is treated
- failing eyesight or hearing
- increase in postural sway so that acute illnesses may present as falls
- impaired central control of bladder function so that acute illnesses may present with urinary incontinence
- perhaps most importantly, an accumulation of other diseases; for example, a fairly trivial acute illness may arise in a person already compromised by heart failure and further limited by impaired mobility following an operation for a fractured neck of femur.

Acute illnesses in old people often arise in a situation of precarious social circumstances in which the support network for the individual is already stretched. Such illnesses are often partly or wholly related to drug therapy.

The paramedic called to an emergency must be aware that an apparently minor illness in an old person can have very different consequences from the same illness in a young person. Consider two patients, one young and one old (Figure 39.1).

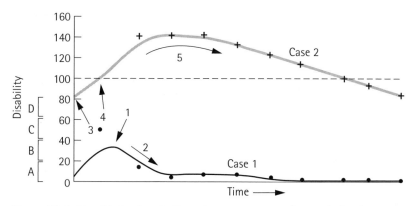

Figure 39.1 The effects of acute illness in a young person (lower plot) and an elderly person (upper plot). Disability is on an arbitrary scale; 100 is the threshold for hospital admission. The elderly person's starting disability of 80 is due to arthritis of the knees (A), poor eyesight (B), cardiac failure (C) and carer stress (D)

CASE 1

A young man of 25 years old, previously fit, develops a runny nose which progresses to laryngitis and acute bronchitis with a painful hacking cough. The course of his illness is illustrated in Figure 39.1 (lower line) which plots his illness in terms of "disability". Because he feels unwell, has a fever and is in some pain from his coughing, he takes to his bed. However, being otherwise fit, he is able to get up to the toilet and to move around in bed. His wife is able to go to the pharmacist and gets some aspirin to relieve his symptoms. She is able to provide him with food and drinks and over a period of 48 hours he improves and is soon up and about. The maximal level of his disability (1 in Figure 39.1) is reduced by the lack of other illnesses (co-morbidity) and the presence of his wife to look after him. His quick recovery (2) is due to his general good health and a responsive immune system. He may never reach his doctor's attention and will not reach the "disability threshold" for admission to hospital.

CASE 2

An 85-year-old widow lives alone in a warden-controlled flat because of previous falls due to a combination of poor eyesight, osteoarthritis of her knees and cardiac failure. Her daughter has felt obliged to visit every day and especially in the evenings and at weekends when there is no warden on duty. The background problems impose a level of disability illustrated by A–D in Figure 39.1. Thus even at her best she has a precarious existence close to the threshold for hospital admission (3 in Figure 39.1). Now follow her illness in Figure 39.1 (upper line). She develops a similar illness to Case 1 on Saturday afternoon and takes to her bed. Her legs, already stiff, seize up and she is unable to go to the toilet, gain access to food or fluids or contact the warden who is off duty. Her daughter arrives to find her lying in a wet bed, acutely embarrassed and with a hacking cough. She is complaining bitterly of pain in her knees and her daughter is unable to

move her, thus her level of disability rises further (4) to the point at which she requires emergency admission to hospital. Thereafter, the slower recovery (5) is due to the secondary effects of the respiratory infection on her mobility and her cardiac failure.

MAJOR MEDICAL PROBLEMS IN OLD AGE

The effects of ageing and acute or chronic illnesses often manifest as conditions best described as "functional failure", as described above. Professor Bernard Isaacs, one of the first generation of academic geriatricians, characterized these common manifestations of illness in old age as the "giants of geriatric medicine".

- Intellectual disorder (dementias and acute confusional states)
- Immobility, incontinence and instability (a tendency to fall)
- Visual and hearing impairment
- Depression
- Adverse drug reactions (approximately 10% of acute admissions to geriatric wards are as a result of adverse drug reactions).

Multiple ailments – so common in old people – often result in multiple drug therapy, thus increasing the risk not only of adverse drug reactions but also of potentially serious drug interactions.

INTELLECTUAL DISORDER

Some impairment of memory and concentration is so common in later life as to be considered normal and not indicative or predictive of dementia. This thought is a great relief to its victims, but occasionally is responsible for a delay in diagnosis of genuine dementia. This type is seldom in any way disabling. In simple terms, intellectual disorder is of two types: due to disease outside the brain (extrinsic) and due to intrinsic brain disease (dementia).

Extrinsic causes

Mental impairment may be caused by drugs, infections, hypoxia, dehydration, electrolyte disorders, disturbances of carbohydrate metabolism and renal and hepatic failure. Hypothyroidism and vitamin B_{12} and folate deficiency very rarely cause intellectual impairment, although they may be found in association. Head injury with or without intracranial haemorrhage may be included in this category. The intellectual dysfunction associated with these extrinsic causes is usually short-lived, unless there is coexisting intrinsic brain disease.

Two cardinal features distinguish this type of mental disorder from dementia:

- acute onset (and usually rapid resolution)
- disturbed or fluctuating conscious level.

Intrinsic causes

Dementia is a pathological state characterized by diffuse loss of brain tissue. When brain tumour and other focal conditions have been excluded, the usual causes are Alzheimer's disease, multifocal vascular disease and a mixture of the two. Dementia also occurs in Parkinson's disease, Huntington's chorea and other rarer brain diseases.

Alzheimer's disease is a slowly progressive disease with a 10-year course on average. While some cases can present in the fifth and sixth decades, most appear in the eighth and ninth decades.

Vascular brain disease, also called multiinfarct dementia, occurs in hypertensive patients who suffer progressive loss of brain tissue, with or without focal neurological signs. The course of this disease is more rapid than that of Alzheimer's disease and many patients die from cardiac disease or stroke.

The history

Patients may give a very misleading history of the illness as they are unable to assess their current state, but may be able to talk convincingly and positively of their past life. Patients have considerable skills of deception. Be very wary of patients who make even the slightest lapse from consistency

of accuracy in answering questions and seek information from relatives who have watched them over a period of time. Tell-tale signs are:

- an increased use of the telephone, especially in the middle of the night
- frequent losses of key, pension books, money, jewellery
- accusations that others have stolen these
- burning out kettles
- leaving the gas on unlit
- resistance to bathing and changing clothes
- changes in sleep-wake patterns
- soiling of clothes and neglect of personal appearance
- leaving the house and getting lost
- repeatedly asking the same question
- misidentifying or failing to identify near relatives
- speaking of the past as if it were the present and of dead people, for example parents, as if they were still alive.

Eventually a crisis occurs which carers can no longer accept and this fracture of sound support may masquerade as a medical emergency.

IMMOBILITY

Immobility can be defined as an inability to occupy space (the life-space, ranging from anywhere in the world to the confines of an upstairs bedroom). From a clinical point of view, however, it can be considered as a restriction of everyday activities.

How commonly does restricted mobility occur?

An investigation in the UK by Age Concern in 1978 of people past retirement age revealed that about 40% had no difficulties getting about. In the remaining 60%, difficulties with hills and ramps were the most commonly reported (31%), while others were traffic and road crossing (23%), uneven pavements (16%) and steps and kerbs (4%).

What are the barriers to maintaining mobility in old age?

Physical barriers (often more than one):

- joint problems, especially osteoarthritis of knees and hips
- neurological deficit: impaired balance, stroke, Parkinson's disease
- previous falls
- sensory deprivation: deafness, impaired vision
- cardiovascular and respiratory diseases.

Mental barriers:

- reduced expectations of an active life
- loss of adaptability and creativity
- introversion with reduced social contact
- anxiety and fear of going out (or of allowing others to).

Box 39.1 Extrinsic causes of mental impairment

- Drugs
- Infections
- Hypoxia
- Dehydration
- Electrolyte disturbances
- Carbohydrate metabolism disturbances
- Renal and hepatic failure
- Hypothyroidism
- Vitamin B_{12} and folate deficiency
- Head injury

Social barriers:

- retirement brings with it dangers of reduced social contact and a drop in income. The retired person may regard a motor car as an unnecessary expense but many regret having got rid of their car
- living alone: an epidemic problem in ageing women
- nowhere to go – insufficient outside interests or activities.

What are the consequences of immobility?

Loss of choice:

- being able to go where we want to be and thus be able to do what we want to do
- being alone or with others
- having the TV on or off (look around any hospital ward or old people's home).

Loss of capability:

- getting to the toilet in time, answering the door or getting upstairs
- social responsiveness
- worsening physical dependency.

An old person's world may thus contract and after becoming housebound he (or more often she) then becomes restricted to the lower half of the house and eventually perhaps to one room.

INCONTINENCE

Anyone can become incontinent if not able or not allowed to have access to proper toilet facilities. The elderly are more vulnerable because of poor mobility and frequency and urgency of micturition. Any acute illness is likely to be associated with deterioration in continence but usually this is transient. Likewise, any change of environment such as admission to hospital may also lead to a temporary period of incontinence.

Extrinsic causes

One common cause for incontinence in old people is faecal impaction. It is easily diagnosed by rectal examination and quickly cured by enemas. Those suffering from chronic brain failure are more likely to develop difficulties with incontinence, which is partly due to a diminished response to sensation of bladder filling. Similar difficulties arise following the removal of indwelling catheters and continence may not be regained for several weeks in some cases. Finally, urinary tract infection may occasionally cause incontinence.

Drugs such as diuretics may exert adverse effects on an older person's bladder by their mode of action. Hypnotics and sedatives may lead to incontinence, especially at night. Anticholinergic drugs such as antidepressants, antiparkinsonian drugs and verapamil can lead to urinary retention with overflow.

Intrinsic causes

Intrinsic causes include disorders of the bladder, sphincter or their nerve supply.

Incontinence may be caused directly because of over- or underactivity of the bladder itself or the sphincter.

INSTABILITY

Balance

Balance is a set of biological strategies designed to maintain the body in the erect posture. Mechanisms involved include ocular, vestibular and proprioceptive (position sense) receptors found in the neck and elsewhere, especially in the weight-bearing joints and in the tendons and ligaments of the trunk. Under normal circumstances, the body undergoes oscillations around a fixed point known as the "sway path". As these balance mechanisms deteriorate with increasing age, sway increases.

Ocular mechanisms

Under normal circumstances, visual cues are constantly used to correct minor deviation from the fixed point. In old people visual acuity is frequently reduced, as is the threshold for light stimulation.

Vestibular mechanisms

The vestibular apparatus is mainly involved with rotatory movements of the head and neck, whereas the otolith organ is involved with acceleration and deceleration. With advancing age, these mechanisms are relatively inefficient. Vestibular mechanisms may be implicated in walking over uneven ground or have some part to play in instability during rising from a chair.

Proprioceptive mechanisms

Position sense is important for maintaining balance. Sensory information from proprioceptors in the spine and major weight-bearing joints may be impaired with ageing and arthritis. Failure of these mechanisms leads to an increased likelihood of falls.

Falls

How common? Very common! About 20% of elderly men and 40% of elderly women will give a history of a recent fall and the liability to fall rises with age, the probability going up from 30% chance of falling at 65 years to 50% at 85 years. The majority of falls are not reported and only about 3% of elderly people who fall sustain an injury that requires medical attention. Nevertheless, in an average-sized health district of 250 000 people, with about 37 000 people over 65 years old, between 16 and 20 beds will be occupied by patients admitted as a direct result of a fall. It is one of the most common causes of emergency admission to an acute geriatric ward, often after a prolonged period lying on the floor unable to get up.

Where and when do falls occur?

Most falls occur indoors or very close to the house, in the daytime. Falls on stairs are more likely to occur when the person is descending.

What are the clinical features?

Falls may be divided into two broad categories: extrinsic and intrinsic. *Extrinsic* falls are those in which an external factor is responsible, for example tripping or accident. This type of fall occurs in a younger, fitter person and the vast majority are unreported and cause no serious injury. The consequences are slight with no restriction in activities or loss of confidence. In *intrinsic* falls the dominant cause is failure of balance for the reasons described above and in which one or more precipitating factors (described below) may play a part. In this case the patient is older and more frail and typically the consequences are much more serious regardless of physical injury: loss of confidence, restriction of activity and a loss of mobility may all result in fear of going out of doors unaccompanied.

Precipitating causes

Change of posture

Getting out of a chair, an unstable situation requiring strength and coordination in antigravity muscles, is a typical precipitating cause. The reason is rarely postural hypotension, an uncommon cause of falls although much loved by medical students and doctors!

Extended movement

In falls due to extended movement the person reaches out or up, which puts the centre of gravity outside the ground base but owing to a slowing of postural reflex movements is unable to compensate by moving the feet quickly enough to prevent a fall.

Illnesses

Any acute illness such as cardiac disease or arrhythmias may lead to a fall, as may poor vision.

Drugs

Diuretics, hypnotics and drugs for hypertension are particularly implicated in falls in the elderly and reducing multiple drug therapy is the most powerful preventive measure which can be taken.

Consequences of falling

The consequences in older people can be serious and far-reaching. Although less than half do not cause serious injury nor referral to health services, for those who are referred the consequences can be catastrophic.

- Fractures (7–10% of falls), usually wrist, hip, pelvis, upper humerus and ribs. The most serious, proximal hip fracture, has a mortality up to 40% and serious morbidity including loss of mobility in survivors.
- Other injuries: soft tissue injuries (5–10% of falls), including bruising, subdural haematoma and dislocations, can occur. Inability to rise from the floor after a fall can result in pressure sores, incontinence and hypothermia and even death.
- Psychological effects: fear of falling often results in delay in reestablishing mobility and a resetting of postural mechanisms which cause a temporary tendency to fall backwards after standing up.
- Institutionalization: recurrent falls are a particularly powerful reason why patients may lose the confidence to live independently.

What is the prognosis?

Falls in the very old often indicate serious underlying disease and have a gloomy outlook. About a quarter will die within a year of their index fall. If they have lain for more than an hour, half will be dead in 6 months.

VISUAL IMPAIRMENT

A few generalizations can be made about the special problems old people with failing vision may encounter.

- The additional burden of other handicaps
- Less opportunity to manipulate their physical and social environment to their needs
- Fewer advantages than younger people in seeking registration as either blind (acuity worse than 6/60 – unable to read top line of Snellen chart) or partially sighted (no better than 6/60 – able to read the top line).

Thus, visual handicap remains grossly underreported both to doctors and registering authorities.

The ageing eye

The following changes are seen in the ageing eye.

Cornea

The cornea becomes more opaque with slight scattering of light and reduction in light transmission, especially at the ultraviolet end of the spectrum. Specific diseases rather than age itself are responsible for any visual handicap.

Lens

The largest contribution to the visual consequences of the ageing process is made by changes in the lens: it becomes thicker, stiffer, denser and more yellow (filtering out blue and violet). The main consequence is presbyopia or reduced ability to accommodate.

Ciliary apparatus

Thickening of the ciliary apparatus may lead to closed angle glaucoma (see below).

Retina

The blood vessels of the retina become narrower. Macular deterioration reduces spatial discrimination, black and white contrast and colour perception.

Eye diseases

Most people enter retirement with some form of corrected optical problem (usually presbyopia and astigmatism). All elderly people with visual disability (worse than 6/36) have a disease, *not* simply the effects of normal ageing.

Most of the major eye diseases encountered are progressive but amenable to treatment, so accurate diagnosis is essential. The four major diseases of the eye in old age are:

- cataract (clouding of the lens of the eye)
- macular degeneration (deterioration in central vision)
- glaucoma (increase in pressure of fluid within the eye)
- diabetic retinopathy (visual failure due to small vessel disease of the retina).

HEARING IMPAIRMENT

Deafness is a common problem in the elderly which increases in prevalence with age, 30–40% of people over 75 years having some degree of hearing loss.

Pathology

Acquired causes are either conductive or sensorineural deafness and are superimposed upon an age-related sensorineural hearing loss termed *presbyacusis.* Presbyacusis is characterized by a predominantly high-tone hearing loss caused by degeneration and atrophy of the sensory cells and neuronal connections within the cochlea.

Symptoms

Difficulty understanding speech is the most distressing and common consequence of hearing impairment. High-tone hearing loss particularly affects consonant as opposed to vowel sounds. Since much of the information in speech is encoded in consonant sounds, when these are imperfectly heard, speech is almost unintelligible. Frequency discrimination, sound localization and reaction time are also impaired. In some patients distressing tinnitus (whistling or ringing) and abnormal loudness perception may add to their problems.

Social consequences

In most elderly patients difficulty in hearing speech is first noticed during group conversation. As with many other disorders in old age, this inability to communicate effectively often leads to loss of independence and social isolation. In some individuals irritation and unhappiness caused by deafness may progress to clinical depression. Alternatively, others may feel "left out" and if unable to lip-read in group discussions, may become suspicious and harbour paranoid ideas.

Hearing aids

Hearing trumpets are still available and, although they may appear outdated, are still effective. Postaural and body-worn aids are readily available; these aids have a volume control and settings marked "O" for off, "M" for on (microphone) and "T" for use with telephones fitted with an induction coupler (telecoil) loop, which cuts out background noise. Some public buildings and phones are also fitted with coupler loop systems. Bone conductor aids are available to patients with severe middle ear disease causing profound conductive deafness.

A hearing aid is most useful in face-to-face conversation when lip-reading augments the comprehension of speech. Group discussions are still difficult owing to amplification of ambient noise and reverberant sound which interferes with what the patient wishes to hear.

DEPRESSION

Depression is both a subjective mood state and an objective psychiatric illness. It is important to distinguish one from the other.

The psychiatric illness of depression is characterized by low mood, unaffected by external circumstances, feelings of unworthiness and helplessness. Suicidal ideas may be present. The future looks bleak. There is appetite disturbance, usually leading to weight loss. Sleep disturbance, characteristically early morning wakening, occurs. Concentration is poor, there is a decrease in normal interests, even in family and friends. In a severe illness, psychotic phenomena may be present, i.e. delusions and hallucinations. Delusions are usually of poverty or are nihilistic (thinking things have disappeared, never to exist again). Hallucinations are usually of a second person who makes derogatory statements, for example "You are dirty", "You should be dead". In elderly patients with depression hypochondriacal ideas are more often present, for example worries about heart disease or cancer. This is often in the setting of real illness which is then exaggerated by fears and worries.

In summary, depression in the elderly is characterized by:

- appetite disturbance
- weight loss
- sleep disturbance (early wakening)
- poor concentration
- decrease in normal interests
- delusions and hallucinations
- hypochondriasis.

Masked depression

Hypochondria or anxiety symptoms predominate and there is no complaint of depression, although symptoms are present and can be revealed by questioning.

Pseudodementia

Pseudodementia is the term given to a syndrome that presents with poor self-care and poor cognitive ability. This change in function is brought about by a retarded depression. All the features mentioned above may be present; lack of interest will result in poor self-care and cognitive function. These patients will often answer "don't know" to questions rather than confabulate. The history of onset of the illness is weeks or months rather than years as in a true dementia. There may be a family or previous history of affective disorder.

Prevalence of depression

A study of prevalence of depression in a community survey amongst elderly people conducted in the UK and USA in 1976 showed that 22% were possibly depressed, 13% had a minor depressive disorder and 1.6% had a major depressive disorder.

> Depression is a major health issue in people over the age of 65

ADVERSE DRUG REACTIONS

Table 39.2 indicates the common culprits that cause problems in old people. The paramedic called to see an old person should (with permission) search for all medications (both prescribed and "over the counter") and bring them with the patient to hospital. They may be crucial in assisting diagnosis, especially when the patient is unable to give an accurate history.

Table 39.2 Drugs that may cause problems in elderly patients

Drug group	Symptoms and signs
Diuretics	Falls, confusion, dry mouth, dehydration, postural fall in blood pressure, urinary incontinence
Compound analgesics	Drowsiness, confusion, falls, constipation
Tricyclic antidepressants	Greater risk of anticholinergic effects: urine retention, constipation, dry mouth, postural hypotension and confusion
Digoxin	Reduced renal excretion. Increased risk of side-effects such as sickness, diarrhoea, slow pulse rate and other heart rhythm disorders causing dizziness, fainting or falls
β-blockers	Falls, confusion, heart failure, slow pulse, postural hypotension, asthma attacks, cold limbs
Hypnotics	Increased and prolonged effects. Confusion, drowsiness, staggering and falls (especially at night)

COMMUNICATING WITH OLD PEOPLE

Problems such as impaired hearing, anxiety, neurological problems (stroke, dementia, depression) and the effects of social isolation may cause problems in communicating with old people. Simple measures such as ensuring that a hearing aid is switched on and that dentures are worn may make a huge difference. In people with impaired hearing, ensuring good lighting and that the patient can see your face clearly may assist with lip-reading, at which many old people are extremely adept. Further tips to assist with communication and obtaining a reliable history are given below.

1. *Introduce yourself.* Patients do not know who you are and it is a simple courtesy to tell them.
2. *Shake hands.* This friendly action provides information on the patient's vision (does the patient see and attend to the hand? Does he miss it when he reaches out his own hand?) and on the strength of grip, the temperature and moisture of the palm and the general feeling of eagerness or apathy.
3. *Sit down close to the patient.* It is off-putting to be asked questions by someone who is towering over you. Get down to the patient's level both physically and psychologically. Speak clearly, have your face in a good light and never put your hand over your mouth.
4. *Don't waste questions.* Have a clear purpose in mind with every one you ask.
5. *How well does the patient hear you?* Watch the movement of the head, the facial expression and the response to questions,

rather than directly asking if the patient hears you. Further guidance is given in the section on impaired hearing.

6. *How credible is the patient as a witness?* Begin by asking name, address, date of birth and current age. Check these against your own information. Discrepancies are very significant.

7. *How good is the patient's memory?* Avoid or postpone "formal" tests of cognitive function. You will obtain just as much information, without risking upsetting the patient, by asking about family: the name of spouse (including wife's maiden name where appropriate), the names of sons, daughters, sons-in-law, daughters-in-law and grandchildren.

8. *How well is the patient oriented?* Establish first orientation by saying, "You know who I am, of course, don't you?" and following with, "Well, who am I?" and "What is my job?". If you are still in doubt about orientation continue with, "You know what place this is, don't you?". Orientation for time is best tested by asking about the month or the time of year, rather than the day of the week. Knowledge of the time of day is also a good guide; but do not ask more questions than you need.

THE HOME ENVIRONMENT: CLUES TO AID DIAGNOSIS AND MANAGEMENT

The paramedic may be in a unique position as "Sherlock Holmes" when called to attend an old person at home. The major illnesses of old age often leave environmental clues to give assistance to the hospital or primary care team. This investigative role of the paramedic is especially crucial when the patient is a recluse, perhaps not well known to neighbours or to the primary care team, or is reluctant to go to hospital and may deny that problems exist.

A useful starting point is to consider who initiated the emergency call; was it:

- the patient? (probably wants help – consider fear and loneliness as well as genuine illness)
- a neighbour? (consider antisocial behaviour or genuine concern about failure of the patient to cope)
- relatives or carers? (consider severe dependency and carer stress. Has the general practitioner been involved? If not, why not?)

Once the paramedic has arrived at the patient's home, careful observation of the following can help in assessing the patient.

1. *The garden and outside of the house* – is it well maintained? If so, by whom? If not, is this because of low income, lack of interest or lack of ability?

2. *Access to the house* – if this is difficult, is the patient a voluntary recluse or socially isolated or is it because of neglect of maintenance, fear of assault or burglary? Check with neighbours.

3. The patient who is *slow or unable to answer the door* may be deaf, immobile or ill. Alternatively, the doorbell may not work.

4. *The letterbox test* – lift the flap and sniff! If the smell is unpleasant, consider severe neglect, urine or faecal incontinence of cats or dogs as well as humans.

5. *The general state of repair, maintenance and cleanliness* inside will give clues to the person's general level of household competence. Is the house well heated? If there is central heating, is it used? If the house is clean and tidy, who does it? At the other extreme, the visitor's feet may stick to the carpet and there may be extreme neglect and squalor. An interesting and not uncommon condition is what geriatricians call the "senile squalor" (or Diogenes) syndrome. An elderly person (or occasionally a young person) lives in utter squalor, often surrounded by piles of junk or magazines to the extent that movement within the house is almost impossible. Surprisingly the person is not demented or ill and may often have a middle-class background and have lived alone for many years. Usually they function reasonably well. People with long-standing psychiatric problems or alcoholism may also live in such squalor.

6. The *life-space* (see section on immobility) – how much of the house does the person occupy? Are there walking aids or grab rails? Does the person go upstairs? Where are the toilet and bathroom? Are they used? Is there a commode? Does the person sleep in a chair? Can they get up and walk safely? Problems in these areas point to difficulties with mobility, recent or previous falls.

7. The *kitchen* – is there food around? Is there a refrigerator? If so, is there fresh food in it? Has the person been eating? Who prepares the food? Is the person capable of using the kitchen?

ABUSE OF OLDER PEOPLE

There has been increasing interest and concern about this important topic. Abuse may be physical, sexual or financial; it may be due to neglect by relatives, carers or (it could be argued) by the welfare state which leaves many old people on very low incomes or insufficiently supported in their own homes.

Paramedics should be trained in recognizing the signs of non-accidental injuries. Much attention has been paid to this topic in children and adults in violent households but only recently in elderly people. Injuries such as finger-mark bruising (especially on the upper arms), cigarette burns (which may not be self-inflicted), bruising around the head and neck and on non-extensor surfaces may be due to assaults and should be carefully documented. Usually they are blamed on falls and in direct confrontation the old person will often deny abuse, which is often from a stressed carer on whom the old person depends. Physical abuse most often occurs within a caring relationship in which the carer, often inadequately supported, is dealing day and night with a person who is mentally or physically very dependent. Management of the situation demands care and treatment not only for the abused person but also for the carer.

CONCLUSION

An understanding of the nature of illness in old age and especially the ways in which acute illness has to be considered in the context of social, physical and mental frailty is essential to the paramedic faced with the difficult task of dealing with the emergency in an old person's home. This important and fascinating area forms an ever-increasing proportion of emergency work.

FURTHER READING

Bennett GJ, Ebrahim S 1992 Health care of the elderly. Edward Arnold, London

Pathy MSJ (ed.) 1992 Principles and practice of geriatric medicine. John Wiley, Chichester

Pitt & Brice 1982 An introduction to the psychiatry of old age, 2nd edn. Churchill Livingstone, Edinburgh

Section 7

7

THE HOSTILE ENVIRONMENT

Chapter **40**

Hypothermia

INTRODUCTION

Hypothermia is a more complicated topic than is frequently appreciated and its presence complicates the pathophysiological effects of trauma. Hypothermia is defined as having a core temperature below 35°C. Clinically, it can be divided into three categories:

- mild: 32–35°C
- moderate: 30–32°C
- severe: below 30°C

and into three groups according to circumstances:

- immersion
- dry
- urban.

These descriptive categories are not strictly delineated and the underlying clinical effects are broadly the same for each group. There are, however, some differences in treatment.

TYPES OF HEAT LOSS

Heat loss occurs from the body in four ways:

- conduction
- convection
- radiation
- evaporation.

CONDUCTION

Conduction is heat loss due to direct contact with the body's immediate surroundings, i.e. the ground, air or water. The speed with which heat is lost to the environment depends on three factors.

1. The temperature difference between the body and the surrounding environment: the greater the temperature difference, the greater and quicker the heat loss.
2. The specific heat capacity of the substance in contact with the body. Dense materials such as stone and metal conduct heat well, which is why they feel cold to the touch. They also take more energy to heat them up; for example, water takes about 240 times more energy to heat than air. Thus, when a body falls into water, rapid heat conduction means it cools very quickly. The low conductance of air as compared with water is why low *still* air temperatures are tolerated much better than immersion in cold water.
3. The surface area over which heat is lost. Children have a larger surface area for their weight than do adults and hence tend to lose heat more quickly.

CONVECTION

Convection is in essence a form of conduction in which air or water that is cooler than the body moves over the body surface. While in contact with the skin it is warmed and as it moves away new air comes in which is warmed in turn. As the rate of heat loss is highest when the temperature difference is at its greatest, this causes a more rapid heat loss than simple conduction. It is this mechanism which explains why coffee is cooled by blowing on it.

The importance of convective heat loss is not great once a casualty is removed to a shelter but is highly significant when the person is exposed to wind. This is the "wind chill" factor. The heat loss increases in relation to the square of the wind speed so a wind speed of 8 mph will remove four times as much heat as a wind speed of 4 mph. This relationship holds until the wind speed reaches 30 mph (13.5 m/s), at which stage the air is moving so rapidly that it is not in contact with the skin for long enough to be warmed to skin temperature and so heat loss increases little at winds over this speed.

RADIATION

Radiation generally contributes most to the overall heat loss in the outdoors. All solid objects, including the human body, radiate heat when not absorbing heat from the sun. The degree of radiant heat loss depends on the difference in temperature between the two substances and the emissivity of the surface (a black surface causes greater loss than white). The majority of this radiant heat loss is in the form of infrared radiation – hence the use of infrared detectors in searching for bodies.

Radiant heat loss is much more significant in the outdoor environment than in hospital, as in the latter the surrounding solid objects are at a much higher temperature (namely room temperature). Radiant heat loss to a mountainside with a temperature of 0°C is highly significant, as the loss is proportional to the fourth power of the temperature difference.

EVAPORATION

Under normal conditions, evaporation is responsible for 20–30% of heat loss from the body. Approximately two-thirds of this occurs as sweating and one-third takes place through the air passages (inspired air needs to be both warmed and humidified before reaching the small airways). Evaporation of 1 g of water takes 0.6 kcal and it is this high energy usage which explains why sweating is such an efficient means of cooling the body.

Evaporative heat loss is increased in the cold environment as cold air is often dry. Thus heat loss from sweating and from humidifying inspired air is increased. At high altitudes, where the air is thin, respiration increases in frequency and depth. As a result up to 4 litres of water a day are required to humidify the inspired air. This results in a heat energy loss of 2400 kcal. Evaporative heat loss due to evaporation from wet clothing can also be significant.

OTHER FACTORS AFFECTING HEAT LOSS

In addition to the above-mentioned problems there are several other factors that will also affect heat loss. These include immobility (often secondary to injury or collapse) and hypothyroidism.

CONTROL OF HEAT LOSS

PHYSIOLOGICAL

The temperature of the human body is normally regulated within strict limits around an average core temperature of 37°C and does not usually alter by more than half a degree. The regulatory centre for this control lies within the hypothalamus at the base of the brain. On detecting a drop in the temperature of the blood reaching the brain or on input from other sensory areas such as the skin, mechanisms to reduce heat loss and increase heat production are activated.

Reduced heat loss

Heat loss is reduced by:

- stimulation of the sympathetic nervous system, causing constriction of blood vessels to the skin
- curling into a ball, thus reducing the surface area of the body
- abolition of sweating (although some evaporation will continue to occur).

Increased heat production

Heat production is increased by:

- shivering – it should be appreciated that this results in an increase in energy and oxygen consumption by the body
- an increase in activity, (e.g.) running on the spot, foot stamping
- eating
- metabolic heat production secondary to release of adrenaline and noradrenaline.

NON-PHYSIOLOGICAL

Non-physiological methods of reducing heat loss include seeking shelter (possibly with a heating source) and the application of clothing. Protective clothing is a topic in its own right, but a few important principles are considered below.

Materials protective against heat loss

Many materials can be used in the production of cold-weather clothing. A problem with some is that their insulation abilities are dramatically reduced when wet (for example, down has only about 10% of its dry thermal insulation value when it is wet). Wool remains one of the best materials in that it retains about 80% of its dry protective value when wet. Synthetic fibre-pile materials are nearly as good.

Other "breathable" fabrics are now available which transmit water and sweat away from the skin to the exterior, thus stopping evaporative heat loss from the skin. These are usually worn as a combination of "thermal" undergarment, an insulating mid layer and a breathable outer garment. Most heat loss protection from clothes comes from their ability to reduce conductive and convective heat loss. Little protection from radiant heat loss is available, although microfibre materials are claimed to be effective.

The fingers are especially susceptible to heat loss because of their thin, cylindrical shape. Wearing mittens significantly reduces heat loss by effectively reducing the surface area of the fingers by combining them into a single unit.

Blood flow to the brain is large and the skull is a good conductor. The scalp has little fat for insulation and its blood supply is not reduced in response to cold in the same way as other areas of the skin. Covering the head is therefore essential to reduce heat loss and a material such as wool is ideal.

The thermal or "space" blanket is designed to protect against radiant loss and will also give some convective heat loss protection; it is therefore probably of more use in the pre-hospital setting as radiant heat loss is less in a warm room (although it is still present). The space blanket must not be used in isolation, however, as its conductive heat loss protection is very limited. There is no evidence to show whether the space blanket should be used on the outside or inside of an ordinary blanket. It should also be remembered that use of the blanket will reduce radiant heat absorption from the sun, which can be significant even in a cold environment.

TYPES OF HYPOTHERMIA

IMMERSION HYPOTHERMIA

A person who falls into water rapidly becomes hypothermic owing to the high heat capacity of water (see above). It is important to realize that the person will continue to cool when removed from the water owing to ongoing evaporative and convective heat loss (Figure 40.1).

Diving hypothermia is similar to immersion hypothermia, but relates to deep diving. At depth, the type of gases breathed and their density mean a tremendous amount of heat is lost through the respiratory system.

DRY HYPOTHERMIA

Dry hypothermia (or exposure, in lay terminology) is in fact rarely dry, the term being used to distinguish the condition from immersion. This is the type of hypothermia found in people who are exposed to wind, rain and low air temperatures. The heat loss is usually slow and occurs as a result of

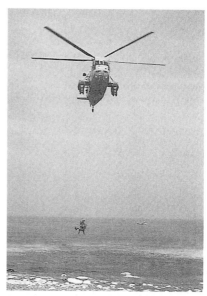

Figure 40.1 Continued cooling after removal from the water in immersion hypothermia

all four forms of heat dissipation. There is usually a degree of exhaustion in addition to the heat loss.

URBAN HYPOTHERMIA

Urban hypothermia is similar to dry hypothermia but results from neglect, immobility or another medical problem. It is frequently seen in the elderly who fall and sustain a fractured hip, lying on the floor overnight; it also occurs, for example, following a stroke or in a drunk who falls and is rendered immobile. In this case the underlying medical problem is as important as the hypothermia.

This form of hypothermia also occurs in the victims of road traffic accidents, where the immobility enhances the other heat-losing processes. This is an underrecognized problem and compounds the effects of hypovolaemic shock in that it increases oxygen requirements.

It should be remembered that severe hypothermia can be protective to the brain but mild to moderate hypothermia is not.

CLINICAL EFFECTS OF HYPOTHERMIA

Hypothermia has a number of effects on the body, irrespective of its cause (Figure 40.2).

Some effects of the cold start as soon as the core temperature begins to drop, before true hypothermia has developed (Table 40.1).

MUSCLES

As cooling occurs the muscles become stiffer and uncoordinated and there is involuntary shivering. As the temperature drops further there is a reduction in the speed of nerve impulses to muscles. This results in increasing weakness and

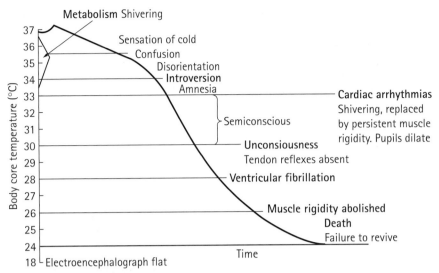

Figure 40.2 Effects of hypothermia (reproduced with permission from Eaton CJ 1992, essentials of immediate care. Churchill Livingstone, Edinburgh)

Table 40.1 Clinical features of hypothermia

Core temperature* (°C)	Clinical feature
36	Sensation of cold, stumbling, personality changes, mild confusion
35	Slurred speech, incoordination. Amnesia of events (on recovery)
34	Development of arrhythmias – typically atrial fibrillation
33	Shivering lost – replaced by muscular rigidity
31	Pupils become dilated. Loss of consciousness
30	Insulin ineffective. Risk of spontaneous ventricular fibrillation – often unable to defibrillate
26	Major acid–base disturbance
24	Significant hypotension
23	Apnoea
18	Asystole

* These temperatures are a guide and will vary between individuals

incoordination of movement. Shivering also depletes the muscle stores of glycogen and causes the accumulation of lactic acid and other metabolites. It also results in a marked increase in oxygen consumption by the body.

As the core temperature reaches 33°C, the shivering response is lost and replaced by persistent muscular contractions. This is less efficient than shivering as a means of heat production and results in the individual becoming literally "stiff with cold".

CARDIOVASCULAR SYSTEM

As cooling sets in there is an increase in heart rate which directly relates to the increase in muscular activity (shivering). It is only as the core temperature drops significantly (below 32°C) that the heart rate starts to drop. The heart, being a muscle, suffers in the same way as other muscles as the temperature drops: it becomes stiffer and less efficient. As the heart cools it also becomes "irritable" and is prone to developing arrhythmias. Blood as it cools becomes more viscous and is more difficult to pump around the body. The oxygen dissociation curve is shifted to the left, causing oxygen to be held more avidly by haemoglobin and therefore not given up in the tissues (it becomes a less efficient transporter).

Hypothermic patients develop a degree of dehydration. This is a complicated phenomenon, due in part to increased urine production (cold-induced diuresis) and complicated by fluid loss prior to the development of hypothermia and a reduced intake once it has developed. A redistribution of fluid also occurs, with intravascular fluid leaving the circulation for the extravascular compartment. This potentiates the increased viscosity of the blood.

BLOOD CHEMISTRY

Acute hypothermia is usually associated with raised glucose levels due to catecholamine-induced glycogenolysis. Prolonged hypothermia results in glycogen depletion leading to hypoglycaemia. The signs of hypoglycaemia will be masked by the hypothermia.

BRAIN

With mild hypothermia brain function becomes slower. An early change in personality can occur; for example, a quiet person becomes noisy or an extrovert becomes withdrawn.

Disinhibition may also occur. As the temperature falls, confusion and disorientation set in. On further temperature reduction these symptoms become worse with increasing lethargy, leading to eventual unconsciousness. This train of deterioration is almost identical to that seen in other conditions where brain function is decreased, for example, in hypovolaemic shock.

The pattern of deteriorating brain function with falling temperature is therefore:

● personality change
● confusion
● disorientation
● lethargy
● unconsciousness.

CLINICAL RECOGNITION OF HYPOTHERMIA

The diagnosis of hypothermia in the field is frequently difficult and often missed as attention is paid to the more obvious injuries. Cases will be missed unless specific consideration is given to its possible presence. It should be remembered that where hypothermia has occurred in one member of a party, the others will also be at risk and further cases may occur unless corrective action is taken.

HISTORY

The history frequently gives an indication of the likely presence of hypothermia and may well be the only indicator. The following questions should be asked.

● Has the patient been immobile for a prolonged period (after a fall or entrapment)?
● Is the patient wet (rain or immersion)?
● Are they adequately clothed for the conditions?
● Has the patient been exposed to the wind?
● Has the patient got open wounds, increasing heat loss?

It should be remembered that temperatures do not have to be freezing to cause hypothermia.

EXAMINATION

There are few consistent signs other than the patient's skin feeling cold. Taking the temperature of the patient is the only conclusive guide but this can be difficult and unreliable in the field. If a temperature is taken it should be performed with a low-reading thermometer. Oral temperatures can be difficult and dangerous to take in an unconscious or confused patient. Axillary temperatures are unreliable, but will at least give an indication of the degree of hypothermia. The best guide is a rectal temperature, which is usually not practical. If a mercury thermometer is used, it must be kept in position for 3 minutes. The answer to this problem may lie with the infrared tympanic thermometer which can give accurate readings within 1–2 seconds. Unfortunately, these devices are expensive and not widely used in prehospital care.

Other signs include:

● *shivering* – disappears around 33°C
● *pulse* – initially raised, then falls (but other factors interfere, e.g. hypovolaemia and raised intracranial pressure). The pulse is difficult to feel and weak. It may be irregular owing to cold-induced arrhythmias
● *breathing* – slow and shallow (although initially the rate may be raised)
● *breath* – fruity, acetone smell due to incomplete metabolism
● *mental state* – confusion through to unconsciousness (but other factors interfere, e.g. hypovolaemia and raised intracranial pressure).

The patient who is thought to be hypothermic must be examined for signs of injury or medical illness which may be masked by the effects of the hypothermia. Hypoglycaemia should be specifically excluded by carrying out a reagent strip blood test.

TREATMENT

PREHOSPITAL

The initial management of the patient is aimed at reducing further heat loss. The patient must therefore be provided with protection against the elements. This involves insulating them from the ground using a foam mat, replacing wet clothes with particular attention to the head insulation, applying blankets (including a "space" blanket) and providing a windproof outer layer. Shelter can vary from a nearby building to a tarpaulin rigged over a vehicle by the fire service at the scene of a road traffic accident. Group bivouac shelters (e.g. *Blokka-bag*) provide lightweight, portable protection for use in the hills.

If the patient is conscious warm drinks will help, but alcohol must be avoided as it causes a peripheral vasodilation.

Useful actions include:

● Insulation from the ground using a foam mat
● Removal and replacement of wet clothing
● Application of blankets
● Provision of a windproof outer layer
● Provision of shelter
● Warm drinks (if conscious).

The patient should be handled carefully, as sudden manoeuvres can precipitate cardiac arrhythmias. Insertion of an oral airway should be performed with care since the vagus nerve tends to be sensitive and stimulation can result in a severe bradycardia or asystolic arrest.

> Careless handling of hypothermia victims may precipitate fatal arrhythmias

Oxygen should be administered wherever possible, especially if injuries are present, and ideally it should be warmed and humidified.

Warmed intravenous fluid should be administered, as this not only aids rewarming but replaces some of the fluid loss. Wherever possible, a fluid warming device should be used. Intravenous fluids should be stored at room temperature and not left in cold medical packs.

The main prehospital danger is that the patient may suffer a cardiac arrest. This is most likely to be due to ventricular fibrillation. The protocols for treating arrests should be followed, but it must be appreciated that it may be impossible to defibrillate successfully if the core temperature is below 30°C. The relative protective effect of severe hypothermia on the brain gives rise to the edict that "no one is presumed dead until they are warm and dead". Thus resuscitation should be continued until the patient is adequately rewarmed.

> **No one is dead unless they are warm and dead**

No attempt should be made to actively warm the hypothermic patient prehospital by other means, such as hot-water bottles or heaters. This causes peripheral heating, with opening of the skin and splanchnic blood vessels, resulting in the washing out of metabolites that have built up in the hypoxic tissue. When these arrive at the cold and "sensitive" heart they can induce fatal arrhythmias.

IN HOSPITAL

Hospital care is only briefly covered as it falls outside the remit of this chapter, although some of these techniques can be used in prehospital care, especially if long transit times are anticipated.

The prehospital measures are continued, with appropriate attention being paid to injuries or medical problems. Further evaluation of the patient is undertaken, including ECG, chest X-ray, serum electrolytes, serum glucose, amylase, blood gases and a full blood count. The patient can then be managed by either active rewarming or passive rewarming.

Passive rewarming

In passive rewarming the patients are allowed to warm up on their own. Bringing a patient into a warm room does not actually warm the patient, it simply reduces heat loss and allows the patient to recover and warm up by their own metabolic efforts. This process is safe, although monitoring of electrolytes needs to be continued.

Active rewarming

Active rewarming involves actively reheating the patient. There are a number of methods that can be used.

Warm humidified oxygen

It is the humidification that is primarily beneficial as it reduces evaporative heat loss (air transfers little heat).

Warmed intravenous fluids

These fluids should be administered at a temperature of 37–39°C if benefit is to be obtained.

Thoracic cradle heating

Heat is applied to the thoracic region to achieve central warming. This can be done with a cradle of lights, although this method is being superseded by a warm air blanket system.

Peritoneal lavage

A peritoneal dialysis catheter can be inserted and warmed fluids instilled into the abdominal cavity to cause central warming.

Oesophageal warming

A closed circuit tube is inserted into the oesophagus and a warm fluid circulated through it. This causes central warming in a similar way to peritoneal lavage.

Extracorporeal rewarming

A cardiopulmonary bypass machine can be used to reheat the blood.

Immersion hypothermia

Patients who have undergone immersion hypothermia can be rapidly rewarmed by placing them in a bath at 40°C with their legs and arms dangling out. This is permissible as the patient has been rapidly cooled and does not run into the same physiological problems as other hypothermic patients. This is discussed further in Chapter 41.

FURTHER READING

Gunn D 1994 Outdoor first-aid and safety manual. British Association of Ski Patrollers.

Langmuir E 1995 Mountain craft and leadership. Edinburgh.

McInnes H 1998 International mountain rescue book. Constable, London.

Steele P 1999 Medical handbook for walkers and climbers. Constable, London.

Chapter 41

Near drowning

INTRODUCTION

Drowning is a common cause of death in the UK, being the fourth leading cause of death in men under the age of 35 years and the second leading cause of death in children, with 40% of all drowning deaths occurring in children under the age of 5 years. Alcohol and drugs are significant predisposing factors. "Near drowning" is the term applied to a survivable drowning episode.

Death by drowning can be "wet" or "dry". In "wet" drowning, the individual aspirates water into the lungs, after an episode of breath holding until the victim cannot hold the breath any longer. On inspiration much of the water is probably swallowed, but a proportion is inhaled. This inhaled water blocks the airways, only a proportion of it getting as far as the alveoli. The result is hypoxia which after a short period results in hypoxic cardiac arrest and hence death. It only requires 10 ml of inhaled water per kilogram of body weight to be fatal (Figure 41.1).

> "Near drowning" is the term applied to a survivable drowning episode

Fresh water in the alveoli is absorbed, resulting in haemolysis of red blood cells and haemodilution. Sea water, being hypertonic, causes withdrawal of water from the blood and no haemolysis. The changes that occur are of interest to the pathologist but not to the paramedic.

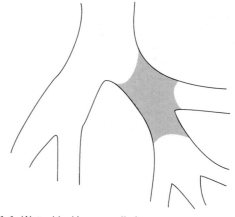

Figure 41.1 Water blocking a small airway

In "dry" drowning no (or very little) water actually enters the lungs. This may be because of laryngeal spasm but is more likely to be because of primary cardiac arrest due to stimulation of the vagus nerve by cold water. It is this mechanism that causes the death of people who drop into cold-water. It is likely that this is the cause of death in "spray drowning", deaths that occur in people on the surface of rough water. Vagal sensitivity is increased by hypothermia which occurs rapidly in cold-water immersion.

"Dry" drowning accounts for between 10% and 25% of drowning deaths, depending on the source of the information. The percentage would seem to be higher in cold-water drowning and this would fit the proposed mechanism.

PATHOPHYSIOLOGY

IMMERSION IN COLD WATER

When a body is immersed in cold water a number of effects occur, as described below.

Body temperature

When a person falls into cold water the body temperature rapidly starts to fall unless he is adequately protected (see Chapter 40). If the water temperature is much below 10°C it is very difficult for the body to generate sufficient heat, even if actively exercising, to prevent this temperature fall. The symptoms and problems related to hypothermia thus develop.

Respiratory system

Cold water has several effects: there tends to be a large intake of breath and breathing tends to occur at the maximum lung capacity, the breaths being rapid and shallow. This has the advantage of increasing the buoyancy of the individual but this form of respiration is both inefficient and hard work, causing the subject to tire rapidly.

When water temperatures are very low (5°C or less) the ability to hold the breath dramatically reduces, maximal times being of the order of 5 seconds.

Cardiovascular system

Water exerts a pressure on the body and in the upright position gives an effect similar to applying a pneumatic anti-shock garment (PASG). This principle is easily understood if one appreciates that there may be a difference of 1.3 m between the neck at the surface and the soles of the feet. A height of 1.3 m is equal to 130 cm of water pressure, which equates to approximately 100 mmHg (mercury is 13 times as dense as water). This hydrostatic pressure effect is very important when removing patients from the water; if they are removed in the upright position there will be a sudden drop in blood pressure similar to that occurring on sudden deflation of a MAST (PASG) suit (Figure 41.2).

Immersion in cold water also results in peripheral vasoconstriction due to the cold and the other changes that occur with hypothermia (e.g. reduction in circulating volume and fluid shifts between compartments).

The diving reflex

The diving reflex occurs in many mammals but its significance in adults is doubtful. It does seem to be more developed in children and probably explains why young children can survive prolonged cold-water immersion.

A reflex bradycardia occurs when cold water stimulates areas of the face and neck. This bradycardia, associated with the rapid cooling caused by cold-water immersion, can be protective of the victim by rapidly reducing the oxygen

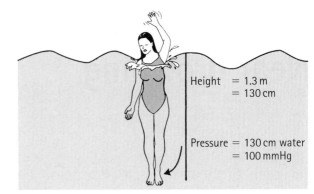

Figure 41.2 MAST effect. Pressure of water at the feet is approximately 100 mmHg. This reduces to zero at the surface

requirements of the brain and other tissues with a high metabolic requirement.

Other effects

The cold water, partly by producing hypothermia and partly by a direct cold effect on the pharynx, causes intense vagal stimulation which results in a severe bradycardia or asystole. For this reason manipulation of the airway in a near-drowned person can cause cardiac arrest.

EFFECTS OF NEAR DROWNING

The effects of near drowning are variable and depend on a number of factors: the temperature of the water, the length of time immersed and the amount of inhaled water. There is little difference between salt and fresh water.

Initial (primary) effects

The initial problem that occurs is hypoxia; the victim becomes confused, then lethargic and eventually unconscious, although patients frequently report that they experience a "high". Several divers have described this phase as being "pleasant", in that they no longer cared what would happen to them. If the hypoxia continues then cardiac arrest will occur as a result of hypoxic myocardium. The victim will also suffer the associated problems of hypothermia and the loss of hydrostatic pressure (as described above). In very cold water an asystolic arrest can occur owing to intense vagal stimulation.

Delayed (secondary) effects

Water inhaled into the lungs causes damage; this is multifactorial and includes the development of pulmonary oedema and a reduction in the amount of surfactant. As a result the subject may initially have few symptoms but may develop marked respiratory problems over several hours (usually 4–8). This problem is known as *secondary drowning*.

The other secondary problem is infection. Victims will have swallowed and inhaled water that may well contain microorganisms from sewage effluent or rat urine contamination (common in canals). Thus consideration should be given to the development of illness such as Weil's disease. Prophylactic antibiotics have not been shown to be of use.

DIAGNOSIS

The diagnosis would seem to be easily deduced from the circumstances; however, the picture is more complex, as the patient is likely to be hypothermic and may have other injuries associated with a fall or dive into water or sustained while in the water. The classic injury to the cervical spine occurs in the person who dives into shallow water thinking that it is deeper than it actually is.

The clinical picture may vary from a cardiac arrest (which may be ventricular fibrillation or asystole) to a conscious patient with few signs or symptoms but who is at risk of secondary drowning.

AIRWAY

Airway findings are variable. It may be totally patent, it can be obstructed by the tongue owing to unconsciousness or it may be obstructed by water in the oropharynx.

BREATHING

Breathing may be normal, but the chest should be auscultated as the presence of crepitations may indicate that secondary drowning is likely to occur. Breathing may be absent, either with or without cardiac arrest.

CIRCULATION

The pulse is highly variable; many of the changes will be cold related. A profound bradycardia may occur in relation to vagal stimulation.

TREATMENT

REMOVAL FROM THE WATER

It is very important that the patient should be kept as horizontal as possible when removed from the water because of the loss of hydrostatic pressure to the body (Figure 41.3). This is especially important if the patient is hypothermic and it is this combination that frequently led to deaths in the past; in World War II it was found that many shipwrecked sailors who were alive in the water had died by the time they were brought on deck.

AIRWAY AND BREATHING

The airway should be checked and cleared with care being taken to maintain the neck in midline immobilization, as a

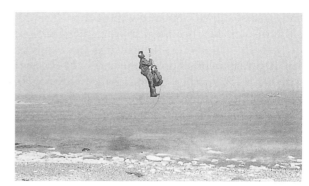

Figure 41.3 Removal from the water

cervical spine injury may have occurred on the fall or dive into the water. A cervical collar should therefore be applied unless cervical spine injury can be definitely excluded (e.g. in a swimmer who has got into difficulties). In the absence of a history of events it is safer to assume cervical spine injury. Protecting the neck is difficult while in the water but an inflated life-jacket (not a buoyancy aid) gives some neck protection.

On attempting to clear the airway, suction of the oropharynx should be used, although it must be remembered that in the hypothermic patient, any airway manipulation could cause vagal stimulation or laryngeal spasm. It is impossible to remove water from the smaller airways because of the capillary attraction between the wall and the water. This water will be absorbed if the patient survives. The patient should not be put in the head-down position as this does not help remove water from the lungs and will raise the intracranial pressure, which may already be elevated from the preceding cerebral hypoxia.

Chin lift and jaw thrust should be used but head tilt avoided, in view of the risk of neck injury. Guedel or nasal airways can be used, but care is needed as vagal stimulation can occur.

In the apnoeic patient ventilation should be commenced. This is best undertaken via an endotracheal tube or laryngeal mask, as bagging via a mask tends to blow air into the stomach, which usually contains water, and thus increases the risk of regurgitation of stomach contents.

The breathing patient may be placed in the recovery position if spinal injury is excluded, the combination of hypoxia and swallowed water being a good stimulus for vomiting.

CIRCULATION

In the absence of a palpable central pulse, cardiopulmonary resuscitation should be commenced and the appropriate cardiac arrest protocol followed. It should be appreciated that ventricular fibrillation may not be "shockable" if the core temperature is below 30°C. Cardiopulmonary resuscitation on its own can occasionally cure the patient by correcting the hypoxia (this has been recorded a number of times in children).

Bradycardias should be treated with caution. If caused by vagal stimulation their treatment improves the situation, but in the severely hypothermic patient it is frequently detrimental. A variety of other arrhythmias may be present due to hypothermia. Hypothermia, the loss of hydrostatic pressure and the presence of other injuries all contribute to a relative hypovolaemia. Intravenous access and warmed fluids are therefore required.

HYPOTHERMIA

It is clear from the preceding text that the near-drowned patient is frequently hypothermic. Once the patient is out of the water, wet clothes should be taken off as early as possible, otherwise continued heat loss will result from evaporation. First-aid measures must be aimed at preventing further heat loss.

ASSOCIATED INJURIES

The possibility of injuries must be considered and appropriate measures taken. The presence of hypovolaemia from a significant haemorrhage considerably complicates the clinical picture.

FURTHER TREATMENT IN HOSPITAL

In the patient with cardiac arrest, continued resuscitation will take place until the patient is warm but still not responding. Immersion hypothermia can be treated by rapid rewarming, in which the patient is placed in a bath at 40°C with legs and arms dangling out. This should only be done where the cooling has been rapid (see Chapter 41). This treatment is only practicable and safe if the patient is conscious and sufficiently alert to cooperate. It should not be used for the unconscious patient. If a bath is unavailable a shower is an alternative, but is less efficient and requires even greater cooperation from the patient.

The successfully treated patient will require the following investigations:

- chest X-ray
- blood gas analysis
- full blood count, urea and electrolytes.

The patient should be kept under observation owing to the risks of secondary drowning and should not be discharged home unless the blood gases and chest X-ray are normal and the patient is free from any symptoms, with a clear chest on auscultation.

Chapter 42

Heat illness

CHAPTER CONTENTS

INTRODUCTION

In the UK heat illness is not a significant problem in civilian practice; it does, however, occur in the summer months and is frequently associated with strenuous activities such as sport or military exercises. Cases of heat illness do occur in other individuals such as labourers working outside in hot, humid conditions or workers in industries such as steel manufacturing, where the working environment is hot.

As with other environmentally produced disorders, there is a range of problems progressing through minor conditions (e.g., muscle cramps) to the life-threatening illness of heat stroke.

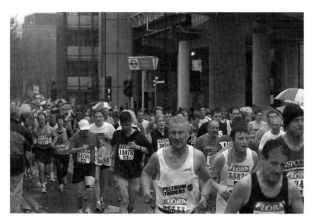

Figure 42.1 Even in the UK, overexertion may result in heat stroke in hot weather

PHYSIOLOGY

In humans the core temperature is regulated to remain constant at around 37°C. The centre for this regulation is sited in the hypothalamic region of the brain. Heat is produced through metabolism, either as a byproduct (e.g., of muscle contraction) or directly as a heat-producing mechanism. Heat loss occurs via a number of mechanisms and a fuller account is given in Chapter 40.

When excessive heat production occurs or the environmental temperature is raised, the hypothalamus detects a rise in the temperature of the blood passing through it and initiates heat-losing mechanisms. The vascular beds in the skin are opened in an attempt to lose heat by convection and conduction. Sweating is stimulated and the evaporation of this water causes significant heat loss via the energy required to cause the change of water from liquid to vapour – the latent heat of evaporation (0.6 kcal/g). In extreme conditions 1.5 litres of sweat may be produced in an hour.

In the exercising individual the respiratory rate is increased, resulting in further heat loss through the evaporation associated with respiration.

There are two types of sweat glands in humans: the *apocrine glands*, which are concentrated in the axilla, and the *eccrine glands*, which are the primary sweat-producing organs. Eccrine sweat is colourless and odourless (unlike that produced by the apocrine glands) and the salt content can be varied depending on the amount of the hormone aldosterone which is produced.

Table 42.1 The physiological response to heat

System	Effects
Respiratory	Increased respiratory rate – with increased fluid loss*
Cardiovascular	Dilated skin capillary beds Increased heart rate* Increased cardiac output* Relative or actual hypovolaemia Reduced renal blood flow
Fluid and electrolytes	Dehydration Hyponatraemia (especially if fluid loss replaced by water only)
Skin	Warm and red – increased blood flow Increased sweating
Other	Decreased liver function Impairment of coagulation

*Exercise-related condition.

The redistribution that occurs in an attempt to lose heat results in a marked increase in the blood flow to the skin and a reduction in the splanchnic and renal beds. This increased skin flow with the increased supply to muscles, in the exercising subject, results in a marked increase in cardiac output and produces a tachycardia. If the situation is prolonged then fluid loss from sweating and respiration results in a reduction in circulating volume.

The physiological effects are summarized in Table 42.1.

ACCLIMATIZATION

Prolonged exposure to a hot environment results in acclimatization. Many of the changes that occur with this process are an attempt to reduce salt loss. The concentration of sodium in sweat is considerably reduced and the kidneys increase reabsorption of sodium. This process is the result of aldosterone secretion and possibly growth hormone release.

TYPES OF HEAT ILLNESS

In order of increasing seriousness, illness due to heat exposure can be divided into:

- heat cramps
- heat syncope
- heat exhaustion
- heat stroke.

HEAT CRAMPS

Heat cramps usually occur in the muscles of the lower limbs and are related to exercise. They occur in people in whom significant fluid losses due to sweating have been replaced with fluid with an insufficient salt content. As a result the individual becomes hyponatraemic and it is this electrolyte disturbance that is thought to cause the muscle cramps.

In the UK this has been recognized as a problem in certain industries such as mining and steelworks. Experience has shown that adequate salt replacement relieves the problem.

HEAT SYNCOPE

Fainting related to the heat is not infrequently seen in A&E departments during hot weather. Elderly people seem particularly prone to this condition. The likely mechanism is a degree of dehydration from sweating, combined with peripheral vasodilation. If the person then stands for a long period, there is pooling of blood in the lower limbs (loss of the calf muscle pump) resulting in a drop in blood pressure and a subsequent syncope. Injuries can occur as a result of the fall. The condition is self-limiting as the supine position restores the circulating blood volume, but the patient should be rested and provided with an oral fluid intake. In the elderly patient this diagnosis should only be made after other, more serious, diagnoses have been excluded.

HEAT EXHAUSTION

Heat exhaustion is a condition caused by water or salt depletion. It typically occurs in subjects who are not acclimatized and who undertake vigorous exertion, for example in military training.

Symptoms and signs

The following symptoms and signs may develop.

- Headache
- Dizziness
- General weakness
- Fainting
- Normal or mildly elevated core temperature (less than 40°C)
- Tachycardia
- Orthostatic hypotension.

It is very important that the patient is treated at this stage as, if left untreated or allowed to progress, heat stroke (see below) will occur.

Treatment

The patient should be placed in a cool environment and an oral electrolyte solution provided. Care needs to be taken when cooling the patient as the traditional tepid sponging and fanning can increase core temperature by causing capillary shutdown in the skin and by stimulating a shivering response. This is a particular problem with younger children. Cautious cooling with a fan is appropriate.

In patients who have significant symptoms, intravenous fluid and electrolyte replacement is required.

HEAT STROKE

Heat stroke is a serious life-threatening condition and requires rapid treatment. The condition normally occurs in hot, humid conditions where there is little wind and it can occur in the absence of exercise. It has been seen in the UK under unusual circumstances such as people exerting themselves while wearing dry (diving) suits.

The condition occurs when the heat-regulating systems fail to keep up with heat production, are unable to function effectively or fail (e.g. loss of sweating).

It is recognized that there are two clinical forms of heat stroke: classic and exertional. Classic heat stroke occurs during a period of sustained high environmental temperature and humidity. It tends to occur in older or debilitated people. Exertional heat stroke is caused by overproduction of heat as a result of exertion and occurs primarily in young, fit subjects. Some people seem to be more prone to this condition than others and the identification of these individuals is currently an area of interest to the military.

Exertional heat stroke differs from classic heat stroke in that rhabdomyolysis and hypoglycaemia are a frequent problem. From the prehospital perspective, the conditions are very similar.

Symptoms and signs

The diagnosis is primarily clinical. The symptoms and signs are:

- temperature usually 41°C or greater
- skin is hot and dry, although sweating may still be present
- weakness
- nausea and vomiting
- confusion progressing to lethargy and eventual coma
- tachycardia and hypovolaemia
- clotting abnormalities, including disseminated intravascular coagulation
- hepatic damage – jaundice seen after 24 hours.

Treatment

Early initiation of treatment in the prehospital phase is very important as heat stroke, if not corrected, will result in rapid death due to damage to the central nervous system. This has been likened to frying eggs – the heat causes the protein to be denatured and irreversibly changed.

The patient should be cooled with care. Clothes should be removed. If there is likely to be a significant delay in transfer of the patient to hospital, then immersion in cool water should be considered. Otherwise rapid cooling can be commenced after urgent transfer to hospital. Emersion rapidly cools the individual owing to the high specific heat capacity of water (its ability to remove heat rapidly). Care needs to be taken if the conscious level of the patient is altered and in the unconscious patient protection of the airway is mandatory while performing this procedure. It is important to avoid the production of hypothermia.

Oxygen is required at high concentration and if the conscious level is altered, airway protection is necessary. There is usually a degree of dehydration and therefore intravenous fluid is required.

Blood glucose levels should be checked using a reagent strip and hypoglycaemia corrected. Fits can occur and treatment is primarily aimed at airway control and maintaining oxygenation.

Hospital management is usually undertaken on an intensive care unit. Cooling needs to be continued and electrolyte levels and the clotting status monitored.

CONCLUSION

Although serious or life-threatening heat illness is rare in this country, milder forms are common and likely to become more so as outdoor leisure activities become increasingly popular. The paramedic should be able to recognize the signs and symptoms and likely progression of these potentially serious conditions in order to ensure prompt and effective treatment.

Chapter 43

Electrocution

INTRODUCTION

The frequency of accidental death by electrocution is about 0.54 per 100 000 population per year in the USA; approximately 20% of reported electrocution injuries are fatal. Generated electricity accounts for over 90% of the deaths, the rest being due to lightning strike. Low-voltage electrical injuries (<1000 volts) are common in the home and the workplace and are responsible for half of the deaths; high-voltage injuries occur in industrial settings. Lightning strike kills approximately 200 people annually in the USA, more than most other natural disasters combined. Children account for 33% of all victims of electrical injury.

PATHOPHYSIOLOGY

Electricity flows from the point of contact to the ground, producing heat directly proportional to the distance between these two points and the resistance of the tissues in between. The effects of electrical passage are generally worse with alternating current (AC) than with direct current (DC). The current follows the line of least resistance within the body. Skin has a high resistance when dry, followed by bone, muscle, blood vessel and nerve. The higher the resistance, the greater the damage produced.

Alternating current is generally more dangerous than direct current at any given voltage because it is more likely to induce ventricular fibrillation.

As current increases the following may be seen.

- *Above 10 mA* tetanic contractions may make it impossible for the patient to release the electrical source
- *Above 50 mA* tetanic contraction of the diaphragm and intercostal muscles leads to respiratory arrest

- *Above 100 mA* primary cardiac arrest may be induced (defibrillators deliver approximately 10 A)
- *Above 50 A* massive shocks cause prolonged respiratory and cardiac arrest and severe burns

The points at which the electrical energy actually enters and leaves the body are marked by burns: the *entrance* and *exit wounds*. These are local lesions with a central charred region, an intermediate zone of whitish coagulation necrosis and an outer area of brighter red, oedematous damaged tissue.

Alternating current in the domestic setting produces entrance and exit wounds of approximately the same size. In industrial environment direct current is the most common cause of injury and produces a small entrance wound and a much larger exit wound.

The greatest threats to life following electrical injury are a consequence of tissue damage, resulting in the release into the circulation of potassium and a product of muscle breakdown, myoglobin. These may cause cardiac arrhythmias and renal failure respectively.

When attending a patient who has suffered electrical injury, it is vital to remember the possibility of secondary blunt injury which may have resulted from the victim being thrown by the electrical contact. In any unconscious patient, therefore, cervical spine injury must be assumed and closed head injury suspected.

Suspect cervical spine injury in electrocution incidents

AT THE SCENE

The scene of an electrocution is a hazardous environment for the rescuer: *are you safe to save?*

When dealing with electrical injury, the first consideration in the rescuer's mind must be personal safety. A rescuer unaware of the potential risks is in considerable danger and if injured, will become a liability and worsen the situation.

It is essential to ensure that the current is switched off before attempting to touch the victim or remove the victim from the electrical source. If possible, the current should be switched off at its source. The rescuer may have to separate the victim from the current using a non-conductive object, such as a dry broom handle. A victim may be unable to release an electrical source because currents in excess of 10 mA will cause tetanic muscular contractions to occur (see above). The only course of action will be to interrupt or discontinue the source of electricity, since separation of the victim from the source will be impossible.

In electricity pylon accidents it will be necessary to telephone the electricity board to prevent them reconnecting an interrupted source, which they will do as a matter of routine after only 20 minutes since the cause of most temporary interruptions is bird strike, which is generally not investigated.

When a worker on a utility pole is electrocuted, expired air ventilation can often be initiated by rescuers on the pole, with chest compressions if needed as soon as the victim can be lowered to the ground. In this situation, even if there is no loss of consciousness, a victim of high-voltage electrical shock should receive cardiac monitoring and transport to hospital because of the danger of delayed cardiac arrest from life-threatening arrhythmias.

RAILWAY ACCIDENTS

Many electrical injuries occur on railways, a significant proportion of which are suicide attempts. Railway-related electrocution may be AC or DC; many lines are electrified on the 25 000 volt AC overhead system, whereas others are electrified on a 750 volt DC third rail system or the 630 volt DC fourth rail system which is used by the London Underground.

The railway is a hazardous environment; it is important not go onto a rail track unless you have to. One should be aware of warning signs which indicate "Reduced Lineside Clearance" or "No Refuge". At all times, one should face oncoming traffic and a high-visibility tabard must be worn.

Telephones are clearly marked at crossings and signals and provide direct communication with Network Rail Control. Permission must be obtained from Network Rail before going on to the track and an official railway lookout should be requested using the trackside phones or through your ambulance control. Overhead line structure numbers, signal numbers or mile-post numbers can be used to identify the exact location.

Using the lineside phones, the current isolation procedure and procedure for stopping trains is as follows.

- State:
  1. "Emergency call"
  2. Name
  3. Location
  4. Why the current needs to be switched off
- Then wait for assistance!

It is important to assume that the electricity supply (whether overhead or a third or fourth rail system) is live until definite assurance that it has been switched off has been received from Network Rail. It is said that if the victim and the rescuer can remain more than 1 metre below the overhead wire at all times, it is not essential for the current to be switched off!

If a major incident occurs a Railtrack incident officer will be appointed.

MANAGEMENT

After the safe extrication of the patient at the scene of an injury, immediate management follows basic principles with an evaluation of:

- airway with cervical spine control
- breathing
- circulation.

Emergency intervention and resuscitation will occur as for any victim of trauma, to achieve and secure an airway, establish adequate ventilation and provide fluid resuscitation. Accepted conventional algorithms for cardiac resuscitation should be followed in the case of cardiac arrest following electrocution.

Electrical shock victims with no signs of life should receive the most immediate treatment. This triage priority is different from priorities in non-electrocution cardiac arrest situations because respiratory arrest may be prolonged beyond cardiac arrest, with little actual tissue damage in an individual who probably has no preexisting cardiac morbidity. Virtually all victims who do not experience cardiac or respiratory arrest survive; therefore, casualties who appear clinically dead should be treated before other victims who show signs of life.

The possibility of blunt trauma should be considered and must be assumed to be present in any unconscious patient who has been electrocuted; the cervical spine should accordingly be immobilized and the patient placed on a spine board until spinal injury can be excluded.

Oxygen should be administered immediately and intravenous access obtained via a large-bore (14 or 16 gauge) cannula in the antecubital fossa en route to hospital. If there is any suspicion of tissue damage, in the absence of intrathoracic or abdominal bleeding a fluid bolus of 2 litres of normal saline (20 ml/kg in children) should be given. If non-compressible haemorrhage is also suspected, IV fluids should be restricted to 250 ml aliquots titrated against the maintenance of a radial pulse. Intravenous fluids are essential to treat shock (from the burn or an associated secondary injury) and to optimize renal perfusion in the face of subsequent renal insult from myoglobin released from damaged muscle.

Cardiac monitoring is essential as there is a significant incidence of delayed arrhythmias following electrocution. Cardiac monitoring is generally continued in hospital for 24 hours in serious incidents.

A brief search should be made for any entrance or exit wounds, which should be covered with a clean, simple dressing during transfer to hospital.

Note that there is a high incidence of foetal mortality following electrocution in pregnant casualties. All pregnant electrocution victims should be transferred urgently to a hospital with obstetric facilities, regardless of the type, voltage or ampage of the shock.

LIGHTNING STRIKE

Unlike other forms of electrical injury, lightning strike rarely produces exposure long enough to cause breakdown of the skin, the primary insulator of the body to current flow. The current instead passes over the outside of the body: the "flashover" phenomenon. The majority of the current thus passes outside the body. If the victim is wet, the flow of current may cause secondary burns as the fluid is turned into steam. Because of the flashover phenomenon, true entrance and exit wounds are uncommon.

The almost universal cause of death is respiratory arrest. Lightning acts as a massive DC countershock, sending the heart into asystole that is normally temporary in the otherwise healthy young adults that are most often its victims. Unfortunately, the respiratory arrest that often accompanies cardiac arrest may last significantly longer than the cardiac event and ventilatory support will be required in these patients.

Patients who do not arrest immediately have an excellent chance of recovery: the victim who is moaning and groaning has a degree of stability of the vital signs and recovery is the rule.

Chapter 44

Chemical incidents

CHAPTER CONTENTS

"Then all over the underground system people began collapsing. The commuters suffered bleeding from the nose, choking, loss of vision, burning in the throat. Several victims reported seeing brown plastic containers, like lunch boxes, wrapped in newspaper on the train floor, leaking a transparent liquid."

The Tokyo underground gas attack (*Daily Express*, 22 March 1995)

INTRODUCTION

The above newspaper description of the chemical gas attack on a Japanese underground train in Tokyo in March 1995, which killed seven people and resulted in more than 4000 attending various hospitals, graphically illustrates the hazards of chemical poisoning, irrespective of whether it is a deliberate terrorist attack or an accidental release. Many chemicals are unseen and the risks are not perceived until disaster strikes. Even then, the symptoms caused by chemicals may not be immediately recognized in the victims until the rescuers develop similar symptoms. In the United Kingdom there are approximately 1300 chemical incidents annually, usually as a consequence of accidental release, the majority involving less than 10 chemically contaminated casualties.

BACKGROUND

THE CHEMICAL CASUALTY

Chemical casualties can be generated from a wide range of incidents including explosions, fires, leaks, spills or through the ingestion of contaminated water. This can result in casualties potentially suffering from a multitude of injuries such as burns (thermal, chemical or both), trauma, environmental effects (hypothermia) and acute poisoning. The effects of fire and explosion are well recognized and the management of these injuries is covered in other chapters. However, the direct effects of exposure to chemicals may result in:

- acute or chronic poisoning from the absorption of the chemical through the lung, skin or digestive tract (for example, having a cigarette without decontaminating the hands!)
- direct tissue damage to the skin or lungs
- a combination of both the above.

The severity of these injuries will depend on a number of factors such as the strength of the chemical, the prevailing environmental conditions and the length of time an individual is exposed the chemical. Therefore, a major component of the therapeutic approach to the management of chemical casualties is firstly to remove the casualty from the main area of chemical exposure (the hot zone) and then secondly to decontaminate the casualty as quickly as possible.

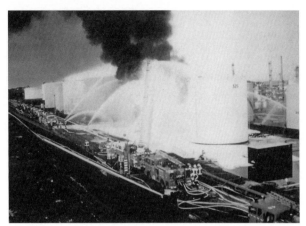

Figure 44.1 An industrial complex where hazardous chemicals are employed

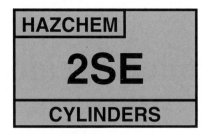

Figure 44.2 Conventional hazard warning symbols

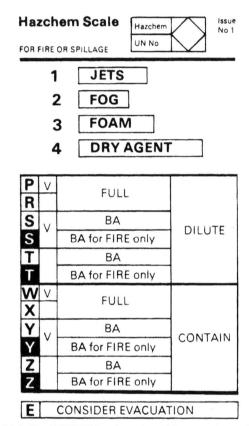

Figure 44.3 The HAZCHEM code system aide-memoire card (front)

THE CHEMICAL HAZARD

There are a variety of regulations in the UK that govern the operation of sites handling dangerous substances. The most important of these are the Notification of Installations Handling Hazardous Substances Regulations 1982 (NIHHS), the Control of Industrial Major Accident Hazard Regulations 1984 (CIMAH) and the Control of Major Accidents Hazards Regulations 1999 (COMAH). Application of these regulations to an industrial site will ensure that in the event of an accident, chemical spill or toxic release, the agents involved and all necessary arrangements for the management of the incident will have been the subject of previous planning (in an ideal world). The emergency services should therefore be aware of the chemicals involved and any special hazards or action which will be necessary to combat the incident.

It is in the realm of transport accidents that uncertainty most often arises. Many thousands of potentially toxic and hazardous loads are carried on UK roads every day. When one such load is involved in an incident it is essential that the attending emergency services can obtain information about the chemicals involved. There are a number of hazard warning systems that are of assistance to attending emergency services.

Hazard warning symbols

The standard diamond-shaped hazard warning symbols indicate to both the emergency services and the public the primary hazard present. Symbols represent hazards such as flammable solids or liquids, flammable or toxic gases, compressed gases, oxidizing agents and corrosive substances, amongst others. On multiloads the hazard warning diamond simply contains an exclamation mark.

The HAZCHEM action code system (Fig. 44.3 and 44.4)

The HAZCHEM code system is a set of code numbers and letters displayed on a vehicle carrying hazardous substances

which gives information about the appropriate fire-fighting methods and personal protection needed to deal with a spill.

HAZCHEM also gives guidance as to whether or not the substance can be safely washed into drains and whether evacuation of surrounding areas should be considered.

The HAZCHEM plate displayed on vehicles (Figure 44.5) will also show the diamond warning sign, the United Nations (UN) number for the chemical carried and a contact number for specialist advice from the manufacturer.

ADR Kemler code

The ADR system is the European road transport system of hazardous load markings. Vehicles must bear a 40 cm × 30 cm label on both front and rear. The label is in two parts: the upper bears the Kemler code and the lower the UN substance number (Figure 44.6).

Notes for Guidance

FOG
In the absence of fog equipment a fine spray may be used.

DRY AGENT
Water **must not** be allowed to come into contact with the substance at risk.

V
Can be violently or even explosively reactive.

FULL
Full body protective clothing with BA.

BA
Breathing apparatus plus protective gloves.

DILUTE
May be washed to drain with large quantities of water.

CONTAIN
Prevent, by any means available, spillage from entering drains or water course.

Printed for Her Majesty's Stationery Office by Trafford Press
Dd 0239720 C250 10/86
**25p per copy; £1.50 per 10 copies; £5.50 per 50 copies;
£10.00 per 100 copies. Exclusive of Tax.**
ISBN 0 11 340752 1

Figure 44.4 The HAZCHEM code system aide-memoire card (back)

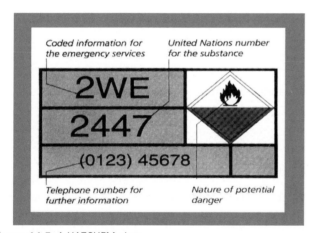

Figure 44.5 A HAZCHEM plate

The Kemler code comprises two or three digits which indicate the properties of the load carried. The first digit describes the primary hazard and the second and third digits the secondary hazards (Table 44.1). If the same number is repeated this indicates an intensified hazard. An "X" in front of the UN substance number indicates that it must not be brought into contact with water. There is no provision in the ADR system for any words to be placed on the warning plate.

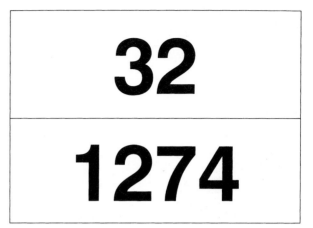

Figure 44.6 A Kemler plate

Table 44.1 The Kemler code

First digit – primary hazard	Second/third digit – secondary hazard
2 Gas	0 No meaning
3 Inflammable liquid	1 Explosion risk
4 Inflammable solid	2 Gas may be given off
5 Oxidizing substance	3 Inflammable risk
6 Toxic substance	5 Oxidizing risk
7 Radio-active substance	6 Toxic risk
8 Corrosive	8 Corrosive risk
	9 Violent reaction risk
	X Do not use water

Transport emergency cards

Transport emergency (TREM) cards exist for road and rail transportation of hazardous loads. For road transport the TREM card is a standard A4 size; it is kept in the cab of the lorry and should be changed each time the load is changed. This card gives details of the hazard, protective clothing necessary and action to be taken in the case of spillage or fire. The card will also carry first aid information for contaminated casualties and specialist contact details. The carriage of TREM cards is not mandatory in the UK road haulage industry at the time of writing.

The information gathered at the scene from the above hazard warning systems can be supplemented and verified by the use of CHEMDATA. This is a database of many thousands of chemicals and their emergency actions provided by the National Chemical Emergency Centre at Harwell. The majority of UK fire brigades now have computer links from their

Transport Emergency Card (Road) Applies Only During Road Transport

LOAD   **PHOSPHORIC ACID**

Classification code 8
UN number 1805
Odourless, colourless or yellow green liquid

NATURE OF THE DANGER
Corrosive: Causes severe damage to eyes on contact
Irritant effect on skin
Causes severe damage on inhalation or ingestion.
Attacks many metals with liberation of hydrogen which is flammable and forms   explosive mixtures with air
Dangerous to aquatic life in high concentrations

PERSONAL PROTECTION
Put on protective equipment before entering danger area
Goggles giving complete eye protection
Plastic or synthetic rubber gloves. Apron or other light protective clothing. Boots.
Eyewash bottle with clean water

GENERAL ACTIONS TO BE TAKEN BY THE DRIVER
Stop the engine of the vehicle.
No naked lights. No smoking
Warn other road users and pedestrians of the danger and to keep upwind
Notify police and fire brigade as soon as possible

ADDITIONAL ACTIONS TO BE TAKEN BY THE DRIVER
Only take action if without personal risk
Avoid direct contact with substance
Stop leaks if without risk
Prevent acid entering water courses and sewers. If this is not practical contain liquid with earth or sand barrier. Consult an expert.
If acid has entered a water course or sewer or contaminated soil or vegetation, advise police.

FIRE
Do not attempt to deal with any fire involving the load
If safe to do so tackle any small vehicle fire with suitable fire extinguishers

FIRST AID
If acid has got into the eyes, immediately wash out with plenty of water. Continue treatment until medical assistance is provided.
Remove contaminated clothing immediately and wash exposed skin with plenty of water.
Seek medical treatment immediately when anyone has symptoms apparently due to inhalation, swallowing or contact with skin or eyes.

INFORMATION FOR EMERGENCY SERVICES
Heating will cause pressure rise with risk of bursting
Keep containers cool by spraying with water if exposed to fire
Extinguish with waterspray, foam or dry chemicals
Do not use water jet

ADDITIONAL INFORMATION
EMERGENCY TELEPHONE:
Revised Aug 2002

Figure 44.7 A TREM card

control rooms to Harwell to ensure that accurate information is relayed to the fire officer in charge at the scene of the incident within minutes. With modern data modems and printers it is now possible to have hard copy information provided at the scene via a fax machine in the ambulance incident control vehicle.

THE ROLE OF THE FIRE SERVICE

Most fire brigades now have specialized vehicles and personnel trained in the management of chemical incidents. They will have appropriate gas-tight clothing and breathing apparatus to allow them to work in a toxic and contaminated area. The fire brigade will also provide decontamination facilities for their personnel, usually in the form of portable showers.

THE ROLE OF THE AMBULANCE SERVICES

As a result of an agreement between the Home Office and the Department of Health, ambulance services now have responsibility for the decontamination of chemical casualties. All UK ambulance services therefore must have rapid access to personal protection equipment (PPE) and decontamination equipment suitable for use on contaminated persons who are not wearing personal protective equipment. The Fire Service have equipment for the decontamination of large numbers (>50) of *uninjured* survivors.

MANAGEMENT

The management of hazardous materials (HAZMAT) incidents is generally dealt with under the following headings.

- Prevention
- Preparedness
- Response
- Recovery.

PREVENTION

The responsibility for prevention of chemical incidents normally lies outside the ambulance service, although senior management will normally have been engaged with the risk assessment process within their own service area. This is necessary in order to ensure that the appropriate plans have been made to deal with such an incident and that the appropriate level of protective equipment is available and the training required to deal with the most likely problems has been carried out and is regularly updated.

PREPAREDNESS

The paramedic dealing with such incidents must be confident about the use of PPE and undertaking clinical procedures, including decontamination whilst wearing these systems. This can only come through effective and regular training and exposure.

RESPONSE

Command and control

For these types of situations the incident area will be divided into a series of zones.

Hot zone

The hot zone is the area where the bulk of the contaminant is located and only those personnel with the right level of PPE and training will be allowed to enter; normally this is the fire service. Exceptionally and at the request of the fire service, paramedic or medical personnel may be required to enter this hot zone; this must only occur under fire service supervision and with the correct level of PPE.

Warm zone

The warm zone extends from the hot zone to the inner cordon and is an artificial area created by the emergency services to provide a location for the triage and decontamination of casualties and decontamination of all emergency service personnel.

Cold zone

This final zone extends out from the inner cordon to an outer cordon (this will be put in place by the police) and, if the procedures by the fire service are effective, is an area free from contamination. Whilst direct contamination should not be a hazard in this zone, vapour, particularly if the wind direction changes, may cause a problem and therefore respiratory protection (only) may be required by personnel working in this area.

Information gathering

At the scene of any incident involving chemicals it is important to gather intelligence about the chemicals involved, their quantities, toxicity and the countermeasures that may be necessary. This information is normally obtained by the fire service, although paramedics, through interpretation of the hazard information outlined in the early part of this chapter, should be able to gain enough information to determine whether special chemical precautions are required.

Safety at the scene

In relation to the hazard information, the appropriate level of PPE should be worn. If there is any doubt it is important to start with the maximum level of protection and work downwards as more information becomes available. It should be remembered that while a liquid chemical spill will be easy to see (and hopefully contain), a toxic chemical gas cloud is no respecter of a police cordon tape. Therefore rescuer safety consists of ensuring that:

- the appropriate level of PPE is worn (this will be dictated by local policies) and once a task is finished effective personal decontamination takes place
- casualties are appropriately decontaminated (this stops further injury and prevents contamination of other healthcare personnel)
- in the case of an incident with an unknown chemical, a maximum level of PPE is the most appropriate initial response which can be downgraded as more information becomes available.

Triage of chemical casualties

Chemical incidents may produce a large number of casualties with a wide range of problems, but they tend to produce patients in the ratio of:

- seriously injured (P1) 10%
- moderately injured (P2) 20%
- mildly injured/worried well (P3) 70%.

The triage process should use a modification of the triage sieve (see Figure 44.8). Walking casualties should be moved upwind near the inner cordon emergency service entry/exit gate whereas P1/P2 stretcher casualties should be taken to the casualty decontamination area (see Figure 44.9).

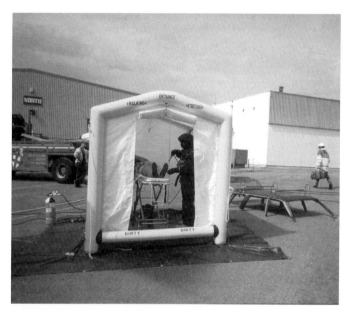

Figure 44.8 The triage sieve at a chemical incident

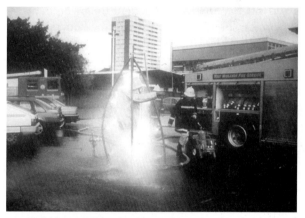

Figure 44.9 Decontamination in action

The priority for decontamination will be a balance of severity of injury against level of contamination. For example, a casualty with a large quantity of an actively caustic substance on his skin will need decontamination before a more seriously injured casualty with a small level of contamination as the former casualty will rapidly become more severely injured if decontamination is not undertaken quickly.

Treatment

The treatment of casualties will depend on the operating location within the zones.

Hot zone

This is not normally a location for paramedics. The fire service will extract casualties rapidly to the triage area whilst providing rudimentary airway protection.

Warm zone

Once a casualty has been triaged:

- P3 casualties should be encouraged to self-decontaminate (which is achieved by simply removing the clothes in most cases) and receive further management within the cold zone
- P1/P2 (stretcher) casualties should be taken to the patient decontamination area and simultaneously the:
  - face should be rapidly decontaminated by washing with water and detergent followed by the appropriate management of the airway using simple airway techniques
  - the patient should receive 100% oxygen via a mask with a reservoir
  - rest of the casualty should be decontaminated using the technique described in the section below
  - patient should receive any other basic life support procedure which is necessary, such as the control of external haemorrhage.

Cold zone

The casualty, once decontaminated, should then be handed over the inner cordon onto a patient trolley and any scoop stretchers (or similar devices) should be handed back into the warm zone. Full resuscitation techniques can now be used. Although the use of antidotes at this level is questionable, the exception being if a specific acute poisoning (or poisonings) is clearly recognized and the antidotes are easily to hand.

Patient decontamination

Decontamination of chemically contaminated casualties should be viewed as part of the initial treatment, not as an additional process, and should occur as soon as possible, within the warm zone and *prior to transport to hospital*. Avoid taking contaminated casualties to hospital as this may well necessitate the closure of an emergency department to all other casualties! The decontamination team carrying out decontamination must wear appropriate PPE. All items of clothing and personal effects must be removed from chemically contaminated casualties prior to decontamination, unless medically contraindicated. Attention should be paid to the prevention of hypothermia and the preservation of dignity at all times. Current evidence suggests that water with detergent is the decontaminant of choice for most chemicals. The "rinse–scrub–rinse" approach to decontamination should be used as summarized Box 44.1.

Evacuation

If the procedures outlined above have been followed, the casualties in the cold zone should be a minimal contact hazard. However, chemicals may continue to be "off gassed" from the casualty's skin or hair or exhaled from the lungs. It would therefore be prudent to ensure that there is effective

---

Box 44.1 Chemical decontamination

The following equipment is required:
- a water source, preferably warm, but with no delay if warm water cannot be found
- a bucket
- detergent, approximately 10 ml to one 10 l bucket of water
- a soft bristle brush.

The decontamination procedure is as follows.

1. If the casualty is non-ambulant he should be placed on either a spinal board or aluminium scoop stretcher.
2. Decontaminate the facial area before any ventilation equipment is applied. Once the airway is secured, should this be required, the remainder of the acute care procedures can be carried out.
3. Remove all items of clothing unless medically contraindicated. Clothing and valuables should be retained in a sealed plastic bag and the police service consulted regarding their evidential value before disposal.
4. Having exposed the patient, rinse the affected areas. This first rinse helps to remove particles and water-based chemicals.
5. "Scrub" the affected areas with a soft brush using the detergent solution. This first wipe helps to remove organic chemicals and petrochemicals that adhere to the skin.
6. Rinse for a second time. This second rinse removes the detergent and the chemicals. The whole process should not take longer than 5 minutes.
7. Repeat steps 5 and 6.
8. When decontaminated, the casualty should be passed over the clean/dirty demarcation line onto a clean trolley. Any equipment used during the decontamination process should not pass over the demarcation line.

---

changeover of air within the back of the ambulance; for some chemicals, respirators may have to be worn.

The accident and emergency department

Accident and emergency departments should also be capable of handling contaminated casualties (since these may self-evacuate from an incident) and both appropriate clothing for staff and a decontamination facility should be available. Each department should have identified areas for contaminated casualties but allow decontaminated casualties immediate access to the department.

RECOVERY

Following a chemical incident and in particular if individuals are transiently exposed to the chemical (or chemicals), then they should be followed up in the emergency department and subsequently by the service's occupational health system.

All equipment used in the warm zone will need to be thoroughly decontaminated or destroyed (if decontamination is not an option). Finally, the incident should be internally reviewed and the lessons learned used to change local standard operational procedures and protocols.

CONCLUSION

Chemical incidents are thankfully rare in the UK and if they do create casualties, these are few in number. However, when they do occur they can be managed with confidence if ambulance personnel have the appropriate PPE and the training to undertake clinical procedures within the warm zone. Like most situations, the secret of success is to learn and follow simple protocols and to avoid unnecessary risks.

Chapter 45

Nuclear incidents

INTRODUCTION

In the emergency response to an incident involving radio-activity the principles of casualty care remain the same – rapid assessment, administration of life-saving procedures, followed by stabilization and transport to a hospital able to deal with a radiation casualty. All of these procedures should be carried out without risking the safety and health of the paramedic team.

Incidents involving radio-activity are fortunately rare but whether it be an injury or illness occurring in someone working with radio-active materials or the result of an accident involving the unplanned release of radiation, the response team is unlikely to have had any training in this field, have no special protective clothing and no access to radiation meters. Nevertheless, paramedics will be expected to act rapidly and with their usual confidence. They therefore must be sure that they are not placing themselves or the casualty at unnecessary risk – or that the risk is acceptable.

The hazards to which paramedics may be exposed are the effects of penetrating radiation and contamination. Ionizing radiation cannot be detected by the human senses but at the levels likely to be encountered in plausible accidents, there is little risk and simple precautions will promote safe management of the radiological aspects of the injury. It is more likely that a threat will be posed by other hazards at the scene of the incident.

THE HAZARDS

Radio-active sources are widely used in the UK throughout industry, in hospitals and in further education establishments. Large amounts of radio-active materials are present in nuclear power stations, research establishments and military bases. Nuclear materials are transported by air, road, sea and rail and X-ray generators are used in industry and medical care. A radiation incident could, therefore, occur virtually anywhere in the UK.

Where radio-active materials are processed on a large nuclear site, there will be contingency plans in the event of an accident, which may require the support of ambulance, fire and local authority agencies as well as the employer's own response team. On the other hand, an incident may occur in an area where there is no local support and an ambulance is requested before radiological assessment. Radio-active materials may be discovered and cause concern at the site of an accident such as a building, fire or road traffic accident.

In this chapter, "radiation" means ionizing radiation, that is, the form of electromagnetic radiation that can produce charged particles (ions) in material with which it interacts and thereby produce in human cells short-term or long-term deleterious health effects. It excludes microwaves, ultraviolet and infrared radiation and radiowaves.

The effects of high doses of ionizing radiation are well known from accidental exposures in the past. The effects at low levels are less certain and have to be deduced from epidemiological studies. However, the risk of injury at the low doses to which paramedic personnel are likely to be exposed is very small indeed.

> Substances are said to be radio-active when they give off radiation.

TYPES OF RADIATION

The types of radiation relevant to paramedical workers are shown in Figure 45.1.

α Radiation

In α radiation a small, positively charged particle called an α particle is emitted; it travels a very short distance in air and is stopped by a sheet of paper, clothing, blood or dressings. It may just penetrate the superficial layers of the skin without any health effect. It is therefore not considered a hazard when outside the body but ingestion or inhalation must be avoided as the particles can damage more sensitive internal organs. Examples of substances that emit α particles are uranium, plutonium and radon.

β Radiation

β Radiation is the emission of a small, negatively charged particle which travels a few centimetres in air but is stopped by a thin sheet of aluminium or heavier clothing. It can penetrate the skin surface and therefore damage the epidermis and dermis to produce radiation burns. The hazard is greatest when the β emitter is in direct contact with the skin, as may occur where clothing is saturated with a solution containing β particles. Examples are iodine and tritium.

γ Radiation, X-rays and neutrons

γ Rays, X-rays and neutrons all travel great distances in air and are only stopped by thick concrete or lead. These forms of radiation can pass through the body, depositing energy and causing damage as they proceed. They are therefore still a hazard at some distance from the casualty or incident. Examples are industrial radiography sources, caesium and cobalt.

RISKS OF EXPOSURE

Ionizing radiation can affect a part of the body or the whole body, causing localized effects (radiation burns) or systemic effects (radiation syndrome). It is more likely that the dose received will not cause any visible signs or reportable symptoms but if any are present, they are very significant and must be recorded accurately.

Of more concern to the paramedic will be the presence of loose particles of radio-active material. This is known as contamination and is defined as the uncontrollable spread of radio-active material usually in the form of a dust, aerosol or liquid. The material will emit radio-activity but in

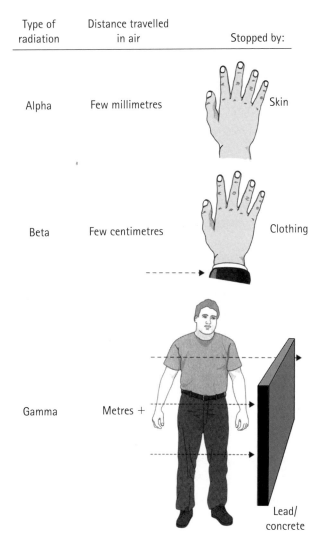

Type of radiation	Distance travelled in air	Stopped by:
Alpha	Few millimetres	Skin
Beta	Few centimetres	Clothing
Gamma	Metres +	Lead/concrete

Figure 45.1 Types of radiation

addition it can easily be inhaled or ingested and precautions are needed to prevent this.

There are therefore three scenarios involving exposure to radio-active materials that the paramedic will have to consider in the immediate care situation.

- The exposure to γ rays or X-rays from a source near to the patient
- The presence or spread of contamination onto skin, hair and clothes of the patient
- The inhalation or ingestion of contamination by the paramedic or patient during rescue, resuscitation and removal.

In each case simple precautions can be taken to reduce the risk to paramedic personnel and patients.

TYPES OF ACCIDENT

In an incident involving radio-activity, the treatment of life-threatening injuries or acute illness is more important than any concern about exposure to radiation. Radio-active

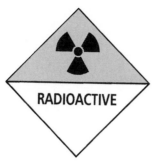

Figure 45.2 Nuclear hazard symbol

materials may be present at road traffic accidents or construction work accidents and the risk of further non-radiological injury should always be evaluated. There may also be chemical hazards or other environmental dangers. The paramedic must consider safety a priority and this is more important in the first few minutes than any concern about radiation exposure.

As a general rule, human beings cannot detect ionizing radiation but there may be useful clues available such as a radiation identification mark on package or vehicle (Figure 45.2), bystander knowledge or an unusual military or police presence. Such clues should alert the paramedic to the possibility of the release of radio-active materials; however, it is more likely that there will be no prior knowledge. The principles that are worth stating at this stage are:

- any radiation dose to the attendants is likely to be small
- simple precautions will reduce risk to personnel.

The principles of ABC (airway, breathing and circulation) still apply and must not be delayed on account of possible radiation exposure. Only when ABC has been completed and life-saving procedures initiated should the possibility of radiation injury be considered.

OVEREXPOSURE TO PENETRATING RADIATION

You may be called to attend a patient who has been exposed to a large dose of penetrating radiation, such as may arise through overexposure to X-rays or γ rays. It is important to realize that this patient is not radio-active (just as patients who have had a clinical X-ray are not radio-active) and therefore *presents no hazard to the medical personnel*. Such an incident may arise with exposure to an industrial radiography source.

EXTERNAL CONTAMINATION

If there has been a spread of radio-active materials, then the patient may be contaminated; this contamination may present a hazard to the patient and the paramedic, so it has to be dealt with safely. Such a release of contamination could arise in medical or research establishments from the rupture of a container or from acute illness in an employee when working with radio-active materials. Most of the contamination is likely to be on the patient's clothes.

INTERNAL CONTAMINATION

There may have been a release of radio-activity which the patient has inadvertently swallowed, inhaled or absorbed through the skin. It may arise if the casualty has been prevented from leaving a contaminated area or has been exposed to smoke in a fire involving radio-active substances. This is unlikely to prove hazardous to attendants but simple procedures can be used to protect both paramedic and patient.

CONTAMINATED WOUND

A patient may have an open wound which is either contaminated by radiation or has a piece of radio-active material in it. Treatment of the injury and associated bleeding is of prime importance, but care must be taken to avoid spread of contamination around the site of the wound.

DEALING WITH A NUCLEAR INCIDENT

There are several types of accidents to which a paramedic may be called. In order to reduce potential exposure to external penetrating radiation and reduce contamination, some simple procedures need to be followed.

- Assess the risks from other hazards, e.g. buildings, traffic, smoke or chemicals, just as you would in any incident.
- Position the ambulance upwind from the accident site, thereby ensuring that any contamination from a ruptured radio-active source or contaminated smoke does not pass over the ambulance.
- Carry out the initial survey, check ABC, institute immediate care and prepare the patient for movement.
- Assume contamination is present and reduce the risk of self-contamination by following the guidelines below.
- Keep the time at the accident scene to a minimum.

If there is a continued risk from radiation exposure the patient should, after resuscitation, be moved at least 10 metres from the source to reduce the dose to an acceptable level. If this is not possible, paramedics or other ambulance staff can take it in turns to monitor the patient, thereby sharing any radiation dose. If this is not possible either, an attempt should be made to reduce the level of radio-activity coming from the source. This is known as *shielding* and can be achieved by using lead or concrete but if these materials are not available then rubble, heavy stones, sand or earth can be used.

PROTECTION

In the emergency situations outlined above it is quite possible that personnel will have no prior knowledge of the presence of radio-active materials, but simple precautions of the type used against chemical or biological hazards will help to reduce the spread of contamination and subsequent risk to personnel.

1. Always assume that contamination is present when dealing with a casualty affected by an incident involving radio-activity.
2. Wear a simple surgical face mask and gloves. This will prevent spread of contamination to hands and face. If the clinical condition permits, a face mask can be placed on the patient.
3. Keep disturbance to the area to a minimum as this reduces the likelihood of airborne contamination. This should not, however, interfere with resuscitation and other emergency procedures.
4. If possible, cover open wounds with simple dressings. This prevents contamination entering wounds or contaminated blood spreading from the wound onto surrounding skin.
5. Remove external clothing (leaving underwear) carefully, if practicable, and place in large, sealable plastic bags. Wrap the patient in a blanket or contamination control envelope as this helps to prevent spread of radio-active materials.
6. Do not eat, drink or smoke until checked for contamination by medical physics personnel.

The above measures will help to keep spread of contamination to a minimum. It is probable that 90% of contamination will be removed with the patient's clothes and the likelihood of spread to attendants will then be significantly reduced.

MANAGEMENT OF PATIENTS

Whether or not the patients have been exposed to radiation, it is likely that they will be concerned and anxious and therefore reassurance is an essential part of care in this type of incident. Employees who regularly work with radio-active materials are just as likely to be affected in this way.

In all the above accidents, overexposure to penetrating radiation is unlikely to result in any specific symptoms and other injuries will dictate the management. However, the paramedic needs to know what to look for. The onset of nausea or vomiting may indicate a significant overexposure and the accurate recording of the time of onset is important for future hospital management. In addition, erythema may be visible on exposed skin and its distribution should be noted. The symptoms of the life-threatening complications of radiation exposure will not occur for days or perhaps weeks and therefore do not affect the initial management of the patient.

The police will be able to give information on the availability of hospital advice on irradiated or contaminated casualties under the National Arrangements for Incidents Involving Radio-activity (NAIR). The NAIR scheme is coordinated by the National Radiation Protection Board (NRPB) to provide advice in the event of a nuclear incident if advice from major plant operators (British Nuclear Fuels Ltd, Scottish Nuclear and Nuclear Electric) is unavailable.

Finally, it is most important to take the patient to the right hospital. A list of hospitals in the area prepared to accept contaminated casualties should be available to the paramedic. However, the clinical condition of the patient may make it necessary to go to the nearest accident and emergency department and then it is essential that warning is given so that suitable preparations can be made.

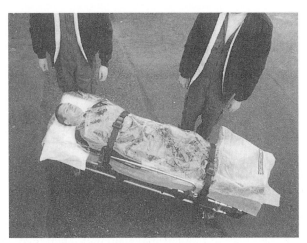

Figure 45.3 A contamination control envelope

Movement in the ambulance should be kept to a minimum and staff can expect to be directed to a specific parking area for unloading, where they should remain until screened for contamination, a task likely to be undertaken by medical physics personnel. As part of the protection available, it is recommended that ambulance crews use a contamination control envelope (Figure 45.3), thereby allowing containment of any residual contamination on the patient while permitting observation of wounds, dressings, skin colour and bruising.

FOLLOW-UP

After the patient has been transferred to hospital it may be discovered that the emergency personnel are contaminated with radiation. Decontamination is a simple process, but may need to be carried out in a special area. This could cause concern to some individuals and requires explanation.

First, contaminated clothing is identified and discarded in sealable bags. All clothing is then removed and monitoring carried out by medical physics personnel using radiation monitors (Geiger counters). Areas of skin contamination are identified by skin markers and decontamination is carried out by washing with soap and water. Areas of contamination that are difficult to remove will require a mild abrasive such as dry soap powder or industrial skin cleanser of the type commonly used in engineering workshops. Continued cleansing of the skin must be done with care to avoid inflammation and must therefore be supervised by medical or nursing staff.

If contamination is present on the face or it is known that airborne spread is a possibility then it is necessary to check for inhalation and this is normally done by checking counts on nasal swabs or nose blows. In addition, personnel will be asked to produce biological samples (faeces and urine) which will be monitored for radio-active substances or alternatively, they may be monitored at a local hospital.

If it is suspected that any intake has occurred it is likely to be small and would probably not require treatment, but therapy does exist and has been used for many radio-active substances: examples are diethylenetriaminepentaacetic acid (DTPA) for plutonium exposure, Prussian blue for caesium exposure and potassium iodate for iodine exposure.

Potassium iodate tablets are sometimes referred to as "radiation pills" and would be recommended by public health officials in the event of a release of radio-active iodine such as might occur in an accident at a nuclear power station. The tablets provide a large amount of iodine which is taken up by the thyroid gland, blocking absorption of any radio-active iodine which is then passed out in the urine and not concentrated in the neck.

Staff who are concerned that they may have received a significant exposure to penetrating ionizing radiation may take a simple blood test. Radiation causes damage to chromosomes, which can be examined within 48 hours using cultured lymphocytes from a 10 ml sample of venous blood. In the majority of cases it is expected this test will serve to exclude rather than confirm exposure.

CONCLUSION

It is unlikely that paramedic workers will be involved in an accident involving ionizing radiation. If they are, then the principles of emergency care should be followed. The paramedic who is exposed to significant amounts of ionizing radiation will be followed up by medical physics personnel and close monitoring will establish whether any specific treatment or further examinations are necessary.

FURTHER READING

Health and Safety Executive 1994 Arrangements for responding to nuclear emergency. HMSO, London

IAEA 1978 Manual on early medical treatment of possible radiation injury. Safety Series No. 47. International Atomic Energy Agency, Vienna

IAEA 1988 Medical handling of accidentally exposed individuals. Safety Series No. 88. International Atomic Energy Agency, Vienna

IAEA 1986 What the general practitioner (MD) should know about medical handling of overexposed individuals. International Atomic Energy Agency, Vienna

ICRP 1978 The principles and general procedures for handling emergency and accidental exposure of workers. ICRP Publication 28. Pergamon, Oxford

NHSE 1992 Planning guidance for the NHS in Scotland: incidents involving ionising radiation. NHS, Edinburgh

Chapter 46

The sports arena

INTRODUCTION

In today's affluent society there is more opportunity than ever before to participate in an ever-growing range of conventional and unconventional sports. Although there has been a trend away from violent contact sports towards more individual pastimes, it is still contact sports that attract the greatest number of players and spectators. It is important, therefore, that the risks involved in sport are identified, so that when called upon to help, paramedic personnel can provide the best possible care. Increasingly, athletes expect their medical and paramedic attendants to be fully conversant with the immediate treatment of sport-related injuries.

THE SPECTRUM OF SPORTS INJURY

SPORT-RELATED DEATHS

Many of the deaths that occur at sporting events are from natural causes. Examples include the spectator getting overexcited at the Cup Final or the golfer having a myocardial infarction on the 18th green. Others include the tragic deaths of youngsters who have congenital heart diseases such as hypertrophic cardiomyopathy. Many, however, arise directly from participation in sports and, furthermore, often occur in sports not usually recognized as dangerous (Table 46.1).

SPORT-RELATED INJURIES

Sports injuries keep the ambulance services and the accident and emergency departments of Britain busy every weekend of the year. There are approximately a million reported sports injuries per year in Britain. Contact sports have the highest injury rate, followed by cricket and cycling (Table 46.2). This reflects the large number of participants. Other pastimes such as riding and cycling have a relatively low injury rate but when an injury occurs, it tends to be more serious.

The factors influencing sports injuries can be classified as *intrinsic* or *extrinsic*. Intrinsic factors include:

- age
- sex
- physical fitness
- history of previous injury.

The age of an athlete influences the type of injury that develops; for example, younger athletes can develop stress fragmentation of bony epiphyses and sustain avulsion of

Table 46.1 Fatal accidents in sport
(UK statistics for 1 year)

Sport	Fatalities per year
Air sports	13
Horse riding	12
Mountaineering	11
Motor sports	10
Ball games	6
Water sports	6
Winter sports	5
Athletics	4
Cycling	1
Shooting	1

Table 46.2 Sports injuries

Sport	Percentage of all sports injuries	Estimated no. of participants (000s)
Association football	41.7	388
Rugby	9.4	87
Roller/ice skating	5.5	51
Cricket	3.6	34
Riding	3.1	29
Swimming/diving	2.9	27
Netball	2.5	23
Gymnastics	2.4	22
Combat sports	2.3	21
Hockey	2.2	21
Basketball	2.1	20
Skiing	1.8	17
Athletics	1.6	14
Others	19	177

sexes overall but boys over 14 years old are three times more likely to be injured than girls of the same age. Physical fitness is important in reducing the number of injuries: unfit participants are more likely to be injured because they do not warm up properly and many suffer knee injuries because quadriceps muscle bulk, and hence the power to maintain stability in the knee joint, is not sufficiently developed. However, experienced athletes are more prone to recurrent sprains and strains as a result of overuse.

Previous injury predisposes to further injury and people who continue to play sport despite injuries are prone to exacerbate their problems and develop further injuries as their technique is likely to be affected.

Extrinsic factors in sports injury include:

- the type and nature of the sport
- the sports venue
- equipment
- the weather
- the control and conduct of the event.

The nature of the sport clearly affects the injury rate. Contact and combat sports by their very nature predispose to injury. Sports that involve the elements, such as scuba diving, carry risks inherent in the hostile environment whereas a gentle, non-contact sport such as bowls is very much less likely in itself to provoke injury.

The venue for sports predisposes to certain injuries. Football players suffer more superficial injuries when playing on artificial turf than when playing on grass. A hard, frosty pitch may lead to a greater knee injury rate as players are unable to manoeuvre and change direction as freely as on a normal soft grass surface. Additionally, poor safety standards at grounds may lead to major problems for crowds of spectators, as evidenced by a number of major incidents at football grounds. Following the Taylor Report (see Chapter 60), stringent regulations have been introduced to ensure that safety is improved and that adequate medical cover is available at mass gatherings.

Equipment such as rackets and hockey sticks can cause severe injury to the head and face; eyes are especially prone to injury in games using small balls, such as squash. Equipment failures, such as a collapsing bar in gymnastics or a frayed rope in climbing, also predispose to injury. A lack of proper protective clothing for goalkeepers, for instance in hockey, puts them at increased risk. The weather can catch out mountaineers and hill walkers, the sea cruelly changes to endanger sailors and runners can suffer heat exhaustion on hot summer days.

Finally, the control of a sport, or lack of it, can affect the safety of players. The control and conduct of a poorly refereed rugby match can result in minor disagreements spilling over into foul play and fist fights with resultant severe injury; a poorly organised cross-country ride can mean dangerous jumps and more falls from horseback, and intrusions from

bone around the hip and pelvis as a response to excessive strain, whereas older athletes tend to develop tendon tears. Additionally, younger, less experienced athletes tend to take greater risks, with a consequent increase in injury rate. No clear difference in injury rate is observed between the

missile-throwing football hooligans endanger professional footballers.

NATURE OF INJURIES IN SPORT

The huge majority of sports injuries are soft tissue injuries. Injuries to the lower limbs are most common, followed by the upper limbs, head and face, and finally the chest and abdomen. The majority are minor and self-limiting; however, serious injuries such as ligament and tendon tears, fractures, spinal and head injuries and damage to viscera do occur and paramedics must be alert to the possibility of their presence. Paramedics must be able to decide whether the problem must be dealt with in hospital immediately or whether the patient can be left to arrange independently for treatment at hospital or by a general practitioner later in the day. Many injuries do not require medical intervention and can be readily treated with rest, ice, compression and elevation (RICE), plus analgesia.

- Rest
- Ice
- Compression
- Elevation

Certain sports predispose to a particular profile of injury. Some of these are detailed below.

ATHLETICS AND FIELD SPORTS

The majority of athletes suffer soft tissue injury and sprains. Overuse predisposes them to chronic muscle and ligament problems that may be suddenly exacerbated in competition. High jumpers and pole vaulters are liable to neck injury (Chapter 28) if they land badly. Spectators are at risk from flying missiles such as hammers, shots and javelins which can cause severe injury. Heat exhaustion is a worry in warm conditions (Chapter 42). Concomitant medical problems are also common sources of illness.

COMBAT SPORTS

Of greatest concern in combat sports are head and neck injuries as a result of direct blows (Figure 46.1) or from falls following throws. Facial fractures and eye injuries are also common (Chapter 24). Injuries to the hands and arms can occur and in some sports involving the use of feet, they too can be injured. Soft tissue injury and fractures are features of the martial arts.

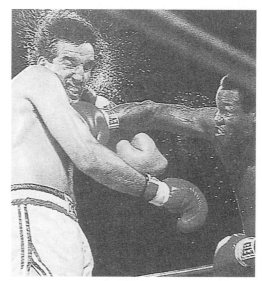

Figure 46.1 Injury in combat sport

FOOTBALL

The majority of association football injuries are to soft tissues, with strains and complete tears of leg muscles and tendons being most common. Severe knee and ankle injuries occur less frequently and fractures to the lower limb are relatively rare. Head and neck injuries can occur in bad falls or clashes of heads.

HOCKEY

Hockey players are prone to the same injuries as footballers; they also run the risk of being hit by a stick or a very hard ball travelling at high speed. Facial injuries are commonly caused by follow-through of a stick. Fractures to the maxilla, mandible and nose are often seen in these circumstances. Goalkeepers are prone to soft tissue injury and if not wearing protective face masks, their facial features may be suddenly altered by a ball at over 150 km/h.

HORSE RIDING

Falls and head injuries may lead to as many as 50% of riding-related deaths (Figure 46.2). Kicking injuries and involvement in road traffic accidents also cause serious injury. Severe injuries to the head, neck and spine are common. Maxillofacial injuries arising from kicks can be severe and airway care may pose major problems. Crushing injury can occur if a horse rolls onto its rider, causing severe blunt chest and abdominal injury. In recent years, the cross-country phase of three-day eventing has been associated with a number of fatalities.

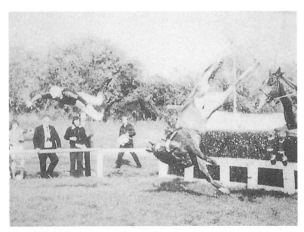

Figure 46.2 A typical equestrian accident

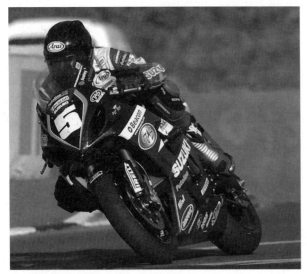

Figure 46.3 Competing in the TT races

MOTOR SPORTS

The speeds involved in motor racing and motorcycle racing can lead to life-threatening multisystem injury. Deceleration injury must always be considered as, although car safety improvements have led to the reduction of direct trauma, there is little that can be done about the deceleration forces resulting from direct contact with a brick wall or other immovable object. Track safety improvements have helped, but in many cases of racing on public roads, as in the Isle of Man TT races (Figure 46.3), little protection is offered to the wayward rider. Burns, fractures and head and neck injuries are common and crash-helmets can lead to problems with management (Chapter 28). Spectators are at great risk from flying debris and wheels or from direct contact with vehicles whose drivers have lost control. Rescuers too are at risk as, unless the track is dangerously affected, the race will continue.

MOUNTAINEERING AND HILL WALKING

Strains, sprains and minor fractures are the most common injuries in these sports. They take on a greater significance when they occur many miles from help in hostile terrain. The weather poses significant problems and the risk of hypothermia and frostbite (Chapter 40) is ever present. Falls can lead to significant multiple injuries. Hill walkers often have medical conditions and the most common cause of death on the hills is myocardial infarction rather than trauma.

> **Remember intercurrent medical illness**

RACKET SPORTS

Soft tissue sprains and strains are the most common injuries. The upper limb is more often injured in these sports. Facial injury from contact with a racket can occur. Of greatest concern in this group is eye injury. Squash balls and shuttlecocks can produce severe damage if they strike a player's orbit at close range. A familiar scenario is the unfit, middle-aged squash player collapsing on court as he attempts to recapture his youth.

RUGBY FOOTBALL AND AMERICAN FOOTBALL

The patterns of injury in rugby and American football are very similar. Players suffer upper limb problems with fractures to the hand, arm and clavicle; lower limb problems include meniscal tear and knee ligament injury, ankle ligament damage (sprain) and fractures of the tibia and fibula. These fractures are often spiral, resulting from a twisting injury on a planted foot. Head injury with lacerations and fractures to the facial bones can be associated with concussion and loss of consciousness. Neck sprains are common and severe neck injury can occur. The majority of severe neck injuries occur in collapsed scrums or in head-on tackles where hyperflexion of the neck combined with axial loading of the spine is common (Figure 46.4). Crush injury in the regular "pile-ups" of rucks and mauls may also occur with resultant damage to chest and abdomen (Chapters 25 and 26).

SCUBA DIVING

The main risks to scuba divers are from faulty equipment, faulty diving practices and hypothermia (Chapter 40). Equipment can fail at depth, causing panic and a dash for the surface. Sudden pressure changes can then lead to major problems with barotrauma or the "bends" (decompression sickness). Faulty technique on descent can lead to significant ear problems, with rupture of the tympanic membrane: cold water rushes into the middle ear and disequilibrates the balance mechanism and as a result the diver loses all sense of direction, with drowning being a real risk. Too

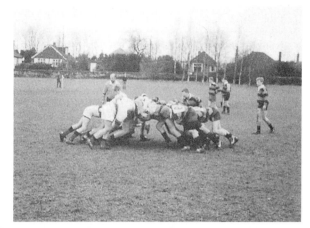

Figure 46.4 Collapsing rugby scrums may result in cervical spine injuries

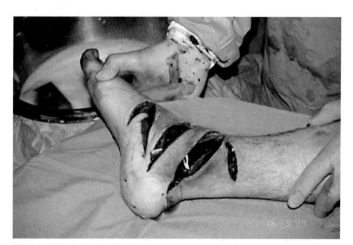

Figure 46.5 A propeller injury

rapid an ascent can lead to overdistension of the lungs and air spaces, resulting in barotrauma to these areas, as the enclosed air expands rapidly with the reduction in ambient pressure. Pulmonary barotrauma can lead to pneumothorax. Air embolus can also occur.

Decompression sickness (Box 46.1) develops because nitrogen bubbles are released from solution in the blood when a diver ascends too quickly. The bubbles can block capillary blood vessels and cause pain, especially in the joints. Itchy skin (the "creeps") and headache are early features. The larynx can be affected, leading to the "chokes", when the diver has the feeling of being strangled. In severe cases the circulation to the spinal cord can be disrupted, leading to a "spinal bend" (the "staggers") and resultant neurological damage. Nitrogen narcosis, characterized by euphoria and loss of judgement, occurs in air divers who go too deep: the mechanism is unknown.

Divers can develop the bends many hours after a dive, especially if they fly in an aircraft, when the ambient pressure is further reduced. This results in an enhanced release of dissolved nitrogen; any diver who exhibits strange symptoms after a flight that closely follows a dive should be viewed with concern. Helicopter aeromedical evacuation poses theoretical risks to injured divers, although with transport at altitudes less than 1000 feet the pressure changes will not be clinically relevant.

WATER SPORTS

Hypothermia is possibly the greatest risk in water sports in the UK. Many sailors, windsurfers and canoeists are ill prepared for sudden changes in the elements. Drowning is an ever-present risk. Head and neck injuries are common in those who dive into shallow water. Sailors can receive head injuries from flailing booms and suffer limb injuries in falls on wet decks. The new sport of jet-skiing predisposes to head and neck injury as a result of high-speed falls and collisions. Power-boat racing poses similar risks to motor racing with multiple injuries and the extra risk of drowning for unconscious or incapacitated drivers. Water-skiers are liable to develop severe rectal and vaginal lacerations when they fall as a result of forceful injection of water into those orifices. Propeller injuries are rare but can be very severe (Figure 46.5).

THE MANAGEMENT OF SPORTS INJURIES

The most important aspect of the management and treatment of sports injuries is to recognize the mechanism of injury and the likely problems which might result. An accurate history must be obtained not only from the patient, but when possible from spectators and fellow participants. The mechanism of injury will lead to the diagnosis in most cases. A thorough examination is important in order to detect hidden or latent injuries. The calculation of the Glasgow Coma Scale score and, if appropriate, a Triage Revised Trauma Score will be helpful in further evaluations (see Chapter 23 and Appendix D).

It is vital that paramedics maintain a high index of suspicion

It must always be remembered that athletes will often make light of their injuries in an attempt to continue with the game. If serious injury is suspected the player must be strongly

---

Box 46.2 Priorities in the management of sporting injuries

- Safety
- Airway and cervical spine
- Breathing with oxygen
- Circulation and haemorrhage control
- Disability
- Exposure

Table 46.3 Banned products

Type of drug	Examples
Stimulants	Ephedrine and pseudoephedrine in cold products
	Adrenaline
Narcotics	Co-proxamol
	Codydramol
	Nalbuphine
	Diamorphine and morphine
	Kaolin and morphine
Anabolic steroids	
β-Blockers	
Diuretics	
Peptide hormones	Corticotrophin (ACTH)
	Human chorionic gonadotrophin
	Erythropoietin

Box 46.3 Restricted products

- Alcohol
- Marijuana
- Local anaesthetic agents
- Corticosteroids (inhaled, topical or intra-articular administration is allowed)

---

advised, despite his protestations, to leave the field of play and be taken to hospital for further assessment.

Many patients with soft tissue injuries may require no more than advice in accordance with the RICE principle. The application of cold compresses may help considerably. If there is any doubt as to the exact nature of an injury, particularly if it involves a joint, the patient should be taken to hospital for medical assessment. Dislodged teeth should be kept in milk since they can be reimplanted if stored appropriately. The patient should be advised to seek medical care if the injury deteriorates or does not resolve quickly.

Refusal against advice to attend hospital for assessment or treatment should be recorded and signed by the patient. A witness should also sign.

All suspected head and neck injuries should be dealt with in the normal manner. In-line immobilization, a cervical collar and, where appropriate, an extrication device and a spinal board should be used. There is no excuse for treating a patient with a suspected cervical injury – or indeed any other spinal injury – in any other way. It is vital not to be fooled into allowing patients who have had a blow to the head to continue to compete; they may well be concussed or be in the latent phase after a serious head injury. The patient must withdraw and go to hospital.

All injuries, whether they are head or neck injuries, fractures or haemorrhage, should be treated in accordance with normal practice: *the tenets of basic life support and advanced trauma life support must NEVER BE IGNORED.* Airway care, the support of breathing and the maintenance of a satisfactory circulation must take priority over all other treatments. Extreme care must be maintained when head or neck injury is suspected. If these basic procedures and principles are followed then victims of injury and illness in the sports arena will have a good prognosis.

Evacuation and transportation of casualties from remote areas often cause difficulties (Chapters 29 and 47). Aeromedical evacuation may be appropriate (Chapter 48), especially when dealing with spinal injuries in remote locations. A helicopter flight may be considerably smoother and faster than a long, bumpy road journey over rough terrain.

DRUGS AND THE ATHLETE

Many competitive athletes are governed by strict rules about the use of drugs. Considerable publicity is given to those drugs that are banned and advice is available to most athletes from their sport's governing bodies. It is incumbent upon medical personnel who attend competitors to ensure that they do not inadvertently provide them with banned substances in the course of treating an injury or illness. It is conceivable that athletes may sue if they are banned after being wrongly advised by their attendants. Banned and restricted drugs are listed in Table 46.3 and Box 46.3.

The majority of banned substances do not come into the province of the paramedic, but painkillers and asthma treatments used by paramedics could affect athletes. A certificate is required from the administering doctor in the case of local anaesthetic agents and corticosteroids. If in doubt, a drug should not be administered unless it is clear that an athlete will not continue in that competition.

CONCLUSION

Sporting injuries are increasingly common but the paramedic does not need an encyclopaedic knowledge of individual sports and their injuries. The key to successful management is careful application of basic principles and strict adherence to guidelines. At the scene of an injury, acquisition of information regarding its causative mechanism will be of inestimable help to hospital personnel. In the majority of cases, injuries are likely to be minor. If these patients can be transported safely to hospital without worsening their injury and with the provision of appropriate analgesia, more detailed assessment can be performed in optimum circumstances.

Section 8

RESCUE

Chapter 47

Rescue from remote places

INTRODUCTION

A remote place may be defined as an area where rescue time is likely to exceed the "golden hour" because of geographical isolation, hazardous terrain or transport difficulties. In most instances medical resources are limited and rescue requires the assistance of specialist teams whose training, skills and equipment are geared towards working in such areas (Figure 47.1).

This chapter covers the following topics:

- mountain rescue
- cave rescue
- ski patrolling
- the lifeboat service
- search and rescue helicopters
- remote industrial sites
- expeditions.

The categories of rescue work discussed in this chapter are carried out by teams who have specialist training, equipment and physical conditioning for working in the remote or austere environments in which they operate. Unless paramedics possess (or are prepared to acquire and maintain) the knowledge, skills and physical attributes of these individuals, under no circumstances should they attempt to participate in their rescue activities. Safety under such circumstances is paramount, so that paramedics must be fully trained team members, otherwise they may become a liability, placing the other team members at risk. At other times, such as on expeditions, paramedics may have to work alone using their own

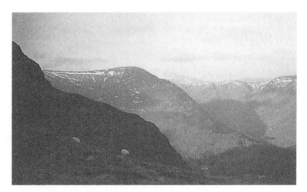

Figure 47.1 Remote terrain

resources and on extended rescues, a varying repertoire of medical skills will be required.

> Your medical skills are of value only if your physical fitness and specialist training are appropriate

This may seem obvious with regard to mountain rescue but it applies equally to the other services. An example is the Royal National Lifeboat Institution, where someone who is unused to travelling in a small boat in rough seas may not be able to cope, may therefore not be able to contribute to patient management and may themselves have to be looked after by a member of the crew, thus preventing them from carrying out their normal duties. Those involved in prehospital care are not encouraged to attempt rescue from such areas without the use of designated specialist teams and should not attempt to provide a replacement service.

Box 47.1 Conditions commonly seen in remote rescue situations

- Environmental injuries: hypo- and hyperthermia
- Dehydration
- Fatigue
- Any physical illness including myocardial infarction
- Near drowning
- Multisystem trauma resulting from falls
- Limb fractures and knee/ankle sprains
- Spinal fractures
- Skull fractures
- Burns

Box 47.2 Planning factors in rescue situations

- Command and control
- Safety
- Communication
- Assessment
- Triage
- Treatment
- Means of evacuation (transport)

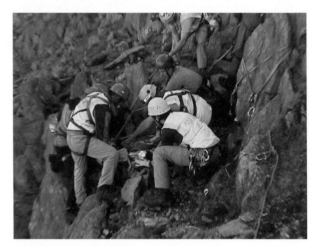

Figure 47.2 A mountain rescue team at work

A more likely scenario is one where the paramedic will be located at the rendezvous point to link up with a rescue team, so that ongoing treatment during the transportation of the victim to hospital can be provided.

Topics that are particularly relevant to remote rescue are helicopter operations and procedures (a Scottish study has shown helicopters to be involved in 59% of all mountain rescues), the use of radio/satellite communications, map reading and familiarity with global positioning system (GPS) equipment.

PLANNING

As Box 47.1 demonstrates, a wide variety of injuries and illnesses will be encountered; however, a risk analysis and review of any previous audit or reports will help to identify the most common problem areas that a paramedic may face. This will also provide the basis for planning appropriate drugs and equipment scalings, an area of vital importance where weight and bulk minimization is paramount.

As with all prehospital care, preparation for a rescue will include the collection of as much information as possible about the mechanism of injury and vital observations taken at the initial assessment on scene. The resulting outline strategy will also take into account factors such as access, extrication difficulties, weather and the severity of the casualty's injuries. The following areas are of particular note in these circumstances:

- the precise location of the incident
- the type of incident and its cause
- any potential or real hazards
- access to the casualty with possible approach routes
- number of casualties.

Much of the planning process used in the MIMMS system of incident management is applicable to remote rescue and Box 47.2 provides an outline of these planning factors.

It is important not only to focus on trauma but to consider all possibilities, as almost any kind of medical emergency can occur in outdoor situations, with asthma attacks and myocardial infarctions being especially common.

MOUNTAIN RESCUE

Mountain rescue in this country is undertaken by teams of volunteers, many of whom will possess advanced first-aid skills. At present there is no unifying standard and the level of training will often depend on the enthusiasm of the team leader and medical advisor. The doctor may or may not take part in the actual rescue work but will frequently provide advice to the team via radio. It can therefore be expected that the patient will have had advanced first-aid procedures performed before arrival at the roadhead or helicopter landing site.

The physical environment, weather and terrain together with the limitations of transport for evacuation can greatly restrict the procedures that can be performed, but should not be allowed to impede initial assessment and monitoring, nor the application of cervical, full-spinal and limb splints. It can also be expected that the team will have gained intravenous access, that external haemorrhage will have been arrested and wounds dressed. Spinal boards, vacuum mattresses and cervical collars are now universally employed and the better trained teams are able to provide enhanced levels of care with sophisticated monitoring, pulse oximetry and warmed IV fluids and oxygen. In areas where cardiac problems are commonly encountered (e.g. the Lakeland fells) ECG traces can be faxed from the scene to a nearby accident and emergency department where they can be interpreted and advice and authorization for drug administration relayed back to the

(a)

(b)

Headboard

Stretcher bed in
elevated position

Chest harness

Locking pins

Helicopter lift cables

Locking pins

Spring loaded
transverse
shafts

Side bearer straps

Patient straps

Holes on runners
for carrying strap
clips

(c)

Slots for shoulder straps for stretcher transport
to accident. Bottom end of these shoulder straps
anchor with clips through holes on edge
of stretcher bed

Helicopter lift wires

Head protector

Wheel frame hook bolts located
in blind holes on runners

Telescopic shafts locked with pins

Locking pin and swivel plate for
holding the two stretcher sections
together

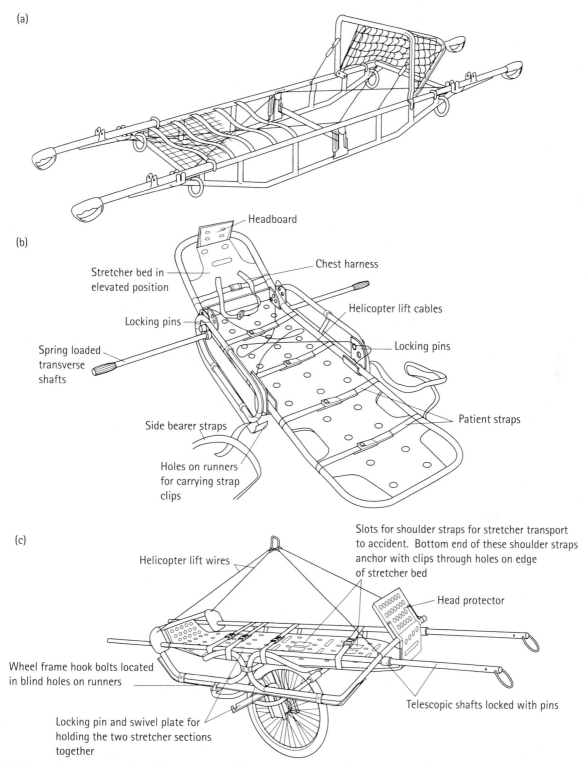

Figure 47.3 Mountain rescue stretchers. (a) Bell stretcher; (b) McInnes stretcher; (c) McInnes stretcher with wheel attachment

scene. Modern communications and the advent of mobile phones have allowed remote care standards to advance considerably in recent years, in tandem with patient expectations and demands, and have helped provide more reliable, albeit insecure, links with the emergency services.

Whenever conditions permit, the patient will be evacuated on a special mountain rescue stretcher; UK devices include the McInnes mark 5 and Bell stretchers (Figure 47.3). These are designed to provide easy transportation whilst ensuring that the harness holds the patient securely when traversing difficult ground or being winched into a helicopter. The newer MIBS stretcher is also finding favour because of its portability and relatively compact design. If the team carries a vacuum mattress the patient should be enclosed in this before being put into the mountain rescue stretcher. This makes the removal of the patient from the stretcher safer and easier and the casualty should remain in the vacuum mattress until arrival at hospital (and probably until after X-ray examination).

The handover to the ambulance crew will be the first opportunity for a more detailed patient survey. Special consideration should be given to the possibility that the patient may be hypothermic, since rough handling can induce a cardiac arrhythmia. Sufficient clothing should only be removed to allow the necessary examination, lest further lowering of core temperature results. It is important to remember that a hypothermic patient cannot be certified dead until they have been taken to hospital and rewarmed.

Hypothermia in mountain rescue deserves special consideration as it is cited as the cause of 13% of all mountain rescue incidents. It is important to remember that hypothermia can occur in both summer and winter and that in addition to air temperature, wind chill and the presence of wet clothing can be contributory factors. It has been suggested that where measurement of the patient's core temperature is impossible, shivering should be used as a differentiating factor. If the patient is shivering, then hypothermia can be considered to be mild and the patient passively rewarmed and evacuated. If the patient is considered to be hypothermic and not shivering, then they are severely hypothermic and must be evacuated and actively rewarmed as soon as possible. This is considered further in Chapter 40.

Most members of mountain rescue teams will carry aspirin, glucose and possibly tablets of a non-steroidal antiinflammatory drug. There will also be a team first-aid pack which is likely to contain morphine for intramuscular injection, salbutamol and an antihistamine. Thanks to the efforts of a Manchester surgeon (Wilson-Hay) in the 1960s, mountain rescue teams in the UK have the facility to keep and administer morphine.

An analysis of mountain rescue figures shows the following distribution of injuries:

- lower limb injuries – 46%
- bruising – 19%
- head injuries – 21%.

An analysis of fatalities shows the following:

- 38% were due to head injuries
- 15% were due to multiple trauma
- 18% were due to medical conditions.

CAVE RESCUE

Many of the difficulties encountered in mountain rescue also apply to cave rescue. Additional complications arise because of the physical environment: narrow tunnels, waterfalls, sumps, flash floods and underground lakes. These dangers, combined with navigation difficulties, low temperatures and the total absence of ambient light, make cave rescue especially hazardous. Common problems include falls and the medical complications of diving.

Even if skilled medical attention in the form of a doctor or paramedic can be delivered to the site of the injured caver, the only procedures that can be adequately undertaken are basic airway maintenance measures, pain relief, splinting of fractures and patient monitoring. It is unlikely that bulky equipment could be brought to the patient and CPR in such a confined space would prove impossible.

The previous advice with regard to hypothermia applies and patients should be left in their wetsuit and wrapped in an exposure bag before being put on a suitable stretcher such as a Stokes litter or a Neil Robertson stretcher (Figure 47.4). It is important to remember that an injured person who has been diving should not be given nitrous oxide/oxygen mixtures (Entonox).

> **The injured diver must never be given Entonox**

SKI PATROLLING

The first layer of planned medical provision on ski slopes is provided by ski patrollers. In the UK such persons may well be members of the British Association of Ski Patrollers and this organization runs courses in advanced first aid. It is likely that the injured person will be brought to an ambulance rendezvous point by the ski patrollers, probably towed on a sledge or riding by skidoo. Hypothermia and fractures and soft tissue injuries of the lower limb are prevalent. It is important to remember that patient packaging and insulation is of critical importance in these subarctic conditions and extremities showing signs of possible frostbite should not be actively rewarmed during the transportation phase.

THE LIFEBOAT SERVICE

Rescue around the coasts and seas of the UK and Ireland is efficiently organized by a combined operation involving statutory organizations, voluntary bodies and the armed forces. A major contributor in this area is the Royal National Lifeboat Institution (RNLI), which responds to approximately 6000 calls per year.

Each lifeboat station has a lifeboat doctor known as the station honorary medical adviser (SHMA). The SHMA undertakes a variety of duties, including advising on the health of the crew and first-aid training, and is encouraged to attend regular exercises and go to sea as part of the lifeboat crew in

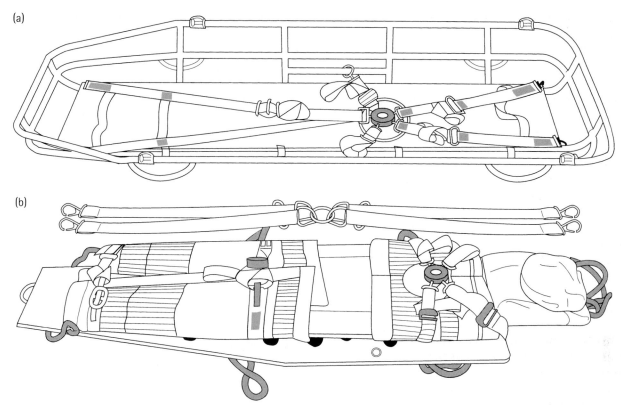

Figure 47.4 The Stokes (a) and the Neil Robertson litter (b)

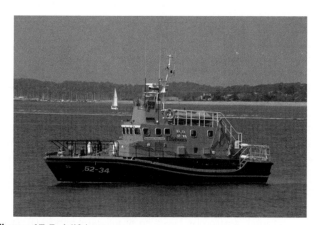

Figure 47.5 A lifeboat rescue

instances where the requirement for medical help is anticipated. The RNLI estimates that in 10% of its calls the rescue will require medical attention and that in 1% a doctor will go to sea with the lifeboat. If the situation warrants it the SHMA can be requested to give medical advice to the lifeboat crew via the radio.

Provision is also made for any member of a lifeboat crew who has paramedical skills to have access to appropriate equipment and to make use of these skills when on a rescue. All crew members are encouraged to attend first-aid courses run specifically for lifeboat crews by the RNLI, which include instruction on the use of oxygen, Entonox and special techniques for airway maintenance and patient immobilization where lack of space may prohibit traditional techniques. Special reference is given to prolonged care and monitoring of the rescued as it may take a considerable time for such persons to reach hospital. Lifeboats usually carry a basket stretcher and a Neil Robertson stretcher.

SEARCH AND RESCUE HELICOPTERS

Search and rescue (SAR) helicopter services are provided in the UK by the Royal Navy and Royal Air Force, although in some areas civilian authorities will be involved; these are generally helicopters supplied by private companies and painted in a coastguard livery. Requests for helicopters are usually made via the police. The crewman and winch operator will have had advanced first-aid training. Increasingly a military doctor with anaesthetic skills or a paramedic will be deployed but weight limitations on fuel-critical missions may preclude this. When carrying out SAR over mountainous terrain helicopters may be used to deliver mountain rescue personnel to the accident location.

An extensive range of equipment is stowed aboard each helicopter, including a first-aid kit, drug box, Laerdal suction apparatus, a pneuPAC-type ventilator, nitrous oxide inhalation (Entonox), traction splints and a pneumatic anti-shock garment (PASG). It is important to remember that a PASG must not be deflated until the patient reaches the operating department.

REMOTE INDUSTRIAL SITES

Certain types of work such as quarrying, oil drilling, fish farming, forestry and estate management may now take place in remote areas, requiring a lengthy journey to hospital. Such activities frequently involve the use of heavy mechanical equipment, hence there is always a risk of serious injury. Fire is an ever-present hazard.

Regulation 3 of the Health and Safety (First Aid) Regulations 1981 requires employers to make provision for first aid in the workplace. This involves providing equipment, facilities and suitable persons to give adequate and appropriate first aid to employees who are injured or become ill at work. These regulations are implemented to different degrees by employers, so that some sites will be totally dependent on the emergency services while others will have appropriate equipment for rendering first aid and staff who have undertaken a standard certificate first-aid course. Sites with special hazards, for example oil rigs, will have a nurse or paramedic with extended skills directed to the particular problems of their working environment. These sites will have access to equipment such as survival bags, stretchers, splints, rigid cervical collars, resuscitators, nitrous oxide (Entonox), oxygen and manual suction equipment. If cyanide is used a dicobalt edetate (Kelocyanor) kit should also be available.

EXPEDITIONS

PREPARATION

Preparation for the expedition must include contingency planning for rescue and, equally importantly, repatriation from developing countries, where medical provision does not meet Western standards. The most crucial aspect lies in obtaining specialized insurance cover prior to departure which specifically permits helicopter evacuation. Where the expedition is located away from hospital facilities a full range of medical supplies will have to be carried. These may be subdivided into individual first-aid kits, the paramedic's medical pack and a base medical kit which is furnished for all possibilities. Items should be broken down and packed in robust, waterproof containers.

The expedition medic may wish to train another team member to act as his or her assistant and ensure that all others have at least a rudimentary knowledge of first aid.

RISK ASSESSMENT

A wide array of dangers will be encountered and the team leader must always consider the unexpected. One of the

paramedic's roles will be to provide input to this process, so that a realistic appraisal may be reached and risks kept to an acceptable level.

EVACUATION FROM REMOTE LOCATIONS

When an accident or illness requiring evacuation occurs, the following chain of events should be followed.

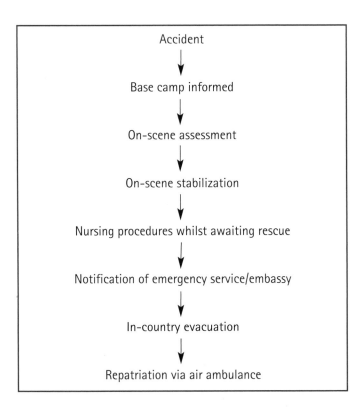

Communications form an essential part of the rescue process. They may consist of an IMMARSAT satellite system, radio, telephone, distress beacon or dispatching a runner, depending on the circumstances. Some remote regions will have access to rescue services, for example the Denali National Park in Alaska and the Himalayan Rescue Association in Nepal, which is staffed by Western physicians and local paramedics. In all cases, however, the expedition must be prepared to rely on self-help.

Rescue may be coordinated either from the base camp or by a local agent or from a distant site by an expedition representative or an emergency centre in the home country. The entire process is likely to take 24–72 hours and this can prove a testing time for those providing care in the field.

Rescue services abroad often will not act unless there is prepayment of costs and full patient details are available, so the following documentation is essential:

- passport
- copy of insurance policy
- credit cards
- local currency or US dollars

- next of kin details
- contact details of handling agent
- blood group.

Failure to provide these at the onset will lead to unwanted delays.

Providing medical cover to an expedition is a potentially demanding undertaking and the reader is directed to *Expedition medicine* (see below) for a fuller account and suggested kit lists.

FURTHER READING

Gunn D 1994 Outdoor first-aid and safety manual. British Association of Ski Patrollers

Langmuir E 1995 Mountain craft and leadership. Edinburgh

McInnes H 1998 International mountain rescue book. Constable, London

Steele P 1999 Medical handbook for walkers and climbers. Constable, London

Warrell D, Anderson A 1998 Expedition medicine Royal Geographical Society, London

Chapter 48

Aeromedical evacuation

CHAPTER CONTENTS

INTRODUCTION

Aviation and medicine may be combined in a number of different ways which encompass a complex range of treatment and transport systems. Historically, this has included the use of hot-air balloons and placing hospital beds on transport aircraft. Medical aviation is now extremely sophisticated and can be conveniently divided into *primary casualty evacuation* and *secondary patient transfer*. The expertise and equipment required for each are different.

Primary casualty evacuation (Figure 48.1) is the transport of a patient from the site of injury to a receiving hospital. This requires a medical crew which is expert in resuscitation, familiar with prehospital hazards and practised in cooperation with other emergency services. Equipment must be robust and specific for urgent interventions which may be required. The level of medical expertise determines the range and type of possible medical intervention. This, in turn, determines the nature of the medical equipment carried and varies greatly between systems. The flexibility of a helicopter system makes it ideal for the primary role, allowing the medical team to take the best possible medical care to the patient's side. The helicopter can be reconfigured to take account of the specific requirements of its role.

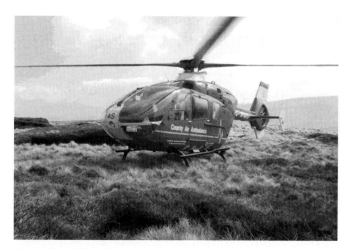

Figure 48.1 Primary casualty evacuation

> **PRIMARY CASUALTY EVACUATION: transport of a patient from the site of injury to a receiving hospital**

Secondary patient transfer is the movement of a patient between hospitals (Figure 48.2). This requires a medical crew expert in the use of intensive care equipment, monitoring and drugs. Often transfers occur over long distances and it is

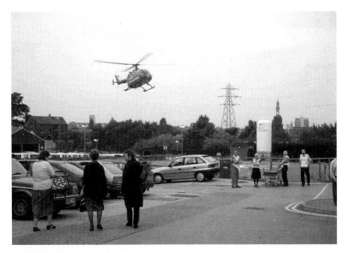

Figure 48.2 Secondary patient transfer

usually quicker and more cost effective to use fixed wing aircraft rather than helicopters for this purpose. This is a specialized subject suited to the intensive care physician and is not normally the province of the paramedic.

> **SECONDARY PATIENT TRANSFER: the movement of a patient between hospitals**

These two types of aeromedical system can coalesce during urgent interhospital transfer of an accident and emergency department patient from a non-specialist hospital to a specialist centre. However, this situation has to be planned with care as there is the potential for role confusion, conflicting priorities and medical skill mismatch (e.g. when the doctor escorting the patient has no training in aeromedical evacuation or a paramedic is asked to escort a patient who requires an intensive level of care).

PRIMARY CASUALTY EVACUATION

It is a common mistake to regard all helicopter systems as a single entity. In fact, many types of aeromedical system provide this type of service but diversity makes comparison of systems difficult and causes much controversy. Before any judgement of value or cost effectiveness can be made, an analysis of the aims of each system and the extent to which these aims are fulfilled is necessary in order to avoid misleading conclusions. The major objectives are discussed below.

TRANSPORT

The emphasis is on moving the patient from one location to another. Usually the casualty requires transfer from an incident scene that is remote by virtue of distance or terrain. There may be little medical expertise available (or required by the patient) and the system is cost effective because it obviates the use of long and difficult land transport. An example of this type of service is the evacuation by an RAF search

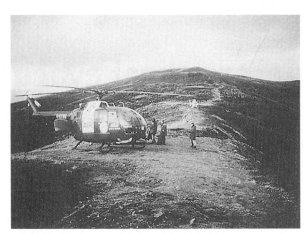

Figure 48.3 Helicopter rescue from remote terrain

and rescue helicopter of a walker with a broken ankle from a mountainous area (Figure 48.3). There is no clinical imperative to use air evacuation, but it is logistically cheaper and more comfortable than the alternative: a long overland evacuation requiring time and a large number of personnel.

In areas with scanty ambulance cover owing to long distances and a diffuse population, helicopter evacuation of patients with minor illness or injury may well preserve ambulance cover and maintain response times. For other patients this type of helicopter system may be a valid use of air transport solely because of the prohibitive cost of staffing and equipping the number of vehicles that would be required to provide the same response times using a land-based alternative. The process of care may be improved but this is a logistic rather than a clinical benefit.

TREATMENT

Most emergency calls to ambulance services are for relatively trivial conditions and most of the small number of truly urgent calls can be dealt with by ambulance personnel with advanced training. However, a small number of patients, particularly following injury, require immediate medical intervention beyond the ability of the paramedic. The patient who sustains a severe head injury (Glasgow Coma Scale score of 8 or less) urgently requires definitive airway management, yet cannot be intubated without muscle relaxants and anaesthesia. The provision of advanced medical prehospital life support is a scarce resource, which must be matched with a rare event – the injured patient whose treatment requires more complex medical intervention than ambulance service skills allow. A helicopter can bring together the rare event and the care provider, combining high-quality prehospital care with advanced medical skills, delivered by experienced doctors and paramedics.

TRIAGE

Medical services have seldom been planned logically according to the needs of the resident population. Specialist units may have arisen as a result of historical accident or the enthusiasm of individuals. The result is a hotchpotch of service provision in which highly specialized units may be on different sites from local district general hospitals. Of more significance is the rarity with which full multidisciplinary provision is available at the centre of a population mass. Bizarre geographical locations for specialist units require the prehospital medical team to exercise ingenuity and a high level of medical skill to determine the hospital best suited for a patient's injuries. This triage decision often taxes the trauma system and cannot usually be achieved by the ambulance service alone.

Matching the patient to the correct hospital can result in unnecessary transport of patients to specialist hospitals (*overtriage*). Most prehospital triage protocols "play safe" by taking the patient to a multidisciplinary centre when in doubt. Transport to a specialist centre may increase the time before hospital arrival in patients with critical conditions but decrease the time to definitive intervention. This apparent conflict is resolved if a prehospital medical team is able to treat critical conditions at the scene and during transport to definitive care.

If a correct triage decision is made at the first point of contact, then the patient can benefit from being taken directly to the "right" hospital. This reduces the time to definitive management.

CONCENTRATORS

Rare conditions benefit from being seen and treated by a small number of clinicians who become expert by virtue of this exposure. A helicopter covers large distances rapidly and can bring patients to specialist skills from a wider area than would otherwise be possible. The patient benefits by being treated by clinicians whose skills are maintained by constant practice. The occasional practitioner of advanced techniques will be unlikely to perform as well.

MATCHING THE RESPONSE TO THE NEED

With the increasing sophistication of the ambulance services there are now a number of possible responses to an emergency. Standard ambulances, rapid response vehicles, motorcycle paramedics and helicopters are all used in a stratified fashion throughout the UK. Each of these resources must be precisely targeted at the appropriate patient. Unfortunately, response capability has developed faster than the command and control systems which target them. The emergency service response for each and every situation must be matched to the medical need of the patient. This can only be achieved with a sensitive dispatch system based on medical priority. The helicopter provides an additional resource but will only be effective if targeted to the appropriate patients.

PRESTIGE

In some parts of the world, especially in the USA, helicopters are used as statements about hospitals or ambulance services.

The expense of the helicopter system speaks of the prestige of the hospital or ambulance service and is often a "loss leader" when considered against financial remuneration. This is not an efficient use of resources. In the UK this is less of a problem, but can still be a risk if helicopter systems do not identify their primary aims or have a robust system of clinical audit.

CLINICAL INDICATIONS FOR THE USE OF AIR TRANSPORT

Clinical indications for the use of a helicopter as a response to an emergency must be considered separately from logistic indications. Many conditions (e.g. cardiac arrest or diabetic coma) are unlikely to have any better outcome when treated by a helicopter system. All paramedics ought to be well practised in treating such conditions, so there is no additional clinical benefit to be gained from helicopter transport of another paramedic (or a doctor) to the scene. Most hospitals are able to manage the full range of medical emergencies, so taking the patient by helicopter to a more distant hospital is unlikely to improve outcome. There may be logistic reasons for using a helicopter, for example a remote location, but medical benefits will be rare. Dispatch and triage protocols must be based on a clear rationale.

HELICOPTER SYSTEMS

A helicopter system comes into its own if it can provide solutions to relatively uncommon situations which require high levels of judgement and skill. The most obvious example of this sort of situation is multiple trauma.

There is still debate about the role of a helicopter in trauma management and recent studies of efficacy have produced conflicting results. It is impossible to isolate the effect of the helicopter from the effect of the rest of the trauma system and so it is difficult to identify which part of the system bestows the health benefit. Furthermore, different systems use differing levels of medical, paramedical and nursing skills, making comparison of results between different systems extremely difficult. Some studies have shown an improvement in outcome, particularly with early advanced treatment followed by rapid transport to definitive care. Although lives can undoubtedly be saved, there is a cost and the society which benefits from such a system must decide whether or not it is prepared to pay for the helicopter and all the additional facilities such as intensive care beds and rehabilitation centres that are required. In the UK, the value of a life was estimated by the Department of Transport at £860 000 (in 1995) when designing roads to reduce accidents. The London helicopter service has been shown to save 13 lives a year for about the same amount. The Department of Health would be unlikely to allow purchasers of healthcare such an exuberant expenditure on an individual patient basis. The value of human life is fundamental to the economic analysis of helicopter systems but it is essentially an imponderable philosophical question, the answer to which is usually based on willingness to pay by the purchaser, arguably because a similar sum spent on an alternative health care intervention may provide an even greater benefit.

In the future there is likely to be a move towards the establishment of regional trauma systems (or regional emergency care systems) with the better integration of helicopter transport with the rest of the emergency care system.

THE MEDICAL CREW

The most important factor in determining clinical outcome is the medical treatment given to the patient rather than the type of vehicle used. The composition of the helicopter medical crew is therefore of vital importance, because there is no point in using such an expensive means of transport if it does not produce the desired clinical outcomes.

The medical team must be experienced and safe in the hostile prehospital environment. They must be trained to cope in unusual situations, including prolonged entrapments and confined spaces. There is no "ideal" medical crew for a helicopter system, as the crew required depends on the aims and use of the system. No single individual is likely to possess all the required attributes; however, a team including an experienced doctor and paramedic will generally provide all the skills required. The inclusion of a paramedic contributes an experience of safety in the prehospital environment, familiarity with other emergency services and their procedures and experience in providing medical treatment outside hospital. The inclusion of an appropriately trained doctor contributes advanced assessment skills and allows critical interventions that may be instantly required to treat the patient, including advanced anaesthetic and surgical skills. Any other combination of medical personnel leaves gaps in the range of skills provided. Many American systems use flight nurses, but this is not a model that has been taken up in the UK. A medical team without ambulance personnel (doctor only or doctor and nurse) may have the high level of medical skills required but will be vulnerable to the prehospital environment and may have difficulty in coordinating with other emergency services. There may also be a tendency to apply inappropriate in-hospital procedures to prehospital situations. Conversely, a "paramedic only" team is unable to provide all the critical interventions that may be necessary. Furthermore, the paramedic may identify a problem that requires advanced medical treatment but is frustrated by restrictive protocols from performing the procedure required.

The paramedic and doctor combination of medical crew gives a medical specification which caters for almost all eventualities and brings the hospital to the accident site. It provides concentrated experience of trauma management to the paramedic and concentrated experience of prehospital care to doctors, encouraging ever closer links between hospital and prehospital services.

SAFETY IN HELICOPTER OPERATIONS

All personnel involved in helicopter operations must be trained to move safely around the aircraft and obey the accepted conventions when in the vicinity of the aircraft. Any ambulance personnel who find themselves in this environment should not put themselves in a position in which they might be exposed to danger. Don't pretend to know if you haven't been taught! The primary danger when working close to a helicopter comes from the moving blades of the main rotor and the tail rotor. The tail rotor is not easy to see and is usually set at a height that makes resuscitation futile. The distance from the ground of both the main rotor blades and the tail rotor varies between helicopter types, with some helicopters having blades that dip at the front and do not allow access.

> **Never approach a helicopter from the rear**

The main rotor height is very variable depending on wind, how fast the blades are turning and resonance. The rule is that a *helicopter should only be approached when the rotor blades have completely stopped turning*. The correct approach is to stand apart in front of the helicopter and wait for the "thumbs up" signal from the pilot before approaching.

If a helicopter must be approached while the rotor blades are still running, it is mandatory to wait well outside the reach of the rotor blades for a direct and unequivocal instruction from the flight crew. Duck while approaching and do not hold any object such as a drip above shoulder height or carry anything that might blow away. During starting or slowing of the rotor blades there is less centrifugal force. The blade tips tend to droop closer to the ground and this effect may be enhanced in high winds. This is always dangerous and a helicopter should never be left or approached during this time. Unequivocal instruction from the pilot is essential. If a helicopter is on a slope the rotor blades are closer to the ground on the uphill side.

Rotor wash is a further hazard, throwing dust and debris into the air and blowing over light objects.

> **If you are standing within the rotor wash, turn away and close your eyes**

The medical team can assist the pilot in maintaining aircraft safety during flight and landing by watching out for hazards. Dark wires stretched across a dark background are particularly difficult to see. The more pairs of eyes that are on the lookout, the better.

Medical teams must be well versed and practised in aircraft safety and evacuation. They must wear suitable fire-retardant clothing and approved flight helmets. Seatbelts or harnesses must be worn throughout the flight and only released when the pilot gives the medical team clearance to leave the aircraft.

In some countries medical helicopters have a dismal safety record, with a reputation for being dangerous for patients and lethal for the medical and paramedical crew. This often stems from a desire to "push on" in marginal circumstances. The natural enthusiasm to reach and evacuate a patient must be restrained, remembering that adding your names to the list of casualties is foolish. A separation of medical and aviation information can be useful, allowing the pilot to make decisions in an atmosphere that is detached from any emotional pressure arising from the incident. The medical crew must never express criticism when a pilot decides that circumstances preclude a mission. The pilot must weigh up the pros and cons of mechanical failure or poor visibility within the constraints of safety. Disappointment in such cases is natural, allowed and probably mutual but criticism or shroud waving from the medical team can undermine the pilot's confidence and lead to an unsafe decision on the next occasion.

TRAINING OF PARAMEDICS FOR HELICOPTER OPERATIONS

Medical helicopter operations are controlled (since 2000) by the European Joint Aviation Authorities (JAA), with the Civil Aviation Authority (CAA) administering the Joint Aviation Requirements (JAR) in Britain. These regulations state that a paramedic can act either as a "HEMS crew member" or a "medical passenger". If the paramedics assist the pilot with any part of the operation of the helicopter, such as navigation or using the airband radio, they must be classified as a "HEMS crew member". If they play no active role during the helicopter flight they are acting as "medical passengers". This distinction is important, as each of these roles requires a different standard of training.

Under JAR-OPS 3 (the HEMS operations section of JAR) "HEMS crew members" have to undergo specified annual training. This must include the following subjects.

- Duties in the HEMS role
- Navigation (map reading, flight planning, navigational aid principles and use)
- Operation of radio equipment
- Use of onboard medical equipment
- Preparing the helicopter and specialist medical equipment for subsequent HEMS departure
- Basic understanding of the helicopter type in terms of location and design of normal and emergency systems and equipments
- Crew coordination
- Practice of response to HEMS callout
- Conducting refuelling and rotors running refuelling
- HEMS operating site selection and use
- Techniques for handling patients, the medical consequences of air transport and some knowledge of hospital casualty reception
- Marshalling signals
- Underslung load operations as appropriate
- Winch operations as appropriate

- The dangers to self and others of rotor running helicopters, including loading of patients
- The use of the helicopter intercommunications system.

All single-pilot medical helicopter operations will have to train their paramedics to these standards if the paramedic is to continue to assist with the navigation.

Medical passengers do not have an active role during flight and so have a smaller training requirement. Subjects that must be covered are:

- familiarization with the helicopter types(s) operated
- entry and exit under normal and emergency conditions for both self and patients
- use of the relevant onboard specialist medical equipment
- the need for the commander's approval prior to use of specialist equipment
- method of supervision of other medical staff
- the use of the helicopter intercommunication systems
- location and use of onboard fire extinguishers.

In addition to the standards required by the CAA, the paramedic has to acquire the skills required for safe and effective patient care in the aeromedical environment. Training must cover safety, advanced patient assessment, advanced paramedical interventions, coordination with other emergency services, rescue in special situations (e.g. confined spaces, entrapment, construction sites) and, if working with a doctor, the indications, rationale and technique used for medical interventions.

The training period should include realistic scenarios which enable individuals to practise with a real prehospital team and plausible physical surroundings. This also helps a prehospital medical team to work together and allows the patient to benefit from a blend of jointly practised skills. This is especially important for the doctor–paramedic team because it is likely that both of these individuals will be used to a high level of autonomy and control.

Time spent flying as an observer with an experienced medical crew is highly desirable, providing space will allow. In a busy system 2 weeks is sufficient, but in a system with few calls observer time needs to be correspondingly longer.

AVIATION MEDICINE

The parts of aviation medicine concerned with the effects of pressure changes (e.g. exacerbation of pneumothoraces, expansion of endotracheal tube balloons) have very little relevance to the sort of systems that most paramedics will encounter. Helicopter systems involved with primary casualty evacuation in the UK are unlikely to fly at more than 450 m and at this sort of altitude pressure changes have few clinical effects. Some transport systems do go through large altitude changes, under which circumstances the medical crew must be appropriately trained (e.g. to fill endotracheal tube balloons with water and to treat air-filled cavities prior to flying) and know and watch for the effects of pressure changes. This is a specialist area (usually involving fixed wing repatriation flights) which is usually practised by an intensive care doctor.

Many subtle physiological changes are produced when a patient travels by helicopter, mainly in the cardiovascular system. In practice, these changes do not affect standard patient monitoring or treatment protocols. The loading of a patient may be affected by the nature of their injuries. A helicopter flies "nose down", which has the effect of raising the patient's feet if loaded with the head forwards. This may increase intracranial pressure, therefore head injury patients may be best transported with their feet forwards, to elevate the head.

WORKING IN THE HELICOPTER

A number of environmental factors make a helicopter a difficult place to work in compared with a road ambulance. The noise and motion of a helicopter can be very disorienting owing to an overload of information reaching the brain from ears, eyes and the vestibular apparatus. It takes training and experience for a paramedic (or any other member of the medical crew) to develop "air sense", in exactly the same way as it takes time to develop "street sense". Some people cannot or will not adjust to this environment and may remain extremely fearful of flying. It is wise for them to be channelled into other areas of work without fuss or condemnation. The major differences from working in a conventional ambulance are discussed below.

Internal space

Many helicopters used in the medical role have limited internal space, which restricts access to the patient. This can make assessment and intervention difficult (Figure 48.4). The Euro-copter 135 has 162 cubic feet of internal space, the MD 902 Explorer has 172 cubic feet, the Augusta 109 Power has 160 cubic feet and the Dauphin has 176 cubic feet, compared to 250 cubic feet in a typical ambulance. The internal configuration must be meticulously planned to provide the best possible utilization of the room available.

Noise

The noise level inside a helicopter is usually 90 decibels or more, a level that will damage hearing over time. This is not solely a risk to the health of the crew – it also gives rise to problems of communication. All crew members must wear approved ear protection. It is essential that helmets include headsets and microphones to allow free communication between members of the team. When conscious patients are being transported, it is essential that the medical crew are able to communicate with the patient, to deliver explanation

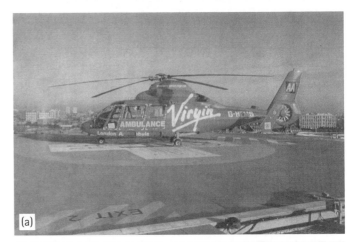

(a)

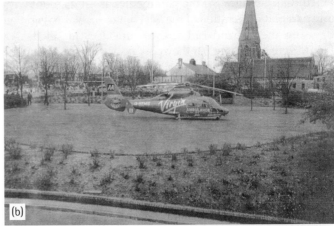

(b)

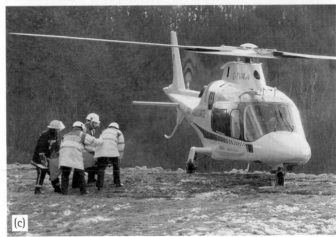

(c)

Figure 48.5 Different types of helicopter

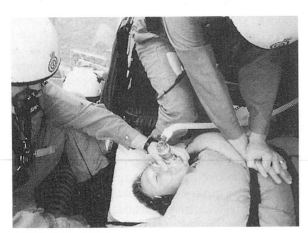

Figure 48.4 Working inside a helicopter

and reassurance. Some operators play music to their patients. Noise precludes the use of auditory alarms on monitoring equipment so visual alarms and persistent close observation are required. Training is required as personnel who normally rely on audible alarms have to readjust their visual and auditory senses.

Vibration, movement and air sickness

Vibration inside a helicopter is extremely variable but can be marked. This may reduce the signal quality of some monitoring systems. In general there is less sudden movement in a helicopter than in a land vehicle. The continual movement as the helicopter assumes different attitudes tends to cause crew fatigue as little-used muscle groups are continuously recruited in order to brace the body against a new and unnatural force.

Air sickness is closely related to movement. The vestibular apparatus of the inner ear gives dynamic and static positional information to the brain which is routinely processed to maintain balance. With movement in three planes, a mismatch of these signals with visual information will almost inevitably give rise to a feeling of nausea. Rough weather adds to the disruption and misinformation given to the brain by the position sensors, making vomiting more likely. Nausea may be exacerbated by strong smells and in particular incompletely burned fuel in exhaust fumes which are drawn into the cabin. The addition of the smell of vomit from a patient may precipitate waves of nausea. Air sickness can be minimized by adjusting air vents to give a supply of cool, fresh air. Starting at a fixed point may help but frequent changes of height may conspire to make the eyes change position, readjusting the way the object is observed. Flying with a full stomach is unwise if one is prone to air sickness and antiemetic medication, particularly cinnarizine (Stugeron), may be of great help to those who are prone to nausea. Frequent flying leads to some habituation and a decrease in the severity of air sickness, although some victims of air sickness cannot be desensitized.

Strength of vehicle

Helicopters are not built to the same rugged internal cabin specification as ambulances. The materials used in helicopter construction are strong where strength is of paramount importance and the ability of the airframe and other parts to take loads is strictly defined by the CAA, but in other areas light materials are used which tend to be fragile and do not stand up well to heavy handling by the medical crew. Helicopter doors, for example are lightweight and can be damaged by a minor knock from a stretcher on loading the patient or even by closure in the wrong way.

MEDICAL MANAGEMENT DURING HELICOPTER TRANSPORT

A helicopter in stable flight is possibly a less difficult place than the back of an ambulance in which to perform medical interventions. The movement does not involve the sudden turns and violent up-and-down forces encountered during road transport. There is undoubtedly advantage to moving a patient by air before critical interventions have been performed. However, even if air evacuation is more rapid than ground evacuation, it may still be too long for the hypoxic, hypercapnic or hypotensive patient to be transported without critical interventions being performed at the moment of first medical contact. The quickest way to correct such physiological abnormalities is for the helicopter medical team to have the skill to perform any treatment that may be needed.

The patients who are most likely to be sensitive to prehospital interventions and who stand to benefit most are those with severe head injuries. To correct hypoxia and hypercapnia in these patients, the prehospital medical team needs to give general anaesthesia with muscle relaxants. Unless the patient is already virtually dead, most will maintain laryngeal reflexes and will not accept an orotracheal tube without gagging and raising their intracranial pressure. Blind nasal intubation by paramedics without anaesthetic drugs is routinely used in America but has failed to win general acceptance in Britain (see Chapter 7). If the helicopter medical team does not have the skills to complete the "AB" of the primary survey in the trauma patient, and in particular the ability to give a general anaesthetic, a "scoop-and-run" policy is mandatory. It seems logical that if one cannot perform the critical intervention required then the patient must be moved to someone who can.

A fundamental precept of all medical treatment is to do no further harm to the patient. The patient therefore needs to be "packaged" before transport by air. Every patient must be firmly secured and protected with spinal immobilization from further harm during transport. This can be achieved by using a vacuum mattress to enclose the patient in a rigid shell. It would also be possible to use firm strapping to secure the patient on a long spinal board (although this method is not currently allowed by the CAA). A particular worry with the use of a long spinal board is that the smooth surface may allow the body to slide while the head is strapped in a secure position, so causing movement of, or traction on, the neck. This can be prevented by using two straps crossing diagonally over each shoulder to the opposite hip; one strap laterally across the hips; and a fourth strap from the lower legs in a figure of eight around the bottom of the feet.

At the time of writing military helicopters are not allowed to carry a vacuum mattress, since rupture of the mattress with release of the enclosed polystyrene beads could cause severe damage, resulting in helicopter grounding.

SELECTION OF RECEIVING HOSPITAL

A helicopter gives the prehospital medical team a wider choice of destination. Hospitals have evolved with different ranges of specialties and vary from the multidisciplinary unit with all the services on one site to single-specialty units such as burns centres. All hospitals are not therefore equal in their ability to deal with particular conditions. As the helicopter can cover large distances in a short time the prehospital team are able to pick the most appropriate hospital destination for each patient. If the prehospital team cannot perform the necessary critical interventions then this choice may not apply, as the priority is to move the patient to someone who can perform the required interventions. This leads to a conflict between the patient's immediate need (critical interventions), and longer term need (specialist treatment that may not be available at the local hospital).

There is good evidence that the sooner a head-injured patient receives surgery, the better the outcome (particularly in the case of traumatic extradural and subdural haematomas). The speed of a helicopter allows patients with isolated head injury to be taken directly to neurosurgical centres, decreasing the time to definitive neurosurgical intervention. Patients with multisystem injury should not be taken to specialist units where the facilities and personnel for general trauma assessment and management are unavailable.

AUDIT

Continuing constructive criticism of helicopter operations is essential. Medical audit is an accepted and valued way of assessing medical systems. This concept is not widely used in prehospital care, but is an invaluable way of examining the performance of a helicopter system. Audit should be concentrated on medical rather than logistic endpoints and so needs the supervision of a senior clinician with experience of prehospital care.

PSYCHOLOGICAL EFFECTS

As a helicopter system acts as a "concentrator", personnel working within the system will be exposed to a large number of seriously ill or traumatized patients. This method of organization makes medical sense (as outlined above), but is stressful for the staff involved. A debriefing system and regular rotation to more routine duties is essential to prevent "burnout", posttraumatic stress or elitism.

CONCLUSION

Aviation and medicine may be combined in a number of different ways: paramedics are most likely to be involved in helicopter primary casualty evacuation. Analysis of the effects of a helicopter system involves a complex mix of medical and logistic considerations and there is no evidence of medical benefit from a helicopter service for non-trauma patients.

The helicopter environment is very different from a ground ambulance. Before working with a helicopter system, comprehensive training is essential in order to ensure safety and to adapt existing medical skills to the new situation. To provide the best and most efficient treatment, the helicopter medical crew must be able to perform all the medical interventions that the patient requires and be able to decide on the most appropriate destination for each patient. Without integration into a comprehensive medical system, a helicopter cannot provide medical treatment and becomes merely an expensive status symbol. As part of a medical system with the correct staffing, training and tasking, a helicopter can be a valuable additional resource.

Chapter **49**

The paramedic in a hostile environment

INTRODUCTION

With the increasing use of international air travel, the world seems to be getting ever smaller: it is possible to travel thousands of miles in a few hours, from the comfort of home to the centre of the Himalayas without time for a sleep in between. The cheapness and availability of long-haul travel, and the increasing trend to explore remote and far-flung corners of the world, have led to a huge expansion in the requirement for medical skills in places far removed from everyday life.

One of the advantages of a shrinking world is that aid can be provided where it is needed within hours of a disaster. Earthquakes, volcanoes, floods, famine and warfare dominate the lives of many in Third World countries (and are not unknown in the West). When disaster strikes, international aid organizations and non-governmental organizations (NGOs) provide relief in many forms. One of the key components of this aid is medical care and the skills of UK paramedics are often called upon.

Medical care in these situations is often referred to as disaster medicine. The purpose of this chapter is to prepare the paramedic not just for disaster relief work but also for any situation where he or she does not have access to modern-day medical facilities. This may involve being the medical cover on a ship at sea, in a mountaineering party or on

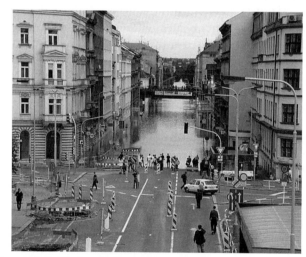

Figure 49.1 The Prague floods, August 2002

an overland trip through Africa: the principles remain the same.

The situations where one's skills will be needed are different from everyday practice, constrained by limited resources, poor communications, extremes of weather and threats from the environment. To practise effectively in these conditions, the deploying paramedic must be prepared for any situation that may be faced.

BEFORE DEPLOYMENT

As in all aspects of life, *"Failing to plan is planning to fail"*. A properly prepared paramedic will cope better with harsh living facilities, extremes of weather, limitations of kit and all else that is thrown at him.

> Failing to plan is planning to fail

Planning before leaving has two parts:

- personal
- medical.

PERSONAL PLANNING

There are many questions to be answered before leaving the comfort of home and a familiar working environment, for the uncomfortable and possibly dangerous area that will be visited. The sooner one deals with these issues, the less stressful and more successful the deployment is likely to be.

General information

The more that one knows about the area to be visited, the better prepared one will be. It is essential to start reading at the earliest opportunity. Travel guidebooks are indispensable, providing information on the history of the area, the people, climate, fauna and flora and often a medical section to warn of the likely health problems. Some of the better books have regular updates on their websites. Suggested guidebooks are included at the end of this chapter.

Legal issues

If working in a disaster relief capacity, it is essential to be accredited to a recognized body, otherwise entry to the country or region is unlikely to be successful and the risk of adverse events after arrival is correspondingly increased without appropriate support. The large NGOs and well-established relief agencies will help to smooth a paramedic's passage into the disaster area by alerting airports and essential local officials of his arrival. It should be remembered, however, that in most disaster relief situations the need for medical care is a much lower priority than provision of food and shelter and this is where initial resources will be concentrated.

Adequate personal identification documentation is essential and most organizations will insist on a photo card ID: precise requirements should be established early.

Everybody travelling outside the European Union requires a full 10-year passport, which must be valid for at least 6 months after returning to the UK. Passports take at least 2 weeks to be issued: the website for the UK passport agency can be found at the end of the chapter. Post offices will now check applications for errors, reducing the likelihood of rejection. This service carries a small fee.

Box 49.1 Key legal issues

Possession of a valid 10-year passport
Appropriate visas
Identification cards

The Foreign and Commonwealth Office (FCO) will provide information about visa requirements, which frequently change in some regions. Occasionally, if a situation in a region is deemed too unsafe, the FCO will place restrictions on travel in that area. Travelling in restricted areas may lead to problems if trouble is encountered whilst away. The FCO website can be found at the end of the chapter.

Locally, obtaining permission for the deployment and time away from work may be problematic. Some paramedics regularly deploy as part of high-profile international rescue teams and have agreements with their ambulance trusts to leave work at short notice. This is not as straightforward for the majority of UK paramedics and entering into discussion well in advance of expected travel dates is advisable.

Adequate travel insurance is essential and not just for belongings. Particular attention must be paid to the level of medical cover as many expedition activities will be classified as hazardous and may need separate cover.

> Do not forget travel insurance

It is essential (although rather sobering!) to write a will before departure: it is the only way to ensure that one's family are protected in the event of something happening whilst deployed. A properly drawn up will is essential and the fee usually small.

Personal kit

It is not possible to produce a single list that will cover requirements for all possible expeditions or deployments; however, the items in Box 49.2 should be considered essential and those in Box 49.3 may be useful as comforts. Some items are relevant for expeditions, where the team will be constantly moving around. Many aid organizations will provide basic living amenities at a disaster relief site where little home comforts can make a big difference to quality of life.

Clothing has not been listed. The requirements will vary depending upon the deployment, but the climate that is likely to be faced is clearly the most important factor. It should be remembered that even in the hottest countries, the nights can be very cold and it is important that *precise* information is obtained about such variations. Assumptions are usually wrong. Other items of kit will depend upon the situation: mountaineering trips will require extreme cold-weather clothing and shelter but these are likely to be of little use for disaster relief in central Africa. Footwear considerations are also important.

Box 49.2 Essential equipment

Passport
Photocard ID
Driving licence
Credit cards
Spare passport photographs
Large grip/backpack
Smaller daypack
Waterproofs
Washing & shaving kit
Sleeping bag (bivvy bag)
Sanitary supplies, including contraceptives
Toilet roll
Spectacles (if worn) and spare pair
Personal medication as required, plus spares
Paracetamol
Blister kit
Water bottle and purification system
Sunscreen
Insect repellent
Reliable watch
Head torch
Spare batteries
Electrical adaptors
Matches
Penknife
Paper and pens
Compass
Mosquito net

Box 49.3 Comforts

Camera, film and spare batteries
Mobile phone and charger (on international band)
Playing cards
Portable CD/cassette player and batteries
Hangers for clothes
Kettle and cup
Photo of your partner/family/dog
Reading books
Pens, paper, envelopes

Packing is something that improves with experience: a useful approach is to pack everything, then unpack, removing up to half of the items and trying again. It should be remembered that everything will have to be carried for at least some of the time so weight should be kept to a minimum. However, it is advisable to make room for some of the comfort items when being deployed in a hostile environment, even for a short period, as this can be physically and mentally exhausting. Having small items to improve one's level of comfort or to help relaxation may seem extravagant at first but is likely to be quickly appreciated. Needless to say, all kit preparation is subject to weight limits imposed by airlines and other carriers.

All belongings should be clearly and indelibly marked with name and postcode.

Vaccinations

All relevant vaccinations must be up to date. It is essential to establish which vaccinations will be required for the area to be visited. Useful sources of information include the family GP, MASTA or British Airways travel clinics: contact details are given at the end of the chapter.

It is important to remember that some vaccinations need to be given several weeks ahead of the date of travel, whilst others need at least two doses to be effective. Where possible, medical advice should be sought 6 weeks before travel. There are a number of combination vaccines now available that can help to reduce the time required to complete all essential immunizations.

Routine immunizations for most travel destinations include polio, tetanus, typhoid, hepatitis A and all childhood vaccinations (TB, pertussis, MMR).

Other vaccinations may be required for certain at-risk areas, including Japanese encephalitis, rabies and meningococcal meningitis.

Yellow fever vaccination is mandatory for some countries, particularly parts of Africa and South America, and a certificate of vaccination will need to be produced at customs points. Only approved centres can undertake yellow fever vaccinations in the UK. Advice on malaria prophylaxis is offered later in this chapter.

MEDICAL PLANNING

Medical assessment

Whether a paramedic is to form part of a four-man ascent of K2 or be one of numerous medical staff at a desert refugee camp, it is essential that he undertakes an assessment of the medical requirements before leaving home. This may simply take the form of talking to people who have done similar trips before, reading at the local medical library or surfing the Internet. For disaster relief organizations, it is vital that a member of the medical team undertakes a thorough assessment on the ground before committing any staff or kit to the work.

The assessment process involves finding out about the landscape, climate and environment where the team will be working, and preparing for the particular problems that this entails. Some specific issues are dealt with in the next section. Useful sources of medical information are listed at the end of the chapter.

If one is deploying for disaster relief purposes, large numbers of refugees (persons who have been forcibly displaced from their homes and have crossed an international boundary) or displaced persons (forcibly removed from their homes but in their own country) should be expected. These people suffer a high mortality and morbidity rate and one needs to be prepared to deal with the biggest killers: malnutrition, measles, respiratory infections, diarrhoeal illnesses and malaria.

Medical equipment

One cannot expect to deliver the same level of care whilst deployed that people receive at home: knowledge will inevitably be restricted and getting advice can be difficult due to communication problems, although telemedicine links are now available in some areas. Even if one knows what to do in a situation, it is not possible to have at hand every drug or piece of medical equipment for every conceivable problem. The medical kit that is taken on deployment should aim to cover common minor conditions, some emergencies and any specific predictable problems (e.g., acute mountain sickness on a mountaineering trip).

On expeditions, the group will have to carry the medical kit, in addition to personal kit, and therefore size and weight will be very restricted. In disaster relief, more equipment can be provided but the logistics chain will inevitably limit what arrives safely at the disaster site.

The Major Incident Medical Management and Support (MIMMS) structure can be used to break down the general equipment that will be required. As before, specific items for specialized trips are beyond the remit of this book but such things as hyperbaric bags for mountaineering trips will need to be considered.

Command

If entering a disaster area, mass casualty situations are a very real threat. Excellent field aide-mémoires are available, such as the Major Incident Management Master (see Further reading), which are weatherproof and contain useful information on managing multiple casualties.

Action cards for specific jobs may be useful, as may staff identification tabards.

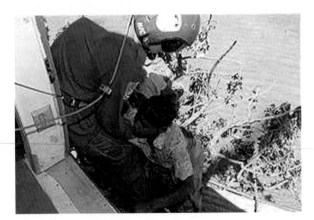

Figure 49.2 Medical disaster relief in operation

Safety

The 1-2-3 of safety (self, scene, casualties) should always be followed. This applies regardless of the number of patients: an injured paramedic is of no use to the patients that he should be treating.

To do one's job safely, key body areas must be covered appropriately (allowing for weather conditions). Box 49.4 lists recommended personal protective equipment (PPE).

Communications

Hostile environments, by their very nature, produce communication difficulties. The following communication methods are available.

Radio   Very high frequency radios will transmit over long distances but are large and bulky and are usually mounted in a vehicle. Mountainous terrain will interfere with their transmission.

Ultra high frequency radios are very useful for communicating over short distances (up to a few hundred metres) and are generally available in cheap hand-held models. However, terrain and weather conditions may interfere with their function.

Mobile telephones   Most people in the UK now own a mobile phone: the fact that they are cheap and generally reliable adds to their attractiveness as a method of communication. However, UK networked phones will need to be activated for overseas use – this is done through the network administrators. It is important to be aware, though, that calls become very expensive, sometimes resulting in a very nasty shock on returning home. Furthermore, many of the hostile environments that paramedics may deploy to will have no cell coverage, rendering a mobile phone useless.

Box 49.4 Personal protective equipment

Head
Goggles
Ear muffs
Helmet with visor +/− torch
(Face mask)

Trunk
Reflective jacket/tabard (appropriate for weather)

Hands
Latex gloves
Heavy-duty gloves

Legs
Reflective trousers (appropriate for weather), preferably with knee pads
Boots – heavy duty

Calls through mobile phones are unmonitored. Care must be taken not to pass delicate or sensitive information to others if this method of communication is used.

Satellite telephones Inmarsat is a global satellite system that is available in many countries throughout the world. Relief organizations will often have a satellite telephone set up on site. Apart from a slight delay in speech, they work very well but calls are very expensive.

Triage

If one deploys as part of an expedition or small team, mass casualties are highly unlikely and packing space is better given over to other equipment. However, for the paramedic deploying to a disaster relief situation, mass casualties are a very real possibility, either from the original disaster (usually trauma victims) or from medical problems following in the wake of the disaster.

Effective triage ensures that limited medical resources are used most effectively: overtriage will tie up valuable resources on patients who do not really need them while undertriage misses seriously ill or injured patients.

Many methods are available for triage. For trauma patients the sieve and sort approach should be used (see Chapter 59).

Whatever method is employed to sort patients, they must be clearly marked so that the treating or evacuating team can identify those at highest priority. There are a multitude of triage labels available for such a purpose. Whichever one is chosen should be clearly visible, have a method of fastening to the patient, be changeable (single coloured card systems are not recommended) and have a space for writing in the patient's details.

Consideration should be given to taking an aide-mémoire to help with triage. With limited resources it is often possible to train a non-medical person to undertake triage and an aide-mémoire will facilitate this process.

Treatment

The list of possible medical conditions and injuries that can occur in remote locations is endless and one cannot expect to pack for all eventualities. However, some problems may be predicted, such as frostbite in Arctic expeditions, altitude sickness if mountaineering and malaria if travelling through endemic areas. It is essential to pack accordingly for these specific conditions: details can be found in the relevant chapters in this text.

Proper preparation by acquainting oneself with the likely problems will allow directed packing of the medical kit for treatment. Box 49.5 lists suggested items for all expeditions. Disaster relief work will have its own unique problems, dependent on the type of disaster and region affected, and an appropriate scale of kit should be decided in conjunction with the authorities and relief agencies.

Transport

One of the main problems facing a paramedic deployed in a hostile environment is that many casualties cannot be properly treated in the location in which they are found. At some point, evacuation up the medical chain must be considered.

In many cases, evacuation will be possible through an ordered system, using land or air transport. In this case, one can expect that most equipment necessary for transport will be provided. However, for the lone paramedic evacuation of a single casualty can be very challenging.

There are many considerations in the preparation for, and undertaking of, evacuation. The patient must have all treatment that he will need during the trip and spares in case of problems. Any items that are used for the transport should be replaced locally when possible: they may be needed again and it is unrealistic to carry duplicates of everything.

Stretchers come in many forms: there are specialized versions for helicopter transfer, search and rescue, and use in ships. Familiarity with the version in the area where the paramedic will be working is essential. If on expedition, improvisation will be necessary.

Specialized equipment for specialized situations should be investigated. A portable hyperbaric bag will allow safe treatment of an altitude sickness case whilst evacuating the patient to a lower level.

DURING THE DEPLOYMENT

There will be many challenges to be faced during the deployment: not all of them can be planned for and no attempt is made to discuss every potential issue here. However, awareness of the likely problems that one will encounter will help to smooth the trip to some extent.

ENVIRONMENTAL

Weather

There can be no guarantees regarding the weather to be faced whilst operating in hostile climes, but most weather patterns can be predicted and prepared for. Seasonal variations should be allowed for when planning: many regions alternate between hot, dry weather and torrential rainfall. There may be dramatic variations in temperature between day and night.

Personal discomfort aside, weather can bring many logistical and medical problems. Communication and transport chains may break down in adverse weather conditions, as may any reliable food and water supplies. A paramedic may find himself without back-up for days and must be able to cope in such a situation.

Medically, the main problems come from weather extremes. Everyone can be considered at risk of either heat

Box 49.5 Recommended equipment and drugs for expeditions

TRAUMA CARE
AIRWAY
Laerdal face mask
Oropharyngeal airways, assorted
Nasopharyngeal airways, assorted
Stiffneck collars, tape

BREATHING
Oxygen, regulator and tubing
Reservoir masks
Chest drain kit

CIRCULATION
Fluids – crystalloid and colloid
Giving sets
Cannulae, assorted 14 g, 18 g, 22 g
NaCl 0.9% 5 ml vials
Needles, assorted
Syringes, assorted

OTHER
Stethoscope
Sphygmomanometer
Pen torch
Inflatable splint
SAM splint
BM sticks
Thermometers

WOUND CARE
Bandage, triangular
Bandage, crepe
Micropore tape
Elastoplast tape
Plasters, assorted
Melolin dressings
Mepore dressings
Steristrips
Gauze swabs
Tincture of iodine BP
Sterile dressings packs

SURGICAL KIT
Gloves, sterile
Examination gloves
Fine suture set (forceps, needle-holder & scissors)
Sutures, assorted
Small sharps bin

DRUGS
ALTITUDE
Acetazolamide 500 mg SR
Nifedipine 10 mg
Dexamethasone 8 mg IM/IV
Dexamethasone 4 mg

ANAESTHETIC AGENTS
1% lignocaine with adrenaline
1% lignocaine

ANALGESIA
Morphine 10 mg IV
Naloxone 0.4 mg
Paracetamol 500 mg
Ibuprofen 400 mg
Diclofenac sodium 100 mg SR
Codeine phosphate 30 mg
Aspirin disp. 300 mg

ANTIMICROBIALS
Augmentin 375 mg
Ciprofloxacin 250 mg
Metronidazole 500 mg
Erythromycin 250 mg
Mebendazole 100 mg

ALLERGY/ANAPHYLAXIS
Salbutamol inhaler
Piriton 4 mg
Piriton 10 mg IV
Adrenaline (1 in 1000) IM
Hydrocortisone 100 mg IV

DERMATOLOGICAL
Calamine lotion
Athlete's foot powder
Canesten HC cream

ENT/EYES
Amethocaine eyedrops
Fluorescein eyedrops
Chloramphenicol ointment
Sofradex eardrops
Menthol crystals
Bradosol lozenges
Pseudoephedrine 60 mg

GASTROINTESTINAL
Anusol ointment
Gavison chewable tablets
Metoclopramide 10 mg
Stemetil 12.5 mg IV
Ranitidine 150 mg
Loperamide 2 mg
Senokot tablets
Oral rehydration sachets

DENTAL
Clove oil
Temporary dressings
Cotton wool rolls
Dental mirror & probe

MISCELLANEOUS
Small pill bags
Alcohol swabs

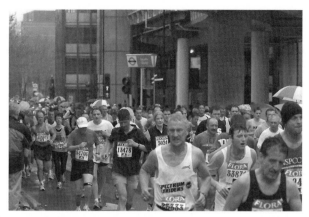

Figure 49.3 Exertion in hot conditions poses a serious threat of heat illness

or cold illness and one important role for the paramedic is to educate those working or on expedition with him as to the signs and symptoms. All of these conditions are easy to prevent and much easier to treat if picked up early. A buddy scheme may be useful, with buddies keeping a check on each other for the early signs.

Heat illness (discussed in Chapter 42) may affect anyone and one must always be alert to the early signs. The temperature does not need to be excessively high; work rate and the amount and type of clothing worn are also important in determining susceptibility. Prevention is much better than cure and regular monitoring of personnel is essential in order to detect those at risk. Frequent breaks should be insisted on for those working in hot weather and a plentiful supply of fluids ensured. If symptoms develop, the paramedic who spots this early will be able to effect treatment with oral fluids and rest only: more advanced cases require active cooling and intravenous fluids.

At the other extreme, cold-related illness is a potential problem in many areas of the world, and is discussed in detail in Chapter 40. Even short exposure to very cold temperatures can put one at risk of freezing cold injury (frostnip and frostbite), whereas prolonged exposure to relatively cool temperatures can lead to non-freezing cold injury (trenchfoot). Once again, prevention and early detection are the cornerstones of management. If working in such conditions, the paramedic must ensure that all personnel wear adequate clothing, keep their extremities warm and dry and take regular hot drinks. Boots must be well fitting but not tight and socks should be removed daily for foot inspections.

Hypothermia may occur from rapid exposure to extreme cold (acute), from long exposure to relative cold (chronic) or from exposure for a relatively short time in someone who is energy depleted – on an arduous mountain climb, for instance. Again, prevention and early detection are the keys. One of the first detectable signs may be erratic behaviour and the paramedic is not immune to this. Regular intakes of hot fluids will help to keep the body temperature up and these must be factored in to any timetable.

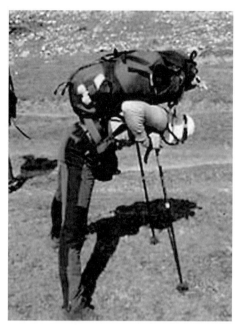

Figure 49.4 Altitude sickness is common in high-altitude expeditions

Altitude

For the paramedic deploying to altitudes of 10 000 feet (3000 m) and above, altitude sickness is a potential problem. There are many excellent texts on the subject and only the basics will be covered here.

Prevention is easy to achieve and the paramedic should be actively involved in the planning of trips to altitude. The rate of ascent should be no more than 300 m (1000 feet) per day, preferably with a rest day every 3 days. The aim is to climb high during the day and sleep low. If chemoprophylaxis is desired (and expert opinion varies on whether it should be used or not) then acetazolamide (Diamox) should be taken, 250 mg slow release daily. Paraesthesia is a common side-effect.

There are three forms of high-altitude illness: acute mountain sickness (AMS), high-altitude pulmonary oedema (HAPE) and high-altitude cerebral oedema (HACE). There is considerable overlap between the three but HACE can be considered the endpoint of untreated AMS. HAPE is usually considered a separate illness, but can be preceded by AMS.

AMS commonly affects otherwise fit and healthy individuals who ascend rapidly to altitude. Typically it presents as a collection of symptoms including:

- headache
- nausea
- vomiting
- lethargy
- disturbed sleep.

The incidence of AMS primarily depends on the rate of ascent and the altitude reached. In the Mount Everest region of Nepal the incidence of AMS has been reported to be between 30% and 50% in trekkers who travel to altitudes above 4000 m. Generally the symptoms will disappear after 5 days provided no further ascent is made.

HAPE occurs in up to 10% of those ascending very rapidly to 4500 m. It typically presents with dyspnoea on exertion and reduced exercise tolerance. Symptoms may progress to dyspnoea at rest and particularly at night.

AMS precedes HACE and the typical feature is ataxia and confusion. Any ataxic and unwell person at altitude should be considered to be suffering from HACE until proven otherwise.

If altitude sickness is suspected, no further ascent should be made. Typically, symptoms settle after 24–48 hours of rest. If symptoms progress or there are any symptoms of HAPE, descent is essential. Oxygen, nifedipine, dexamethasone and recompression bags all have a useful place in management, but descending back below the level at which symptoms began is the only effective treatment.

FOOD AND WATER

One of the main medical problems that a paramedic is likely to face is ill health from local food and drink, either in himself, members of his team or in the patients that he is treating.

Food

A few simple hygiene rules can make a big difference in prevention of gastroenteritis. Hands should ALWAYS be thoroughly washed before handling food and all food must be carefully washed and adequately cooked. Fruit and vegetables should be peeled. Only appropriately treated water must be used for food preparation. In some areas safe bottled drinks are readily available.

Field purification of water

Without potable and hygienic drinking water, it is not possible to function effectively in role. In many hostile environments, the water supply is not fit for consumption even at the best of times: an earthquake, flood or mass casualty situation usually renders even good water unsafe. Box 49.6 defines some important terms with regard to water treatment.

Box 49.7 lists the various treatment methods that are available in the wilderness.

Heat

Boiling any water for 30 minutes will kill all organisms and render the water safe to drink. It will also produce water suitable for use in surgery and wound care. However, due to the amount of fuel required to carry out this procedure, it is often not practical. Water will be safe to drink if brought to the boil and then cooled, but will not be suitable for other purposes.

It is important to remember that water must be stored in clean containers after it has been boiled.

Box 49.6 Important terms in water purification

- *Sterilization*: inactivation of all disease-forming organisms
- *Disinfection*: inactivation of infective organisms
- *Clarification*: removal of debris
- *Potable*: safe to drink
- *Palatable*: pleasant to drink

Box 49.7 Water purification methods

Heat
Filtration
Halogenation

Altitude reduces the temperature at which water boils: at 10 000 feet it is only 90°C, with reduction in the effectiveness of this treatment modality.

Filtration

Filter systems remove debris and large organisms from water: the size of organisms that remain depends upon the size of the filter pores. Viruses will remain behind. For drinking purposes, filters need to be at most 0.4-micron diameter. This size of filter needs a pressure gradient to effect the filtration process, and most commercial filters have some form of pump to generate this pressure. Filters do little to improve the taste of water.

Halogenation

Chlorine and iodine kill viruses, enteric bacteria and protozoa, but do not kill all eggs and parasites. If the water supply is at risk, use of a cheap, large-pore filter prior to halogenation is recommended to remove any eggs or parasites. Chlorine is very effective in low concentrations but has a nasty taste that is hard to disguise. Its effect is directly related to its concentration and the temperature of the water: cold or cloudy water needs higher concentrations or a longer contact time before the water can be safely used. Chlorination tablets are available from outdoor stores.

Iodine is a better chemical, being more effective under the same temperature range and having a better taste. Nearly all traces of the taste can be removed by use of ascorbate powder, which is often sold with iodine as part of a kit. Iodine is available as drops or tablets from most outdoor stores. If only tincture of iodine (2%) is available, four drops per litre of clear water are used and the water is left to stand for 30 minutes.

MEDICAL PROBLEMS

The main threats to health in any hostile environment come from the lack of hygienic food and water, as discussed above.

However, each specific region visited will have its own threats.

Hygiene

Disaster relief areas usually suffer from lack of adequate sanitation and hygiene facilities: a priority for aid agencies is the supply of fresh water and toilet facilities. A simple step that can make a big difference to the amount of faecal–oral spread of disease is the provision of soap. Locals must be educated about the value of hand washing as in disaster conditions, disease spreads rapidly through overcrowded living areas.

Traveller's diarrhoea

This is usually a self-limiting illness of mild severity, acquired through food or water. The most common identified cause (most cases are not investigated) is enterotoxigenic *E. coli*. The illness usually lasts 3–5 days, with watery diarrhoea, vomiting and abdominal cramps. Antimotility agents such as loperamide may be used if travel must continue despite the illness, but they are generally best avoided. Oral rehydration is recommended, either with commercially available powder or salt and sugar in clean water (1 teaspoon of salt, 1 tablespoon of sugar in 1 litre water).

If the illness is protracted or if it interferes excessively with the expedition or work, then antibiotics (such as co-trimoxazole) may be used.

Malnutrition

Failure of crops may be the instigating cause of the disaster which leads to a paramedic's deployment or a disaster may interrupt the flow of food to the local populace. Either way, provision of adequate calories is a major challenge in many disaster scenarios. This leads to undernourishment and malnutrition, often on a large scale. Malnutrition is one of the major killers in disaster situations. The very young and very old are at highest risk. The World Health Organization recommends a minimum intake of 2000 kilocalories a day for an adult.

Provision of adequate food is beyond the remit of the paramedic, but he must be aware of the problems that can arise as a result of malnourishment, from reduced immunity to infection to marasmus and kwashiorkor (forms of protein-energy malnutrition) in children.

Trauma

A paramedic may face trauma cases (with which he is likely to feel more comfortable than many of the tropical illnesses that he will see) from a wide range of different causes. In a natural disaster situation, there are often many dead and injured. As the aid response is likely to be delayed by hours (if not days), by the time a medical team arrives these casualties may have died or suffered complications from their injuries, making management more difficult.

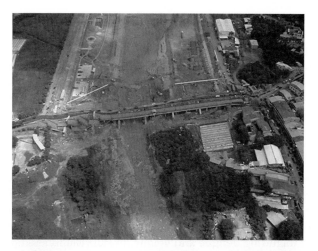

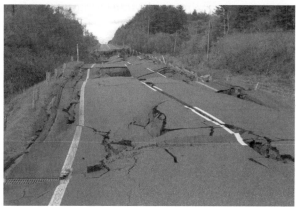

Figure 49.5 An earthquake in Japan

Fresh trauma cases often arise from violence in the disaster zone, as stresses and tensions begin to run high, or from transportation with large volumes of traffic moving on unfit roads.

Earthquakes produce roughly three times as many injured as dead, with fractures and crush injury being common. The deploying paramedic is likely to deal with these patients hours or days later. Aftershocks may cause new injuries and knowledge of the management of crush injury is essential. The chance of survival of trapped casualties decreases with the duration of entrapment and survival longer than 48 hours is unusual.

Volcanoes may produce burns in those that survive the initial eruption, but the main problems arise from the aftereffects of the ash and gas clouds. Eye symptoms are common, as are upper respiratory tract infections. Exacerbations of asthma may be precipitated by atmospheric ash.

Childhood problems

In a disaster relief operation, children often constitute a large proportion of the patient caseload. In addition to the effects of malnourishment and trauma, one is likely to be responsible for their ongoing healthcare. This will include "everyday" acute paediatric problems such as viral illnesses and rashes, in addition to chronic problems such as asthma and epilepsy.

Diarrhoea and vomiting are common in such situations and, like upper respiratory infections, will spread rapidly through a camp. Where possible, dehydration should be corrected by oral rehydration therapy unless intravenous fluids are essential.

Tropical medical problems

Specific illnesses are common in particular regions and most good travel medicine guides will give reliable information on the illnesses to be faced. Likely problems include arthropod-borne diseases (malaria being the commonest, but also including dengue and yellow fever), viral illness (such as Japanese encephalitis and viral haemorrhagic fevers), water-borne infections (including schistosomiasis) and bites from assorted venomous animals. One cannot expect to be fully prepared for all eventualities, but time spent learning about the particular risks in the area to be visited will allow appropriate reading before deployment as well as the provision of any appropriate medications. Most people take the time to discover whether malaria will be a problem in the area that they are visiting, but few check whether their area is at risk of typhoid, anthrax or diphtheria. Time spent on this aspect of predeployment planning will help to prevent unexpected problems later.

Malaria

Malaria is a parasitic infection transmitted by mosquitoes. The most common presenting feature is fever, which may follow a pattern or be irregular. Rigors, shivering and sweating occur. Other features include haemolytic anaemia, splenomegaly and jaundice. The most serious form of malaria is that due to *Plasmodium falciparum* (one of four causative organisms) which, in addition to the above, also causes cerebral malaria, abdominal pain, renal failure, severe anaemia, haematuria, renal and cardiac failure. Diarrhoea, hypoglycaemia and pulmonary oedema may also occur. Cerebral malaria presents with confusion, coma and focal neurological signs.

Malaria is a problem affecting many developing countries. Chloroquine resistance (especially in South America, Oceania, South East Asia and sub-Saharan Africa) means that prophylaxis and treatment regimes vary from area to area: up-to-date advice can be obtained from many of the sources listed at the end of the chapter.

Chloroquine and proguanil offer good prophylaxis in non-resistant areas: chloroquine (once weekly) and proguanil (daily) must be started one week prior to arrival in area. Options for chloroquine-resistant regions include mefloquine (weekly, starting one week pre-entry), which has had a lot of bad press as it causes anxiety and nightmares in a small percentage of users, doxycycline (daily, starting one week before entry) and malarone (a combination of proguanil and

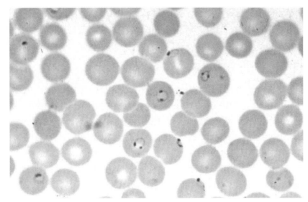

Figure 49.6 *Plasmodium falciparum* malarial parasites on a thick blood screen

atovaquone) weekly and which only needs starting the day before entry. All chemoprophylactics should be continued for 4 weeks after leaving a malaria area, with the exception of malarone, which only needs to be continued for one week.

Chemical prophylaxis is not the only measure in safeguarding against malaria: wearing long sleeves and trousers and applying an effective insect repellent are also essential. Other useful measures include mosquito nets for sleeping, mosquito coils and electrical repellents. These also help to prevent other vector-borne disease such as yellow fever or dengue.

The treatment of malaria depends in part on the specific *Plasmodium* involved but in general, starting treatment with quinine is effective (oral dose 600 mg 8 hourly) until further advice can be sought regarding ongoing care.

Sexually transmitted diseases

Developing countries suffer a much higher incidence of most sexually transmitted diseases than we encounter in the UK, particularly HIV/AIDS and syphilis. Awareness of the signs and symptoms of the more common STDs may be of use in a disaster relief situation where the paramedic is involved in providing ongoing healthcare for the affected persons. However, it is important to be aware that members of the travelling team are also at risk, and appropriate advice should be provided to all group members regarding safe sex practices.

HIV prophylaxis

Following exposure to potentially infected body fluids, appropriate first aid should be undertaken (encouraging bleeding, washing under a running tap). Chemoprophylaxis should be offered in the case of a significant exposure to blood and other high-risk body fluids (or any other body fluid if visibly blood-stained) from a patient known to be HIV positive, or considered to be at high risk but where HIV infection status cannot be determined (see Dept. of Health, 2004). A suitable regime is shown in Box 49.8.

Box 49.8 Postexposure prophylaxis for HIV infection

Zidovudine 300 mg b.d.
plus
lamivudine 150 mg b.d.
plus
Nelfinair 1250 mg b.d.
(see Dept. of Health, 2004)

The dead

Contrary to popular belief, dead bodies generally do not result in outbreaks of disease. They may, of course, be a source of vermin infestation with the resultant problems that this brings.

Bodies should be removed to a temporary mortuary area whenever possible. Here they should be identified and then disposed of according to local custom, as discussed later in this chapter.

CULTURAL

One of the fastest ways to make life difficult for oneself in a foreign land is to be disrespectful of local customs. Once again, preparation prior to departure will help to avoid difficulties.

Time taken to learn a few words of the language (greetings, please and thank you as a minimum) helps to ingratiate one with locals. Although outsiders may not agree with the ruling methods of the country's incumbent government or may have strong opinions on how to alleviate the poverty seen there, these opinions should be kept to oneself. Locals generally do not take kindly to foreigners (particularly from the affluent West) lecturing them on what is right and wrong. It is vital to be respectful of locals and particularly of their religion, which is taken much more seriously in many countries than we are used to in the UK.

In many countries women are treated as second-class citizens. Again, opining loudly on this subject is likely to cause problems for the visiting paramedic. At all times it is essential to try to remain respectful of the culture, regardless of one's own thoughts on the matter.

In many cultures, the left hand is used for cleaning after defecation and eating and greetings are all done with the right hand: offering to shake with the left hand is insulting. In many Eastern countries shoes should be removed at the door to a house; the same holds for places of worship, where one should be appropriately covered up without bare legs or other inappropriate show of bare flesh.

In many societies a great emphasis is placed on the correct handling of dying patients and the dead, in the belief that preparation for an afterlife is all-important. Insensitive or inadequate attention to local custom can affect a bereaved relative forever. Once again, taking the time to learn the local custom (if one is likely to be dealing with the dead and dying) will help to avoid problems.

OTHER MISCELLANEOUS PROBLEMS

The media

Handling the media is a specialized skill in itself and is beyond the remit of this book. However, disasters generate huge media interest and one may be asked to comment on the medical side of a disaster relief project. If this happens, a written statement should be prepared and stuck to. One should be prepared to take questions but must not stray into passing comments on aspects of the relief work other than those for which one has been responsible. Opinions regarding blame or causation should be avoided and questioning should firmly but politely be brought back to the medical work. Always use press statements as an opportunity to praise rescue workers.

Relationships with the military and police

In many regions, the military and police are badly organized, poorly paid (if at all) and have poor control structures to moderate their activities. It is not unusual to be asked for money to make up for "incorrect paperwork" or to be allowed to pass a "checkpoint". Whilst seen as bribery by many in the UK, without money from affluent Westerners many military or police personnel would receive no payment. That is not to condone their action but rather to put it into perspective. Initially it is probably best to try to refuse politely, always being firm but courteous. However, if pressed it is better to part with a small amount of money than to spend time in custody for one's "crime".

Photography

Some areas are off limits for photography: the military and police are particularly reluctant to allow pictures of their personnel or buildings. A much televised court case in Greece highlighted the danger of photographing military installations, with imprisonment for a group of British "plane spotters".

AFTER DEPLOYMENT

Returning home from an overseas deployment is often one of the most difficult problems to be faced. Dependent upon the length of time spent away from one's home and family and the degree of stress experienced through the deployment, problems may occur in readjusting to a more "normal" home-based lifestyle. Organized groups which have worked together in stressful and unpleasant circumstances should ideally not be immediately broken up at disembarkation. A short period of time in which experiences can be discussed with those who have shared them is invaluable and may reduce subsequent adverse effects of deployment.

RETURN TO FAMILY

If one has been away for many weeks or months, returning to the family home can be a particularly difficult experience. While the paramedic is away, loved ones develop their own coping mechanisms and routines. It is difficult for all concerned to readjust to new routines and demands, and the first few days after return can be trying for all concerned. A few days at home with no plans, spending time learning to live together again, will help considerably.

ILLNESS

Many tropical diseases can present after the return home. However, that does not necessarily mean that any illness suffered after return from abroad is tropical in nature: colds and chest infections are just as likely to cause problems.

If a paramedic develops a febrile illness on return to the UK, then medical attention is advised at an early stage. It is essential to provide the doctor with full travel details, including the malaria prophylaxis regime followed. Unfortunately malaria is still a possibility even though prophylaxis has been taken.

Diarrhoea and vomiting can present after return, from infection with *E. coli*, *Salmonella*, *Shigella*, *Giardia* and viral infections. Haematuria may indicate *falciparum* malaria or schistosomiasis.

DEBRIEFING

If one has been deployed as part of a NGO or similar aid agency, then a formal debrief is likely to be required. This may take the form of a written report or group meeting. Useful items that need feeding back are related to the positive and negative aspects of the deployment.

- Did the transport chain work?
- Was there sufficient medical equipment, and were the use-by dates acceptable?
- Did communications function?
- Did the team function together?
- What specific medical problems were seen during the deployment (a medical register should be kept)?
- Was there an outbreak of any specific illness or infection?

A less formal debrief is also recommended. This should involve members of the team or expedition getting together for drinks or a meal, to discuss any burning issues or problems.

Debriefs are ideally held after a short "cooling off" period, to allow some degree of normality to return, but close enough to the time of deployment for events to be fresh in the mind. They are intended to be a constructive means of learning what went well and what could be done better by people in similar situations in the future: they should not be seen as a complaint session or a chance to get at one particular person. Specific issues should be dealt with more formally by written communication.

POLITICALLY SENSITIVE DISCUSSIONS

Some topics of discussion are not appropriate after return from deployment. Disaster relief often occurs in unstable, poor countries and spreading news of their problems to friends and family will help no-one. It is important to be respectful of the people whose hospitality one has enjoyed when recalling stories at home.

Discussion of specific issues relating to local military and police is generally considered inappropriate and most international aid bodies would not appreciate "bad mouthing" by those who have worked for them. If one has a specific issue or complaint, the same advice holds: it should be channelled formally through the correct procedure.

CONCLUSION

Overseas relief work or acting as medical assistance on an expedition is becoming increasingly common. If sensible precautions are followed and adequate preparation is carried out before departure, such activities have the potential to be hugely rewarding, if stressful and tiring. If preparations are inadequate and behaviour inappropriate, there are few situations in which things can go so badly wrong. Good advice is widely available and there is a great deal of experience which can be tapped into. If the approach outlined in this chapter is followed the chances of significant problems will be reduced to a minimum and a rewarding experience will result.

USEFUL CONTACTS

Altitude-related illness: www.gorge.net/hamg/ (AMS score sheets are available on this site)

British Airways travel clinics: www.britishairways.com/travelclinics

Centers for Disease Prevention and Control (USA): www.cdc.gov/travel

Foreign and Commonwealth Office for general advice on travelling (also some health advice): www.fco.gov.uk

International Society of Travel Medicine: www.istm.org

MASTA (general travel health advice): www.masta.org

NHS advice for travellers and healthcare workers: www.travax.scot.nhs.uk

UK Passport Agency: www.ukpa.gov.uk

WHO vaccination requirements: www.who.int/ith/ and disease outbreak reports: www.who.int/disease-outbreak-news/

FURTHER READING

Lonely Planet guidebooks (from all good bookstores): www.lonelyplanet.com

Medical books

Baskett P, Weller R 1988 Medicine for disasters. Butterworth, London

Bodiwala GG, McKaskie AW, Thompson MM 1993 International translation guide for emergency medicine. Butterworth-Heinemann, London

Department of Health. HIV post-exposure prophylaxis. Guidance from the Chief Medical Officers' Expert Advisory Group on AIDS. Available at URL <http://www.dh.gov.uk/assetRoot/04/08/36/40/04083640.pdf> [accessed 31st May 2005.]

Grant IC, Guly HR, Thompson L 2001 Kurafid: the British Antarctic Survey Medical Unit handbook. BOE, Blackpool

Greaves I, Porter K 1999 Pre hospital medicine. Arnold, London

Hodgetts T, Porter C 2002 Major Incident Management Master. BMJ Books, London

Ryan J, Mahoney P, Greaves I, Bowyer G 2002 Conflict medicine: a handbook for aid workers. Springer Verlag, London

Stewart E 1990 Environmental emergencies. LWW, Baltimore

9

PREGNANCY AND CHILDBIRTH

Chapter 50

Childbirth

CHAPTER CONTENTS

INTRODUCTION

Childbirth is a normal, natural phenomenon and not an illness. For the paramedic confronted with a woman in labour, the fear caused by dealing with the unfamiliar can be countered by the knowledge that human beings have reproduced and given birth without interference from doctors, midwives or paramedics for thousands of years. The old adage "meddlesome midwifery" is as true today as it ever was and the labouring mother should, by and large, be left to get on with labour; her attendants (be they paramedics, midwives or doctors) should stand back, not interfere and provide moral and physical support, coupled with informed clinical observation only. The time when a paramedic may have to become involved is established second stage of labour, when the journey to hospital is too long to complete before delivery is expected.

Many of the critical decisions in childbirth relate to timing, the actual clinical execution of interventions being relatively straightforward. In the UK, there will be very few situations where the time to hospital is longer than the time to the baby's birth and even fewer situations where the paramedic is the only medical person present at birth.

In order to make informed clinical observations and, therefore, reasoned decisions, it is necessary to be aware of the salient anatomy and physiology of normal pregnancy and reproduction, together with an understanding of the normal process of delivery. It should be remembered that the aim is to be a safe birth attendant in an emergency situation.

In the vast majority of calls to a pregnant woman in suspected or established labour, the correct response will be to transport the patient safely and swiftly to the appropriate delivery suite. The critical question for the paramedic is, "Can I safely get this woman to definitive care before the conclusion of second stage or delivery of the baby?". In the vast majority of cases, the answer to this question will be yes.

ANATOMY

The external female genitalia are shown in Figures 50.1 and 50.2. The anatomy of the female reproductive organs is shown in Figure 50.3.

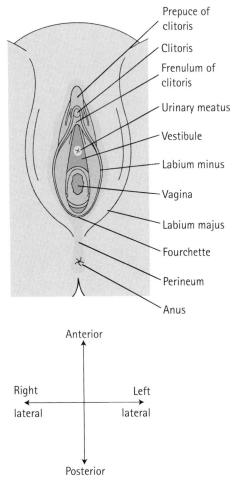

Figure 50.1 The female external genitalia and their orientation in the dorsal position. From Miller & Callander, *Obstetrics illustrated*, 4th edn, with permission from Churchill Livingstone

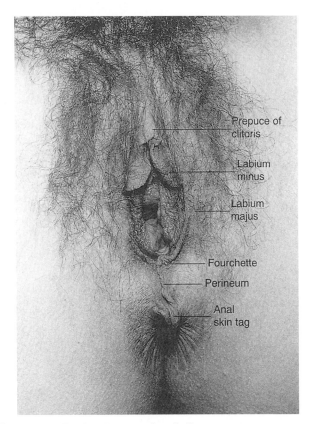

Figure 50.2 The female external genitalia

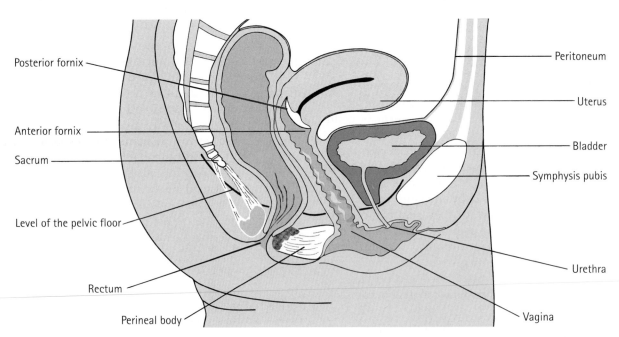

Figure 50.3 The female reproductive organs. From Chilman & Thomas, *Understanding nursing care*, 2nd edn, with permission from Churchill Livingstone

PHYSIOLOGICAL BASIS OF PREGNANCY

To understand the process of conception and pregnancy it is necessary to have a basic knowledge of female reproductive physiology. Full details may be obtained from a textbook of obstetrics or midwifery (see Further reading) – only the information needed for safe, effective emergency care is included here.

Women of reproductive age have monthly periods when the endometrial lining of the uterus is shed because of falling oestrogen and progesterone levels. The first day of bleeding is known as the date of the last menstrual period (LMP) (Figure 50.4).

THE MENSTRUAL CYCLE

A woman has two ovaries, containing a large number of ova surrounded by connective tissue. In the inner part of the ovary are thousands of primordial follicles consisting of an oogonium (egg) plus a single layer of stromal cells called *granulosa cells*. Under hormonal control, just one primordial follicle each month ripens fully to become a Graafian follicle with a proliferation of granulosa cells and an accumulation of fluid (liquor) within the follicle. Some of the stromal cells change to form hormone-secreting cells and, under hormonal influence, the follicle ripens, growing in size from approximately 0.25 mm to 8 mm in diameter. At ovulation, the follicle bursts and the ovum is expelled. Normally this enters the fallopian tube and is carried slowly down the tube, taking 3–4 days to reach the uterus. It is while en route to the uterus that fertilization will occur, provided that coitus has occurred at the relevant time, and it is in the fallopian tube that the majority of ectopic pregnancies arise (Figures 50.4, 50.5).

The remnants of the Graafian follicle develop into the hormone-secreting *corpus luteum*, providing progesterones to stimulate the proliferation of the endometrial lining of the uterus in preparation for implantation by the fertilized

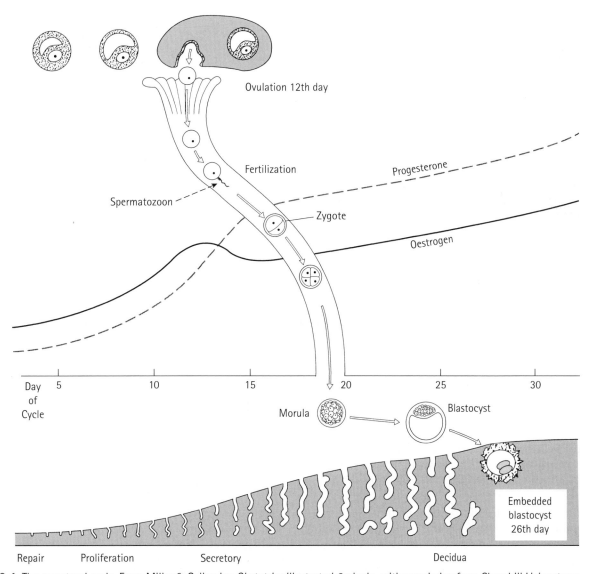

Figure 50.4 The menstrual cycle. From Miller & Callander, *Obstetrics illustrated*, 2nd edn, with permission from Churchill Livingstone

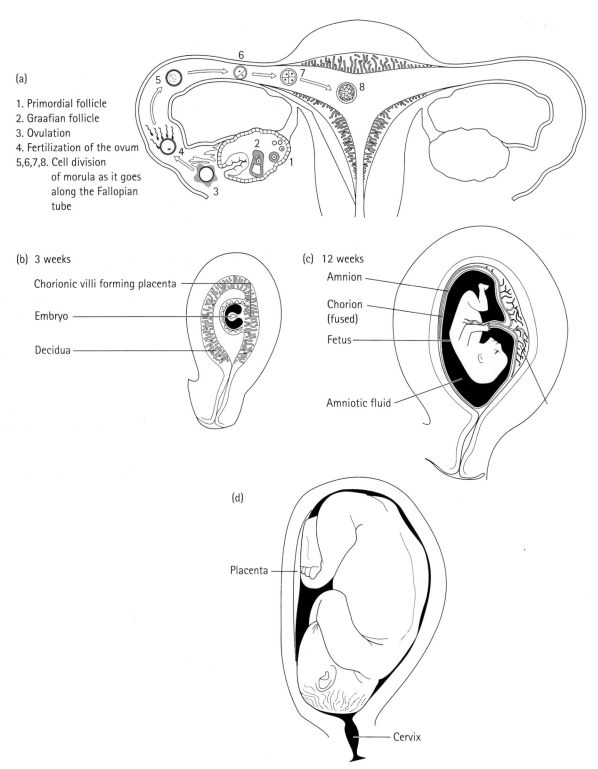

(a)

1. Primordial follicle
2. Graafian follicle
3. Ovulation
4. Fertilization of the ovum
5,6,7,8. Cell division
of morula as it goes
along the Fallopian
tube

(b) 3 weeks

Chorionic villi forming placenta

Embryo

Decidua

(c) 12 weeks

Amnion

Chorion
(fused)

Fetus

Amniotic fluid

(d)

Placenta

Cervix

Figure 50.5 Fertilization, implantation and the development of the fetus. (a) Fertilization of ovum and subsequent cell division; (b) embedding of ovum (3 weeks); (c) 12th week of pregnancy; (d) full-term pregnancy. From Chilman & Thomas, *Understanding nursing care*, 2nd edn, with permission from Churchill Livingstone

egg. If the ovum is not fertilized, then after about 12 days the corpus luteum ceases functioning, progesterone secretion falls and the uterine lining – the *endometrium* – is shed and the cycle starts again. The hormonal mechanisms controlling the menstrual cycle are complex.

When the ovum is fertilized, cell division follows and a *blastocyst* develops and implants in the uterine wall. Part of the blastocyst – the *trophoblast* – invades the uterine wall by forming chorionic villi (finger-like protrusions) which are the forerunner of the placenta.

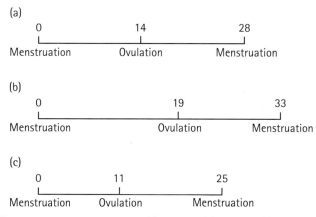

Figure 50.6 Menstrual cycles. (a) 28 days; (b) 33 days; (c) 25 days

GESTATIONAL DATES

Most women have a menstrual cycle of approximately 28 days, although this can vary. By convention and definition, day 1 of the cycle is the first day of the menstrual bleed. The only fixed timing in the menstrual cycle is that ovulation *precedes* menstruation by 14 days. Thus, it is the proliferation phase which varies (Figure 50.6).

From fertilization to delivery is 266 days or 38 weeks and thus the time from LMP to delivery is 280 days or 40 weeks in a woman with a 28-day cycle.

CALCULATION OF ESTIMATED DATE OF DELIVERY

It is important to be able to calculate the estimated date of delivery (EDD), as many management decisions have to be made according to whether the baby is premature (born early) or postmature (born late).

Provided that the mother's cycle length is between 24 and 35 days, she has not been on the contraceptive pill in the past 3 months and she is reasonably certain of the date of her LMP, the EDD is calculated by subtracting 3 months from the date, adding 1 year and then adding 7 days. For example:

LMP:	21 January 1998
Subtract 3 months:	21 October 1997
Add 1 year:	21 October 1998
Add 7 days:	28 October 1998
The EDD is therefore	28 October 1998.

Gestational calculators or even a calendar can be used to calculate the current gestation.

CHANGES TO MATERNAL ANATOMY AND PHYSIOLOGY DURING PREGNANCY

Many changes occur in maternal physiology during pregnancy to accommodate the growth of the fetus and the placenta and in preparation for lactation. During pregnancy the mother's weight may increase by up to 12.5 kg and there are marked changes in maternal metabolism. The most important changes as far as emergency care is concerned are those connected with the cardiovascular and respiratory systems; in short, those that affect the management of airway with cervical spine, breathing with oxygen and circulation with posture.

As pregnancy progresses, the metabolic load increases as the fetus grows. The mother has considerably greater metabolic requirements simply to service the extra 12.5 kg of tissues a full-term pregnancy demands. From the viewpoint of emergency care, the changes in pregnancy are best viewed from the operational priorities list rather than from a formal physiological approach.

ANATOMICAL FACTORS IN PREGNANCY

The anatomical changes in pregnancy affecting the airway are the presence of a relatively short obese neck and engorgement of the breast tissue, especially in the third trimester. These conspire to make airway management more difficult. In addition, the pregnant patient usually has a full dentition. As the uterus rises up out of the pelvis and into the abdominal cavity, especially towards term, it has the effect of splinting the diaphragm in the elevated position and also causes some splaying of the ribs; these effects make ventilation and external cardiac compression difficult.

As the uterus enlarges, especially in the third trimester, the inferior vena cava is compressed when the mother lies in the supine position. Beyond 16 weeks the enlarging uterus has less bony protection and is thus at greater risk from direct trauma or deceleration forces.

In summary, the anatomical factors interfering with resuscitation techniques are as follows.

AIRWAY
- Full dentition
- Short, obese neck
- Breast engorgement

BREATHING
- Splinted diaphragm
- Splaying of the ribs

CIRCULATION
- Vena cava compression
- Breast engorgement (affects CPR)
- Splaying of the ribs (affects CPR)

PHYSIOLOGICAL FACTORS IN PREGNANCY

Airway

The risks of reflux acid regurgitation and aspiration of stomach contents into the lungs is increased because of a relaxed gastro-oesophageal junction, delayed emptying of the stomach and increased intragastric pressure from the compressive effects of an increasing uterine size. This is the rationale behind the recommendation for early intubation in pregnant women.

Breathing

There is an increased oxygen requirement during pregnancy because of the high oxygen consumption rates of fetal tissues and because the hypertrophied maternal breast and uterine tissue also have higher oxygen requirements. As pregnancy progresses and diaphragmatic splinting increases, although the vital capacity is not reduced, functional residual capacity is reduced, chest compliance reduces and so to compensate, there is a 40% rise in tidal volume. In short, just at the time when there is the need to satisfy a high oxygen requirement, the means to deliver this are stretched. While respiration is adequate in the fit, healthy mother, it is easily overtaxed in the ill or traumatized mother. This is the reason for early airway intervention, respiratory support and the provision of high-flow oxygen during emergencies in pregnancy.

Circulation changes

Cardiac output is the product of stroke volume and heart rate and in pregnancy the 40% increase in cardiac output at rest is derived from cardiac muscle hypertrophy, enlargement of the cardiac chambers, giving increased stroke volume, and a rise in the resting heart rate of approximately 15–20 beats per minute. Even greater cardiac output is obtained at term and in labour. Because of decreased peripheral resistance and in later weeks the arteriovenous shunt-like effect of the placental bed, blood pressure at rest drops by 5–15 mmHg. The cardiac enlargement and muscle hypertrophy may produce electrocardiographic changes with evidence of left ventricular strain and, as the heart unfolds on the aorta, inverted T waves may be seen in leads V_2 and V_3. On auscultation, as a consequence of the hyperkinetic and hypervolaemic state of pregnancy, a systolic ejection murmur may be heard, but this is of no significance in prehospital emergency care.

Because of the hypertrophied breast and uterine tissue, the demands of the placental bed and increased renal demands, the circulating blood volume increases by 50%, *but there is no corresponding increase in oxygen-carrying capacity*. There is, therefore, a relative *physiological anaemia* as part of the body's attempt to moderate the increased cardiac demands of pregnancy. The anaemia results in reduced blood viscosity which manifests itself as a reduced peripheral resistance and is reflected in reduced diastolic blood pressure.

In summary, the physiological changes of pregnancy are:

AIRWAY
- Relaxed gastro-oesophageal junction
- Delayed stomach emptying
- Increased intragastric pressure

continued

BREATHING
- 40% increase in tidal volume
- Decreased functional residual capacity
- Increased oxygen requirement

CIRCULATION
- 40% increase in cardiac output
- Tachycardia
- Hypotension (systolic blood pressure reduced by 5–15 mmHg)
- ECG changes
- Circulating blood volume increased by 50%

During pregnancy the normal physiological reserves to cope with stresses are all in action to keep the demands on the heart within manageable limits. Because all the normal compensatory mechanisms are already being used, should the pregnant woman suffer blood loss of any significance, she has little physiological reserve left and will show few premonitory signs before passing very rapidly into often irretrievable grade III or IV hypovolaemic shock.

Within normal limits, according to Starling's law (see Chapter 12), the heart will pump out all that it is presented with. In the third trimester of pregnancy, the gravid uterus presses on the inferior vena cava, reducing venous return to the heart. In the supine position the *inferior vena cava compression syndrome* reduces venous return by as much as 40% and fully efficient basic life support only gives at best 30% of the cardiac output. Thus, the pregnant woman should be nursed in the left lateral position and must be resuscitated in that position. The left lateral position maybe achieved by placing a cushion or pillow under the right hip or by a human wedge (Figure 50.7). The uterus can also be manually displaced to the left.

Other detailed changes in the physiology of the pregnant woman are not relevant to prehospital care, except that renal blood flow rises by 50%, occasionally glucose leaks into the urine and protein in the urine always requires further evaluation.

THE CALL TO A PREGNANT WOMAN

A call-out to a pregnant woman is always more stressful than to a non-pregnant patient because there are two lives at stake – mother and fetus. However, in the vast majority of cases, labour is a normal, natural event which takes care of itself without sophisticated intervention from others, and there is time to transport the patient to definitive care.

The mother is the best and most natural incubator for the fetus and therefore she must always be assessed, managed and stabilized first. The main purpose of the assessment by history, examination and observation is to piece together sufficient information to answer one simple question: *"Is there time to transport the mother to hospital or is delivery so imminent that it will have to be managed without assistance?"*.

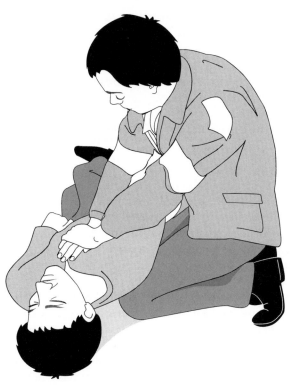

Figure 50.7 The human wedge in use during CPR

Table 50.1 True and false labour

	True labour	False labour
Contractions	Regular	Irregular
Intensity of contractions	Increases as time goes on	Remains at same level of intensity
Contraction-free interval	Gradually shortens	Stays long
Location of pain	Abdomen and back	Lower abdomen only

Table 50.2 The stages of labour

	Nulliparous woman	Multiparous woman
Stage 1	8–12 hours	4–8 hours
Stage 2	1–2 hours	30–60 minutes
Stage 3	A few minutes to 1 hour	A few minutes to 1 hour

The assessment may also give some warning indications of potential complications. General history taking is outlined in Chapter 2, but more focused questions need to be asked in relation to pregnancy. Knowledge of the facts and the general mechanisms of labour will give further information on which to make a balanced, professional but nevertheless critical decision as to whether to attempt transfer or to manage the delivery at the scene.

DEFINITIONS

Parity is the number of times that a woman has carried a pregnancy to 24 weeks. The definition has changed from 28 weeks to 24 weeks, reflecting advances in medical technology which allow many 24-week gestation deliveries to survive in neonatal intensive care units. Similar dating changes have occurred in the definition of stillbirth and the upper limit for legal termination of pregnancy.

Gravidity is the number of times a woman has conceived and been pregnant, regardless of the outcome.

A *primigravida* is a woman who is pregnant for the first time, a *nullipara* is a woman who has never delivered and a *multipara* (or multip) is a woman who has had two or more deliveries.

Other obstetric definitions can be found in the glossary.

THE NORMAL PROCESS OF LABOUR

At any time from 37 weeks to 42 weeks of gestation, labour is said to be at *term*. Prior to 37 weeks the labour is *premature* and after 42 weeks the pregnancy is *prolonged* (*postmature*).

Full term is 40 weeks. There are three phases of labour, but the symptoms of labour can be mimicked by "false labour". It is clearly important to distinguish between the two. The characteristics of each are given in Table 50.1.

DURATION OF LABOUR

Labour falls into three stages (Table 50.2). If the ambulance arrives at the end of the first stage of labour, there is almost always time to transfer the mother to either a consultant-led or midwife-led district general hospital or, failing that, to a general practitioner maternity unit. There will certainly be time to summon a midwife and general practitioner via ambulance control.

GETTING HELP

All NHS general practitioners are required by their terms of service to respond to calls in their practice area for obstetric emergencies. General practitioners rarely practise intrapartum "home delivery" obstetrics nowadays, but will at least provide the assistance of someone who has conducted a reasonable number of normal deliveries. These situations are never ideal and it is important to work as a team, although the general practitioner will carry the ultimate responsibility and therefore the chain of command must be respected. It is likely that both the doctor and the ambulance paramedic will be relieved to see the midwife. Many community midwives still practise intrapartum obstetrics and are required to attend a refresher practical attachment every 12–18 months in an active labour suite, so at least one of the team will have delivered a baby in the past 18 months!

The role of the obstetric flying squad has diminished in recent years. Such squads were initially set up by teaching hospital obstetric units in the 1950s when the majority of births occurred at home. Calls were frequent and teaching hospitals had an abundance of staff to despatch on such calls. Nowadays, most deliveries are planned for hospital or general practitioner maternity units and there are well-established mechanisms to admit women in early labour. Additionally, most district general hospitals usually have only one obstetric team on duty, especially out of hours, and as the normal work of a delivery suite has to continue, a flying squad call simply strips the receiving unit of its staff. Therefore the despatch time for a flying squad can be up to 45 minutes while back-up staff are mobilized, either to form the flying squad or to fill the gaps on the labour ward created by the despatch of the squad. Once the travelling time is added, the flying squad can effectively be discounted in terms of practical help for normal, uncomplicated deliveries. Indeed, many obstetric units only have a flying squad in name, if at all. It is important to be aware of local provision.

THE NORMAL DELIVERY

Unless the baby's head is about to deliver, the first action – assuming that the scene is safe – is to call for help if there is not time to transport the mother to hospital. As in all emergency situations, the fall-back procedure for a clinical situation beyond one's competence is to:

- recognize that fact
- summon help from someone competent
- attend to all those factors that can be effectively dealt with, namely airway breathing with oxygen, circulation with posture, analgesia.

If nothing else, the area can be prepared for immediate delivery, the equipment laid out so that everything is to hand and, as a precaution, at least one intravenous line set up. The biggest threat to the mother is haemorrhage and in this less than ideal environment, the lack of skilled pairs of hands at a crucial time will be most acute.

- ABC
- Posture
- Analgesia with nitrous oxide and oxygen (Entonox)

NORMAL CHILDBIRTH

Normal childbirth occurs through the process of labour which is the expulsion of the products of conception (fetus, placenta and amniotic fluid) from the uterus via the birth canal after the 24th week of gestation. It is achieved via regular and painful uterine contractions accompanied by effacement (see below) and dilation of the cervix, which can only be detected by vaginal examination. Since paramedics do not perform vaginal examinations, in the early stages of labour one's professional role will be to transport the mother to hospital. Any one of rupture of the membranes, loss of the mucus plug from the cervix or a "bloody show" in addition to regular painful uterine contractions constitutes a diagnosis of true labour for the purposes of operational paramedic practice.

THE THREE STAGES OF LABOUR

First stage

The first stage of labour is the longest, during which the cervix (neck) of the uterus effaces and then dilates – a process taking several hours, accompanied by a pink "bloody show" of bloodstained mucus as the plug in the cervical canal is dislodged. During pregnancy the cervix is like a long sausage with a longitudinal canal through it. *Effacement* is the process where, as the uterus changes its shape during contractions, the sausage-shaped cervix becomes compressed in its longitudinal axis and then, in the later stages of effacement, begins to dilate. Full dilation is 10 cm and marks the end of the first stage of labour. As this happens the amniotic sac containing fluid bulges through the widening cervical os; the forewaters then rupture (if they have not already done so), liberating 50 ml or more of watery fluid.

During the first stage of labour, the pain of contraction becomes greater and the contractions increase in frequency, rising from one every 20 minutes to one every 4 or 5 minutes. During the latter half of the first stage of labour, the fetal head begins to descend into the pelvis (Figures 50.8, 50.9).

A useful analogy in visualizing uterine activity in the first stage and early second stage is to think of a chef icing a cake using an icing bag. As he ices the cake, he twists and screws up the top half of the bag in his hand, gathering up the emptying bag in his hand as the icing is expelled through the funnel and nozzle.

Second stage

The second stage of labour lasts from full dilation of the cervix (Figure 50.9) to delivery of the baby. During the second stage of labour the baby's head descends into the pelvis where space is at a premium and towards the end of the second stage of labour, the birth canal is fully formed, but the canal outlet is at 90° to the inlet. In a brief description of labour such as this there is no place for discussion of all eight of the different presentations of the vertex (head). Suffice it to say that the shape and layout of the pelvic floor musculature cause the baby's head to flex and then to internally rotate, bringing the occiput anterior (face posterior) and then allowing the head to extend at birth. All of these movements cause considerable displacement of the pelvic floor musculature, which manifests itself externally as "crowning" (Figure 50.10a).

The occiput is the first part to deliver, followed by the vertex, forehead and then face. Just after delivery of the face, the head "restitutes"; in other words, the neck untwists

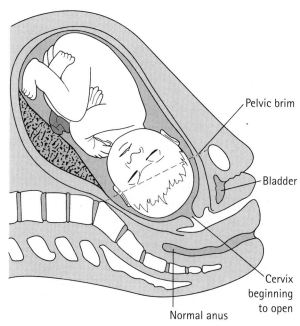

Figure 50.8 Birth canal, early first stage of labour. From Miller & Callander, *Obstetrics illustrated*, 4th edn, with permission from Churchill Livingstone

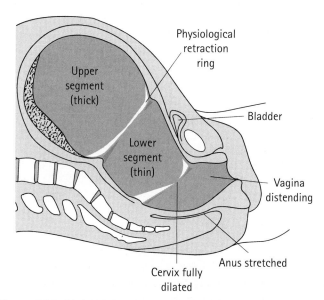

Figure 50.9 Birth canal at the beginning of the second stage of labour. From Miller & Callander, *Obstetrics illustrated*, 4th edn, with permission from Churchill Livingstone

itself so that the head is in the neutral position relative to the shoulders (Figures 50.10b, 50.11). As the shoulders deliver, so the second phase of rotation occurs. The anterior shoulder is the first to deliver followed by the posterior shoulder (Figure 50.10c). The rest of the trunk follows on by lateral flexion of the spine (Figure 50.10d).

Third stage

The third stage of delivery is from the delivery of the baby until delivery of the placenta is complete. Following the vacation of the uterus by the fetus, the uterus contracts in size very markedly in comparison with the placenta, which stays the same size. Hence, the placenta is stripped off the uterine wall and expelled. It is at this stage that the greatest risk of haemorrhage occurs.

MANAGEMENT OF LABOUR

On first attending a woman in labour, it is important to obtain a brief general history by asking appropriate questions. An early request to see her maternity cooperation card can pay dividends, as it may possess much of the information required to decide whether there is time to reach hospital or whether delivery is imminent. Many women now carry their own complete maternity record with them. The layout varies from district to district, so it is important to be familiar with the local one.

The woman should be asked the date of her last normal menstrual period and what her EDD is (the two may not tally, in which case the EDD should be believed). She should be asked whether her waters have gone or whether she has had a bloody show (signs of early labour). Details of her pains should be sought, asking specifically:

- How long have you had the pains?
- Where are the pains?
- Are the pains getting worse or staying the same?
- Are the pains becoming more frequent. If so, how frequent are they?
- Are the pains lasting longer each time there is a pain?

According to the answers, it will be possible to determine whether she is in true labour and, if so, for how long and what stage she is at. Any urge to defecate indicates rectal compression from late second-stage labour.

It is important to enquire into the woman's past medical and obstetric history, specifically asking about:

- previous caesarean sections – indicative of previous delivery problems
- previous precipitate labours – indicative of very rapid labour (compare her answers with the times given in Table 50.2)
- problems with this or other pregnancies.

Clues can be obtained as to whether or not this will also be a complicated pregnancy. Permission should be sought to examine the woman's abdomen and to inspect (*not* palpate) the woman's perineum, whilst giving an explanation of what is going on (e.g. palpation of the abdomen for contractions and observation of the perineum for evidence of the waters having gone or any evidence of crowning). Auscultation of the fetal heart is almost impossible in a noisy environment, and difficult to undertake successfully without regular practice.

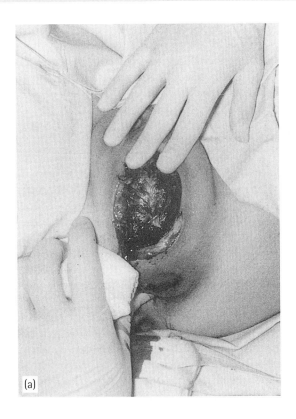

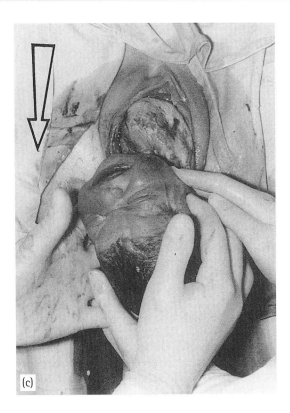

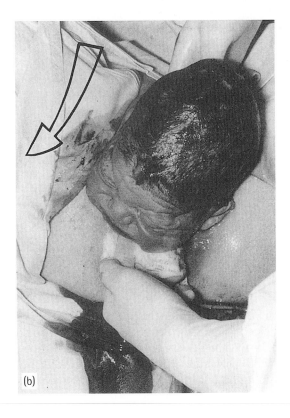

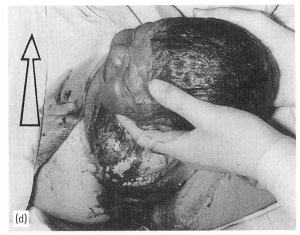

Figure 50.10 The second stage of labour. (a) Normal delivery in the lithotomy position (this patient has, in fact, had an episiotomy, but this is not necessary for all deliveries). (b) The head is born. The perineal pad is protecting the face from faecal contamination and restitution of the head has undone the twist on the neck. (c) The anterior shoulder is being released from beneath the symphysis pubis by directing the head and neck posteriorly. A midwife or doctor may apply gentle traction also at this stage, but paramedics and others without extensive formal training should not apply traction. (d) The posterior shoulder is then delivered by lateral flexion of the trunk in an upward direction. This is achieved by elevating the baby's head, neck and shoulder girdle as one fixed unit in an anterior direction. Do not apply any traction

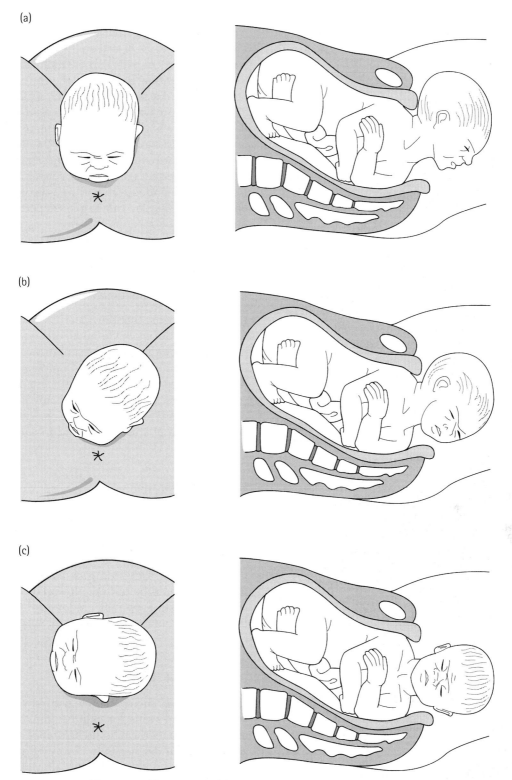

Figure 50.11 Delivery of the head. (a) Delivery; (b) restitution; (c) external rotation. From Miller & Callander, *Obstetrics illustrated*, 4th edn, with permission from Churchill Livingstone

Unless the woman is in the later stage of labour, arrangements should be made to transport her to hospital swiftly in the left lateral position. Clinically, the order of preference for places to deliver is:

- district general hospital labour suite
- general practitioner/midwife-led labour suite in a community hospital
- an accident and emergency department
- a community hospital minor injuries department
- the woman's home, if enough help can be mustered in time
- a general practitioner's treatment room
- the back of an ambulance
- a public place.

Most types of helicopter ambulances in the UK are not suitable places for delivering a child, as access to the mother's pelvis is difficult, if not impossible. In remote situations it is important to think laterally. There may be alternatives to delivering in the back of the ambulance, so call for help and arrange an alternative destination as soon as possible if there is sufficient time to move the mother but not enough to reach a district general hospital. There are many possibilities for providing somewhere in which to conduct a delivery that is more spacious, warmer and better lit than the back of an ambulance. There are also many potential sources of experienced staff. Medical and midwifery back-up should be arranged via ambulance control.

PREPARATION FOR DELIVERY

If forced to conduct a delivery, there are five phases to the preparations if sufficient time is available. If delivery is really imminent with the head crowning, it is far more important to control the delivery than to worry about sterility and there may only be time to put on a pair of gloves, grab a piece of gauze and place the pad over the anus with the palm of the hand, holding the gauze pad with the thumb and forefinger pressing in the skin crease of each groin. The palm of the other hand is laid upon the crowning head, very gently providing upward pressure to encourage the head to extend and deliver. The rest of the delivery sequence is as outlined below.

If there is sufficient time, preparations should be as described below.

Call for help

It is vital to call for help and back-up or, if necessary, to send a reliable person with a written message to read over the telephone. Under normal circumstances a call over the ambulance radio is the most effective and rapid method.

Preparation of the environment

Ideally, the delivery should take place somewhere warm and private, preferably with a bed or stout table on which the mother can lie. The maternity pack should be brought from the vehicle, together with a sheet and absorbent pads. The sheet should be placed on the bed or table, then covered with the absorbent pads and the mother asked to lie on it in the supine position. She should then be covered with a blanket. A towel to dry the baby should be available and preferably a second towel to wrap the baby in after drying. Additionally, if the delivery is going to take place in a public place, the crowds should be moved away. Wherever the location, if possible one or two level-headed adults, preferably female, should be selected, one to act as chaperone and cheerleader for the mother and the other to act as "gofer". If the woman's partner is present, he can be the chaperone and comforter, but if he is too anxious to be of assistance he should be despatched to occupy himself doing something useful such as looking after the other children.

Preparation of the equipment

It is vital to ensure that the maternity pack, paramedic case, oxygen and nitrous oxide inhalation equipment (Entonox) have been brought from the ambulance. Everything must be to hand and the oxygen and Entonox cylinders must be full and turned on. The paramedic case should be laid open so that helpers can retrieve from it any items which may be required when trained staff are gowned up. It may be advantageous at this stage to cannulate the mother and have in situ an IV line in case of problems later.

Personal preparation

Rings, wristwatch, jacket, jerseys and other heavy clothing should be removed as well as keys and coins from the pockets. The hands should be thoroughly washed, including the forearms. A colleague should be asked to break open the maternity pack. Depending on the contents of the pack, the gown should be put on. Nowadays few people bother with the mask, especially under field conditions, unless they have a cold or other infection. Surgical gloves should be used.

Preparation of the mother

If there is time, the chaperone should wash the perineum with soap and water, or chlorhexidine 0.1% and water, if available. The mother should be draped with sterile towels, placing one under her buttocks in a double fold. Another towel is placed with its edge just above the vagina with the towel lying across her abdomen. Many modern maternity packs no longer contain legging towels, but if available they may be put on. The ideal is to have sterile towels over all the field except the vagina and perineum. A colleague can give the mother a brief tutorial on the use of the Entonox and she should be encouraged to use it at the beginning of each pain, since then the analgesic effects will be maximal at the time of maximum pain.

THE DELIVERY

As an inexperienced practitioner, one's aim is simple: to achieve a safe delivery with controlled delivery of the head.

Every time the woman has a contraction she will tend to hold her breath and bear down. While preparing, and in order to slow the delivery, the woman should be instructed to pant like a dog during pains, as this will prevent her from bearing down. In the early stages the head will come down, bulging the perineum, during contraction, but then recede during relaxation. Once the head no longer recedes during relaxations, the head has passed through the level of the pelvic floor and delivery is imminent (Figure 50.10a). If at this stage delivery of the head is not controlled, there is a risk of perineal tears. Because of the pain the woman should be encouraged to use the Entonox. It is at this stage that a doctor or midwife may consider an episiotomy, to prevent what might be an uncontrolled tear of the perineum, to protect a premature fetus or for the aftercoming head in breech births. Tears are much more likely to occur in uncontrolled, rapid births and the risk of tears is reduced by performing episiotomy, thus increasing the size of the aperture for the head to deliver. However, episiotomy should *not* be performed by healthcare professionals without formal training in midwifery.

The mother should be instructed to pant during delivery; if she wishes to use her hands to pull her knees back onto her chest, this can be beneficial.

Taking a gauze pad, preferably soaked in antiseptic, in one's right hand if working from the right side of mother, the pad should be held with the palm of the right hand against the anus, allowing the first web space of the right hand to support the perineum with the thumb and forefinger each lying in a groin crease. Careful gentle pressure on the perineum will allow the head to deliver in a slow, controlled manner with the aim of the head delivering between labour pains. A doctor or midwife at this stage may apply pressure upwards using the palm of the free left hand to encourage the extension of the head on the neck to allow greater control of delivery of the head. Such additional manoeuvres are undertaken on the basis of greater experience and, often, a formal vaginal examination. Paramedics should not utilize such manoeuvres. The procedure outlined above involving only pressure on the perineum is something of a compromise in a difficult situation, but for an inexperienced practitioner with only minimal obstetric and midwifery training, it is safe and allows nature to take its course.

Once the head has delivered, it should be quickly supported and one's fingers slipped into the vagina in order to feel whether the umbilical cord is wrapped around the neck. If it is, the first thing to do is to try to slip the loop of cord off over the head. If this fails, the cord should be clamped twice, cut between the clamps and unwound from around the neck.

Whilst continuing to support the head, taking care not to put any traction on it, the baby's nose should be wiped and fluid mopped from the mouth, clearing the face except the eyes. At the next contraction the baby's head should be gently guided downward towards the bed without putting any traction on the baby. This is more of a lowering manoeuvre, causing the anterior shoulder to deliver. Then, the baby is raised and the posterior shoulder will deliver rapidly, followed by the rest of the trunk and legs. The baby should be allowed to lie on the bed and be wrapped in a towel. Once the baby has cried and the cord has ceased pulsating the umbilical cord is clamped twice and cut between the clamps, close to the introitus (opening of the vagina). If the baby requires resuscitation, this should be carried out immediately (see Chapter 53). If the baby is pinking up well and breathing, it must be dried off to prevent heat loss, wrapped in a dry towel which covers the head and given to the mother.

At delivery of the anterior shoulder, provided it is not a multiple pregnancy, a doctor or midwife will usually give syntometrine intramuscularly to the mother. Paramedics who have completed emergency domestic obstetrics training may also administer this drug. Syntometrine contains oxytocin 5 units and ergometrine 0.5 mg. The oxytocin provokes marked uterine contraction after approximately 3 minutes but is short-lived, and as its effects begin to wear off the ergometrine begins to act and provides longer-lasting uterine contractions, reducing the risk of postpartum haemorrhage.

MANAGING THE THIRD STAGE

The third stage of labour is from the delivery of the baby to delivery of the placenta and usually takes 5–20 minutes. A delay beyond 1 hour is by definition a retained placenta, which is an obstetric emergency requiring a transfer to an obstetric unit where anaesthetic services are available. In the absence of syntometrine following delivery, the uterus will cease contracting for a few minutes and then start contracting again regularly as the placenta separates from the vaginal wall. Often, there is a small gush of blood and the visible length of umbilical cord will increase. The mother will then expel the placenta which should be put into a polythene bag for inspection by the doctor or midwife or at hospital, who will check to confirm it is complete. It is at this stage that the risk of haemorrhage is greatest in the absence of syntometrine administration, and that is why a paramedic is advised to have an IV line in situ.

Doctors and midwives now manage the third stage actively, using syntometrine, application of artery forceps on the umbilical cord and placement of the operator's hand just above the symphysis pubis. The cord is drawn taut, but not actively pulled, using the right hand. The uterus is pushed up gently and then the left hand is pushed down onto the uterus until the placenta is seen at the introitus. The uterus is then pushed upwards and the placenta membranes will slip out of the vagina. This technique is only for experienced operators as the risks of cord avulsion or even uterine eversion are real and potentially life threatening. As a paramedic, one must let nature take its course pending the arrival of a doctor or midwife and, in the meantime, maintain a watch for haemorrhage, acting by instigating rapid IV infusion, if indicated. Early infusion is the watchword.

After the placenta has delivered, bleeding may occur from either the uterus or the perineum or from damage to other structures in the birth canal. A clean pad should be placed over the vagina. If the arrival of a doctor or midwife is not imminent, there is a clear case for moving the woman to hospital but there is no great urgency unless she continues to bleed.

Should the mother continue to bleed after delivery, but before the placenta delivers, an attempt to rub up a contraction of the uterus, by vigorously massaging the uterus in a circular motion just below the mother's umbilicus, is appropriate. Syntometrine should be administered as it is an effective method of haemorrhage control. A call for assistance should be put out and an intravenous infusion commenced. In the event of a retained placenta or massive haemorrhage, urgent transfer to hospital will be required, although if transfer time is likely to be prolonged, medical (or midwifery) assistance (if available) might be appropriate first.

OTHER BIRTH PRESENTATIONS

By far the most common presenting part at birth is the head, but about 3% of all deliveries are breech (bottom first), and these are more common in preterm deliveries. About 0.3% of all deliveries are shoulder presentation; another 0.3% are face presentations and 0.1% are brow presentations. Given that the involvement of paramedics in childbirth is rare, and having to manage a delivery alone is even rarer, it is not necessary to learn the management of malpresentation in detail; such cases almost always require the skills of an obstetrician.

BREECH BIRTH (FIGURE 50.12)

Just occasionally, one may come across a breech birth in the second stage of labour. As indicated earlier in the chapter, when confronted with a clinical situation to which one cannot contribute decisively, the key is to attend to those areas where one can contribute – general patient welfare, reassurance, making preparations and assisting with the maintenance of airway, breathing and circulation. Having called for help, two intravenous lines should be inserted and the mother helped into the supported squatting, kneeling or standing position, because the aim is to allow gravity to assist a much more exhausting process of delivery. If left to nature the baby will normally deliver quite easily and should not be interfered with except to support it when free of the birth canal. A watch must be kept for a prolapsed cord where the umbilical cord drops out ahead of the baby. Alternatively, the mother may wish to labour lying down, in which case she should be manoeuvred so that her buttocks are at the edge of the bed. Her legs can be supported by assistants or, if there is no one else available, by resting them on one's shoulders. The baby should be allowed to deliver without interference until the nape of its neck clears the pubic arch. The baby is then grasped by the feet with one hand and lifted vertically upwards and the head will deliver. The baby is then laid on the mother's abdomen. Following this, the cord can be double clamped and then cut.

The method used by a midwife or doctor to conduct a breech delivery is not described, as it involves a generous episiotomy, rotation and traction of baby with Lovset's manoeuvre (see obstetric glossary) and the application of forceps to the aftercoming head, and is beyond the scope of this book.

MULTIPLE DELIVERIES

Multiple deliveries are not uncommon. Twins occur in about 1 in 80 pregnancies. With modern antenatal care, a surprise twin diagnosis at confinement is generally a thing of the past.

Over 50% of multiple pregnancies go into premature labour and eclampsia is three times as common, as is prolapsed umbilical cord and postpartum haemorrhage. Every effort should be made to transport the mother to a consultant obstetric unit or the flying squad should be called. If the first twin is delivering, then it should be delivered as in a singleton pregnancy and an intravenous line should be set up at the earliest opportunity. If no assistance has arrived, the next stage is to wait for the second twin to deliver and then – and only then – attempt to deliver the placentae. Syntometrine should *not* be administered until the second twin delivers.

PROLAPSED UMBILICAL CORD (FIGURE 50.13)

Prolapsed umbilical cord is an obstetric emergency and occurs when the cord drops out of the uterus into the vagina or even outside the body ahead of the presenting part. Occasionally, the cord prolapses ahead of the presenting part with the amniotic membranes intact. Under these circumstances, there is no immediate danger. More usually, cord prolapse occurs for one of the following reasons.

- Unusual fetal presentation, for example footling breech or transverse lie
- Premature or abnormal fetus
- Multiple pregnancy
- Polyhydramnios (a condition where there is excessive amniotic fluid)
- Placenta praevia (see Chapter 51)

The cooling and drying effects on the umbilical cord, coupled with handling, can provoke spasm in the cord, thus cutting off the placentofetal blood supply. Occasionally, the presenting part can crush the umbilical cord against the mother's bony pelvis with a similar outcome. Out of hospital

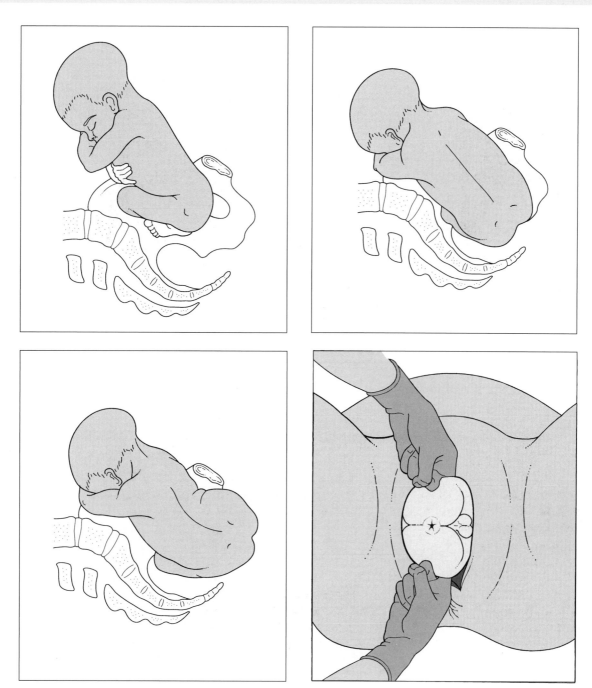

Figure 50.12 A breech birth

there is only one realistic course of action and that is to obtain either gauze pads or towels soaked in warm saline and gently replace the cord as far into the vagina as possible, with the minimum of handling. This is easier if the woman adopts the knee–elbow position. However, it is quite impossible to transport a woman in this position in a moving ambulance, especially as it is necessary to keep a gloved hand in the vagina in transit to prevent prolapse recurring. Thus, the most practical manner of transportation will be with the patient in the left lateral position. The hand must be maintained in the vagina at all times and this means the practitioner will have to jam themselves for transport in any

position they can as long as their hand remains in the appropriate place. If time permits, an intravenous line should be inserted.

SHOULDER DYSTOCIA

This is a very serious but fortunately rare adverse event that can occur during the second stage of labour. Following delivery of the head, labour fails to progress and the neck and shoulders do not become visible.

This is a time-critical emergency, as the baby can die within 10 minutes if delivery cannot be completed. It

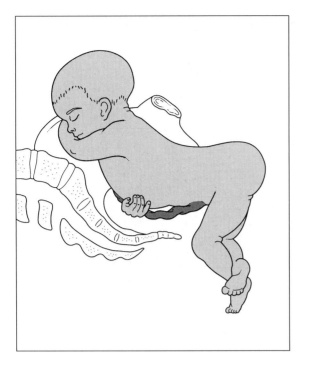

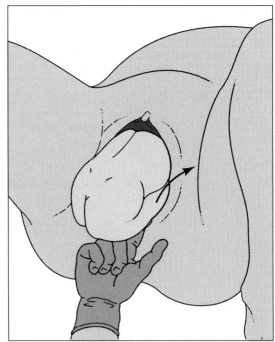

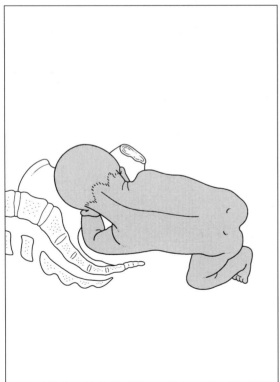

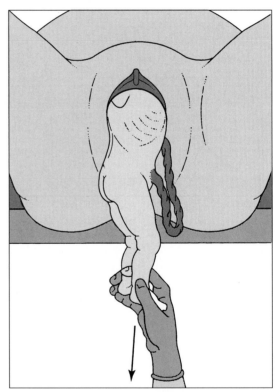

Figure 50.12 *Continued*

should be managed according to "the rule of two's" with respect to the number of contractions between each step. If delivery of the shoulders does not occur within *two* contractions of delivery of the head:

1. Contact the *senior* on-call obstetrician and inform him that you are managing a patient with suspected shoulder dystocia.

2. Ensure a midwife and/or GP are en route to you.
3. Place the patient on her back with her knees drawn upwards as far as possible and turned outwards (McRobert's position).
4. If the delivery does not progress after *two* contractions in the McRobert's position, apply suprapubic pressure with the aim

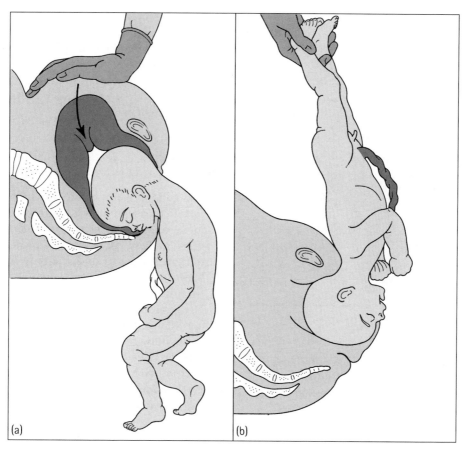

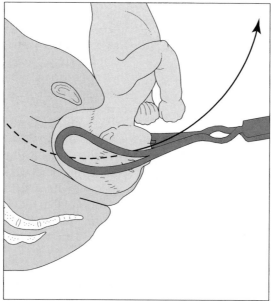

Figure 50.12 *Continued*

of pushing/rotating the anterior shoulder under the pelvic arch:

(a) Keeping the mother in McRobert's position, position yourself vertically over the patient's abdomen at their left side

(b) Keep your elbows locked straight, with the heel of one hand over the symphysis, with the other hand on top

(c) Push down firmly and away from you (but do not administer a blow)

(d) Discontinue suprapubic pressure if labour does not progress with *two* further contractions maintain McRobert's position.

5. You must now decide on the most rapid way for getting skilled obstetric help for the mother—either transportation to the

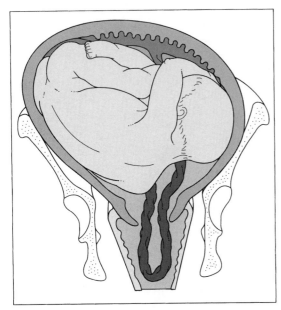

Figure 50.13 Umbilical cord prolapse

hospital or waiting at scene for the midwife/GP. Regardless of your decision, contact the *senior* on-call obstetrician for further advice, en route to hospital if necessary.

SHORT CORD

This is an umbilical cord of less than 40 cm, which may be too short to allow delivery of the baby without pulling on the cord. This risks a cord tear and consequent haemorrhage or premature separation of the placenta, also risking haemorrhage and/or fetal distress.

During delivery of a baby with a short cord, avoid any traction. If necessary, double clamp and cut the cord to facilitate delivery.

CORD RUPTURE

Cord rupture can result in an exsanguinating haemorrhage for the baby. Prevention, through careful handling of the cord (including avoiding pulling on it) is the preferred treatment! If a rupture does occur, place a cord clamp between the tear and the baby. If this is not possible apply direct pressure over a sterile dressing. Give oxygen and consider the need for fluid replacement.

PRIMARY POST-PARTUM HAEMORRHAGE (PPH)

Primary Post Partum Haemorrhage is defined as blood loss of 500 ml or more within 24 hours of delivery. It occurs most commonly with delivery of the placenta. The common causes of PPH are atony of uterine muscle, which prevents the process of vascular constriction after separation of the

placenta; retained placenta (or placental parts) and trauma to the genital tract.

Tears should be managed by direct pressure. If bleeding is severe and is secondary to uterine atony or suspected retention of placental tissue, give syntometrine. High concentration oxygen should be administered and IV fluid replacement considered.

CONCLUSION

The incidence of obstetric incidents in prehospital care is certain to rise in the UK, partly as the result of the government report on *Changing childbirth*, which gives women much more freedom to choose where they deliver and gives the green light to midwife-only maternity units, and also because of the increasing trend towards earlier discharge from hospital. Additionally, because of the changes in the NHS concerning the free market, the purchaser–provider split and changes in hospital staffing patterns, hospital trusts are less willing and less able to provide obstetric flying squad services. General practitioners are rarely involved in intrapartum care, and apart from the time demands of such work, many are wary of undertaking work with such high medicolegal risks, especially as the falling birth rate means that even willing general practitioners will have insufficient experience of intrapartum obstetrics.

Paramedics by default are likely to transport an increasing number of obstetric cases, but the actual number requiring intervention will be small. Such is the nature of obstetric work that the only realistic approach to paramedic involvement in intrapartum care is to "let nature take its course". It is neither appropriate nor possible for paramedics to take any other approach to the problem at current resource and demand levels.

As with other areas of paramedic activity, true professionals will take the trouble to read beyond the level of their permitted practice to better understand the rationale behind that practice. Reference to an undergraduate obstetric or midwifery textbook will pay dividends and reinforce the concept that for the inexperienced *practitioner*, the policy of letting nature take its course, coupled with skilled observation, is the only realistic approach to childbirth.

FURTHER READING

Drire J, Magowan BA 2004 Clinical obstetrics and gynaecology. Saunders, London

Miller A and Callender R 1994 Obstetrics illustrated, 4th edn. Churchill Livingstone, London

O'Reilly B, Bottomley C, Rymer J 2005 Pocket essentials of obstetrics and gynaecology. Saunders, London

Chapter 51

Emergencies in pregnancy

INTRODUCTION

Pregnancy should be considered in any woman of reproductive age. For various reasons, including fear, denial or social stigma, not every woman will admit, or even realize, that she is pregnant.

Pregnancy itself is not an illness, but there are medical conditions and emergencies specific to the pregnant state which must be considered in the context of prehospital care, as well as general emergencies such as asthma or epilepsy that can occur in any patient, which may have their assessment and management altered by pregnancy.

The most common reasons for calling the emergency services in early pregnancy are vaginal bleeding, abdominal pain, or both.

VAGINAL BLEEDING AND ABDOMINAL PAIN IN EARLY PREGNANCY

A history should be taken by the attending paramedic to corroborate the possibility of pregnancy in any woman complaining of abdominal pain or vaginal bleeding. The conventional limits to child-bearing age can be relied on less than was previously the case. A high index of suspicion can be gained simply from finding out the date of the last menstrual period (LMP). Any regularly menstruating woman whose LMP was more than 4 weeks prior to the current date

is likely to be pregnant. If the LMP was normal and occurred more than 4 weeks prior to the onset of the current problems, the patient should be considered to be pregnant until proved otherwise.

Once the possibility of pregnancy is suggested by the history, or confirmed by the patient, vital signs should be measured (pulse, blood pressure, respiratory rate) to assess whether the patient is clinically hypovolaemic. If any signs suggest that hypovolaemia is present, then intravenous access should be obtained and fluid infusion started.

The most frequent cause of vaginal bleeding, with or without abdominal pain, early in pregnancy is miscarriage. The most dangerous cause of vaginal bleeding and abdominal pain is ectopic pregnancy and this should be considered in any woman of reproductive age complaining of abdominal pain, especially if this is associated with collapse.

> Abdominal pain and vaginal bleeding in early pregnancy: think of miscarriage and ectopic pregnancy

MISCARRIAGE

Approximately 10–15% of confirmed pregnancies end in miscarriage. This occurs most often at either 8 weeks or 12 weeks from the first day of the LMP. There are several postulated causes of miscarriages, but most are due to a genetic defect in the fetus or to uterine abnormalities. Many threatened miscarriages may settle spontaneously and lead to a normal pregnancy and subsequent delivery of a normal infant. Miscarriage may, however, cause significant uterine bleeding, resulting in hypovolaemic shock.

Terminology

Any form of miscarriage is a stressful and distressing experience not only for the mother but also for the father. It is important not to make the situation worse by using the term *abortion*. There are a number of different types of miscarriage, although these cannot always be distinguished without vaginal examination. Clearly the prognosis is better with threatened abortion and it is important not to be over-specific about prognosis (either in terms of inappropriate reassurance or unnecessary pessimism) unless it is absolutely clear that the products of conception have been lost.

Threatened miscarriage

In threatened miscarriage, vaginal bleeding is associated with cramping abdominal pain; the cervix remains closed and pregnancy may progress normally.

Incomplete miscarriage

In incomplete miscarriage, vaginal bleeding may be heavy, the cervix is open and abdominal pain is caused by uterine contractions, which have begun to expel the products of conception.

Complete miscarriage

In complete miscarriage the products are completely expelled through an open cervix. The symptoms usually then settle.

Symptoms and signs

The patient may be known to be pregnant or admit to being late with a period. There may be a history of previous miscarriage; she will be complaining of vaginal blood loss and may have lower abdominal cramping pain.

There may be obvious external signs of vaginal bleeding associated with varying degrees of shock. Measurement of pulse, blood pressure and respiratory rate is mandatory.

Management

Most women will naturally be anxious at the prospect of a miscarriage and gentle handling and reassurance are very important during the initial assessment and transfer to hospital for more detailed examination and management.

If signs of hypovolaemia are present or there is a history of significant blood loss, high-flow oxygen should be given and fluid infusion started.

On arrival in hospital the patient will be assessed fully by the receiving doctor. This will include vaginal examination and ultrasound scanning, to confirm pregnancy and determine the viability of the fetus.

ECTOPIC PREGNANCY

Ectopic pregnancy is the most life threatening of the early complications of pregnancy. The incidence of ectopic pregnancy is approximately 1% of all pregnancies and is increasing. Ruptured ectopic pregnancies account for 13% of maternal deaths and are the leading cause of maternal death in the first trimester, although the death rate is falling due to improved awareness, early diagnostic facilities and improved management.

An ectopic pregnancy normally occurs in one or other of the fallopian tubes; predisposition will occur in women with a history of pelvic inflammatory disease, previous ectopic pregnancy, previous fallopian tube surgery and in those who use the intrauterine contraceptive device (IUCD or "coil").

Symptoms and signs

Most tubal ectopic pregnancies present 5–8 weeks after the LMP. Pain is typically the first symptom, occurring in up to 95% of patients, and 75% complain of abnormal vaginal bleeding (such as "spotting"). The pain is felt in the lower abdomen and may be localized to one side early in the condition (Table 51.1).

If the pregnancy causes rupture of the tube, the condition's most dramatic form, the patient may present in a state of collapse secondary to hypovolaemic shock: the diagnosis must be considered in any woman of reproductive age who presents in this way. More commonly, the patient exhibits less marked degrees of shock, including tachycardia and tachypnoea, with or without hypotension. Pallor may be prominent. There will be abdominal tenderness and a reluctance to move, since movement will exacerbate the pain.

Management

Ectopic pregnancy is a gynaecological emergency. The patient must be transferred as soon as possible to hospital for further assessment by the receiving doctor.

Table 51.1 Differential diagnosis of miscarriage and ectopic pregnancy

	Miscarriage	Ectopic pregnancy
Timing	5–12 weeks	5–8 weeks
Abdominal pain	Central and cramping	May be unilateral
Relation to bleeding	Follows	Precedes
Vaginal bleeding	Frank May be heavy	Normally scanty Dark brown
Haemodynamic status	Shock rare	Shock common

Shock should be treated aggressively: oxygen should be administered, two large-bore (14 G) intravenous cannulae inserted into the antecubital fossae, and fluid resuscitation commenced.

On arrival in hospital, the patient's pregnancy will be confirmed by clinical examination and ultrasound scan: definitive management is surgical.

VAGINAL BLEEDING AND ABDOMINAL PAIN IN LATER PREGNANCY

Third-trimester vaginal bleeding (antepartum haemorrhage) is bleeding that occurs after 28 weeks of pregnancy. It occurs in approximately 4% of pregnancies; the two most common causes are placental abruption and placenta praevia. All patients with antepartum haemorrhage must be assessed in hospital.

> Abdominal pain and vaginal bleeding in later pregnancy: think of placental abruption and placenta praevia

PLACENTAL ABRUPTION

Placental abruption is the separation of a normally located placenta before delivery of the fetus. Bleeding occurs and the blood is initially confined between the placenta and the uterine wall (Figure 51.1).

Symptoms and signs

Placental abruption may present in its most severe form with painful vaginal bleeding associated with a tender, contracting uterus, shock and fetal compromise. Most women, however, do not present with so dramatic a picture; they complain of abdominal pain, usually of sudden onset, with or without vaginal bleeding.

Management

Any woman in the later stages of pregnancy with abdominal pain and vaginal bleeding should be considered to have a placental abruption, since this diagnosis is potentially dangerous for both mother and baby. Urgent transfer to an obstetric unit or hospital is appropriate.

Vital signs must be measured: it is important to remember that vital signs will not suggest shock until it is too late, so a high index of suspicion is required and treatment should be aggressive. Oxygen should be administered and fluid resuscitation commenced.

The stable patient will be fully assessed on arrival in hospital and continued observation may be appropriate. If the patient is shocked or has deteriorating vital signs in transit, appropriate warning to the receiving obstetric unit or hospital should be given, enabling staff to prepare for urgent delivery of the baby.

PLACENTA PRAEVIA

Placenta praevia occurs when the placenta is implanted in the lower uterine segment (Figure 51.2), and subsequent

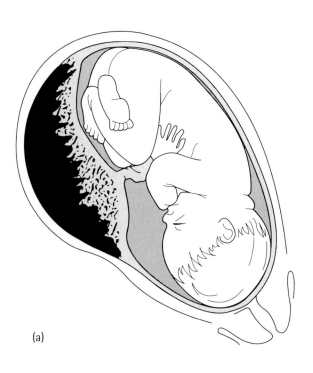
(a)

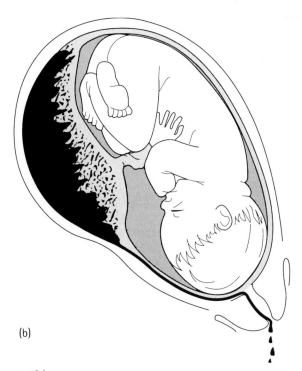
(b)

Figure 51.1 Placental abruption: haemorrhage may be concealed (a) or revealed (b)

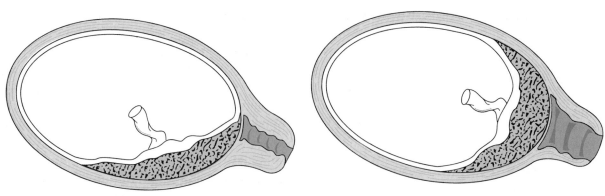

Figure 51.2 Placenta praevia: the placenta may partly or completely cover the uterine opening

separation will cause blood loss into the vagina. Patients present with vaginal bleeding, which may be heavy, but may have little or no abdominal pain. The patient should be transferred urgently to hospital for full assessment. The need for fluid resuscitation in transit will be determined by the amount of blood loss and the vital signs.

HYPERTENSIVE EMERGENCIES IN PREGNANCY

ECLAMPSIA

A degree of hypertension occurs in approximately 8% of pregnancies but the most severe manifestation is *eclampsia*, in which a combination of hypertension, cerebral oedema, intracerebral haemorrhage and seizures may be fatal for mother and baby. Eclampsia results in the death of about 1000 babies and 10 women each year in the UK.

Symptoms and signs

The clinical features of eclampsia are listed in Box 51.1.

Patients usually have a known history of hypertension earlier in their pregnancy. Prior to the onset of seizures there may have been headache, visual disturbance, abdominal pain, weight gain and swelling of the peripheries. On examination, the patient may be fitting, will be hypertensive and will have peripheral oedema.

Management

Urgent transfer to hospital is essential, since definitive treatment requires urgent delivery of the baby. If there is fitting, the first priority is to establish an airway and ensure that the patient is adequately oxygenated for transfer to hospital. In a fitting patient, often the most practical means of achieving an airway is via the nasopharyngeal route.

Oxygen should be administered via a face mask with reservoir bag. Intravenous or rectal diazepam (10 to 20 mg) should be given in an attempt to terminate the seizures. The receiving obstetric unit or hospital should be alerted so that an appropriately experienced team can be awaiting the arrival of the patient.

Box 51.1 Clinical features of eclampsia

- Hypertension
- Cerebral oedema and haemorrhage
- Seizures
- Headaches
- Visual disturbance
- Weight gain and peripheral oedema
- Abdominal pain

COMMON GENERAL MEDICAL EMERGENCIES IN PREGNANCY

A pregnant woman may have preexisting illness that presents acutely with an exacerbation while she is pregnant; examples include asthma, epilepsy and diabetes mellitus. It is always important to bear the pregnancy in mind when managing these emergencies but common sense and first principles apply and these are the same whether the patient is pregnant or not.

ASTHMA

The effect of pregnancy on asthma is variable. The majority of patients experience less frequent attacks, but a few experience more frequent attacks. Asthma has no effect on the course of pregnancy. The management of an acute exacerbation is the same as in a non-pregnant woman, with oxygen, nebulized salbutamol and transfer to hospital for assessment.

EPILEPSY

Seizures may occur in pregnancy unrelated to hypertension, simply as a manifestation of preexisting epilepsy. Treatment regimens may have been modified prior to or early in pregnancy in order to avoid fetal damage, and control may have been lost. Management of seizures is conventional and consists of prevention of harm to the patient during a seizure, attention to the airway, administration of oxygen, diazepam if the fit is prolonged, and transfer to hospital.

DIABETES MELLITUS

When a diabetic woman becomes pregnant, close attention is required to maintain good control of the disease throughout the pregnancy. Hypoglycaemic and hyperglycaemic emergencies may occur and will be rapidly identified clinically using a glucose reagent strip. Standard protocols for control of hypoglycaemia should be followed (Hypostop gel, IV glucose, IM glucagon). Patients with hyperglycaemic emergencies should receive oxygen and fluid resuscitation with normal saline, and be transferred immediately to hospital.

CONCLUSION

Emergencies in pregnant patients always cause anxiety. In reality, there are relatively few diagnoses that are specific to pregnancy and the gestational age will usually offer a clue as to the most likely possibilities. The most dangerous potential diagnoses should always be considered and appropriate treatment commenced until the diagnosis is confirmed or excluded in hospital. The key to the management of these, as of other life-threatening problems, is attention to ABC. The prehospital management of coincident medical problems in pregnancy is not affected by the pregnant state.

FURTHER READING

Baskett TF 2004 Essential management of obstetric emergencies (4th edn). Clinical Press, London

Cox C, Grady K, Johanson R, Howell C 2003 Managing obstetric emergencies and trauma: The MOET cause manual. RCOG Bookshop, London

Stevens L, Kenney A 1994 Emergencies in obstetrics and gynaecology. Oxford University Press, Oxford

Chapter 52

Trauma in pregnancy

CHAPTER CONTENTS

INTRODUCTION

A full understanding of the management of trauma in pregnancy requires complete familiarity with the anatomical and physiological changes that occur during pregnancy, and the ability to integrate the consequences of these changes into the philosophy of the consistent pattern of care expounded throughout this book: personal safety, scene safety, victim safety, primary survey and resuscitation according to ABC protocols, and constant re-evaluation en route to hospital. Because many of the physical signs of shock and haemorrhage only present late in the pregnant woman, a thorough understanding of the mechanism of trauma and a proper history are vital.

The approach to the pregnant trauma victim is exactly the same as for the non-pregnant trauma victim except that there are two victims – mother and fetus – to consider. The mother is treated directly, the fetus is treated indirectly by optimum resuscitation of the mother. The mother is the best incubator for the fetus and in the prehospital situation, a dead mother almost certainly means a dead fetus. Trauma in pregnancy is always a highly charged emotional situation, but by adhering to the same conventional pattern of care as for the non-pregnant trauma victim, the chances of success are optimized.

According to American studies 7% of all pregnant women sustain trauma, the vast majority resulting from road accidents, followed by falls, penetrating injury and thermal injuries, including smoke inhalation.

The anatomical and physiological changes in pregnancy were outlined in Chapter 50 but they are also crucial to the proper management of the pregnant trauma victim that they are restated here.

ANATOMICAL CHANGES

The anatomical factors in pregnancy include the presence of a full dentition, a relatively short obese neck and engorged breast tissue. Internally there is oedema of the upper airway, increased fat deposition, especially around the face and neck, and increased fragility of the mucous membranes, making them liable to bleed. All of these features conspire to make intubation and airway maintenance more difficult and cause difficulty in the sizing and fitting of cervical collars.

As the uterus enlarges it changes from being a thick-walled organ protected deep within the pelvic cavity before 12 weeks of gestation, becoming progressively more thin-walled as pregnancy advances. Between 12 and 24 weeks the fetus is protected by the relatively large volume of amniotic fluid within the uterus but in the third trimester, as the fetus grows, the relative volume of cushioning amniotic fluid decreases and the uterine wall becomes thinner. Up to 34 weeks, before the fetal head engages in the maternal pelvis, the uterine fundus continues to grow, expanding further and further into the abdominal cavity until at 34 weeks the fundus is some 34 cm above the pubic bone. Under these circumstances the intestines are pushed ever further upwards, the diaphragm becomes splinted because of increasing abdominal cavity volume and the lower ribs become flared out, reducing the functional residual capacity of the lungs

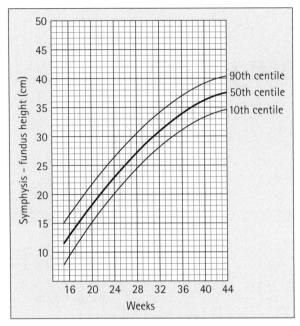

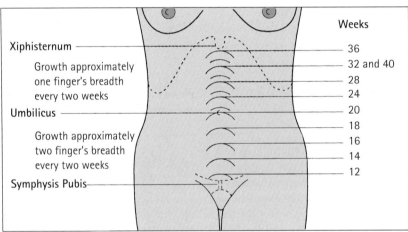

Figure 52.1 The fundal height and gestational age

and the compliance of the chest wall. This splinting of the diaphragm and reduced compliance of the chest wall due to splaying of the ribs make ventilation difficult and, together with engorgement of the breasts, hinder external chest compression.

Other anatomical changes in pregnancy include enlargement of the pituitary gland, which makes it more susceptible to decelerative head injuries, and the urinary bladder is pulled up out of the bony pelvis during the third trimester and is therefore more liable to be damaged.

PHYSIOLOGICAL CHANGES

Relaxation of the gastro-oesophageal junction, delayed gastric emptying and increasing intragastric pressure from the compressive effects of increasing uterine size raise the potential for reflux acid regurgitation with aspiration of stomach contents into the lungs, and are part of the rationale behind

the recommendation to secure the airway definitively by early endotracheal intubation when anaesthetic facilities exist.

Fetal tissue has a high oxygen consumption and maternal oxygen requirements are increased because of hypertrophied breast and uterine tissue, coupled with the need to meet the metabolic requirements of the extra 12.5 kg of tissues of a term pregnancy. However, functional residual capacity and chest compliance are reduced, so demands are met by increased ventilation through a 40% rise in tidal volume, although the respiratory rate remains unchanged. Thus, just when there is a need to satisfy a high oxygen requirement, the means to deliver this requirement are stretched and while adequate in the fit, healthy mother, are easily overtaxed in the traumatized mother. Thus the spontaneously breathing pregnant trauma victim must *always* receive oxygen at as high a concentration as possible, preferably close to 100%, via a reservoir face mask.

> Always administer high–flow oxygen

If there are any doubts as to the adequacy of ventilation or questions of airway compromise, then early intubation and early intermittent positive pressure ventilation are indicated. This is unlikely to be possible in prehospital care unless a doctor with anaesthetic skills and appropriate drugs and equipment is available, or the patient is already moribund. Attempts to intubate patients who are unlikely to tolerate a tube (that is, those with an intact gag reflex) are inappropriate and likely to be dangerous. The altered chest dynamics can make observation of respiratory excursion difficult.

In relation to trauma the most important physiological changes in pregnancy concern the cardiovascular system. The cardiac output rises by 40% through a combination of a rise in resting heart rate of 15–20 beats per minute and by an increased stroke volume achieved by hypertrophy of the cardiac muscle and enlargement of the cardiac chambers.

During pregnancy, the circulating blood volume increases by about 50% to service the increased demands of the hypertrophied breast and uterine tissue, increased renal demands and the enormous low pressure shunt of the placental bed. The placenta itself has a circulatory demand of approximately 600 ml per minute – or 10% of the maternal circulation.

There is thus a physiological anaemia of pregnancy. The anaemia results in reduced blood viscosity which manifests itself as a reduced peripheral resistance (and therefore reduced cardiac work) and is reflected in the reduced diastolic blood pressure.

The normal physiological reserves to cope with stresses are already in action during pregnancy to keep the demands on the heart within manageable limits. Should the pregnant woman suffer blood loss of any significance, she has few physiological reserves to bring into play, and this is why pregnant women show few premonitory clinical signs before passing almost immediately into often irretrievable grade III or IV hypovolaemic shock.

A high index of suspicion for both concealed and revealed haemorrhage is therefore vital, especially because initially vasodilation and increased overall blood volume cause both skin colour and capillary refill to remain within normal limits. Hypovolaemic shock in pregnancy can also cause necrosis of the anterior pituitary gland, giving rise to pituitary insufficiency with multiple endocrine problems which require lifelong replacement of thyroxine and steroid therapy (*Sheehan's syndrome*).

In the third trimester of pregnancy the gravid uterus presses on the inferior vena cava, reducing venous return to the heart, thus reducing cardiac output (Starling's law – see

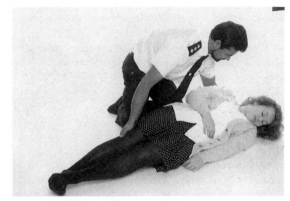

Figure 52.2 Maintaining the left lateral position

Chapter 12) by up to 40% and inducing maternal hypotension. This leads to reduced maternal cardiac and cerebral perfusion pressure and reduced uteroplacental perfusion, compromising the fetus as well. The hypotension so induced also releases catecholamines which further diminish uteroplacental circulation. When maternal resuscitation is attempted it should be remembered that fully efficient basic life support gives at best 30% of cardiac output. Thus resuscitation attempts in the pregnant woman will fail unless caval compression is relieved by nursing the woman in the left lateral or left lateral decubitus position (Figure 52.2).

There are three ways in which caval compression can be relieved:

- manually, by holding the uterus over to the left
- by a sandbag or pillow under the right buttock
- by nursing the patient on a long spinal board tilted 25–30° to the left.

The first method will occupy an assistant who might be useful in other ways; sandbags or pillows may compromise a spinal injury; so use of a spinal board is the method of choice. A scoop stretcher is not adequate for this purpose as it is unable to take the force of external chest compressions should the patient suffer a cardiac arrest. A tilt of 25–30° is required to decompress the inferior vena cava. There is no place for the Cardiff wedge in prehospital care. Where access is difficult, the use of the human wedge can be considered (Figure 52.3).

The patient is log rolled to the left and then one or two rescuers kneel down with their knees a few centimetres away from the patient's right side. The patient is then gently log rolled back onto the laps of the rescuers. It is possible to perform external chest compressions from this position but not effective ventilation, so there would need to be at least three rescuers for this technique to be effective.

The relief of hypoxia and hypovolaemia in the pregnant trauma victim is as urgent as in the non-pregnant victim. However, by the time hypovolaemia manifests itself with clinical signs (30–40% haemorrhage), the fetus will be severely compromised. Losses of only 10–20% of circulatory blood volume markedly reduce uterine perfusion, and the only sign of fetal distress may be fetal bradycardia of 110 beats per

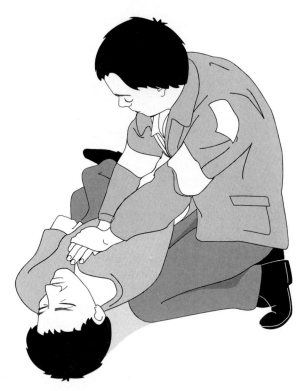

Figure 52.3 The human wedge during CPR

minute or less. Attempting to listen for a fetal heart at the roadside or other noisy environment is unlikely to be helpful. With increasing maternal hypovolaemia, the chances of fetal survival fall rapidly and unless the fetus is delivered by caesarean section within about 20 minutes of the failure of uterine circulation, death of the fetus is inevitable. The practical implication of this fact is that in the severely injured, un-entrapped mother whose survival may be questionable, if a hospital facility able to perform an emergency caesarean section is less than 20 minutes away, the decision must be "load and go". There is no justification whatsoever to "stay and play". Interventions, including cannulation, must be carried out in transit. If intravenous access is established in the prehospital environment (or in transit), the key is to infuse sufficient fluid to prevent maternal hypotension if at all possible.

It is important to radio ahead to the emergency department so that an obstetric team can be ready on arrival should it be needed. Time is of the essence; definitive treatment is not possible in the back of an ambulance and for both mother and baby, the *only* chance is immediate caesarean section once maternal hypovolaemia is established. The clear duty is to get the mother to a surgeon as quickly as possible.

THE APPROACH TO THE PREGNANT TRAUMA VICTIM

The approach to the pregnant trauma victim is exactly the same as to the non-pregnant victim. Once the scene is safe,

during the process of primary survey and resuscitation an accurate history of events should be obtained with special reference to the mechanisms of injury and the sequence of the accident.

The history is important because maternal clinical signs of hypovolaemia and haemorrhage present too late to save the fetus in 80% of cases, and unnecessary damage is caused to the mother while this haemorrhage and hypovolaemia remain unrecognized. The only means of making such a diagnosis in the field is to think of the possible mechanisms of injury and maintain a high index of suspicion. Thus treatment precedes formal definitive diagnosis.

> If there is **ANY** possibility of significant trauma immediate evacuation is essential

The mother is the best and most natural transport incubator for her fetus, but physiologically the mother will always sacrifice the fetus to preserve her own life. Fetal distress will ensue after the loss of only 10–20% of maternal blood volume, as at this point material compensatory mechanisms restrict blood flow to the uterus. Signs of maternal hypotension, however, will only declare themselves suddenly at 35% blood loss. As a consequence fluid administration should be more vigorous and earlier than in the non-pregnant trauma victim. The only indication of fetal distress detectable in the field is a fetal bradycardia of under 110 beats per minute and in a noisy environment this may be difficult, if not impossible, to detect.

Assessment and stabilization of the mother conform to the standard primary survey and resuscitation pattern outlined in Chapters 2 and 21, with particular attention to early oxygenation, intubation if the patient is unconscious, and relief of venal caval compression.

● High-flow oxygen
● Early intubation if unconscious
● Relief of vena caval compression.

As part of the identification of life-threatening haemorrhage, it is useful to inspect the perineum but formal examination must not be attempted. Bleeding or fluid from the vagina or urethra and any signs of bruising or bulging of the perineum should be sought.

It is important to remember that concealed blood loss is common and threatens both the fetus and the mother.

An attempt should be made to palpate the abdomen, checking for fetal parts, movements and the fetal heart rate if possible. Undue time must not be wasted on this part of the assessment. It is vital to remember to ensure relief of vena cava-compression.

It is important to remember that, except in the case of burns, pregnancy itself does not increase maternal morbidity from trauma. It is the consequences of unrecognized haemorrhage, hypovolaemia, hypotension and hypoxia which result from pregnancy masking their normal clinical signs and failure by the rescuer to understand the implications of the altered anatomy and physiology of pregnancy that increase maternal morbidity in the pregnant trauma victim.

CONSEQUENCES OF TRAUMA IN PREGNANCY

This discussion of the consequences of trauma for the pregnant patient is confined to the effects of trauma on the abdomen and pelvis; in prehospital care the treatment of trauma elsewhere in the body is the same as for the non-pregnant patient.

A pregnant woman sustaining *any* trauma to the abdomen and pelvis, however minor, requires specialist assessment and observation at hospital. Even small degrees of abdominal trauma can cause sufficient placental leakage for the maternal circulation to be contaminated by fetal red blood cells. As a consequence, maternal antibody formation against fetal red cells may result in fetal anaemia and problems with future pregnancies. The incidence of fetomaternal haemorrhage is raised fivefold in the face of trauma; this is the rationale behind taking samples of blood for Kleihauer testing for Rhesus status as well as for crossmatching when cannulating.

BLUNT TRAUMA

Blunt trauma to the abdomen and pelvis is more common than penetrating trauma in UK practice, and in the pregnant woman is most often caused by:

- road traffic accidents
- falls
- assaults.

Unsteadiness in late pregnancy increases the risk of falling. There is no doubt that any risk of injury to the pregnant passenger caused by the wearing of a seatbelt is far outweighed by the reduction in risk from ejection or impaction.

In any abdominal injury the concept of concealed haemorrhage must be remembered, be it from ruptured liver or spleen, retroperitoneal bleed or a concealed placental abruption. All these injuries are time critical and need a surgeon urgently.

The three most common pathological mechanisms in blunt abdominopelvic trauma in the pregnant mother are:

- placental abruption
- uterine rupture
- pelvic fracture.

In each of these mechanisms of injury there is the potential for fetal injury and in each, both mother and fetus may die from unrecognized, often concealed, hypovolaemic shock resulting from haemorrhage.

Placental abruption

The uterine wall near term is relatively thin, elastic and muscular; adhering to the inside surface of the uterine wall is the placenta, which is relatively inelastic. Direct trauma to

---

Box 52.2 Symptoms and signs of placental abruption

- History of trauma
- Tender uterus (may feel "woody")
- Steady (usually lower abdominal) pain
- Shock (maternal)
- Vaginal bleeding (variable)
- Fetal distress
- Premature labour
- Increasing fundal height

---

the abdominal wall transmitted to the uterus, or deceleration forces applied to the body as a whole, may cause the placenta to shear off the uterine wall (Figure 52.4). Haemorrhage occurs between the placenta and the uterine wall and may be concealed or revealed (per vaginam). This haemorrhage will strip further areas of the placenta from the uterine wall, thus increasing the bleeding.

Maternal blood flow to the placenta is approximately 600 ml per minute at term or 10% of the mother's circulating volume. At 10–20% maternal haemorrhage, blood flow to the uterus is shut down and time-critical fetal distress ensues. Beyond 20 minutes few babies will survive. At the site of placental abruption, in addition to the possibility of fetomaternal haemorrhage, substances are released into the maternal circulation which will predispose toward disseminated intravascular coagulation. Amniotic fluid embolism is also a recognized complication of placental abruption. The immediate care of both conditions is early, adequate fluid resuscitation.

Placental abruption occurs in as many as 5% of episodes of minor trauma and 50% of major trauma cases, and can present up to 48 hours after trauma. An adequate history and high index of suspicion are vital. Once again, it must be remembered that maternal hypovolaemic shock may only reveal its presence at a late stage, and that vaginal bleeding may be absent. Premature labour may be precipitated by placental abruption.

In the late presentation of placental abruption the mother may report reduced fetal movements or no movements at all. In the short period of prehospital care, the expanding fundal height, which reflects increased bleeding into the uterus, is unlikely to be recognized; however, as a baseline for other carers it is helpful to mark on the abdomen the fundal height at first assessment.

Uterine rupture

Uterine rupture is much rarer than abruption; it requires considerable direct force and will almost inevitably be associated with other life-threatening injuries.

Signs of uterine rupture include maternal shock, fetal bradycardia (or absence of fetal heart sounds) and obvious palpable fetal parts on abdominal examination. There may or may not be vaginal bleeding or abdominal pain.

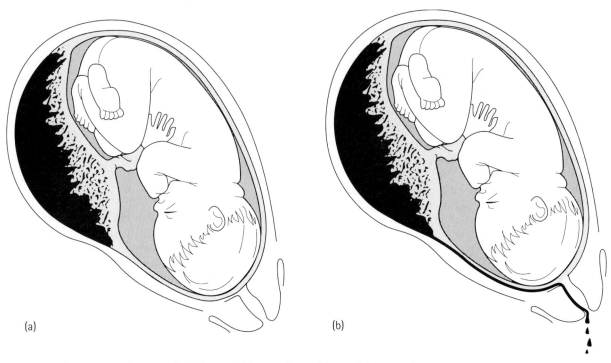

Figure 52.4 Placental abruption (traumatic). (a) Concealed haemorrhage; (b) revealed haemorrhage

---

Box 52.3 Symptoms and signs of uterine rupture

- Maternal shock
- Fetal bradycardia or absence of fetal heart sounds
- Palpable fetal parts
- Vaginal bleeding (variable)
- Abdominal pain (variable)

In the third trimester of pregnancy, stretching of the peritoneum by the enlarging uterus reduces its sensitivity to pain and therefore abdominal pain, particularly in the presence of other painful injuries, may not be apparent.

Pelvic fracture

Even in non-pregnant patients pelvic fractures produce considerable blood loss. In the pregnant state the pelvic venous plexuses are markedly engorged and pelvic trauma may lead to massive bleeding from low-volume capacitance vessels. This type of bleeding is difficult to control. The usual causes of pelvic fractures are falls from a height and road traffic accidents. The signs are those of massive or progressive maternal haemorrhagic shock. This is a desperate situation. Time is of the essence and copious IV fluids will be indicated in order to prevent or reduce maternal hypotension, although transfer to hospital must *never* be delayed while intravenous access is attained. Use of a pelvic splint may also be considered. Definitive surgery is the patient's only hope.

PENETRATING TRAUMA

Penetrating trauma is rarer in Europe than in America. Within the UK penetrating trauma is largely from stab wounds (impalement injuries and road traffic accidents excepted). Gunshot wounds are more common in other parts of the world, and the nature of the injury will depend on the type of missile and its velocity. Nevertheless, the gravid fluid- and fetus-filled uterus protects abdominal viscera and can absorb considerable quantities of kinetic energy. The usual outcome is fetal death with maternal survival.

As far as prehospital care is concerned, the approach is the same as for the non-pregnant woman, with a continuous watch for concealed haemorrhage and the possibility of time-critical but concealed injury to other organs. Attention to ABC and rapid transport are essential.

BURNS

The management of pregnant patients with burns is exactly the same as for non-pregnant patients, except that they must be taken to a facility where caesarean section can be performed. As with all burns, it is vital to check that the environment is safe to approach (remembering the dangers of a noxious atmosphere), ensure that the fire is out, and that any burning or chemically contaminated clothing is removed. Once the patient is removed to a safe environment the use of humidified oxygen and early intubation are essential. It should be remembered that there may have been an explosion during the fire and the patient may also show the effects of blunt trauma. Because of the metabolic and fluid requirements of the pregnant and burnt woman, delivery by caesarean section is often the only option. The mortality rates in pregnant women depend on the body surface area burnt: in those with burns of 33–66% of body surface area, survival will depend crucially on the early management of hypoxia and hypovolaemia.

CONCLUSION

The treatment of the pregnant trauma victim is the same as for the non-pregnant victim, remembering that:

- there are two patients: mother and fetus
- the only way to save both is to save the mother first
- assessment and management of the mother take priority

- haemorrhage is frequently concealed in the pregnant victim and hypovolaemic shock is inevitably severe once the signs manifest
- intravenous fluid therapy should aim to avoid the development of maternal hypotension
- failure to relieve vena caval-compression can kill both mother and fetus
- the pregnant trauma victim should always be considered to have time-critical injuries and be transported to a surgical facility quickly
- obstetric and gynaecological diagnoses need not be made in the field.

FURTHER READING

See Chapter 51

Chapter 53

Neonatal resuscitation and transport

CHAPTER CONTENTS

INTRODUCTION

The paramedic may be faced with illness or cardiac arrest in a neonate (a baby less than 1 month old) in a range of situations: for example, a planned home delivery, an unplanned birth before arrival in hospital or in an infant who has a normal birth and is discharged home (usually after 48 hours in a maternity unit) and thereafter becomes ill. Regardless of the situation, the general principles remain the same: support of airway (A), breathing (B) and circulation (C).

NEONATAL RESUSCITATION

The paramedic faced with a baby born outside hospital has two patients to look after – the mother and the baby. In most instances the baby will not require any advanced interventions. If the baby is active with a normal respiratory rate and heart rate, then the only treatment required will be to dry and warm the baby, and to use suction as required.

However, a small number of babies will require more active resuscitative measures. In practice it is more likely that the paramedic will need to deal with an ill neonate rather than a full cardiorespiratory arrest; this chapter therefore concentrates on the approach to serious illness.

Problems may arise because there has been fetal distress during labour and the amniotic fluid surrounding the baby has become contaminated with meconium from the baby. If this occurs, as soon as the head of the baby is born onto the perineum, suction of the nasal passages and the oral airway should take place in order to remove meconium which could otherwise be inhaled. The baby will require active

and vigorous suction after the body is delivered to ensure that no further meconium is aspirated into the trachea and lower airways, since the morbidity and mortality rates from meconium aspiration syndrome remain high.

In some cases there is no evidence of meconium, but the baby at birth fails to respond properly and has difficulties maintaining respiration and circulation. The Apgar scoring system (Table 53.1) assesses the baby's overall condition at 1 minute and 5 minutes after birth and later if required. Resuscitative measures should be started immediately, however, and not delayed for evaluation of the Apgar score.

If the neonate has obvious cardiorespiratory difficulties or has suffered a full respiratory arrest, then resuscitative measures must begin. If the child has a low respiratory or cardiac rate, the first measure is to stimulate the child. This occurs during drying and warming, and by suctioning of the nasopharyngeal and oropharyngeal passages. This is often enough to increase the child's respiratory rate which,

Table 53.1 Apgar scoring

Sign	0	1	2
Heart rate (beats/min)	Absent	Slow (less than 100)	Greater than 100
Respirations	Absent	Slow, irregular	Good, crying
Muscle tone	Limp	Some flexion	Active motion
Reflex irritability (catheter in nares)	No response	Grimace	Cough or sneeze
Colour	Blue or pale	Pink body with blue extremities	Completely pink

as a result of better oxygenation, increases the cardiac rate. However, if after a short period of stimulation the clinical situation remains grave the next measure is to maintain the airway by placing the baby in a supine position with the neck in a neutral position, thus avoiding hyperextension (a folded towel under the shoulder can facilitate this). At this point supplemental oxygen via a face mask can be applied, with further suction if copious secretions are present (a folded towel under the shoulders confacilitate this). Again, the hoped-for result is improved respiratory effort and consequently increased cardiac output.

If the infant fails to respond to these measures it will be necessary to ventilate the baby using a self-inflating bag and mask. Care needs to be taken not to overinflate the lungs as the infant is at risk of barotrauma, which could lead to a pneumothorax. For the neonate, the smallest self-inflating bag is used, commonly the 240 ml capacity bag. These bags have a pressure-limiting valve and also a special pop-off valve which the operator can override in special circumstances, such as the infant with stiff lungs.

The paramedic should ventilate at a rate of 60 breaths per minute for approximately 15–30 seconds. The pulse is then checked to see if the rate has reached at least 100 per minute. If the neonate again fails to respond (in other words, the brachial or femoral pulse rate remains at less than 60 per minute or ceases), then chest compressions are the next step. These are achieved as described in Chapter **37**, namely two-finger compression using the ring and middle fingers on the sternum of the neonate one-finger breadth below the nipple line. The depth of each compression is one-third of the child's anterior–posterior chest wall distance. An alternative technique for chest compression is to place both thumbs on the middle third of the sternum with the fingers of both hands encircling the chest and supporting the back.

In either event, the sternum should be compressed 100–120 times per minute. The cycle for chest compressions to ventilation is 3 to 1 for a neonate.

> Neonatal CPR: 3 compressions to 1 ventilation

If these measures are unsuccessful and the neonate fails to respond, or indeed goes into full cardiopulmonary arrest, more advanced life support techniques are needed. The paramedic may elect to intubate the child to improve ventilation and to secure the airway against inhalation. The usual size of an ET tube for a term baby is 3–3.5 mm. The next step for advanced life support is to achieve vascular access either through a peripheral vein or by insertion of an intraosseous needle into the tibia of the neonate (Chapter **8**).

> ET tube size for a full-term baby: 3 or 3.5 mm (uncuffed)

Adrenaline is given in asystole or profound bradycardia at a dose of 0.01 mg/kg (0.1 ml/kg) of adrenaline 1 in 10 000 solution intravenously or by the intraosseous route. If the child is intubated then 1 in 1 000 solution at 0.1 mg/kg can be given via the ET tube. This quantity of adrenaline is very small and so to aid its dispersal and uptake within the lung, it is given in 2 ml normal saline solution via a suction catheter placed at the distal end of the endotracheal tube. This helps to produce an aerosol and causes the adrenaline to be widely dispersed throughout both lungs. This dose may be repeated every 3 minutes if required.

> Adrenaline dose in neonates is 0.1 ml/kg of 1 in 10 000 solution IV

Neonates born after showing signs of fetal distress during labour are usually acidotic and may require sodium bicarbonate at 2 ml/kg sodium bicarbonate 4.2% solution. In addition to drugs, it is sometimes necessary to give the neonate a fluid challenge of 10–20 ml/kg of normal saline. This treatment is usually carried out during urgent evacuation to hospital.

It is essential to remember that the neonate has poor mechanisms for maintaining its temperature and will quickly become cold during a resuscitation attempt. This does not aid the chances of successful resuscitation and therefore care should be taken to maintain the child's temperature, for example by using warm blankets. Always remember to cover the head as well as the body.

NEONATAL TRANSPORT

The paramedic team may become involved in the transfer of a neonate from one hospital to another. This commonly occurs where babies born in peripheral units, such as district

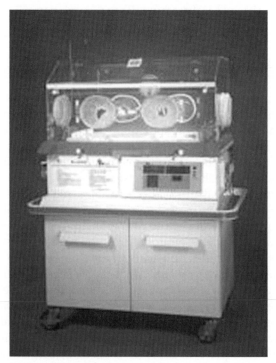

Figure 53.1 A neonatal transport incubator

general hospitals, have to be transferred to specialized neonatal or paediatric units because of the need for intensive care, treatment of congenital heart disease or neonatal surgery, facilities for which are usually sited at larger units in teaching hospitals. In these instances the paramedical team will work in close association with nursing staff and doctors from the peripheral hospital who will usually also travel with the neonate. The most important point is that the neonate should be stable prior to transfer, and the paramedics should work with the medical team to ensure that this is the case. It is also important that the whole transfer should be well planned by the sending and the receiving hospitals, so that it is known in advance to which part of the receiving hospital the child is to be taken. Ideally, these patients should be taken direct to their intended destination, and not to the accident and emergency department.

In most neonatal transfers an incubator rather than an open stretcher is used, chiefly to maintain the child's temperature during the transfer (Figure 53.1). Most modern incubators also allow for ventilation of the neonate. The incubator operates on a battery supply and requires the use of cylinders of oxygen and air for ventilation. When preparing for such a transfer, it is mandatory to check that sufficient oxygen and battery life are available for the intended journey, allowing some leeway for unforeseen delays or detours. Most modern incubators can be plugged into the ambulance electrical system although it is necessary to check that this is the case.

In addition, the transport team must have the necessary equipment and drugs available in case the child deteriorates en route. Mishaps can happen, such as the endotracheal tube being dislodged, so it is necessary for the child to be monitored during the journey, and facilities for procedures such as reintubation and any other resuscitation techniques such as the reinsertion of intravenous access must be available.

The accompanying professionals must be satisfied that there is at least one person who can carry out cardiopulmonary resuscitation of the neonate before embarking on the journey.

FURTHER READING

www.resus.org.uk/pages/nls.htm
www.resus.org.uk/pages/nlsalgo.pdf
Richmond S 2001 Resuscitation at birth: newborn life support provider manual. Resuscitation Council (UK), London

Section 10

PSYCHIATRY

Chapter 54

Substance abuse

CHAPTER CONTENTS

INTRODUCTION

Problems related to the use of alcohol, drugs and solvents are increasingly common in the UK. This reflects both an increase in incidence and greater awareness of such behaviour by medical and paramedical workers and the public. Amongst teenagers the rising incidence of substance misuse is particularly worrying. The problem is exacerbated by the availability of new "designer" drugs, and an increase in the misuse of volatile substances.

DEFINITIONS

Drug dependence is a socio-psychobiological syndrome, the key feature being the priority given to drug-seeking behaviour over other behaviours. Drug or alcohol use does not always lead to dependence and a problem substance taker is someone who experiences social, physical or legal sequelae related to intoxication, excessive consumption or dependence resulting from use of drugs, alcohol or other substances.

ALCOHOL

EPIDEMIOLOGY

Twenty-five percent of men are said to be problem drinkers at some point in their lives and approximately 25% of general medical admissions involve alcohol-related problems. Two percent of the UK population suffer from alcohol dependence syndrome at any time.

Dependence is most common in those aged 40–54 years. There is a sharp drop in heavy drinking in men over 70 years old and in women aged 50–60 years. The male-to-female ratio is 4:1, but the female rate is increasing. Factors increasing risk of dependence include cheap or easily available alcohol, unsupervised work routine, unsociable working hours and work involving separation from family or other stabilizing social constraints. Publicans, doctors, journalists and senior businessmen are most vulnerable. Alcoholism is more likely amongst the divorced and separated as well as amongst those who have never been married.

ALCOHOL DEPENDENCE SYNDROME

There are a number of behaviour patterns which are strongly suggestive of alcohol dependence syndrome.

- Narrowing of drinking repertoire (drinking from a smaller range of alcoholic drinks)
- Salience of drink-seeking behaviour (drinking supersedes other activities)
- Increased tolerance to alcohol (more alcohol is required to produce intoxication or stave off withdrawals)
- Repeated attempts at withdrawal from alcohol that end in failure even with professional help
- Relief or avoidance of withdrawal symptoms by further drinking (responsible for morning drinking)

- Subjective awareness of compulsion to drink (may continue long after cessation of drinking)
- Reinstatement of dependent drinking after a period of abstinence ("perhaps just one drink since we are celebrating").

PHYSICAL EFFECTS OF ALCOHOL

Physically, alcohol dependence causes problems in a number of body systems. These are listed in Boxes 54.1–54.4.

Wernicke–Korsakoff syndrome is caused by deficiency of thiamine (vitamin B$_1$). In acute Wernicke's encephalopathy, symptoms include alteration in level of consciousness, nystagmus, external ophthalmoplegia, ataxia and peripheral neuropathy. The risk of this occurring increases following IV glucose administration to patients with chronic alcoholism or malnourishment Consequently IM thiamine should be given immediately after IV dextrose for this patient group.

PSYCHOLOGICAL EFFECTS OF ALCOHOL

Hallucinations of voices (alcoholic hallucinosis), which are usually derogatory in content, may occur in clear consciousness. Affective symptoms occur in 90% of people with alcoholism and there is a 10–15% risk of completed suicide associated with alcoholism. Pathological jealousy manifests as a morbid delusional belief that a partner is being unfaithful. It is twice as common in men and may put the partner at risk of serious violence.

MEDICAL EMERGENCIES SPECIFICALLY RELATED TO ALCOHOL

Acute intoxication

Acute intoxication may lead to physical injury from trauma or head injury. It is essential always to look for evidence of injury or illness in intoxicated patients before putting their clinical state down to alcohol intoxication. The intoxicated fall and get beaten up. Intoxication may cause hypoglycaemia or metabolic acidosis. Severe intoxication with alcohol can cause death, often from vomiting leading to asphyxiation, but also directly related to alcohol poisoning.

> **Alcohol alone should never be accepted as a cause of reduced or lost consciousness**

Acute alcohol withdrawal

Acute alcohol withdrawal occurs in the dependent state and is characterized by:

- nausea
- vomiting
- tremors
- excessive sweating
- tachycardia.

It may begin within 6 hours of cessation or reduction of alcohol and peaks by 48 hours, subsiding over the next 7 days. It can be associated with withdrawal grand mal epileptic seizures 12–24 hours after drinking.

Box 54.1 Effects of alcohol on the gastrointestinal tract

- Liver damage
- Alcoholic hepatitis
- Fatty liver
- Cirrhosis
- Liver failure and hepatic encephalopathy
- Oesophagitis and gastritis causing vomiting and retching
- Mallory–Weiss tear in lower oesophagus causing haematemesis
- Portal hypertension causing oesophageal varices and possible massive haematemesis
- Peptic ulceration
- Acute and chronic pancreatitis (acute has a mortality of 10–40%)
- Carcinoma of upper gastrointestinal tract

Box 54.2 Effects of alcohol on the cardiovascular system

- Cardiac arrhythmias
- Cardiomyopathy
- Coronary artery disease
- Hypertension
- Cerebrovascular accident

Box 54.3 Metabolic and haematological effects of alcohol

Metabolic
Hypoglycaemia
Ketoacidosis
Haematological
Anaemia
Thrombocytopenia

Box 54.4 The effects of alcohol on the nervous system

- Diffuse brain damage from cortical shrinkage and ventricular dilation
- Alcoholic dementia
- Wernicke–Korsakoff syndrome
- Epilepsy from withdrawal fits

Box 54.5 Psychological effects of alcohol

- Alcoholic hallucinosis
- Affective symptoms
- Suicide
- Pathological jealousy

Delirium tremens

Delirium tremens ("the DTs") occurs on days 3–5 following cessation or significant reduction of drinking in an alcohol-dependent person. It is characterized by:

- confusion
- disorientation
- delusions
- hallucinations
- vivid imagery (often insects but not the pink elephants of popular belief)
- intense tremulousness.

There is often a marked lability of emotions and autonomic dysfunction. There is no craving for alcohol. Admission to a medical ward for rehydration, sedation and nutrition is essential. In 50% of cases DTs are precipitated by an intercurrent infection. The mortality rate is up to 10%.

ABUSE OF OTHER SUBSTANCES

Although the stereotypical image of a drug addict is a dishevelled, unwashed young man with staring eyes and an aggressive manner, people who misuse drugs or other substances come from all walks of life and there is no particular personality profile, ethnic group, class or profession that identifies characteristic substance misusers. Official figures of substance misusers in the UK relate to those seeking treatment or those notified to the Home Office and do not reflect the true extent of use.

Unusual behaviour of any sort could be due to substance misuse and it is important to note that substance misusers will often use more than one substance at a time, causing a mixture of symptoms and signs. When assessing patients whose behaviour is suggestive of substance misuse, it is essential to check their arms and legs for evidence of injection sites. Misusers of volatile solvents often smell of glue or aerosol propellant and may have a rash around their mouth and nose where there has been contact with an inhalation bag. Appropriate precautions against contact with bodily fluids should be taken, as the incidence of human immunodeficiency virus (HIV) and hepatitis B infection is increased in injecting drug abusers.

There are few specific antidotes for most substances of abuse and the basic ABC approach is essential. Specific details of treatment are not given in this chapter unless they can be started during prehospital care.

In the following list of substances, street names of drugs are given, but the names vary in different geographical areas and also change over time, some names becoming more popular than others. If in doubt, it is best to ask for, or suggest, the generic name of the substance and seek confirmation from the patient. It is merely embarrassing to attempt to match the patient in "street cred".

OPIATES

The opiates are a large group of drugs ranging from the natural substance opium to the synthetic substance fentanyl. The duration of action and toxic levels vary from drug to drug. Fatal doses (below) are given for adults: in general the fatal dose for children is unknown but it will usually be less than the mg/kg conversion from the adult dose, since children are more sensitive to opiates. In general, addicts can tolerate higher doses than non-addicts before manifesting the effects of toxicity, but it is important to beware of addicts who have had a period of abstinence (e.g. in prison) and whose tolerance therefore is markedly reduced. In addition, the purity of commercial heroin is variable and deaths have resulted from sudden exposure to much purer heroin than normally abused.

Overdosage or ingestion of opiates is characterized by altered level of consciousness, respiratory depression and pinpoint pupils. Fits occur less commonly. Other signs include a euphoric or stuporous mental state, convulsions, hypotension and hypothermia.

The initial management of an opiate overdose or respiratory depression due to opiate ingestion is maintenance of the airway and oxygenation followed by the administration of naloxone. However, as long as the patient is breathing adequately and can be closely observed, naloxone is probably best left until after arrival in hospital. Unfortunately, all too often, if naloxone is given prehospital, the patient simply absconds on regaining consciousness or becomes aggressive or uncooperative and much more difficult to manage safely and effectively. In addition, in some cases, having left the scene, the patient will collapse again as the naloxone wears off. Simultaneous administration of an intramuscular dose when intravenous naloxone is given may go some way to preventing this. Even in patients with depressed respiration, maintenance of adequate artificial ventilation alone often offers an effective means of managing a potentially volatile situation.

Opium

The fatal dose of opium depends on the preparation and the clinical situation. The amount taken is not usually known.

Box 54.6 Features of opiate poisoning

Common
Altered level of consciousness
Respiratory depression
Pinpoint pupils

Less common
Fits
Euphoric or stuporous mental state
Convulsions
Hypotension
Hypothermia

Street names include: big O, brown stuff, China white and dust.

Heroin

Heroin is produced from morphine which in turn is contained in opium, the dried sap of the opium poppy. Much street heroin is only 10% pure. Daily consumption is commonly in the region of 0.25–0.75 g, although the fatal dose can be as little as 0.2 g. Severe reactions, sometimes fatal, are seen when an unusually "pure" batch of heroin becomes available for sale.

Clinical features and recognition of use

Heroin acts on opiate receptors to produce analgesia, miosis, euphoria, hypotension, bradycardia and respiratory depression. Tolerance to the euphoriant action appears rapidly and dependence may occur in weeks or months.

The withdrawal syndrome appears within 4–12 hours, peaks at 48 hours and is alleviated after 1 week. Symptoms include dysphoria, aching limbs, increased perspiration with "gooseflesh" of the skin (hence "cold turkey"), diarrhoea, dilated pupils, shivering, yawning and fatigue. Insomnia and craving for the drug may persist for weeks.

Street names include black tar, Persian boy, rock, Chinese (rock), smack, dana, stuff, H, TNT, Harry, white elephant, horse, white stuff and noise.

Morphine

The fatal dose of morphine is as little as 100 mg. Street names for morphine include cube juice, dreamer, hard stuff, hocus-morf and morpho.

Methadone

Methadone is a synthetic opiate that can be taken orally or intravenously and has a half-life of 15 hours. This longer half-life increases the time of onset of withdrawal symptoms and when used therapeutically to wean addicts off heroin, methadone is administered as a once-daily dose. Methadone is usually bright green in colour and as a result there have been a significant number of serious and fatal poisonings in children who have gained access to methadone prescribed for a parent or other addict. There is a significant black market for legitimately prescribed methadone.

Street names for methadone include doll, dollies and dolophine.

Dipipanone (Diconal)

The fatal dose of dipipanone is unknown. Diconal is a combination of dipipanone and cyclizine. It produces intense euphoria when used intravenously but presents a danger of arterial closure and gangrene. The commonest street name is dike.

Pethidine

The fatal dose of pethidine is about 1 g.

Fentanyl

The fatal dose of fentanyl is unknown. It is a potent drug with a short half-life and therefore doses near the therapeutic range may be fatal. A common street name is China white.

Dextromoramide (Palfium)

The fatal dose of dextromoramide, which is usually called peach palf, is about 500 mg.

Codeine

The fatal dose of codeine ("schoolboy") is more than 1 g.

Dextro-opoxyphene napsylate (co-proxamol)

The fatal dose is 1–1.5 g.

HALLUCINOGENS

Lysergic acid diethylamide (LSD)

Lysergic acid diethylamide is a synthetic psychedelic drug of low toxicity. Symptoms include confusion, agitation, hallucinations, dilated pupils, and (rarely) coma and respiratory arrest. Supportive measures only are required.

There are many street names for LSD, including acid, beast, blotter acid, blue caps, blue drops, boy, dome (dots), ghost, green caps, paper acid, pink drops, purple haze, sunshine, white lightning, yellow caps and yellow drops.

Psilocybin (magic mushrooms)

Ingestion of magic mushrooms ("Shrooms") is a seasonal problem, usually well known in particular localities where the mushrooms can be picked. Cases may occur in small epidemics. The fatal dose is unknown.

Euphoria, anxiety, depression, illusions and psychosis are all common manifestations. Hyperthermia, tachycardia, tremors and dilated pupils are characteristic. There is no specific treatment in the prehospital setting but efforts should be made to calm the victim by giving reassurance that the effects are self-limiting.

Box 54.7 Effects of LSD

- Confusion
- Agitation
- Hallucinations
- Dilated pupils
- Coma
- Respiratory arrest

Phencyclidine

Phencyclidine is a psychedelic drug, fatal dose unknown. Symptoms include anxiety and psychosis, ataxia, paraesthesia, catatonic movements, fits, coma, hypotension, respiratory impairment, Cheyne–Stokes breathing and respiratory arrest. Treatment is supportive.

Street names for phencyclidine include angel dust, aurora borealis, busy bee, CJs, cycline, dust, embalming fluid, fuel, happy sticks, hog, horse tracks, joy sticks, killer weed, KJ, LBJ, mist, MCP, peace weed, seccies, Sherman snorts, superkool, supergrass, superjoint, superweed, surfer, TAC, TIC, white powder and zoom.

Cannabis

Cannabis is a common drug of abuse considered by many to be a "recreational" drug (without serious consequences from its use). There is, however, good evidence to support an association between the use of cannabis and the development of mental problems, including psychosis. It has also been suggested that many users subsequently "graduate" to "hard" drugs such as heroin. Of relatively low toxicity (unless ingested by children when coma may ensue), it may be smoked or eaten. The symptoms of toxicity include excitement, euphoria, drowsiness, panic attacks, toxic psychosis and, rarely, coma and dilated pupils. No specific treatment is required in the prehospital setting apart from supportive measures.

Street names for cannabis include bhang, dope, ganja, grass, happy sticks, hash (oil), homegrown, joint, joy sticks, Mary Jane (MJ), paki, pot, reefers, resin, roaches, shit, smoke and tea.

Amyl nitrate

Amyl nitrate is toxic by ingestion and inhalation. Its principal mode of toxicity is by the formation of methaemoglobin. The fatal dose is unknown, but even small amounts can cause symptoms. Symptoms occur within a few seconds of inhalation, but may be delayed by ingestion. Headache, nausea and vomiting occur along with sweating and flushing. Tightness of the chest is common as is confusion and occasionally fits. Cyanosis due to methaemoglobinaemia may be found. There is no specific prehospital treatment apart from maintenance of the airway and administration of oxygen to treat cyanosis.

Amyl nitrate is also referred to as poppers, snappers or sweat.

Remember that the presence of methaemoglobinaemia will make pulse oximetry unreliable.

STIMULANTS

Amphetamines

Illicit amphetamine sulphate may only be 20–30% pure. A heavy user may use several grams a day. Dexamphetamine (Dexedrine, "dexies") and amphetamine-like drugs such as methylphenidate (Ritalin) and diethylpropion (Tenuate) are also abused.

The acute effects of amphetamines include euphoria, anxiety, increased energy, miosis and tachycardia. Amphetamine psychosis mimics acute symptoms of schizophrenia and manifests with paranoid delusions, auditory, visual and tactile hallucinations and increased arousal and irritability. Consciousness is impaired. Withdrawal effects include dysphoria, fatigue, lassitude and depression.

There are a number of common street names for amphetamines including A, amphet, speed, STP, sulp, sulphate, uppers, ups, wake-ups and whizz.

Cocaine

Cocaine is a local anaesthetic agent, which is still used in some clinical areas (such as ear, nose and throat surgery). The fatal dose is approximately 1 g when taken orally and 10 mg when injected. Symptoms include tachycardia, sweating, hallucinations, increased respiratory rate, increased temperature, fits, arrhythmias and rarely cardiac arrest. There is no specific treatment; fits should be controlled with diazepam and general supportive measures instituted.

Street names for cocaine include base, bazooka, big C, blow, C, candy, cake, Charlie, coke, crack, dose, dust, dynamite, flake, freebase, gold dust, happy dust, heaven dust, hit, ice, paradise, smack and snort.

Crack is a processed form of cocaine which produces a much quicker "high" which is of short duration. It is much more addictive than cocaine.

Box 54.8 Effects of cannabis

- Excitement
- Euphoria
- Drowsiness
- Panic attacks
- Toxic psychosis
- Coma (rare)
- Dilated pupils (rare)

Box 54.9 Effects of amphetamine

- Euphoria
- Anxiety
- Increased energy
- Miosis
- Tachycardia
- Amphetamine psychosis (paranoid delusions, auditory, visual and tactile hallucinations and increased arousal)

Ecstasy (MDMA)

A semisynthetic amphetamine (3,4-methylenedioxymethamphetamine), Ecstasy has become notorious in recent years as the cause of deaths in otherwise healthy teenagers. Two causes of death are commonly recognized: early deaths are due to arrhythmias and late deaths are due to an effect on muscles associated with a fatal rise in body temperature (a similar condition, neuroleptic malignant syndrome, occurs rarely as a side-effect of antipsychotic drugs). Deaths can occur after exposure to doses previously tolerated and are thought to be due to an idiosyncratic reaction. Symptoms range from mild to life threatening and include muscle spasms, dilated pupils, anxiety, tachycardia, increased temperature, abdominal pain, hypotension, fits, coma and stroke. The fatal dose is unknown, but is near to the "therapeutic" dose. There are no specific treatments other than supportive measures in the prehospital setting.

Street names for ecstasy include acid, Adam, AKA, Bart Simpson, Dennis the Menace, disco biscuits, E, ecsta, red and black, white burger, white dove, XTC and yellow burger.

Ephedrine

Ephedrine (ups or uppers) is a sympathomimetic drug with a fatal dose of 200 mg in children and over 2 g in adults. It causes restlessness, tachycardia, dilated pupils, arrhythmias and hallucinations. Apart from treating fits with diazepam, there is no specific prehospital treatment but supportive measures should be instituted.

Caffeine

Caffeine (also referred to as ups or uppers) has similar side-effects to ephedrine; the fatal dose is 10 g. Treatment is as for ephedrine.

SEDATIVES

Barbiturates

The barbiturates are a group of drugs that include amylobarbitone (Amytal), barbitone, pentobarbitone (Nembutal), phenobarbitone and sodium amylobarbitone (sodium amytal). Overdose of barbiturates is relatively uncommon nowadays, but still occurs occasionally. Symptoms of overdose include ataxia, dysarthria, decreased conscious level, coma, respiratory depression, hypothermia and hypotension.

There are no specific treatments apart from general supportive measures. Withdrawal seizures may occur and should be controlled with diazepam.

VOLATILE SOLVENTS

Glue

Toluene is the most common solvent in glues available over the counter. Effects include excitement, chest tightness, fits, coma, arrhythmias and death. Supportive measures should be instituted with particular emphasis on oxygenation to reduce the likelihood of arrhythmias.

Butane

Butane is a colourless, odourless gas, commonly used as the propellant in "ozone-friendly" sprays but also available in cigarette lighters. It is generally inhaled from a bag. Symptoms include respiratory depression, coma, hypotension and arrhythmias. Treatment is supportive only.

Butyl nitrate

An industrial solvent, butyl nitrate is also used as a room deodorizer. It can be fatal when ingested in even small quantities, but the fatal dose is unknown. Symptoms include flushing, tachycardia, hypotension, confusion, shortness of breath and cyanosis (from the formation of methaemoglobin), coma and fits. Treatment is supportive. Remember that pulse oximetry readings are likely to be inaccurate.

CONCLUSION

Drug abuse is an increasingly common problem for prehospital carers and an aspect of practice which is often frustrating and unrewarding in terms of long-term prognosis and relationships with the patient. It is even more important, therefore, that paramedics follow the most appropriate clinical guidelines scrupulously in order to achieve the best result possible under the circumstances. At the same time, unnecessary risks to the rescuer (the drug culture is becoming increasingly violent, not to mention the risks of transmission of infectious diseases) must be avoided at all costs. However hard it may be, the drug user must be treated the same as any other patient, with the single proviso of the clinician's own safety.

Chapter 55

The uncooperative or violent patient

INTRODUCTION

It is unfortunately the case that ambulance crews are increasingly having to deal with violent or potentially violent patients and members of the public. Not surprisingly, this can be extremely stressful and frightening. Effective education and training in how to deal with these incidents is essential. This chapter focuses on risk assessment at the scene, de-escalation techniques and the legal rights of the patient and ambulance personnel.

Each individual will have his own background, culture, standards and beliefs. These characteristics will affect the manner in which he deals with a situation. It is important to understand what anger, aggression and violence are. Once these are defined, it is possible to look at risk assessment in the field.

WHAT IS ANGER?

Anger is a *"violent passion, excited by real or supposed injury"* (the definitions in this chapter are taken from Collins Dictionary).

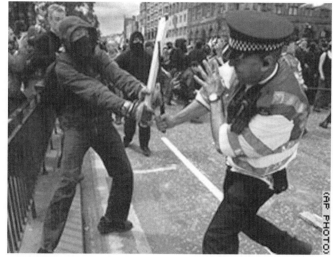

Figure 55.1 A riot

- It is a feeling or emotion.
- It is often a response to something that has happened.
- It is often triggered by frustration of some sort.
- It may lead to aggression, but doesn't always.

Box 55.1 Early warning signs of anger

General agitation (e.g. pacing)	Racist, sexist, defamatory comments
Tone of voice	Invasion of personal space
Volume of speech	Clenching of hands
Verbal threats	Threatening gestures
Use of expletives	

Box 55.2 Levels of intervention in risk management

Primary – is proactive and aims to prevent harm occurring.
Secondary – occurs during and immediately after an adverse incident.
Tertiary – aims to reduce the risks which arise as a consequence of any adverse incident.
Externally imposed – legislation and guidelines may be imposed.

- It may be helpful, in a controlled situation.
- It is often visible: an angry person may look angry.

The early warning signs of anger are listed in Box 55.1.

WHAT IS AGGRESSION?

Aggression may be defined as an *"unprovoked attack"* or *"hostile behaviour"*.

- Aggression is action or behaviour, although it is often associated with an emotion such as anger or frustration.
- It is usually intended to hurt someone in some way.
- It takes many different forms: verbal or physical, including insults, gestures, slapping, kicking and using weapons.

Box 55.3 Factors suggesting the possibility of risk

Geographical location – night club, party, rave, etc.
Historical – is the location known to the crew? Have there been previous problems? Have other crews talked of problems at this location?
Type of call – fighting, stabbing, domestic violence, substance misuse (alcohol and drugs).
Illness related – symptoms such as head injury, pain, abnormal mood, hallucinations, delusions, confusion.

WHAT IS VIOLENCE?

Violence is *"using or marked by physical strength, that is harmful or destructive; aggressive in intent; using excessive force"*.

- The term "violence" is often used when speaking about serious physical attacks.
- Like aggression, it may be directed at objects as well as people.

RISK MANAGEMENT

This should be carried out at every level – management, ambulance control and at the scene. Risk management is everyone's business and should not be seen as an academic exercise. Risk management is the introduction of measures which have a reasonable likelihood of minimizing the risks to personnel and others.

There are four levels of intervention when managing risk, explained in Box 55.2.

Managers and officers in the ambulance service should provide an appropriate level of training for staff in violence management. This should be done in conjunction with trade unions to ensure a minimally acceptable level of training is provided for all staff. This should not be seen as a "one-off" or rare event and it must be reviewed regularly. This can be done by audit or by monitoring incident forms. Trends should be noted; for example, a particular area of operations which is associated with an above average number of incidents or individual staff members who appear to have been involved on several occasions. Evident training deficiencies should also be identified. Regular meetings with staff may help facilitate discussion on violence, whether potential or actual. Support services should be in place (e.g. occupational health) to help staff affected by violence.

Ambulance control should collate as much information as possible about any call they receive. Where is the call to? Who is calling? Are there any risk factors? Guidelines and procedures must be in place which can be activated if there is any suspicion that a crew is being despatched to a potential or actual violent incident. These procedures must be widely distributed and highlighted to all staff. If there is doubt, an ambulance officer should be involved in the case. A safe balance must be achieved between providing emergency care and the safety of the ambulance crew.

Ambulance crews should assess risk en route to the emergency. Close liaison with ambulance control is essential. The factors in Box 55.3 should be taken into consideration in this risk assessment.

There are also a number of factors which increase the actual or potential risk to ambulance service personnel.

- High levels of anger or hostility.
- History of violent behaviour.
- Homelessness.
- Non-compliance with medication.

PRIOR TO ARRIVAL

Information available before arrival at the scene may suggest the nature of the environment which is to be encountered. It is essential that ambulance service personnel take care of themselves in the first instance in order to prevent injury to themselves, colleagues or the patient. It is important to think about equipment that may be used against personnel, for example:

- hand-held radio sets or pagers
- mobile phones
- torches
- equipment bags
- scissors, pens, pencils
- stethoscopes.

All communication equipment, including hand-held devices, must be checked. The last thing one needs is a communications breakdown when help is needed in a violent or potentially violent situation.

ON ARRIVAL

On arrival the initial considerations must include:

- protective clothing – is there a need for a helmet and eye protection? Should high-visibility clothing be worn?
- vehicle positioning – safely with an easily accessible exit
- surveying the scene
- establishing if there are other services present. Who is in charge?
- determining whether support (ambulance officer, police, fire brigade) will be needed
- clearing bystanders.

The patient (or their relatives or friends) may feel that it has taken a long time for help to arrive. As a consequence, feelings which may be encountered will include:

- anger
- fear
- frustration
- joy
- relief.

To deal with these feelings in the best way possible, it is important to remain alert and flexible in one's approach to care.

PRINCIPLES OF ASSESSMENT

As mentioned above, it is essential to complete a brief survey of the scene.

- Is it safe to enter?
- Where is the person? Is he standing, sitting or lying?
- Is the person calm, upset or angry?
- Are there objects nearby he could use to inflict harm? (If there are, they should be discreetly removed to a safe distance.)

> **Box 55.4 Appropriate and inappropriate use of non-verbal communication**
>
> *Appropriate behaviour*
> Expression showing acknowledgement of crisis
> Appearing relaxed, arms by the side
> Standing side-on to the person and at arm's length
>
> *Inappropriate behaviour*
> Laughing inappropriately
> Crossing the arms and legs
> Standing with the front of the body exposed
> Standing within arm's length

It is vital not to rush in and try to "make everything all right". It is more useful to be prepared to spend time with the person whilst ensuring that there is an easily accessible exit in case the situation deteriorates. However difficult the situation, it is important to attempt to treat the person in the same manner in which one would like to be treated oneself, with respect and maintenance of dignity. The person should be addressed as "Sir" or "Madam" until permission is given to do otherwise.

VERBAL AND NON-VERBAL COMMUNICATION

Verbal

When speaking to an aggressive (or potentially aggressive) or uncooperative patient, one should ideally speak more slowly than normal but at a normal volume – *not shouting*. Ideally the pitch of the voice should be slightly higher than normal to increase clarity.

Non-verbal

Non-verbal communication is often referred to as "body language". It is the physical signs and signals that are given out to others. Sometimes it does not matter if people are aware of what we are communicating non-verbally, but at other times it is important to take care. This is especially important when dealing with people in personal crisis. Some of the forms of non-verbal communication are:

- facial expressions
- movement of arms, hands, legs
- body stance
- distance from the other person
- touch.

Appropriate and inappropriate use of non-verbal behaviour is given in Box 55.4.

ESTABLISHING A RAPPORT

Basic skills of communication are vital in establishing a rapport with the person. It is important to encourage reality and orientation; for example, awareness of place, date and time. The first step is to gain eye contact but to avoid staring.

Eye contact should be broken regularly but always keeping the person in sight. An introduction should be offered.

> "Hello sir, I'm a paramedic with the ambulance service."

If necessary, the introduction should be repeated as it may not have been heard the first time. The person should be asked if it is all right to approach. If the answer is yes, the approach should be made slowly, stopping at arm's length. Any closer to the person would be encroaching on his "personal space" and might provoke an aggressive verbal or physical response. If the answer is no, then no approach should be made whilst a discussion of the person's fears or worries is attempted from a distance. It is useful to try to get the person to sit down.

> "Would you like to sit?"

It is important to offer the person choices rather than to give orders. If the person chooses to sit then one should sit as well, positioning one's chair at an angle of 45°, allowing enough room for everybody to stretch their legs.

The next step is to establish ground rules.

> "I am here to help, not to hurt you."

It may be helpful to explain to the person that it is all right to show emotion, for example to cry or scream, but that it is not all right to harm himself or others. It should be clearly stated that one will be honest with him. It is important not to lie! Trust can be lost easily. Confirmation should be sought that the person has heard and understood what has been said.

> "Do you understand what I have said?"

Once again, it may be necessary to reiterate what has been said.

IDENTIFYING THE PROBLEM

Open questions should be used to allow the person to give as much information as possible; for example: "*What has happened to you*"?. Once he has told "his story", more specific questions can be used to extract further information. For example: "*You said you hit your head yesterday. Tell me more about what happened*".

Closed questions (those requiring a response of only "yes", "no" or "I don't know") should be avoided. Firstly, they provide little information and secondly, they cause frustration for the person being interviewed, as well as for the interviewer. It is important not to ask leading questions, as these can give a false reflection of what is happening. An example of a leading question is: "*Is it your neighbour who is causing the problem?*".

It is important not to interrupt but if there are silences, to appear supportive by remaining alert and attentive verbally – "*…and then what happened?*" – and non-verbally – maintaining eye contact, nodding the head. If the person shows emotion, he can be told that it is all right to do so.

> "It is all right to cry."

If necessary, support should be offered, for example tissues or a drink of water. Enough time should be allowed for the person to regain control and composure.

"Telling the story" may be traumatic. It is important to clarify the "story" by repeating key phrases (paraphrasing) and ensuring that it has been properly understood. This demonstrates that one values the person, firstly by spending time with him and secondly by listening to what he has said.

The following steps summarize the systematic approach to the uncooperative or violent patient.

- Maintain safety.
- Introduce yourself.
- Establish a rapport.
- Set the ground rules.
- Seek a history.
- Seek clarification.

Assessment and identification of the problem are vital to:
- provide a clear history
- prevent frustration
- prevent violence and non-cooperation with ambulance personnel and others

---

RIGHTS OF THE PATIENT

Unless the call is to a person placed under the care of the Mental Health Act, all patients must be treated as voluntary patients.

VOLUNTARY PATIENTS

Voluntary patients have the choice of receiving or not receiving care. They should always be given the choice. If the person declines, actions should include:

- giving the person all reasonable help and advice
- informing ambulance control that the person has refused treatment
- asking the person to sign the casualty report form next to the appropriate entry, stating that he is refusing treatment.

It is important to ensure that the patient understands, what clinical harm may come to them as a result of their refusal of care. The information provided should be documented in the patient's clinical record. If the patient's refusal of care appears to leave him at risk, the police should be requested to attend. They have powers to place the person on Section 136 of the Mental Health Act 1983 which allows them to take a person to a place of safety (such as a hospital or a police station) to enable him to be examined by a doctor and interviewed by an approved social worker (ASW).

COMPULSORY ADMISSION

The majority of admissions to psychiatric hospitals are voluntary. Approximately 10% are by formal admission, under the Mental Health Act 1983 (see Chapter 56). This Act sets out first to provide appropriate care for the mentally disordered and second, to provide a safeguard against wrongful detention for those people who are not mentally disordered.

As discussed earlier, the first step (assuming the scene is safe) is to find out who is in charge. This may be an ASW or the responsible medical officer. Talking with the person in charge will help in assessing the situation. It is vital to see all the relevant documentation for the appropriate section. All parts of the forms must be completed satisfactorily. If there is any doubt, advice should be sought from the person in charge or from ambulance control.

The person's rights according to the section that he has been placed under should have been explained to him by the ASW. It must be remembered that during this time the individual is in personal crisis. There may be family or friends involved, who will also be distressed at the situation. Time, patience and diplomacy are vital in caring for these people. In the case of a female patient, a woman ambulance crew member, ASW, doctor or police constable must be in attendance at all times. This also means during transport to the hospital.

If the person wishes to speak then the guidelines for assessment should be followed. It is important not to enter into the person's delusions or hallucinations but to try to maintain reality. If the person rejects reality, then this has to be accepted. If the person chooses not to speak then this should be respected. Conversation should not be forced.

Persons expressing suicidal thoughts should be treated with care. Prehospital assessment is not the time to decide whether or not they are serious. It is important to be aware that they may try to deceive in order to carry out their intentions. These persons should not be left alone but supervised at all times.

If patients refuse to go to hospital, then a minimal amount of force may be used under the Mental Health Act 1983, to transport them safely. If, after assessing the situation, it is felt that the support of the police is required, then an explanation should be given to the family or friends regarding the reasons for this decision.

RIGHTS OF AMBULANCE PERSONNEL

Ambulance service personnel are responsible for their own actions at all times. If an incident takes place, an officer should be informed immediately. The event should be fully documented. If the incident is reported to the police by the patient or a member of the public, a criminal investigation may take place to see if there is sufficient evidence to prosecute.

Prosecution could result in a fine or imprisonment. This in turn may lead to dismissal. In a civil proceeding, action would be undertaken by the person or his relatives. Prosecution could result in payment of damages to the person or the person's family.

If one is the victim of an attack, legal advice should be sought. It may be possible to claim compensation for injuries from the Criminal Injuries Board (Criminal Justice Act 1988).

Dealing with mentally ill persons is part of the job. It is only reasonable, therefore, to expect to be given appropriate training in this area. When dealing with persons placed under Sections 2, 3 or 4 of the Mental Health Act 1983, Section 139 protects ambulance personnel from criminal or civil proceedings, unless it is done without reasonable care.

THE ROLE OF THE POLICE

In all situations, personal safety and that of professional colleagues must come first. There is no point in becoming a further casualty. If the situation appears to be threatening and the police have not been contacted, then a decision must be taken as to whether their assistance is required. The role of the police is to uphold and enforce the law. Good communication skills are vital. Cooperation and respect for each other's role must be maintained. The police may request the transfer of a person from the police station to the local accident and emergency department for treatment. All such persons must be escorted by a police officer.

MANAGEMENT OF VIOLENCE

There are five phases when dealing with violence.

- Trigger phase
- Escalation phase
- Crisis phase
- Recovery phase
- Post-crisis depression phase.

TRIGGER PHASE

This is where the person's behaviour moves away from his normal or baseline behaviour. This may be due to a change of environment, in the way in which he perceives people or in the way he thinks he is perceived. Changes may be demonstrated verbally or non-verbally (or both). Personal safety is paramount. De-escalation techniques should be attempted: it is useful to reinforce the nature of one's role, that one is only there to help. Protective clothing or equipment may be a trigger. It is helpful to decide what is essential and to leave the rest in the vehicle.

ESCALATION PHASE

By this stage, the person's behaviour has moved from the baseline. De-escalation techniques can be effective and prevent violence from being expressed. It is essential to remember to speak slowly, maintaining eye contact and being aware of body posture. If the person is standing aggressively, it is advisable to stand off centre from him, keeping one's hands in front of the body but not crossing the arms. Instructions should be consistent and the patient should not be, or feel, boxed in. The person should feel involved in the decision making and his opinion should be sought regarding potential courses of action. Safety remains paramount at all times. An escape route must be available, as must a contingency plan if the person's behaviour escalates and reaches crisis phase.

People may become violent for a number of reasons.

- Crowd behaviour (e.g. incitement in football gangs)
- Perceived threats (e.g. shooting, stabbing)
- Drug and alcohol abuse (use of or withdrawal from)
- Physical illness (e.g. hypoglycaemia, sepsis, electrolyte imbalance, head injury)
- Mental illness (delusions, hallucinations).

It is essential to be continuously alert for any sign that the situation is deteriorating. Verbal signs of a deteriorating situation include:

- the person's attitude towards other people changes
- the person becomes more demanding
- the volume of their voice rises
- sarcasm features strongly in their conversation
- the person demands help from others.

Non-verbal signs include:

- the person becomes restless, for example pacing the floor, tapping feet, wringing hands
- the person has difficulty in concentration.

CRISIS PHASE

The person is becoming increasingly physically and emotionally aroused. Their control mechanisms over violent impulses decrease and violence is very likely. Interventions (de-escalation) aimed at returning the person to his baseline behaviour are of little value. The safety of anyone under threat is the main priority. Now is the time to escape or implement the contingency plan.

RECOVERY PHASE

The person starts to regain control over his behaviour. The severity of what has happened now surfaces. The person shows signs of remorse and apology. His emotions are extremely labile and may be varied, for example crying. The person is now starting to show signs of being receptive to interactions. This is the time to reinforce one's identity and role. Simple language should be used, avoiding jargon or abbreviations. It is important to be assertive and to give direction. The person will need support and may not be able to function fully. It may be important to act as his advocate with other agencies.

POST-CRISIS DEPRESSION PHASE

The full impact of what has happened now sets in. The person regresses below baseline behaviour. Attention should be paid to his basic needs. Is he warm enough? Has he sustained any injuries? He should be reassured that the incident is over. False promises must not be made as this may led to a further crisis in the future. It is important to be honest. He may ask you "What will happen to me?" and inappropriate reassurance, however attractive it may seem, must be avoided. The information offered should be restricted to areas of ambulance service responsibility. Liaison with other agencies such as the police will be vital. Opinions regarding injuries should be avoided; this is best left to medical staff.

The approach shown in Box 55.5 will help when dealing with a potentially violent patient.

Once a situation has deteriorated into violence, the first priority must be one's own safety and it is essential to call for assistance. Personal heroics are not appropriate. The approach detailed in Box 55.6 should ensure an optimal safe outcome.

Box 55.5 Dealing with a potentially violent patient (summary)

- Remain calm
- Ensure that there is an exit
- Maintain a 2-metre distance from the person and stand side-on
- Maintain non-threatening eye contact
- Seek extra help (in the background, for example in another room)
- Be careful what one says
- Try to negotiate and so defuse the situation
- Not lying, or promising outcomes one cannot keep
- Recognize the need for rapid intervention if the situation deteriorates further

---

Box 55.6 Dealing with a violent patient (summary)

- Immediately call for police assistance
- Use only the minimum of physical restraint to control the situation
- Never restrain a person in a way that could impair breathing, for example pushing the person's face down or sitting on his chest
- Never restrain the person around the neck
- When restraining, use only the legs and arms
- Check pulses in these limbs to ensure circulation
- Reassure the person at all times
- Keeps calm and avoid threats
- Negotiate with the person
- When the person is calm, slowly release the physical restraint
- Liaise with the police to decide appropriate management – hospital care or police custody

TRANSPORTATION OF THE UNCOOPERATIVE OR VIOLENT PERSON

When arranging transport, it is important to consider whether it will be necessary for a police officer to accompany the patient to hospital and to ensure that ambulance control is fully aware of the situation. Before entering the ambulance with the patient, any potentially dangerous objects should be stowed securely away. Once such patients are in the ambulance, if carried on a stretcher, the adjustable straps should be used to ensure that they do not harm themselves during transit. If the patient is sitting, attention should be paid to the seating arrangements, bearing in mind the patient's potential for violence or escape and crew safety. Is an ambulance the safest mode of transport? Is there another type of vehicle that may be more appropriate? It may be helpful to speak to an ambulance officer before transporting the patient. If a patient suffering from a mental illness has been assessed by a doctor as in need of hospital admission and is accepting of admission (a voluntary admission), the questions in Box 55.7 should be asked.

Only when it is clear that one has enough information should a decision be made to transport the patient. It is important not to be rushed into a decision or to presume that things will be all right. People's mental state or symptoms can change very quickly. As a consequence it is vital to have a plan before moving off. Reference should be made to service guidelines and policies on transporting violent or uncooperative patients.

If the person is to be admitted under the Mental Health Act 1983 then all the necessary documents must have been completed. An Application for Admission, including the appropriate medical recommendations, is required for the person to be transported to hospital. The applicant is normally the ASW. Usually the ASW follows in his own transport to the hospital; however, one can insist that the ASW or other approved person travels in the ambulance. If male ambulance personnel are transporting a disturbed woman, then a female chaperone is essential to protect the crew from allegations of misconduct.

WHAT TO DO AFTER AN INCIDENT

After an incident involving violence has occurred, ambulance control must be informed. An officer should attend to give support and guidance regarding any action which might be required. Medical attention should be sought for any injuries and the police will need to be informed.

An incident form should be completed. This is essential; it should not be left to the following day or avoided because "nothing gets done anyway". Without incident forms it is very difficult to take matters any further. Completing the incident form is the responsibility of the staff member involved in the incident.

The facts of what happened at the incident should be documented. This will include the predisposing factors and the action taken then and afterwards (good record keeping helps with debriefing and identifying training needs). Violent incidents can leave people feeling angry, guilty, tired or upset; the policies relating to violent incidents (verbal and/or physical) should be adhered to. Included in such a policy should be a provision for debriefing staff following an incident.

It may be helpful to speak to other professionals involved. Sharing thoughts and feelings can reduce stress (see Chapter 59). Nobody in the caring profession enjoys being involved in violence so it is vital to help and support each other.

CONCLUSION

Dealing with the violent or potentially violent patient or member of the public can be extremely challenging. Risk management is essential, at every level from management to operational staff. A plan of how to approach the scene and an idea of the resources which may be required are essential. If the situation is hostile, deescalation techniques may be of value. It is important to be aware of the rights of the patient and of ambulance service personnel. Consideration should be given to how the patient is to be transported, remembering risk management at all times. Is it safe, is the patient safe?

If one is involved in a violent or potentially violent situation, the line manager must be informed. An incident form must be completed, recording as much information as possible since details fade with time. Reporting of incidents is vital as this will help with strategic planning of the ambulance service and will affect such issues as education and training, guidelines and policies, protective clothing, vehicle design and methods of service delivery.

Box 55.7 Voluntary admission for mental illness: questions to ask

- When did the assessment take place?
- What were the circumstances?
- Is the doctor still present to give you a history?
- Is there a letter?
- Is the patient still happy to be transported to hospital?
- How is the patient now?
- Is there any history of violent behaviour?

FURTHER READING

Wright R 1993 *Caring in crises – a handbook of intervention skills*, 2nd edn. Churchill Livingstone, Edinburgh

Dernocoeur KB 1996 Streetsense: Communication, Safety and Control, 3rd edn. Laing Research Services, Redmond.

National Institute for Clinical Excellence 2005 Clinical Guideline 25. Violence. NICE, London. (Available at www.nice.org.uk/CG025NICEguideline)

Chapter 56

Psychiatric emergencies

INTRODUCTION

Psychiatric emergencies differ from medical emergencies in that admission to hospital is not always indicated. Most psychiatric emergencies are not immediately life threatening and there is usually time in which to plan a coordinated and careful response. Unfortunately, perhaps owing to ignorance, there is a tendency to overreact and to look on hospital admission as the only option; this may result in the unnecessary use of expensive resources but, more importantly, may have a profound and long-lasting detrimental effect on the patient. Prejudice against mental illness remains rife, as does stigma associated with psychiatric hospitals.

Immense efforts are being made in many areas to promote the use of alternative, community facilities for the management of people with mental disorders and it is likely that many people who in the past would otherwise have been admitted to hospital can now be managed at home or in an alternative community facility. Unfortunately community facilities may carry with them the same prejudice that is linked to more traditional psychiatric settings. This applies equally to patients presenting as an apparent emergency, who are often subject to the fear and apparent helplessness of carers or authorities, who in turn may have become blinded by their desire to react quickly and remove the person from the crisis situation without first considering the other options that may be available. On the other hand, severe mental illness must be taken seriously and hospitals are the first choice for those patients who require intensive support, treatment and supervision. Admission to hospital should never be avoided because of ideological considerations.

Most psychiatric emergencies involve patients who are distressed and helpless and who may also appear dangerous or at risk of harm. Most psychiatric patients are not dangerous and it is important to bury the myth that they are.

It is particularly important to be aware that as a result of their behaviour (if they are deemed to be a risk to themselves or others) mentally ill patients may be admitted to hospital involuntarily under the Mental Health Act. This results in loss of liberty and may have a profound effect on how they are treated both immediately and in the long term.

Dealing with psychiatric patients requires important skills of counselling, empathy, negotiation and the ability to liaise with different professional groups (the police, social workers, nurses and doctors). The general public too have a role, as their concerns may have precipitated the response from health or social services and it is especially important to support and inform relatives who are often bemused and upset at the situation. They may harbour strong feelings of anger, guilt and sadness and require reassurance and understanding.

WHAT IS A PSYCHIATRIC EMERGENCY?

A psychiatric emergency can be defined as a situation involving someone exhibiting psychological distress that exceeds the coping strategies of that individual, the carers or society, and that may involve a possible risk to themselves or others.

The causes of psychiatric emergencies are manifold. Some are described below. However, it is important to note that many apparent emergencies can be resolved without resorting to the powers of the Mental Health Act or the facilities of the local hospital. Problems often arise out of particular social difficulties (e.g. financial problems, lack of electricity, homelessness, lack of food), breakdown in relationships or altercations with the police. Some may occur as a result of a physical disorder or be related to medication or the use of illicit drugs. All require an assessment that may be prolonged and may involve psychiatrists, social workers and relatives; at the end of this assessment the result may be the loss of liberty of a person who is admitted to hospital against his will.

ESSENTIALS OF ASSESSMENT

The essentials of assessment of a psychiatric emergency are to engage the patient and to gather detailed information in a sensitive manner; to undertake mental state and physical examinations; to support any relatives or carers; and above all to remain patient and unflustered. Ensuring the safety of everyone involved is paramount and if there is any doubt as to the level of risk towards those undertaking the assessment, no attempt should be made to continue without further assistance.

GATHERING INFORMATION FROM PATIENTS AND INFORMANTS

All psychiatric assessments should begin by gathering as much information as possible about the patient. The nature of presenting symptoms (whether gradual or sudden onset), past medical and psychiatric history, including substance misuse, present medication (both prescribed and non-prescribed) and level of support at home are essential elements of an accurate assessment and should be obtained both from the patient and from an informant.

This initial assessment may not be straightforward. For example, a patient may not allow access to the house. In this

Box 56.1 Important components of the history

- Nature and onset of presenting symptoms
- Past psychiatric history
- Past medical history
- Current medication
- History of substance misuse
- Social support

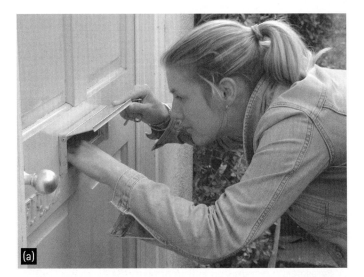

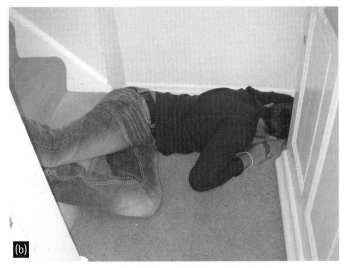

Figure 56.1 Assessment through the letter box!

case it may be possible to conduct a reasonable appraisal of the situation through the letterbox, thereby persuading the patient to open the door or allowing enough information to be gathered to make a decision that there are likely to be grounds for admission under the Mental Health Act. Neighbours can be extremely useful informants who, as well as providing background information about the patient, will often have noticed recent changes in behaviour. Close relatives are often available to give detailed information.

MENTAL STATE EXAMINATION

Mental state examination is the term given to observation of the patient's behaviour, mood and speech in order to gather evidence of mental disorder. It is important that a mental state examination is objective and not subjective or based on supposition. A comprehensive mental state examination should be carried out in all cases. The usual procedure is to subdivide the examination into the following categories.

- Appearance and behaviour
- Speech form (i.e. coherence) and content
- Beliefs and thoughts
- Overall mood state and whether it is congruent with the thought content
- Observable abnormal perceptions or experiences (e.g. hallucinations)
- Assessment of level of consciousness, orientation to time, place and person, concentration and short-term memory
- Presence of insight (the acknowledgement by the patient that there are psychological problems that need to be resolved)
- Suicidal ideation.

PHYSICAL EXAMINATION

A brief physical examination should be carried out in every case, as far as possible, even if there appears to be no apparent physical disorder. Common organic causes of psychiatric emergencies (such as hypoglycaemia, infection, cardiac failure, delirium tremens and subdural haematoma) should be rigorously and systematically sought. Breath odour may reveal solvent or alcohol misuse, ketones or uraemia and recent skin puncture marks suggests drug misuse (Fig 56.2).

PSYCHOSIS: RECOGNITION AND TREATMENT

Psychosis refers to disturbances in thinking and behaviour, usually involving delusions, hallucinations and thought disorder. Where these symptoms are sufficiently recognizable and characteristic, they may be attributable to a diagnosis such as schizophrenia, mania or psychotic depression. However, psychiatric diagnosis is complicated and bedevilled by problems of definition and applicability and it is usually simpler just to describe the symptoms which are expressed and the signs which are observed.

ASSESSMENT OF PSYCHOSIS

Delusions

A delusion is a firmly held but false belief that is out of context with the person's social and cultural background, unamenable to any logical argument that is presented to refute it, and based on spurious and inappropriate evidence. There is often an element of persecution that accompanies the belief, but patients may express delusions that

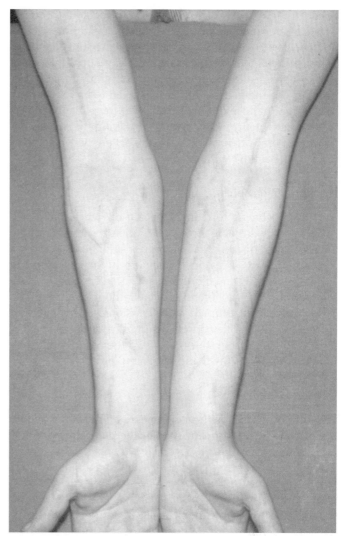

Figure 56.2 Multiple puncture marks due to intravenous injection in a heroin abuser

they have special powers or are invested with great authority or fame. Examples include delusions that they are being persecuted or hounded by others (often the police or other authority figures); that others are watching or listening to them through bugging devices; that presenters on the television are referring directly to them or items in newspapers or the media have special significance to them; beliefs about bodily malfunctions (e.g. bowels seizing up or interference with particular organs); or excessive guilt or self-blame for particular life circumstances. Often it is impossible even to attempt to confront the reality of the belief, and there is a danger of losing rapport with the patient, resulting in argument.

Hallucinations

Hallucinations refer to the experience of perceptions (e.g. hearing voices or noises, seeing vivid images or tasting particular flavours) in the absence of a stimulus causing the perception. They can occur in any sensory modality. They are not imagined experiences and appear real to the patient. Often a delusional explanation of the hallucination may be put forward. For example, voices may be explained in terms of transmitters through the electric cable or bugging devices in the pipes. Hallucinations are often frightening and distressing and the patient may be observed to be responding to apparent hallucinations, especially if the patient appears to be distracted, preoccupied or talking or muttering inappropriately. Rarely, patients may act on their hallucinations in an impulsive manner.

Psychotic behaviour

Psychotic behaviour is often the reason why emergency services have become involved. Patients suffering acute psychological distress may act in unusual, bizarre or even frightening ways. They may shout and swear, gesticulate in a threatening way and indulge in antisocial behaviour. Their speech may be incoherent and their thoughts disjointed. They may be preoccupied with delusions and responding to hallucinations. They may attempt to harm themselves or appear to be endangering others. On the other hand, they may become withdrawn and uncommunicative.

Dangerous behaviour

It is important early in the assessment of a psychotic patient to be aware of any propensity to dangerous behaviour. It is a common fallacy that all psychotic patients are dangerous. While this is not true for the overwhelming majority, a few have a tendency to be violent, usually as a direct consequence of their illness. Part of the initial assessment should include an appraisal of the presence of any such aggressive or violent behaviour. Pointers towards whether a patient is likely to be violent are a past history of violence, whether violence has already occurred, the patient's appearance and behaviour, whether the patient is intoxicated by alcohol or drugs and the content of any delusions. Clearly it is inadvisable to enter a situation that puts the paramedic in physical danger and if there is a likelihood that this will occur, the police should be involved.

As a general rule it is inadvisable to assess an acutely psychotic patient alone because of the risk of unpredictable behaviour that may lead to injury. The assessment should be carried out in an area that is easy to escape from and the paramedic should remain between the patient and the exit (see Chapter 55). Although it is sufficient in many cases to defuse the situation by sitting down, if necessary the interview should be conducted standing up. It should be noted that much aggression in these situations is born out of fear and it is helpful to be as reassuring, empathetic and non-confrontational as possible to try to establish a rapport.

MANAGEMENT OF PSYCHOSIS

The key to managing an acutely psychotic patient is to be able to control behaviour. This can often be achieved by use of good interpersonal skills of empathy, reassurance, a non-threatening posture, an air of calmness and confidence. For any patient – and particularly for patients who are paranoid (believing fervently that individuals or groups are against them), distressed and reacting to threatening hallucinations – the use of inappropriate force, verbal aggression and impatience is distressing and may be seen as confrontational. This may invite retaliation, further compromising any established therapeutic relationship and resulting in a greater use of force. Worse still, the display of aggression by the patient is very likely to be attributable to "illness" and this will colour others' assessment and will label the patient as aggressive and perhaps a troublemaker.

If sedative medication is required this will usually take the form of antipsychotic drugs (also called neuroleptics or major tranquillizers), of which there are several different groups.

Antipsychotic drugs

Antipsychotic drugs have an initial sedative action that precedes any antipsychotic effect. They are not available for use by paramedics and are included here for information. The safest group to inject are the butyrophenones (haloperidol 2–10 mg). It may be necessary to repeat the dose if the initial dose has been ineffective. Haloperidol can be given in doses up to 30 mg for emergency control. Chlorpromazine has been associated with fatal cardiovascular collapse when given by intramuscular injection and should not be given by this route. However, it is the most sedative neuroleptic and effective when given orally in doses of 25–100 mg.

It is important to be aware that neuroleptics can precipitate severe extrapyramidal side-effects in the form of acute dystonia (a bizarre and painful combination of abnormal rigid posturing, eye rolling and pelvic thrusting), tremor, muscular rigidity or motor restlessness. This can be treated symptomatically or prophylactically with procyclidine 5–10 mg intramuscularly.

One rare but potentially fatal consequence of using antipsychotic medication is *neuroleptic malignant syndrome*. This is characterized by a rapid onset over 1–3 days of acute autonomic instability (with marked swings in blood pressure, tachycardia, excessive sweating, salivation and urinary incontinence), hyperpyrexia and muscular rigidity. The mortality rate is 1–15%. Treatment is symptomatic. The patient should be cooled and fluid balance maintained. Often there is an intercurrent infection that should be treated.

PARASUICIDE: RECOGNITION AND TREATMENT

Evaluating suicide risk is one of the hardest yet most pertinent parts of any psychiatric assessment. In an emergency (for example, following a suicide attempt), the first consideration must be safeguarding the physical welfare of the patient and this will usually entail transportation to the nearest accident and emergency department. It is important to be alert to the suspicion of a suicide attempt, especially if the patient has a past history of psychiatric contact, is drowsy or unconscious or is drunk. One should not be deceived by any apparent evidence that only a small quantity of tablets have been ingested or the patient's protestations that the overdose was not life threatening. A significant proportion of those who attempt suicide will make a further fatal attempt and often patients are unaware of the lack of toxicity of the medication that they have taken and believe that the quantity ingested was sufficient to cause death. It is necessary not to be side-tracked by the responses of others who may minimize the importance of a person's actual or threatened attempt at self-harm and give explanations or interpretations of behaviour (most commonly in terms of manipulativeness, acting out or attention seeking). More violent methods of attempted self-harm (e.g. hanging, shooting or deep lacerations) should always be assessed by a psychiatrist. Attempted suicide should be considered as a possibility at any single-occupant road traffic accident where the conditions of the accident are unclear.

It is important to be aware that self-harm is not in itself a mental illness and the majority of people who harm themselves have no psychiatric illness. Moreover, there is no good evidence that psychiatric treatment will prevent the repetition of self-harm behaviour in the absence of psychiatric illness. Nevertheless, the most important intervention in the management of the suicidal patient is the treatment of any psychiatric illness that is present.

If a person has not made an attempt at self-harm but is expressing suicidal ideation then a thorough assessment should be made as outlined above. Risk factors of eventual suicide such as present or past psychiatric illness (especially depression, schizophrenia and eating disorders), personality disorder, family history of suicide, single status, unemployment, social isolation, problem drinking, previous attempts at self-harm, recent "loss" events and older age should be noted. If the person agrees to admission to hospital and this is appropriate then it should be expedited. If the person does not agree, but is detainable under the Mental Health Act, then the appropriate procedures should be followed with the patient being closely supervised until admission takes place. The paramedic has no powers under the Mental Health Act but the police may take an individual to a place of safety (for example, psychiatric unit or police station) under Section 136. Alternatively, the patient's general practitioner can arrange an emergency admission for assessment and treatment under this Act. Before leaving, the paramedic should supervise the patient until an appropriate professional can take over.

If the person is deemed not to be detainable under the Mental Health Act but still expresses suicidal ideation, then there is an ethical dilemma. Strictly speaking, the patient cannot be prevented from leaving. However, persons who appear to be actively attempting to end their own life,

Box 56.2 Risk factors in suicide

- Past or present psychiatric history of depression, schizophrenia or eating disorder
- Personality disorder
- Family history of suicide
- Single status
- Unemployment
- Social isolation
- Problem drinking
- Previous attempts at self-harm
- Recent "loss event"
- Older age

or seem to be about to do so, can be restrained from doing so (under common law), pending a further psychiatric assessment.

DEPRESSION AND MANIA

Suicide is most commonly associated with depression, although people with serious and long-standing mental disorders such as schizophrenia, manic depression, alcohol dependence and chronic anxiety are also at risk. Clinical depression refers to a persistent and debilitating disorder of mood characterized by sadness, an inability to derive pleasure from any activity, low self-worth, lethargy and lack of motivation. Other common symptoms include disturbed sleep and appetite, lack of libido, anxiety symptoms and thoughts of guilt and self-blame. Patients may neglect themselves and become physically at risk through not eating or drinking. Often depressed mood is associated with poor social circumstances and deprivation.

Occasionally patients with a history of depression may become elated and overactive with increased speed of thought and excessive, expansive speech. They may appear to be excessively cheerful or irritable or their mood may swing between the two emotional states. They may express grandiose delusions of excessive self-importance or unwarranted ability, and there is often a history of increased spending (sometimes extravagantly) and sexual excesses or disinhibition. They may see themselves as being famous or having particular powers, and may experience hallucinations which reinforce their behaviour. This is a presentation of mania and is often difficult to manage outside hospital. Such individuals may become so preoccupied with their beliefs and behaviour that they neglect their appearance or dress in florid but totally unsuitable clothing, stop eating and drinking and pay little attention to their living conditions. If their mood state progresses unchecked, they may develop a manic stupor in which they appear mute and motionless, although fully conscious. Stuporous states can also occur in depression.

ANXIETY DISORDERS

Anxiety disorders include anxiety states, phobias and obsessive compulsive disorder. These disorders rarely present as a psychiatric emergency, but anxiety commonly accompanies other psychiatric disorders and may exacerbate a patient's distress. Anxiety can be defined as the combination of psychological symptoms of fearfulness, irritability, difficulty in concentration, sensitivity to noise and feelings of restlessness, with physical symptoms of sympathetic nervous system overactivity such as sweating, increased heart rate, churning stomach and dry mouth.

Acute anxiety is extremely distressing and may occur in normal people, especially victims of (or witnesses to) traumatic events. It is manifested in a psychological and physiological response of which the most important feature is hyperventilation. Hyperventilation is the result of excessive breathing from the upper chest (ribcage) and results in hypocapnia, which causes tinnitus, tetany, tingling, weakness and chest pains. The experience of these physical symptoms may exacerbate the feeling of anxiety, causing more hyperventilation. An explanation of the symptoms and reassurance that the patient will not come to any harm as a result of them is the first step, and may need frequent and authoritative repetition.

Hyperventilation is effectively managed by getting the person to breathe into a large paper bag for several minutes or until the breathing begins to regulate. The patient must be sitting or lying in a supported posture and the need to regulate the breathing by breathing more slowly and taking shallower breaths (not deeper ones), ideally until the patient can breathe through the nose, must be stressed. It may be useful to demonstrate how the patient can breathe using the diaphragm by placing one hand on the chest and one on the abdomen. The hand on the abdomen should move more than the one on the chest. Ongoing explanation for the symptoms should be offered and reassurance given. Always rule out other possible causes of the symptoms (such as an acute coronary syndrome) before treating any patient for hyperventilation.

These measures may obviate the need for pharmacological treatment. If treatment is required, benzodiazepines are the drugs of choice for acute short-term anxiety. The intravenous or rectal route is the most effective for administration. Diazepam should not be given by intramuscular injection because of its variable absorption rate, but can be given intravenously in the form of diazepam emulsion (Diazemuls). Doses vary considerably between patients, with a range of 2–20 mg. Lorazepam (25–30 mg/kg) is a short-acting benzodiazepine and is effective for panic attacks (episodes of acute anxiety associated with overpowering thoughts of dying or imminent physical ill health and desire to escape). Only in the rarest circumstances should anxiety disorders be treated with benzodiazepines out of hospital and only then by a medical practitioner.

PHYSICAL CAUSES OF PSYCHIATRIC EMERGENCIES

There are numerous physical causes of psychiatric emergencies which manifest as an acute toxic confusional state. The cardinal features of this state, also called delirium, are clouding and fluctuation of consciousness (patients have periods of drowsiness, poor concentration and lack of lucidity), increased arousal (often manifested in acute anxiety and fearfulness), disturbances in perception (in the form of illusions or hallucinations) and disorientation to time, place and person. As a result of these experiences a person may become extremely distressed and be liable to misinterpret the actions of others. Often elderly people present as an emergency in this way and it is important to be aware that many drugs to which the elderly are sensitive can precipitate delirium. An elderly person suffering from dementia may develop a toxic confusional state as a complication. Differentiation of dementia and delirium is not difficult – the latter has an acute onset with an abrupt change in behaviour, whereas dementia is altogether a more gradual deterioration in functioning and behaviour and does not fulfil the criteria for delirium.

ALCOHOL AND ILLICIT DRUGS

The assessment and appropriate management of intoxicated individuals pose particular problems for all health service staff. It may not be easy to decide whether an intoxicated individual requires hospital assessment or (if causing a disturbance) whether police custody is more appropriate.

Box 56.3 Symptoms of anxiety states

- Fearfulness
- Irritability
- Difficulty in concentration
- Sensitivity to noise
- Feelings of restlessness
- Hyperventilation
- Sweating
- Increased heart rate
- Churning stomach
- Dry mouth

Box 56.4 Features of acute toxic confusional state (delirium)

- Clouding and fluctuation of consciousness – drowsiness, poor concentration and lack of lucidity
- Acute anxiety and fearfulness
- Illusions or hallucinations
- Disorientation to time, place and person

On the one hand, intoxication is not uncommon, is sanctioned by society and in most cases leads to no harm; on the other, intoxicated individuals may be a considerable risk to themselves, especially if they have a history of alcohol dependence, and may therefore require assessment in a hospital setting. If it is felt that intoxicated patients are likely to suffer from physical effects of the intoxicating substance (e.g. delirium tremens, withdrawal fits or septicaemia) to the extent that they need to be monitored in hospital, then they should be taken to an emergency department. However, as soon as they are no longer at physical risk, they must be allowed to leave unless they are liable for detention under the Mental Health Act.

Admission to a psychiatric hospital may be indicated for assessment of a suspected underlying mental disorder. In this case it may be possible to detain the patient under the Mental Health Act. Certain hallucinogens (such as LSD or magic mushrooms) can trigger off a psychotic reaction in a previously undiagnosed or vulnerable person or may worsen preexisting states of psychosis.

Delirium tremens, which occurs hours or days after the cessation or reduction of drinking, is characterized by tremulousness, disorientation, vivid hallucinations or illusions and autonomic overactivity, is associated with a mortality of 10% and should always be managed in a general hospital. Acute withdrawal can be managed with long-acting benzodiazepines such as chlordiazepoxide. However, it should be noted that many problem drinkers will supplement benzodiazepines with alcohol and only a small quantity should be prescribed at any one time. Chlormethiazole (Heminevrin) should not be used for outpatient detoxification or treatment of withdrawal.

PERSONALITY DISORDER

One of the most difficult categories of patient to assess is those with a diagnosis of personality disorder. The validity and meaning of this term are a matter of some debate and it is often used as a pejorative and demeaning label (along with other discredited terms such as "manipulative", "hysterical", "attention seeking" and "inadequate"). These patients often harm themselves or express suicidal ideation and have often been frequently admitted to hospital. They may be hostile and impatient and lack the ability to form a rapport. They appear to induce feelings of irritability and antagonism in staff and it is easy to lose an objective approach to their problems. This may result in an inadequate assessment and a failure to recognize serious psychiatric illness.

There may be a tendency to minimize these patients' risk of eventually committing suicide because of the number of previous attempts which are often not life threatening. However, a proportion of these patients do succeed in ending their lives and it is important therefore to be aware that personality-disordered patients do develop other psychiatric disorders (e.g. depression) which may predispose them to making a more serious attempt to end their life. Thus it is vital that patients with personality disorders are assessed thoroughly if they are expressing suicidal ideation. Other professionals who may be involved include social workers, community psychiatric nurses and the patient's general practitioner, as well as family and friends or voluntary agencies. It often benefits the patient if these other professionals are involved sooner rather than later, as they are likely to be extremely familiar with the patient's history and may obviate the need for hospital assessment.

THE MENTAL HEALTH ACT 1983

If, after assessment, it is felt that a patient needs to be in a psychiatric hospital, a patient who refuses admission can be admitted compulsorily under the provisions of the Mental Health Act 1983. The sections that are most likely to be used in an emergency are Sections 2, 3, 4, 135 and 136. The section papers must be filled in before the patient is taken to hospital but it should be noted that the section only comes into force when all the forms have been accepted by or on behalf of the hospital managers after the patient arrives in hospital.

It is important to note that the Mental Health Act does not apply to persons who are intoxicated by alcohol or drugs. However, if it is felt that there is an actual or possible underlying mental disorder in someone who is intoxicated, and that person is a risk to self or others, then admission under the Act may be appropriate.

SECTION 2: ADMISSION FOR ASSESSMENT

Section 2 is for assessment in hospital, or for assessment followed by treatment, and it is usually applied when a patient has no past history of mental disorder or is not known to the local psychiatric service. The grounds for detention are that the patient must suffer from a mental disorder that warrants the patient's detention in hospital and that admission is necessary in the interests of the patient's own health or safety or for the protection of others. A specific diagnosis is not a prerequisite for detention – indeed, the reason for detention is to make a diagnosis. The section is valid for 28 days. The procedure requires an application by an approved social worker or nearest relative and medical recommendations by two doctors, one of whom must be approved under the Act (usually a consultant psychiatrist). The approved social worker must have seen the patient within the last 14 days and should, so far as is practicable, consult the nearest relative. The approved social worker can be contacted at the local social services department.

SECTION 3: ADMISSION FOR TREATMENT

Section 3 allows the compulsory admission of a patient and treatment for up to 6 months. It is usually applied when there is a known diagnosis. In order for this longer term order to apply, the patient must suffer from a mental disorder – specified as mental illness, severe mental impairment, psychopathic disorder or mental impairment – that is of a nature or degree which makes it appropriate for the patient to receive medical treatment in a hospital. In the case of psychopathic disorder or mental impairment, treatment should alleviate or prevent a deterioration of the patient's condition. In addition, in all cases, it must be necessary for the health or safety of the patient or for the protection of others that such treatment should be given and that it cannot be provided unless the patient is detained under this section. The application is made by the patient's nearest relative or an approved social worker. The latter must, if practicable, consult the nearest relative before making an application and cannot proceed if the nearest relative objects. The medical recommendations are as for Section 2. In addition, the recommendations must state the particular grounds for the doctor's opinion, specifying whether any other methods of dealing with the patient are available and, if so, why they are not appropriate. The doctor must specify one of the four types of mental disorder (see above).

SECTION 4: ADMISSION IN AN EMERGENCY

If there is difficulty in obtaining a second medical application from an approved doctor to detain the patient under Section 2 and the situation is an emergency, then an emergency order for assessment (Section 4) can be completed by the approved social worker and a doctor who need not be approved under the Act. Application is made by the approved social worker, who must have seen the patient within the previous 24 hours, or the nearest relative. The patient must be admitted within 24 hours of the medical examination or application. The duration of the order is 72 hours and it is expected that it will be converted to a Section 2 order as soon as possible after the patient has arrived in hospital.

SECTION 135

A social worker who believes that someone is suffering from a mental disorder and is unable to care for himself, or is being ill treated or neglected, may apply to a magistrate for a warrant for that person's removal to a place of safety.

SECTION 136

It is possible that some emergency situations (such as road traffic accidents) will necessitate the removal of apparently mentally ill people to a place of safety without the possibility of obtaining applications from social workers or psychiatrists. With Section 136, police constables have the power to remove to a place of safety a person whom they find in a public place who appears to be suffering from a mental disorder and to be in need of care and control for his own interests or for the protection of others. The person should be taken to the nearest convenient place of safety (usually a hospital or police station) to be detained for a period not exceeding 72 hours for the purpose of examination by a doctor and interview by an approved social worker.

COMMON LAW AND INFORMED CONSENT

Any interaction between a health service worker and a patient is assumed to occur with the patient's informed consent. If a patient does not give consent for a particular examination or intervention, however minor, and is capable of consent, then the worker can be charged with assault. If a patient is unable to give consent because of mental illness then a health worker can act against the patient's wishes, but only in certain circumstances: the treatment or investigation must be seen to be life saving or necessary to prevent immediate serious harm to the patient or others, and should be given in good faith ("the doctrine of necessity"). If at all possible, treatment should be given under the provisions of the Mental Health Act 1983. However, in certain circumstances this will not be possible and emergency treatment (usually an injection) can be administered against the patient's will. It is good practice always to make a note at the time as to the reasons for any treatment given without the patient's consent, as well as recording the names of witnesses.

CONCLUSION

Assessment and appropriate management of a psychiatric emergency requires time, patience and common sense. It is a dynamic process in which negotiation and arbitration may have to take place not only between the patient, relative or carer and professionals, but also between the professionals involved. Time should be taken to gather information and decisions should be reached as a result of objective appraisal of that information, as opposed to arbitrary, hasty and ill-informed opinion. A knowledge of psychiatric disorders and the psychopathology that accompanies them, and an understanding of the risk of psychiatric patients losing their right of autonomy and advocacy as a result of misplaced stigma and prejudice, will increase the likelihood of a thorough assessment.

At the end of the assessment, it should be possible to decide whether the patient has an organic, functional or predominantly social problem. The decision then needs to be made as to whether the patient requires further assessment in hospital or a local community facility or whether it would be more appropriate for other agencies (e.g. social services) to review the situation. It may be more appropriate for the patient to make contact with voluntary agencies or self-help groups. These have been established for many of the problems that can present as psychiatric emergencies and include substance misuse groups such as Alcoholics or Narcotics Anonymous and Aquarius; helplines for drug addicts, rape victims or battered wives; church organizations; and marriage guidance (Relate).

Patients who appear to require further assessment and agree to go to hospital should be taken there. Patients who refuse, and appear to be a risk to themselves or others, either can be taken by the police to a place of safety (if they are in a public place) or a Mental Health Act assessment can be arranged by the local social services team. Where patients do not appear to be at immediate risk but remain distressed, it would be appropriate to contact their general practitioner.

FURTHER READING

National Institute for Clinical Excellence 2004 Guideline 16. Self-harm: the short term physical and psychological management and secondary prevention of self-harm is primary and secondary care. NICE, London. (Available at: www.nice.org.uk/(G016NICEguideline)

Chapter **57**

Coping with stress

CHAPTER CONTENTS

Men are not disquieted by things themselves but by their idea of things. Epictetus

INTRODUCTION

This chapter offers practical ways of coping with stress. The origins and evolution of the stress response are outlined, as are the physiological and psychological responses of individuals. An overview of the principles of dealing with excessive stress and a detailed, practical account of stress-reducing techniques are provided. Throughout the chapter it is emphasized that it is not events that are stressful but our reaction to them. Coping with stress involves changing our reactions, thereby altering how stressful we feel. Stress is not all bad – it can have positive effects too.

WHAT IS STRESS?

Stress is a nebulous term. It is subject to individual interpretation and experience and cannot be rigorously defined. However, unless there is common understanding of what stress means, there is little worth in discussing ways of coping with it, because successful stress management starts with its recognition.

When considering "psychological" stress, two themes emerge. Firstly, stress is an experience that occurs when people are faced with situations that they perceive as threatening to their physical or psychological well-being. Secondly, dealing with these situations engenders a degree of uncertainty. The psychological component to stress has its origins in the way the body reacts in response to immediate danger. However, whether this psychological response is activated depends on a cognitive evaluation by the individual of what demands are being made and what resources are available to deal with them.

STRESS AND HEALTHCARE PROFESSIONALS

Healthcare professionals are particularly likely to be affected by adverse stress. The fact that they deal with people in crisis about whom decisions have to be made, often in emergency situations, heightens the degree of pressure upon them. Frequently they have to practise within time and resource constraints, both of which limit their ability to deal effectively with the situations with which they are faced. Most experience an intense sense of responsibility and personal involvement in their work, and all these factors increase stress. However, healthcare professionals also show a remarkable reluctance to seek help when faced with the results of adverse stress. Whether this is due to a sense that they will let themselves or the service down, professional machismo or just plain ignorance has not been established. It is clear that among health service workers there are high rates of substance misuse, psychological distress and suicide. It seems peculiar that in a profession that experiences such a high degree of stress at all levels there is such apathy when it comes to recognizing and dealing with it.

ORIGINS AND EVOLUTION OF STRESS RESPONSE

BIOLOGICAL ADAPTIVITY TO THREAT

The origins of stress lie in the process by which the body mobilizes its capacity for dealing with danger through the "fight or flight" response. When an individual is faced with what is perceived as a threatening situation, that individual can either stay and confront it or make an escape. Both of these options depend on the body's ability to prepare itself for immediate physical exertion. The "fight or flight" response is a description of these physical changes: they include an increase in heart rate, diversion of blood to major muscle groups, dilation of airways with increased rate of respiration, slowing of the digestive system, increased acuity of senses (e.g., pupil dilation) and release of endorphins, cortisone, adrenaline, thyroid hormones and glucose into the bloodstream. Normally a period of intense activity would ensue which would end when the threat was no longer present. The subsequent release of tension at the end of physical exertion comprises the relaxation response. The source of many stress-related health problems is that the "fight or flight" response is triggered many times a day but there is no resulting physical exertion. This results in the production of tension which is not released, the relaxation response is not activated and the body chemistry does not return to normal.

GOOD STRESS AND BAD STRESS

Stress results from the interplay between demands and resources. Tension results from the non-resolution of stress. If the resources are equal to the demands, stress may still be experienced but in a positive way, leading to greater productivity and a sense of satisfaction. Even when the demands increase, provided they are within an individual's capabilities, the stress induced may be pleasurable. Stress that results in better achievement is associated with well-being and satisfactory relaxation. However, if the pressure becomes a little greater, individuals may be pushed beyond their ability to cope and start to become fatigued. Similarly, stress resulting from a situation that is unresolved creates tension that leads to ill health. If a situation has been resolved satisfactorily – or, if not resolved, is accepted as being a satisfactory conclusion – this is a healthy response but if the outcome of the situation is not accepted, this leads to tension that is destructive.

STRESS AND PERSONALITY

Research has shown that certain personality types are more likely to be affected adversely by stress. Individuals known as type A personalities demonstrate behaviour such as having high levels of energy, doing several things at once and being unable to delegate. They have high ideals and expectations and are very conscientious. These individuals are unable to deal with the stress that they encounter and are prone to physical consequences of excessive stress – in particular there is a strong association between heart disease and type A personality.

Burn-out is a phenomenon that describes the fatigue and frustration brought about by devotion to a cause, way of life or relationship that fails to produce the expected reward. Burn-out is also associated with type A personalities.

STRESS AND PHYSICAL ILLNESS

A number of physical symptoms or disorders have been linked with stress. These range from minor rashes and food sensitivities to more disabling and serious conditions such as hypertension, peptic ulcers and irritable bowel syndrome. Musculoskeletal, cardiovascular and gastrointestinal systems can all be affected and there is some evidence that stress and fatigue can weaken the action of the immune system and predispose to the development of cancer, multiple sclerosis and rheumatoid arthritis. Stress-related illnesses comprise almost 75% of conditions for which people seek medical attention.

STRESS AND PSYCHIATRIC ILLNESS

Substance abuse

Individuals who have difficulty coping with stress may resort to artificial relaxants in the form of alcohol or prescribed anxiolytics such as diazepam (Valium). These are central depressants that induce relaxation at the cost of dependence. The cost is high, causing physical, emotional and social damage. Not only do these substances fail to deal with the source of the stress (i.e. the stress-producing circumstances), they also provide extra unforeseen stresses such as physical ill health, employment compromises (e.g., through drinking and driving, accidents, poor work record), relationship difficulties and increased anxiety.

Depression and anxiety

Chronic unresolved stress can predispose to the development of clinical depression. If a situation is habitually interpreted as threatening or the resources for dealing with it as being inadequate, then not only will that situation induce stress but also the ability to deal with the stress is likely to be compromised. This may result in persistent low self-esteem and predispose to the development of a depressive

Box 57.1 Features of posttraumatic stress disorder

- "Flashbacks" (intrusive memories or nightmares of the trauma)
- Numbness and detachment
- Lack of enjoyment
- Heightened anxiety levels
- Avoidance of cues

Box 57.2 Coping with stress

- Recognize tension
- Decide that "something must be done"
- Identify the stressor
- Deal with it

Table 57.1 Signs and symptoms of stress

Signs	Symptoms
Ankle bending or tapping of feet	Headache
Coiled legs	Neckache
Hair twirling	Nausea and vomiting
Arms folded across chest	
Clenched fists with tight knuckles	
Gripped thumbs	
Clenched teeth	
Furrowed forehead	

illness. Similarly, neutral events that are interpreted in a negative way are thought to contribute to the onset of depression. Continued, unresolved stress can predispose to the development of an anxiety disorder.

Posttraumatic stress disorder

Posttraumatic stress disorder is an established psychiatric condition. First recognized in the Vietnam war, this psychological reaction to a horrific, exceptionally threatening and catastrophic situation is not uncommon in both victims and witnesses. The situation can cause pervasive distress in almost anyone and the disorder manifests itself after a short time in "flashbacks" consisting of intrusive memories or nightmares of the trauma, a sense of numbness and detachment, lack of enjoyment, heightened anxiety levels and avoidance of cues that remind the sufferer of the original trauma. The onset follows the trauma usually with a delay of several weeks. The course is fluctuating but recovery occurs in the majority of cases. Most are treated with psychotherapy but it is important to exclude the possibility of a depressive illness.

COPING WITH EXCESSIVE STRESS

The principles of coping with stress (here meaning excessive stress; in other words, stress that is stressful!) are recognition of tension, deciding that "something needs to be done", knowing what is causing the stress, and dealing with it by either taking action against the stressor or, if this is not possible, making a positive decision to ignore it or adapt to it.

RECOGNIZING THE EFFECTS

Signs of bodily tension include ankle bending or tapping of feet; coiled legs; hair twirling; arms folded tightly across the chest with abdomen drawn in; nail biting; tight, hunched shoulders; clenched fists with tight knuckles and a gripped thumb; clenched teeth with jutting jaw; worry muscles of the forehead contracted. Tension may become apparent through the development of symptoms such as headache, neckache or stomach problems (Table 57.1). More serious manifestations such as anxiety, depression or physical symptoms have been described above.

RECOGNIZING THE CAUSES

The most effective way to deal with actual or potential stress is to anticipate it. By looking at the common causes of stress and the effects of particular demands on individuals, it should be possible to recognize the origin of stress. It may be related to the nature of a job or may be closer to home and more personal.

General causes

Many of the general causes of stress relate to how work is structured. Poor organization, lack of appropriate supervision and long or unsociable hours can all contribute to devaluing a person's role at work and chip away at their self-esteem. Frequent changes in policy, lack of communication and a perceived lack of direction from superiors contribute to poor morale, lack of status and job dissatisfaction. The necessity to conform with bureaucratic procedures ("paper pushing") that are inappropriate to the level of training affects performance ("the harder I work, the more I have to do and the less efficient I become"). Poor pay and promotion prospects lead to financial pressures and frustration of ambition.

Life events

Research has shown that stressful events can have both positive and negative effects. In an American study, 80% of those who experienced many dramatic changes in their lives developed a major illness within the next 2 years. They identified and rated 43 changes in lifestyle ranging from

Table 57.2 Life events

Event	Score
Death of a partner	100 points
Divorce	73 points
Marriage	50 points
Minor law violation	11 points

death of a partner (100 points) to minor violation of the law (11 points).

Marriage was set at 50 points, with 73 points for divorce. If the total score was over 300 in 1 year there was likely to be major illness. A score over 100 indicated the need to take some remedial measures. Effects were cumulative such that events from 2 years previously could still produce effects (Table 57.2).

Specific causes

Specific causes of stress at work comprise those factors that relate to how individuals tackle their roles. Uncertainty about one's role causes uncertainty in decision making. There may be problems deciding on how far one's responsibility extends. There may be a conflict of interest regarding patient care and loyalty to colleagues or family. Those with perfectionist and obsessional qualities (clearly necessary to some degree in healthcare workers) may have difficulty knowing when to stop and how to delegate. An inability to influence those making decisions (powerlessness) may produce high levels of frustration. Difficult relationships with colleagues, especially superiors, will be detrimental to performance.

Task-related causes

Being at the forefront of healthcare, especially being first on the scene at emergencies, produces its own problems. Difficulties may arise with patients or their relatives who may be obstructive, violent, verbally abusive or just in need of copious reassurance. An inability to help or act immediately coupled with demonstrable suffering may lead to doubts about professional effectiveness. The responsibility entailed by working in an increasingly litigious health service for an increasingly sceptical, informed and querulous public conscious of their rights may lead to overcautiousness and "defensive" practice. Emotional involvement with patients may colour judgement and compromise objectivity. The requirement to be impartial and avoid being caught up in a patient's distress may be difficult for some individuals.

Stress in the home

Domestic stress is a powerful means of destabilizing efficiency at work, whether caused by a partner, children, domestic arrangements or environmental pressures upon the home (e.g., noisy neighbours, financial worries or insecurity of accommodation).

Personal causes

Stress involves the personal response to a demand or situation. How one reacts when faced with a particular circumstance governs how stressed one feels. The more one knows about one's likely or actual responses, the more feelings of tension can be minimized. Thus becoming aware of oneself, one's personality and one's patterns of reacting to situations and circumstances allows a more appropriate response to demands us. Being aware of one's temperamental characteristics, degree of obsessionality and the extent to which one indulges in risk taking is important in recognizing stressful events. Similarly, unnecessary self-blame for a set of circumstances or overidentification with a particular outcome may be relevant in the development of stress.

MANAGING THE STRESSOR

Once excess stress has been recognized and there is motivation to deal with it, the next step is to make a list of likely causes. Doing this not only entails a process of self-evaluation but also starts a process of solution. Identifying possible stressors allows the possibility of resolution of the stress, and list making in itself seems to reduce tension. Once the list has been formed, the stressor that is easiest to resolve can be chosen and broken down into objective parts. For example, if "unclear role" has been identified as a source of stress, one's present activity should be compared with what one perceives one ought to be doing. The unclear part should be identified, and examples given. If "poor communication" is recognized as being stressful, it is important to work out why this is the case, with whom and in what circumstances.

Having made a list and objectified the problem, it is important to decide whether this requires immediate action or should be left for the future and also whether the circumstance is likely to be resolved or will be impossible to resolve and should be ignored or adapted to (e.g., pay and promotion aspects). It must be realized that choosing to ignore or adapt to stress is a positive outcome. If there is difficulty arriving at a solution creative thinking may be helpful, perhaps putting oneself in the place of some hapless manager and not forgetting to use humour. A lighthearted approach to difficulties can immediately reduce their intensity and threat.

The steps in coping with stress are:

- make a list
- think creatively
- objectify the problem
- use humour
- decide on immediate or future action
- ignore or adapt to the stress.

PERSONAL MANAGEMENT

SELF-AWARENESS

An ability to get in touch with one's physical, emotional and spiritual states is essential or any attempt to modify them will be bound to fail. Self-awareness is the process by which an individual undergoes such analysis. Understanding how we react gives an insight into how others see us and that in itself may go some way to solving hitherto intractable problems.

TIME MANAGEMENT

Much of the cause of non-specific stress lies in personal inefficiency and poor time management. Clearly, there will be unavoidable demands on one's time and the wider organization may be inefficient and time consuming. However, throughout the day there are pockets of time that can be used effectively. Thinking about how one spends one's time and why it is being spend in this way, together with goal setting and planning, listing priorities and being assertive, are all techniques that result in effective time use rather than time wasting. It is important to be aware of the dangers of too many meetings, overavailability on the telephone, poor communication, indecision and lack of self-discipline. These are all potential causes of time wasting.

MEDITATION

Meditation and relaxation are valuable skills to help cope with stress. A full discussion of meditation is beyond the scope of this chapter. However, a simple method is to sit in an upright position, undisturbed, for 5–10 minutes each day. When comfortable, the eyes are closed and attention is focused gently on one's breathing. At the same time any thoughts that arise are denied attention. Attention instead is focused on a particular object or experience, such as the air rushing in through the nostrils or a repeated word or phrase (a mantra). In this way it is possible to train attention and increase control over thought processes. Subsequently there is an improved ability to handle emotions and physical relaxation is more effective.

RELAXATION

The psychological changes that accompany the relaxation response are:

- decrease in muscle tone, heart and respiratory rate, blood pressure, and blood lactate and cortisone levels
- a noticeable decrease in oxygen consumption and carbon dioxide elimination
- increased blood flow to major internal organs
- improvement in peripheral circulation
- a rise in skin temperature
- an increase in basal skin resistance.

One way of measuring the extent of relaxation is by use of biofeedback machines. These monitor the physiological processes within the body that usually are unnoticed (e.g., muscle tension, skin temperature, blood pressure and heart rate) and can give a visual or audible reading of them. The different subjective feelings of relaxation can then be related to the accompanying physiological changes. Moreover, this monitoring of psychological processes helps bring them under voluntary control so that individuals can learn what brings about body relaxation, what disrupts it and how to apply relaxation at times of stress.

There are several different types of relaxation technique. The thread that runs through them all, however, is that they have to be learned to be effective. This requires an effective understanding of the technique to be used, the achievement of satisfactory relaxation on each occasion and frequent (at least daily) practice. It is no good attempting to learn relaxation in an environment that is not peaceful or is liable to interruption or other disturbance. Clearly, once effective relaxation has been learned it is valuable to apply it in any situation.

Types of relaxation include the use of breathing techniques, graded muscle relaxation and graded imagery.

Breathing techniques

Overbreathing is common in anxiety and usually takes place in the upper chest. Breathing exercises are effective in reducing anxiety, depression, irritability and fatigue, and most systems of relaxation include an emphasis on breathing. Breathing exercises can be done either sitting upright on a supportive chair with legs uncrossed or lying on the floor with knees bent and spine straight.

The process begins with scanning the body for tension, especially in the throat, chest and abdomen, and allowing the release of tension. Next, one hand is placed on the chest and one on the abdomen. With slow and deep breathing, the abdomen can be felt to rise with each inhalation. There should be very little movement in the upper chest but plenty in the lower. Exhalations should be slow, allowing the air to leave the body with a slight sigh through the mouth. Inhalation should be through the nose. Focus should be kept on the sound of breath, the slow rhythm of breathing and the gentle abdominal rise and fall. It is important to be conscious of the deepening sense of relaxation and to continue for 5–10 minutes at a time. At the end of each breathing session, one's body should be scanned again for tension and any differences from what was there before noted.

Graded muscle relaxation

Graded muscle relaxation involves tensing groups of muscles and relaxing them, making note of the difference in tension.

Lying on the floor, flat on one's back with feet about 30 cm apart and hands resting by one's sides, the first step is gentle breathing in through the nose and out through the mouth. All attention is now directed to the muscles of the face, screwing them up as tight as possible. This tension is held for just a few moments … then relaxed. The next focus is on the muscles of the shoulders. The shoulders are hunched as high as possible. … and the tension held for a few moments … and then relaxed, allowing the shoulders to drop and to broaden and make greater contact with the floor. Now both fists are tightly clenched … then both arms are stretched downwards, towards the feet. … once again, the tension is held for just a few moments … and the hands and arms are then allowed to relax completely. Attention is then focused on the stomach. A deep breath is taken, and on breathing out, the stomach muscles are allowed to be pulled in. The tension is held for just a few moments … then relaxed completely with normal breathing, allowing a feeling of increasing relaxation. Finally, attention is focused on the legs and feet. Both feet are pointed as far downwards as possible, allowing the legs to push forward as far as possible, and the tension is held for a few moments … then both feet and legs are relaxed. It is vital to allow oneself to completely relax and to feel how much heavier the body feels whilst allowing it to sink further into the floor. One should appreciate what it feels like to have all the muscles relaxed. Breathing gently and easily and remaining in the relaxed position for a few minutes completes the technique.

Graded imagery

Using graded imagery entails closing the eyes, scanning the body for tension and releasing it, and then visualizing a scene that is either well known or can be easily imagined clearly. It should be a pleasant scene in which there is plenty of detail. Examples include a garden, a beach or a picture. Once the vision has been established one must start to envisage details, being as accurate as possible without straining too much. Colours, scents, noises and touch sensations should be picked out in passing through or scanning the vision. The physical sensations associated with it – the warmth of the sun, the gentleness of the breeze, the sparkling of water and the softness of touch and noise – should all be felt. In becoming part of the scene, one becomes part of the tranquillity within it. No deadlines, no demands, no pressures … just the feeling of being at one with peace around and within. One can then stay in this state for as long as is desired, following which one can then gradually sink back into the surface on which one is lying or sitting. The scene is allowed to gently dissolve and then the eyes can be opened and reorientation takes place.

DIET, FLUIDS AND PHYSICAL EXERCISE

Some of the physiological effects of stress result in dehydration. Moreover, people who are stressed tend not to eat or drink regularly, thereby compounding the problem. It is recommended that 4 pints (approximately 2 litres) of fluid per day are taken in addition to that in food and added to cereal. Tea and coffee are diuretics and contain caffeine so they should be avoided. Excessive intake of caffeine during the week can lead to weekend withdrawal symptoms of headache, nausea and tremor.

In order to combat stress the body requires more energy and a healthy diet is important. Fat intake should be reduced, especially saturated fat, for example in red meat, hard cheese, cream, butter and eggs. The quantity of fruit, vegetables and absorbable fibre should be increased and sugar and salt intake reduced. Weight should be watched. It is important to exercise regularly and to remember that each time the body becomes stressed it is gearing itself up for exercise. If this is met by actual physical exercise on a regular basis, the subsequent release of endorphins aids relaxation.

ROLE OF THE TEAM

The team has an important role in helping to cope with stress. By recognizing the signs of stress in team members and being aware of demands on individuals, support can be given to encourage resolution of problems. Group activities such as debriefing and staff councils allow presentation of problems at an early stage. Lines of communication can be drawn up, allowing effective dissemination of news and management changes.

CONCLUSION

Prehospital healthcare workers work in a very stressful environment and recognize that they or their colleagues become stressed and work less effectively as a consequence. Nevertheless, there is an undoubted reluctance to *act* even when the effects of stress are becoming serious. It is vital that professionals look out for the effects of stress in themselves and colleagues and take appropriate action and provide support when they are found. Each individual can also do a great deal using the techniques described in this chapter to recognize and reduce stress in themselves.

FURTHER READING

Dernocoeur KB 1996 Streetsense: Communication, Safety, and Control, 3rd edn. Laing Research Services, Redmond.

National Institute for Clinical Excellence 2005 Clinical Guideline 26: Post-traumatic Stress Disorder (PTSD). NICE, London. (Available at: www.nice.org.uk/CG026NICEguideline)

Section 11

MAJOR INCIDENTS

Chapter 58

The major incident: an overview

INTRODUCTION

Recent events in Britain and elsewhere have highlighted the need for contingency planning and preparation to cope with possible mass casualty situations (major incidents). The world of the 21st century seems less secure than that of the end of the 20th and international terrorism and civil disorder are ever-present threats.

However, the recent history of organized major incident responses might be said to have begun some 20 years ago. In the 1980s the UK suffered a flurry of major incidents, including the King's Cross Underground fire and the Clapham rail crash (Table 58.1). The combined effect of these was to generate a surge of activity in the field of emergency planning. As a result, greater importance was given to the roles of health authority and ambulance service emergency planning officers. Local authority emergency planning departments are now allowed a role in civil emergencies, rather than remaining restricted to their former wartime contingency planning. Practical experience has raised awareness of the need for an integrated interservice cooperation in responding to disasters. The key players from each service must be aware of each other's capabilities and responsibilities and effective lines of communication must be established long before they are put to the test at a major incident.

While these encouraging developments within the emergency services and local authorities have been taking place, the health service has been subjected to considerable organizational restructuring. The development of trusts, for both the health and ambulance services, has fundamentally changed the provision of healthcare. The purchaser–provider split has further confused the ground rules for the response to major incidents. As the statistical chance of a major incident occurring in any given area is remote, it is often difficult to raise the motivation to provide for an adequate response to such incidents. Maintaining stockpiles of equipment that are unlikely to be used does not seem cost effective to a management that is reactive, not proactive.

Lessons of past major incidents are rarely learned and incidents tend to repeat themselves. For the paramedic, the major incident is a challenge. Few are likely to attend more than one in their entire professional career and most will never be involved at all. Despite this, the developing role of paramedics in the modern efficient ambulance service

Table 58.1 Major incidents in the UK in the 1980s

Year	Incident	Total injured and dead	Year	Incident	Total injured and dead
1981	Bombing in Chelsea, London	74	1985	Coach crash on M61 motorway	52
1981	Bombing in Hyde Park, London	25	1985	Football stadium fire, Bradford	308
1982	Gas explosion, Jersey, Channel Islands	10	1985	Train crash at Battersea, London	105
1982	Bombing in Regents Park, London	27	1985	Tottenham riots, London	>70
1982	Explosion at Cardowan mine	40	1985	Ship explosion at Milford Haven	16
1983	Air crash at Aberdeen airport	18	1985	Riot at Luton Town football	16
1983	Bombing at Harrods, London	95	1985	Riot at Birmingham	71
1983	Coach crash, M5 motorway	31	1985	Riots in Brixton, London	>50
1983	Refinery fire, Pembrokeshire	6	1985	Train crash at Haywards Heath	50
1984	Explosion at Abbotstead	44	1986	Train crash at Beverley	47
1984	Train crash at Wembley, London	24	1986	Train crash at Stafford	78
1984	Refinery explosion, Pembrokeshire	20	1987	Kings Cross Underground fire	91
1984	Brighton bombing	34	1987	Hovercraft collision, Dover	43
1984	*Armorique* ship fire, Cornwall	79	1987	Mass shooting, Hungerford	32
1984	Heathrow airport bombing	25	1987	Multiple RTA, M4 motorway	78
1984	Liverpool St station train crash	40	1988	Clapham train crash	123
1984	Train crash in Falkirk	>73	1988	Industrial explosion at Poole	19
1984	Oxford Circus Underground fire	>15	1988	Piper Alpha oil rig explosion	228
1984	Train crash at Salford, Manchester	79	1989	Air crash near Kegworth	126
1984	Multiple RTA, M25 motorway, Surrey	>20	1989	Crowd crush at Hillsborough	240
1985	Air crash at Manchester airport	137	1989	Riverboat sinking, London	131
1985	Coach crash on M6 motorway	45	1989	Train crash at Purley	93

requires them to be prepared to cope with the major incident around the corner. The old saying is as true today as ever: *"Failing to plan is planning to fail"*.

Nevertheless, in the light of recent events, major initiatives are in progress to ensure an effective response to global terrorism and once these have been fully established, the ambulance services will play a major role in their implementation in the event of an incident.

DEFINITIONS

The health service defines a major incident as:

> *"Any occurrence which presents a serious threat to the health of the community, disruption to the services, or causes or is likely to cause such numbers of casualties as to require special arrangements by the Health Service."* (HC90 25)

What is a major incident to one emergency service may not be to all: many major incidents do not produce live casualties. The Lockerbie plane crash, when a terrorist device blew up a passenger aircraft as it flew over a small Scottish border town, caused minimal disruption to the health service. For the police, fire service, military and local authorities the impact was enormous and involvement spanned weeks and months. On the other hand, a food poisoning epidemic would have major repercussions for the health service but little or no effect on the fire service. While all the services are not fully engaged in all major incidents, integrated "all-hazards" planning with the other emergency services may produce a simpler and better definition of what constitutes a major incident:

> *"Any situation which develops or threatens to develop which is beyond the local resources and requires the special mobilization of the emergency services to deal with it."*

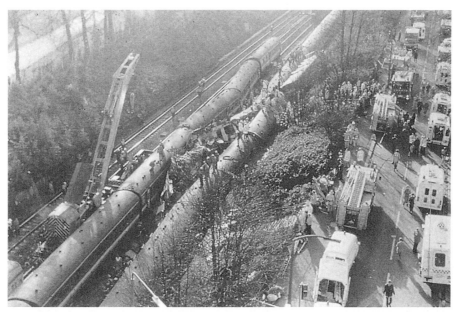

Figure 58.1 The Clapham rail disaster

CLASSIFICATION

Major incidents can be classified into simple or compound, and compensated or uncompensated.

- A *simple* major incident is one in which the infrastructure of the community in which it occurs remains intact, for example a train or air crash.
- A *compound* major incident destroys or damages the infrastructure of the surrounding community, for example the Los Angeles or Japanese earthquakes.
- A *compensated* major incident is one in which there are sufficient local resources to deal with the consequences.
- An *uncompensated* major incident is one where the medical and other responding emergency services are destroyed or totally inadequate.

Almost all British major incidents have been simple and compensated. However, the risks of a major incident on a far greater scale have to be considered from storms, floods, terrorism or disease. Earthquakes, common in some parts of the world, are a remote consideration for Britain. However, teams of British paramedics and other rescuers have attended uncompensated major incidents in other parts of the world and it is useful for training to include these worst-case scenarios. An uncompensated major incident is synonymous with a "disaster".

CSCATTT

The mnemonic CSCATTT (Box 58.1) describes a system widely accepted in the United Kingdom, and now in many

---

Box 58.1 CSCATTT

COMMAND
SAFETY
COMMUNICATION
ASSESSMENT
TRIAGE
TREATMENT
TRANSPORT

Box 58.2 Common aims of the emergency response

- Save life
- Prevent escalation
- Relieve suffering
- Protect the environment
- Protect property
- Rapidly restore normality
- Assist any criminal investigation or enquiry

---

other countries, which is designed to ensure the successful medical management of a major incident with live casualties. It is a hierarchy of actions that help the otherwise potentially chaotic actions of multiple staff to come together into a system.

This sequence can be remembered using the acronym "Command Spells Calm And Time To Treat".

The overriding aim of this approach is to achieve the common aims of all emergency services at a major incident (Box 58.2).

RESPONSIBILITIES OF THE FIRST CREW ON SCENE

The actions of the first ambulance crew on scene will determine the rate at which other resources are mobilized and give receiving hospitals the maximum possible time to prepare. It is essential, therefore, that these actions occur rapidly and efficiently.

These actions revolve around the core principle of achieving early, effective control of the medical response.

ATTENDANT

The attendant assumes the role of *Ambulance Commander*. He will remain in this position until relieved by a senior ambulance officer. He should undertake a rapid reconnaissance of the scene and feed back a situation report to the driver, who can then pass this to control. Declaring a major incident is at the discretion of the attendant and is a heavy responsibility. However, it is of paramount importance that the decision to declare a major incident is taken at the earliest opportunity.

Once he has provided an initial report to the driver, he should continue his reconnaissance, paying particular attention to suitable sites for the ambulance parking point, control point and the casualty clearing station. The *Fire Commander* and *Police Commander* should be identified and contacted at an early opportunity. The attendant must not, under any circumstances, become involved with the treatment of casualties.

DRIVER

The driver is to stay with the vehicle at all times. He will form the communication link between the scene and ambulance control. His first responsibility is to park the vehicle as close to the scene as safety allows and leave the beacon switched on. He should then provide control with a brief report, stating the location and type of incident.

Once he has been contacted by the attendant, it is essential that the declaration of a major incident is made at the earliest opportunity, using the METHANE mnemonic (Box 58.3).

The driver must remain in contact with the attendant at all times and should not leave the vehicle until directed to do so by a senior ambulance officer.

Box 58.3 METHANE	
M	Major incident standby/major incident declared
E	Exact location
T	Type of incident
H	Hazards
A	Access
	Number of casualties
E	Emergency services present and required

COMMAND AND CONTROL (*C*SCATTT)

EMERGENCY SERVICES

Command and control are the cornerstones of major incident management. Command is a "vertical" process, control is a "horizontal" one.

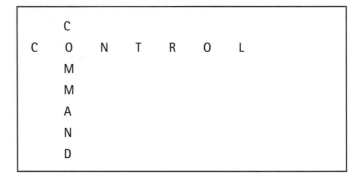

Although individual paramedics are unlikely to be involved in tasks outwith their usual remit of triage and treatment, it is essential to understand the command structures in place at major incidents.

Overall control of the scene is the responsibility of the police, who may be treating the incident as a criminal investigation from the outset. If hazards are present, the fire service will have responsibility inside the inner cordon (the area of hazard) until the danger is controlled.

One of the first tasks the police will undertake is the establishment of cordons: a physical outer cordon and an inner cordon. The outer cordon may consist of police vehicles blocking streets, tape or metal fencing. The outer cordon is usually several hundred metres from the scene and keeps members of the public at a safe distance. There will be a police manned *incident control point* through which all staff should enter and leave: all movements will be logged by the police.

The inner cordon is often not marked, but tape may be used. This marks the area where the rescue operation is taking place. Personnel entering and leaving this area must also be recorded for safety or forensic investigation purposes. Nationally a variety of local systems are used, including cordon control cards which are deposited in a box, the fire service tally system and an armband system. Whatever system is used, it must be possible at all times to know who is inside the inner cordon in case of a secondary incident or a requirement for evacuation.

The incident is broken down into three tiers of command (Figure 58.2). The *bronze* (*operational*) area lies within the inner cordon and is the area where the rescue operation is in place. There will be bronze commanders (*forward commanders*) from each emergency service. *Silver* (*tactical*) command consists of the area within the outer cordon. The commanders from each service will be within this area, although they may move in and out of the bronze zones. *Gold* (*strategic*) command is far removed from the scene – usually in the police HQ or local authority buildings – and is the location where the chief officers from each emergency service meet. Gold control is usually a fixed predetermined facility.

> A note on terminology: the term "commander" has replaced that of "incident officer". Thus the *medical incident officer* is now the *medical commander* (at silver level) and the *forward fire incident officer* is now the *forward fire commander* (at bronze level). The old terms are likely to continue in use for some time.

Each emergency service will have an appointed *silver commander* who is in charge at the scene. This is usually handed over to more senior officers in each service as they arrive on scene. Commanders control the use of the resources at the site: they must not become involved in the rescue or treatment of casualties. It is essential for the smooth operation of the emergency response that there are frequent meetings between these commanders. (Figure 58.3)

These meetings of silver commanders will need to be documented (logged). The first priority is to share intelligence and establish what has happened.

- What are the main priorities for the next hour?
- What difficulties need to be resolved?
- Are other resources required?
- Which are the casualty receiving hospitals?
- Where is the survivor reception centre and who is resourcing it?
- Do any of the services present have particular problems or difficulties that another may be able to help with?

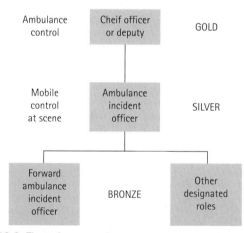

Figure 58.2 Tiers of command

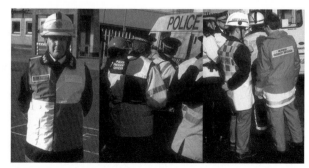

Figure 58.3 The silver commanders

All major incidents are potential scenes of crime. They need to be treated as such, with maximal preservation of evidence. Arrangements need to be made concerning the dead. A body-holding area may be required on scene and a temporary mortuary may eventually be required. Each region usually has predetermined locations for temporary mortuaries.

Commanders must be readily identifiable and will wear appropriate coloured tabards (Table 58.2).

HEALTH SERVICE

The health service response is controlled by the Ambulance Commander (AC) at silver level. His duties are set out in Box 58.4.

The Ambulance Commander may be joined by an appropriately trained doctor who will act as *Medical Commander*; this position is often occupied by a general practitioner from a local immediate care scheme. The primary role of the Medical Commander is to work in close conjunction with the Ambulance Commander and to this end they should usually be found in close proximity to each other. He should also direct medical and nursing resources and establish and maintain contact with the receiving hospitals. The decision to call for specialist medical teams will be his. Of course, many decisions will be taken in conjunction with the Ambulance Commander.

Doctors who turn up or who are plucked out of a local hospital or surgery just because they happen to be on duty may not be properly trained, equipped or in appropriate protective clothing. Such staff should only be used in an appropriate role. Bogus doctors have often been attracted to

Table 58.2 Identifying commanders at scene

Commander	Tabard
Fire	Red/white
Police	Blue/white
Ambulance	Green/white

> **Box 58.4 Responsibilities of the Ambulance Commander**
>
> - Liaise with other commanders.
> - Delegate tasks to other ambulance personnel.
> - Ensure adequate communications for all health service staff.
> - Determine (with the Medical Commander) the receiving hospitals.
> - Determine (with the Medical Commander) where mobile medical teams are drawn from.
> - Establish triage and treatment.
> - Determine appropriate transport routes.
> - Organize replenishment of equipment.
> - Liaise with police regarding the media

the scene of major incidents. If the identity and experience of doctors cannot be verified the ambulance service must decline their assistance and have them escorted from the scene.

There are several key locations that must be determined early in the health service response: these are illustrated in Figure 58.4

A steady green rooflight should identify the *ambulance control point*. All health service staff are to report there on arrival at the scene. The *forward control point* is an area at the scene where the forward incident officers can meet to direct the rescue operation. The forward commanders report to their respective commanders. An appropriate site for secondary triage and treatment of patients must be chosen early – this will be the *casualty clearing station* (CCS). Ideally it will be sheltered, safe, accessible and have electricity and water; however, initially it may be little more than a few fire brigade tarpaulins on the ground.

Ambulances should be parked at the *ambulance parking point* until called forward to the rear of the CCS to receive a patient ready for transport to a receiving hospital: the collection area is known as the *ambulance loading point*.

There are several key roles that must be delegated by the Ambulance Commander.

Communications Officer

The Communications Officer provides and coordinates all on-site communications. He works at the ambulance control point.

Forward Ambulance Commander

The Forward Ambulance Commander manages ambulance resources in the bronze area, to effect triage and removal of patients.

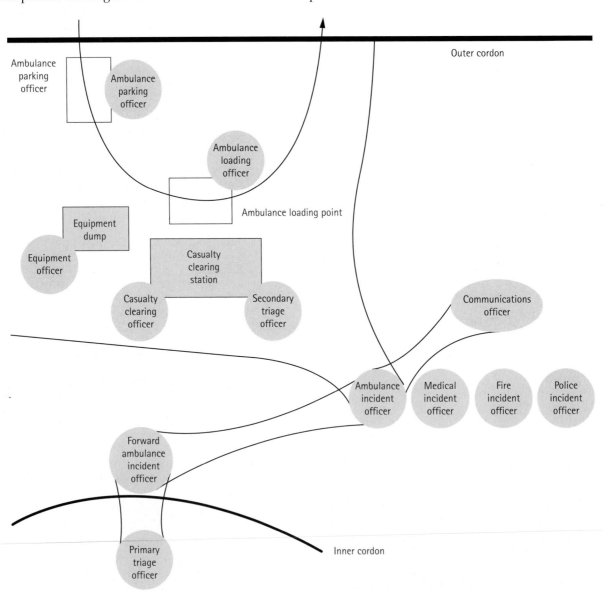

Figure 58.4 Key health service locations

Casualty Clearing Station Officer

The Casualty Clearing Station Officer organizes and manages the CCS, including overseeing secondary triage and further treatment and maintaining equipment levels.

Ambulance Parking Officer

The Ambulance Parking Officer is responsible for managing the ambulance parking point. This is a key role as this officer will ensure that staff report to the Ambulance Control Point rather than rushing into the incident.

Ambulance Loading Officer

The Ambulance Loading Officer works at the ambulance loading point and, in conjunction with the police, ensures a suitable transport route for appropriate patients to appropriate hospitals.

Primary Triage Officer

The Primary Triage Officer is responsible for triaging patients in the bronze area.

Ambulance Safety Officer

See below.

SAFETY (CSCATTT)

Everyone at the scene of a major incident has a responsibility for their *own* safety, the safety of *the scene* and the safety of *the casualties* (the 1-2-3 of safety). The Ambulance Commander will task someone to be *Ambulance Safety Officer*: he will be responsible for overseeing all safety-related matters. Incorrectly dressed or inadequately protected individuals will not be allowed to enter the scene, regardless of who they are. This rule may be relaxed once an adequate casualty clearing station has been established, if the individuals concerned have the necessary skills to be employed there.

COMMUNICATIONS (CSCATTT)

AT THE SCENE

Effective communication is essential to ensure the smooth running of the emergency service response. There are many methods available but commonly two are used: verbal and radio.

Communication at the scene usually relies upon UHF radios: these will be provided by the Communications Officer at the ambulance control point. He will also have radio communication with control (VHF).

To ensure appropriate use of resources and control of the incident, all communication must be passed vertically up the chain of command before moving horizontally to other services.

WITH HOSPITALS

Communications between the scene and hospitals have been a problem area for many years. Traditionally the hospitals have considered their representative on scene to be the Medical Commander. The hospital staff will have a natural curiosity about the scene and want to have as much detail as possible. It is difficult for those not on site to understand the inevitable confusion. Casualty numbers are usually guesses to start with. Important information really needs to flow in the opposite direction. The management team of the Medical Commander (MC) and the Ambulance Commander (AC) need to know the casualty capacity of the receiving hospitals.

- How many theatres can be staffed?
- How many intensive care unit beds are available?
- How many general beds are there?
- Are there adequate blood supplies?
- How many more minor injuries can they cope with in the next hour?

The site management team will use as many receiving hospitals as appropriate. It is inappropriate for one hospital to try to cope with all casualties. The ambulance service should aim to achieve an even distribution of the injured to several hospitals.

To aid communication between hospitals and the scene, the ambulance service should despatch a liaison team to each receiving hospital. One officer should ensure smooth

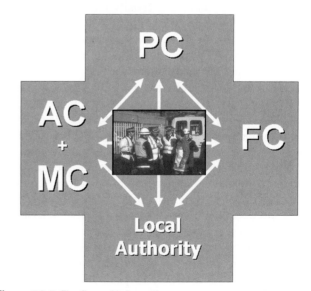

Figure 58.5 The flow of information

turnaround and re-equipping of ambulances and document the number of casualties. The other should join the hospital coordination team to advise and update the hospital staff on progress at the scene. It is vital that these ambulance officers have radio communications to the scene and to ambulance control. Traditionally, hospital beds are freed by the early discharge of convalescent patients. In the 1980s this was easy and produced a substantial number of free beds; however, in today's surgical wards patients are discharged very quickly so the potential pool of available beds has disappeared. While there are often closed wards, they are not staffed and would take a long time to make useable. Moving patients from one hospital to another has transport implications for the ambulance control who may well have to seek aid from neighbouring services and voluntary aid societies. In extreme circumstances military resources might be requested.

Fax machines are a useful means of communication between hospitals and ambulance controls, particularly for lists of casualties. They save air time on radio channels, which are always overloaded and prone to being overheard by scanners used by the media. Mobile phones, on the other hand, are rarely much use as the media reporters overload the cells when they keep lines open continuously. Unless special arrangements are invoked by the police, mobile phones cannot be relied on. These arrangements are known as ACCOLC, or **ACC**ess **O**ver**L**oad **C**ontrol, whereby only mobile phones operating on a protected number of cells will be able to initiate calls. This requires a modification to the phones simm card, which must have been authorized previously by the Home Office.

If the incident scene is complex or extensive, agreement should be reached by all the emergency services on "sectorization". In a rail accident, each carriage might be considered as a sector. If different buildings are involved, again each may be considered as a separate sector. In multiple motorway crashes each vehicle should be allocated a number. The location of each casualty released can then be recorded in terms of vehicle number. As staff become available, each sector can be supervised and the activity to release and remove trapped casualties can be monitored and reported back to the silver control.

Requests for drugs and equipment must be kept under careful control and a clear chain of communication established. Past experiences have shown that messages can easily become duplicated and confused. Often the equipment is already on scene but not identified. An equipment officer can be invaluable in keeping control over the utilization of equipment, the provision of oxygen, nitrous oxide (Entonox), masks and drugs. If controlled drugs are required, careful control and documentation is necessary. If emergency blood is required on scene, requests should always go via the ambulance silver control to the hospitals, with the MC being involved. Independent requests direct to hospitals by mobile phone or via police officers are a recipe for disaster, confusion and duplication.

ASSESSMENT (CSC*A*TTT)

Scene assessment is a dynamic process and regular updates must be fed back from bronze to silver and from silver to gold control and receiving hospitals, to ensure appropriate deployment and use of available resources.

TRIAGE (CSCA*T*TT)

Triage occurs at two places at a major incident scene: *primary triage* occurs in the bronze area and aims to rapidly identify those in need of immediate life-saving treatments. The *triage sieve* is used for primary triage and is illustrated in Figure 58.6. A modified version exists for children.

Secondary triage occurs at the entrance to the CCS, where a more detailed system involving the triage revised trauma score (TRTS) is used (see Chapter 59).

Patients are triaged as:

- delayed (green)
- urgent (yellow)
- immediate (red)
- dead (white).

Occasionally a decision may be made to implement an *expectant* category (*blue*) for those patients whose injuries will use too many resources in a major incident setting and who have a significant chance of dying, despite using resources which might more effectively be directed to patients with a greater chance of survival. The expectant category will only be implemented on the joint agreement of the Ambulance and Medical Commanders.

Once triaged, casualties must be marked so that other personnel can rapidly identify them for treatment. A variety of triage labels are in operation throughout the country and the

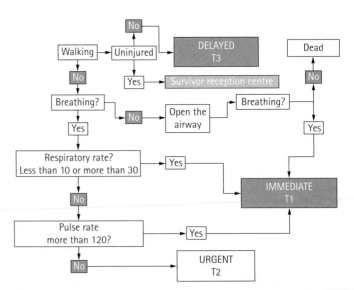

Figure 58.6 The triage sieve

specific card used is irrelevant: however, it is of paramount importance that ambulance personnel know how to use them.

One of the major limitations to effective triage in the past has been the provision of triage labels: they may not arrive on scene early enough. For triage to be performed effectively there must be a supply of labels on every frontline vehicle. It is not satisfactory for them to be kept only on major incident control or equipment vehicles.

Further triage will occur in the decision to transport patients to hospital and again on arrival at the emergency department.

TREATMENT (CSCAT*T* T)

The aim of all treatments is to allow the maximum number of patients to arrive at hospital safely. In the bronze area, unless the patient is trapped, only basic airway and circulation treatments will be undertaken – once their other duties have been fulfilled, fire officers and police may help with this task. In the CCS, more advanced manoeuvres are performed, similar to those that might be undertaken in an emergency department resuscitation room, such as intubation or the administration of IV fluids and drugs.

In specific cases, a *mobile medical team* (MMT) may be called from a local hospital: ideally, this should not be one of the receiving units. The MMT usually consists of two doctors and two nurses and can be used on scene as a unit or broken up and allocated to different areas as appropriate. *Mobile surgical teams* (MST) can also be requested. Usually consisting of a surgeon, anaesthetist, nurse and theatre practitioner, the MST will normally be used for specific procedures on trapped patients under the command of the Forward Ambulance or Medical Commander.

TRANSPORT (CSCATT*T*)

Ambulances are parked at the ambulance parking point under the direction of the Parking Officer. Personnel who are called away from their vehicle must leave their keys in the ignition and should inform the Parking Officer if they have removed important equipment.

A circuit will be established, to allow access to and from the ambulance loading point where appropriate casualties are loaded for transport to hospital. Vehicles must arrive in a steady flow and be able to leave the scene without delay. Ambulances are the only emergency vehicles that need to come and go from the incident. The aim of transport is to get *the right patient to the right place at the right time* – the most severely injured may not necessarily be transported first.

All patients must be adequately packaged for transport, including securing of all lines and tubes, supply of sufficient oxygen and drugs for the journey and provision of relevant paperwork. Casualties requiring specialist centre treatment (e.g., burns or neurosurgery) should be transported directly to a centre providing that speciality, to avoid delays later in secondary transportation. However, patients with multiple system injuries are likely to need assessment and initial management first.

Vehicles other than land ambulances may be used for transport: helicopters have advantages of speed, but can only transport one patient. Patients with minor injuries may be sent to hospital by recruited buses or vans.

CONTROL ACTIVITY

As soon as reports of a possible major incident are received, the ambulance control should automatically bring into action a prepared response to cope with the incident. Once the incident is confirmed as genuine the plan should continue to resource the scene. Initial reports may be very vague and sketchy and later become confused and contradictory. Eventually control will be bombarded with information, which needs careful documenting and coordinating. It is important to remember that control staff are completely blind to the incident. They rely totally on graphic and descriptive reports from personnel on scene: the METHANE format is useful for updates. The media response to a disaster is often rapid. Many controls now rely on television, especially cable or satellite continuous news reports, to obtain a better understanding of the situation at the scene. Accident and emergency departments are also blind to the scene: they too are initially relying on rumours, media reports and impressions from patients and staff arriving at their department.

THE DEAD

In England and Wales the dead are the responsibility of the Coroner and in Scotland of the Procurator Fiscal. In practice, the police act as the Coroner's agents and will control all further management of the deceased. As bodies will provide forensic evidence, liaison with the Coroner's officer will be essential at an early stage. Initially those casualties triaged as dead should be labelled as such and covered with a blanket where they are found.

Dead bodies should be left where they are found during the rescue effort, except in two circumstances: where they will be destroyed (e.g., by fire or chemicals) or where they are blocking access to the living. If they are to be moved, efforts should be made to photograph them first.

Subsequently, when the pressure of the incident is reduced, a doctor accompanied by a nominated police officer should formally confirm death. An attached label should indicate the date and time, location found and the name of the doctor and police officer. Photographs of the body in situ should be taken, before it is removed to a body-holding point or temporary mortuary.

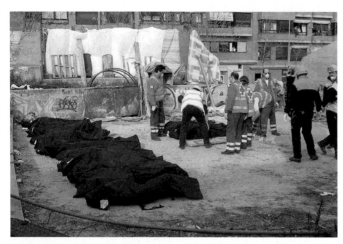

Figure 58.7 A body-holding area

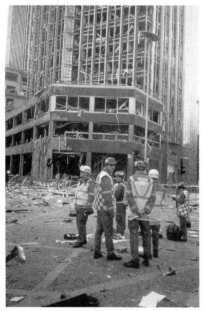

Figure 58.8 The City of London bomb

TERRORIST INCIDENTS

The major incident plan needs to be capable of modification to cope with the specific problems that terrorist incidents can cause. Bomb explosions result in devastation over a wide area (Figure 58.8). Secondary devices are a common hazard and all attending emergency service personnel need to remember the basic rule – *protect yourself*. The location of the rendezvous point for attending vehicles should be chosen with great care. A search of this area to confirm safety is of paramount importance. Use of radios and mobile phones may be restricted as these devices can trigger secondary devices.

A minimal number of personnel should be deployed in the explosion site, at least until safety has been established. The preservation of life and rescue of live casualties has to be balanced carefully with the risks to the rescuers.

Considerable importance is attached to the preservation of forensic evidence after a bomb explosion. The dressings, clothing and other belongings of the casualties may need to be preserved for forensic examination. Pieces of shrapnel must also be preserved. It goes without saying that the scene should be disturbed as little as possible.

CIVIL DISORDER

Civil disorder can present special challenges for the paramedic. The key to a successful operation in a civil disorder situation is neutrality. The paramedic must not take sides with the police or with demonstrators, with left-wing or right-wing political protestors or with racial groups.

Three distinct patterns of civil disorder can occur. Firstly, a prearranged demonstration may have potentially violent overtones. The demonstrators muster at a predetermined point and move along a prescribed route to a known destination. Police intelligence should allow for preplanning and preparation by the ambulance service. Secondly, there can be static confrontation: demonstrators against the police or rival factions with police intervention, usually with an area of conflict which is fairly clearly defined. Advanced warning of such an incident is usual and sensible plans can be prepared to contend with difficulties. The third scenario, with rampaging hordes and no set pattern or direction, is much more difficult to manage. Innocent persons or property may be attacked, with vehicles overturned and set alight. There may be a changing focus of casualties.

With other major incidents the casualties occur all at once and usually in a defined place. With civil disorder, casualties may continue to occur for hours or even days. The point at which it becomes a major incident is debatable. No-one can predict the casualty numbers in the next few hours. Rioting casualties can cause mayhem in accident and emergency departments. Rival groups must be taken to separate hospitals. If the police form a third group then they too must have a dedicated accident and emergency department. In rural areas or small towns this can cause problems but whenever possible, this principle must be adhered to.

Treatment facilities at a static point may avoid the need for a large number of people with minor injuries being moved to hospital. Minor dressings and treatment for strains and bruises should, where possible, be available on site. Additionally supplies of drinking water and minor analgesics such as paracetamol should be available. Paramedics should consider these minor treatments an important part of their role. Seriously injured casualties should be recovered and evacuated to a place of safety. Battlefield medicine principles may apply. Police should recover their own personnel, evacuating them to *paramedic forward aid points*. Full riot protective clothing and in some situations flak jackets may be required by crews. Foot patrol teams are most useful. Ambulances should have a crew of three whenever possible.

The flashpoints and the continuing production of casualties make preplanning difficult. At times it may not be possible to reach an incident safely. An ambulance liaison officer in the police control room is vital in informing paramedic teams of police tactics to ensure their safety when working among demonstrators or rioters. Similarly, ambulance liaison officers have a major role at the receiving hospitals. Hospital staff are often frightened by what is happening in the community and will be seeking advice about safe routes in and out of the hospital. Intelligence reports should be shared with hospital staff. To preserve neutrality it is essential that ambulances are not seen to be used to transport uninjured police officers, even if they are only given a well-intentioned lift from a hospital back to the incident.

UNDERGROUND INCIDENTS

Major incidents underground may present special problems. Communications can be particularly difficult. For caves and coal mines specialist rescue teams are usually available but in the underground railway system, ambulance paramedics will be required to work in conditions of very high temperatures. In the London Underground railway system, temperatures regularly rise to 40°C. Evacuation of trains with over a thousand passengers is often necessary. On occasions the scene may have to be approached from two different stations either side of the incident.

CHEMICAL INCIDENTS

Chemical incidents (see Chapter 44) may also require modifications to major incident plans. The fire service will of necessity take a lead role in ascertaining safety. Only fire officers normally have the appropriate protective clothing and breathing apparatus to enter the contaminated area.

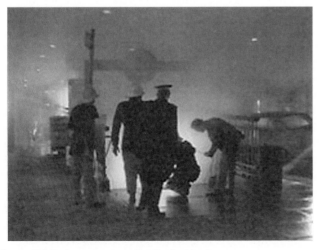

Figure 58.9 An underground major incident

Decisions about evacuation of areas affected by a chemical plume can be very difficult. It may often be preferable to keep members of the public inside buildings with windows and doors closed, rather than expose them in the street to a higher level of contamination while effecting their evacuation.

RADIATION INCIDENTS

Nuclear installations all have detailed on-site and off-site plans to cope with major incidents (see Chapter 45). Considerable fear and anxiety are created by radiation, based largely on ignorance of its nature. It cannot be seen, felt or smelt and is only detectable with sophisticated monitoring instruments. Acute and long-term effects can be considerable. The paramedic needs to understand the nature of radiation, know the details of locally produced plans and be informed about the workings of the National Arrangements for Incidents Involving Radiation (NAIR) scheme as applied locally.

DEBRIEFING

When paramedical staff have finished their duties at the scene of a major incident it is most important that a senior officer takes the trouble to thank them personally and check that they are safe to travel home. Fatigue and soiled or damaged clothing may mean they need assistance to get home. Words of encouragement and thanks and a brief discussion of any obvious concerns go a long way to prevent post-traumatic stress reactions. This *hot debrief* can either occur at the scene or back at a suitable station. It should not last for very long and should be directed towards welfare issues.

Within a few days it is necessary to arrange a more *formal debrief* for those involved. This should be directed towards fact finding. Who did what and when? What went well and what went wrong? What lessons can be learnt and how can the plans be modified for next time? Written reports from all those with a specific role should be requested. A final, full written report can then be prepared for all interested parties. This meeting provides another opportunity to spot those with posttraumatic stress and inappropriate reactions who may need professional support and help. It must always be remembered that these meetings are never for personal recriminations and "mud-slinging". Nobody does less than their best at an incident. Any criticism must be utilized in a positive way to modify and change responses next time.

A further interservice debrief to assess the level of successful integration and cooperation in working together is essential. Similar debriefs with casualty receiving hospitals provide a useful forum for further discussion.

Major incidents will always subject the emergency services to intense public scrutiny. The inevitable public enquiry will follow. Documentation and recording of all times and decisions are essential. Every choice or action made will be dissected with the benefit of hindsight and alternative actions considered. A detailed log must be kept at the ambulance control, at the incident silver command vehicle and at forward bronze controls. All radio messages must be tape recorded and transcribed as soon as possible after the incident.

Pocket tape recorders are useful jotter systems for some officers but it is important to dictate the time of the note for future transcription.

CONCLUSION

Major incident planning for the ambulance service must be based on the question *"What if . . .?"*. Any paramedic could play a part in a major incident response and so requires a detailed knowledge of the local centres likely to be involved. Railway stations, airports, sports stadia, industrial and chemical works, shopping centres and motorway complexes are all potential hazard spots. Each frontline ambulance should carry maps and plans of such locations in their normal operational area. These maps should show normal access and egress routes for ambulances, predetermined rendezvous points and joint emergency service controls.

The clinical care of casualties from a major incident is relatively straightforward, with the paramedics utilizing all their skills to provide the greatest good for the greatest number of patients. The real challenge is in the organizational aspects of command, control and communications.

Regular exercises to test major incident responses should be targeted towards interservice liaison and multiagency working, rather than the clinical aspects that are used every day.

FURTHER READING

All ambulance services, local authorities and hospitals have major incident plans which can usually be obtained on request.

National and local emergency plans for the UK

Ambulance service major incident plans.

County or borough emergency plans.

Local hospital major incident plans.

Health service arrangements for dealing with major incidents. HC90(25).

Home Office 1994 Dealing with fatalities during disasters. The Stationery Office, London

Home Office 1995 Dealing with disaster, 2nd edn. The Stationery Office, London

CIMAH site plans for local installations.

Health service arrangements for dealing with accidents involving radioactivity. The NAIR Scheme. HC(89)8.

Health service responsibilities in civil defence. HC(88)31.

HMSO 1991 Disasters: planning for a caring response. The Disasters Working Party. HMSO, London

HMSO 1994 Arrangements for responding to nuclear emergencies. HSE, London

Ministry of Defence 1989 Military aid to the civil community, 3rd edn. MOD, London

The Responses of the Faith Communities to Major Emergencies: Some Guidelines. (Board for Social Responsibility of the General Synod of the Church of England.)

Advanced Life Support Group 2002 Major incident medical management and support: the practical approach. BMJ Books, London

General reading

Advanced Life Support Group 2002 Major Incident Medical Management and Support, 2nd edn. BMJ Publications, London

Baskett P, Weller R 1988 *Medicine for disasters*. John Wright, Bristol

Hines K, Robertson B 1985 Guide to major incident management. BASICS, Ispwich

Murray V, ed. 1990 Major chemical disasters: medical aspects of management. Royal Society of Medicine Press, London

Chapter 59

Triage

CHAPTER CONTENTS

INTRODUCTION

Triage is the sorting of casualties according to clinical priorities. In multiple casualty situations, it is impossible to match patients with the management they require unless a robust triage system is established. Triage can be used to assess priorities for treatment *and* for evacuation.

Triage should be undertaken whenever the number of casualties exceeds the number of skilled helpers available. Thus a two-vehicle collision involving four people attended by one ambulance with two crew members is just as appropriate a place for the application of triage as a major incident with hundreds of casualties and many paramedical and medical staff.

Triage principles can also be applied to individual patients to assess the urgency of their problem. Specific criteria can be applied to determine where patients should be taken – in particular, the decision about where to take victims of trauma needs to be soundly based if there is tiered care available.

HISTORY OF TRIAGE

The sorting of casualties into priorities considerably predates the use of the word "triage", and there is evidence of the triage process in ancient Egyptian drawings. The term itself is derived from the French word *trier* meaning to sieve or sort. It was used by Surgeon-Marshal Larrey (Napoleon's Chief Medical Officer) to describe a system of sorting wounded French soldiers into priority for treatment; in this case, the minor wounds receiving quick dressings and being returned to combat while the more serious wounds waited.

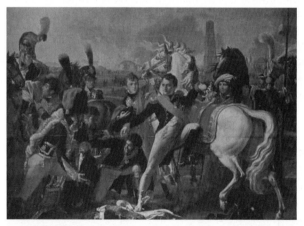

Figure 59.1 Baron Larrey providing care to the wounded during the Napoleonic Wars

The first written English language usage was again military and described the area of an American World War I dressing station that dealt with the sorting of casualties. By common usage it has come to mean the sorting process itself. Triage has been adopted in the day-to-day management of most civilian accident and emergency departments and remains a key element of military medicine.

PRINCIPLES OF TRIAGE

Triage is intended to establish the relative urgency of each casualty. In its purest form the result of the triage process would be an exact ordering of patients by urgency – thus 30 patients would be ordered from number 1 to number 30.

This approach, although superficially attractive, is impractical for a number of reasons. Firstly, it is difficult to establish sufficient information about each casualty to make such a fine judgement about relative order; this is especially so in the chaos of a major incident. Secondly, it is impossible for anyone (however skilled) to collect and collate the available details with any degree of accuracy and this system would require an assessment of every patient before triage priorities could be allocated. Finally, the clinical state of patients is constantly changing, either because of interventions that have been made or because they have deteriorated further. To overcome these problems the end-point of the triage process is not an ordering of patients but the allocation of a triage priority – in other words, the assignment of a patient to a category of urgency. These priorities must be standard and must be assigned according to set criteria. The actual method used to decide the priority will vary according to when and where the decision is being made, and will depend on the skills of the person making the decision.

Triage must reflect the changing state of the casualty and is therefore a dynamic rather than a static process. Casualties may be re-triaged repeatedly at a given stage of care and must be re-triaged whenever they enter a different stage of their care. Thus triage may occur a number of times at the site of an incident and will be repeated on reception at hospital.

It is essential that the current priority of a given casualty is known to the staff making decisions about interventions. To achieve this, there must be an agreed method of indicating the priority. Triage labelling is one method of achieving this.

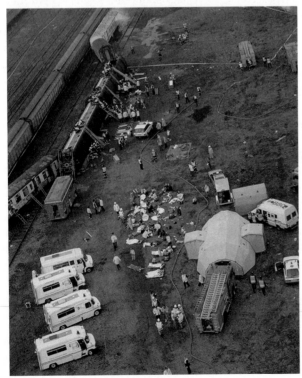

Figure 59.2 Triage at a major incident

PRIORITIES

The end-point of the triage process is the allocation of a priority. This priority is then used in conjunction with other factors to determine optimum care. The systems of priorities in common use are referred to as the treatment (T) system and the priority (P) system (Table 59.1). The words describing the priorities and their associated colours are as important as the numbers. In the past different words have been used to describe priorities, different triage criteria have been applied and different colours have been associated with the categories. These have all now been standardized.

As can be seen from Table 59.1, the only difference between the T and P systems is an additional category (*expectant*) included in the former.

DEFINITIONS

It is essential that at each stage all staff involved in triage use the same criteria for categorizing patients into defined priority groups. Failure to do this can lead to significant errors. An understanding of the definition of each priority category is essential if triage is to be performed correctly. The definitions are deliberately broad, because they must be applicable in a range of situations, from an initial sorting of casualties at the scene of an incident to the allocation of priorities for surgery. The triage category definitions are given in Table 59.2.

Table 59.1 Triage priority systems

Description	Colour	T system	P system
Immediate	Red	1	1
Urgent	Yellow	2	2
Delayed	Green	3	3
Expectant	Blue	4	
Dead	White		

Table 59.2 Triage category definitions

Category	Definition
1. Immediate	Casualties who require immediate lifesaving treatment
2. Urgent	Casualties who require treatment within 6 hours
3. Delayed	Less serious cases who require treatment but not within a set time
4. Expectant	Casualties whose injuries are so severe that either: they cannot survive despite treatment; or the degree of intervention required is such that, in the circumstances, their treatment would seriously compromise the provision of treatment for others

USE OF THE FOURTH CATEGORY

Whether or not the *expectant* category is used is a decision for the senior personnel involved (the ambulance and medical incident officers at the scene and the chief triage officer at the hospital). The decision must be based on an overall assessment of the situation and must take into account both the patient load and the resources available. It must be emphasized that failure to institute the use of this category as soon as it becomes necessary will result in higher overall morbidity and mortality rates. The undoubted difficulty of making the decision to leave seriously ill or injured casualties without treatment cannot be used as an excuse for not making it at all.

Many triage labelling systems do not include an expectant label and a local solution to this problem needs to be found. Standard approaches include using the green (delayed) category and ensuring that the patients are placed in a separate area, using the red (immediate) category and marking the card "hold" or using the Cambridge cruciform card showing green with the corners folded back to reveal red (Figure 59.3). Patients in the expectant category will be treated and transported *after* those in the T1 category but *before* those in the T2 and T3 categories.

TRIAGE METHODS

A sorting of casualties according to an exact description of their injuries with an informed estimation of the overall severity of injury is impractical (and unnecessary) for most triage decisions. The method used for triage must be varied according to the time available for decision making, the location of the patient, the nature of the treatment being considered and the experience of the person performing triage.

It should not be changed to reflect the number of patients, nor the resources available – except that the fourth (expectant) category may come into play as discussed earlier.

The information gathered to make triage decisions will reflect the particular decision being taken; thus primary triage at a major incident will be based on different information from that used to decide whether a patient should be taken to a trauma centre. Decisions about single patient urgency should be based on yet another group of observations. Some situations and the appropriate methods of triage are discussed below.

TRIAGE AT MAJOR INCIDENTS

There may be a large number of casualties at a major incident and thus an enormous number of decisions need to be made as quickly and efficiently as possible. The method used must therefore be fast, easy and safe and must give the same result whoever carries it out. Since the accuracy of any method depends on the amount of information used to reach a decision, and gathering information takes time, there is a trade-off between speed and accuracy. All patients will be re-triaged after the first look and any necessary refinements can then be made.

Triage sieve

The aim of the triage sieve is to convert the chaos of the incident site into some sort of medical order. Since the greatest number of patients are likely to have minor injuries, the most effective first step in establishing order is the separation of the *priority 3* (delayed) patients from the rest (Figure 59.4).

At this stage it is reasonable to assume that patients who can walk do not require urgent or immediate treatment and all such patients are therefore categorized as *priority 3* (delayed). Uninjured survivors are also separated and sent to a survivor reception centre.

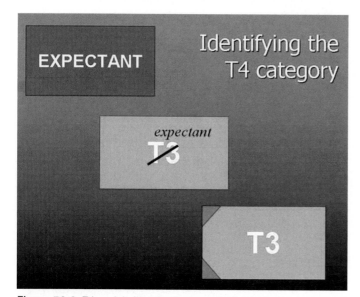

Figure 59.3 Triage labelling for the expectant category

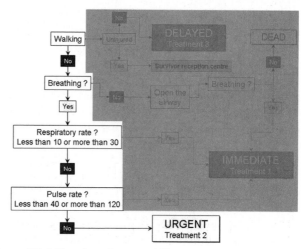

Figure 59.4 The triage sieve – mobility assessment

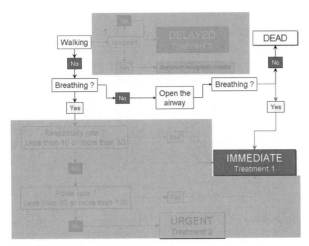

Figure 59.5 The triage sieve – the A component

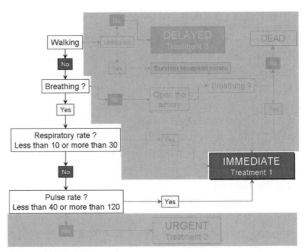

Figure 59.7 The triage sieve – the C component

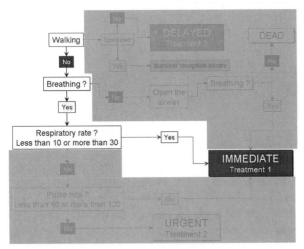

Figure 59.6 The triage sieve – the B component

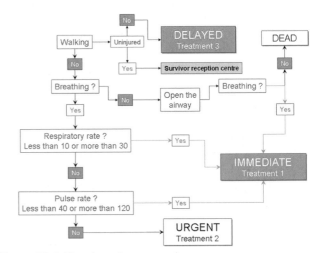

Figure 59.8 The triage sieve – summary

Once this has been done, the state of the airway, breathing and circulation is considered in the remainder of the patients.

Patients who remain after the mobility sieve has been applied must be *priority 1* (immediate), *priority 2* (urgent) or *dead*. They are sorted into the appropriate category by looking at simply assessed aspects of airway, breathing and circulation.

Airway patency (not security) is assumed in conscious patients and is assessed in the unconscious by performing a simple opening manoeuvre (chin lift and jaw thrust) and seeing if breathing occurs. Patients who cannot breathe despite an open airway are *dead*. Some patients may need a simple airway adjunct to maintain airway patency, which can be inserted at this stage. Patients who breathe after their airway is opened are *priority 1*.

Those who are breathing have their respiratory rate counted. If the respiratory rate is low (less than 10 breaths/min) or high (more than 30 breaths/min), then the casualty is *priority 1* (immediate) (Figure 59.6).

If the rate is normal (10–30 breaths/min) then an assessment of circulation is carried out (Figure 59.7).

The cardiovascular component of the triage sieve is an assessment of the pulse rate. The pulse rate is measured and a cut-off of 120 beats per minute used to differentiate between the priorities.

Every effort should be made to stop frank external exsanguinating haemorrhage at this stage. Time is of the essence and this task must be left to follow-up treatment staff if it is not accomplished rapidly.

The triage sieve (Figure 59.8) should take no more than 20 seconds for each non-ambulant patient, and first-look triage can therefore be done very rapidly. This "broad-brush" approach gives some urgently needed direction to the health service response which can then be focused on the *priority 1* patients (Figure 59.9).

Triage sort

Following the triage sieve, on arrival in the casualty clearing centre patients are triaged using a more detailed

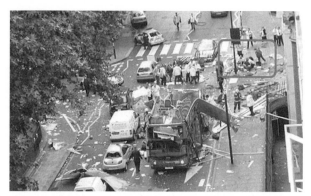

Figure 59.9 Priority 1 patients at a major incident

method. This is the *triage sort* which is based on three parameters:

- respiratory rate
- systolic blood pressure
- Glasgow Coma Scale.

A score for each of these is assigned to the patient (Table 59.3).

The sum of these three scores is the *triage revised trauma score* (TRTS). This method can be used to assign triage priorities (Table 59.4).

A worked example of the triage sort is given in Table 59.5.

It should be remembered that patients can deteriorate – or get better! If this occurs, reassessment of the triage category will be required. Although more time consuming than the triage sieve, the triage sort is more accurate and can be used to prioritize further treatment and evacuation.

Triage is dynamic

CRAMS

An alternative triage system used by some UK ambulance services is the CRAMS system.

> **C**irculation
> **R**espiration
> **A**bdomen and thorax
> **M**otor response
> **S**peech

The CRAMS score is calculated by adding the five values together (Box 59.1).

The triage category is then assigned as shown in Table 59.6.

Triage labelling

It is essential that everyone involved in the response is kept aware of the current triage status of the casualties. This simple measure will reduce needless duplication of effort and will ensure that the overall management plan (which will

Table 59.3 The triage sort 1–1 scoring

Physiological parameter	Measured value	Score
Respiratory rate (breaths/min)	10–29	4
	>29	3
	6–9	2
	1–5	1
	0	0
Systolic blood pressure (mmHg)	90	4
	76–89	3
	50–75	2
	1–49	1
	0	0
Glasgow coma scale score	13–15	4
	9–12	3
	6–8	2
	4–5	1
	3	0

Table 59.4 Triage priorities using the TRTS

Category	Priority	TRTS
Immediate	T1	1–9
Urgent	T2	10–11
Delayed	T3	12
Dead	T4	0

Table 59.5 An example of the triage sort

A 28-year-old male has lost control of his motorcycle and skidded and hit a fence. On arrival he has a respiratory rate of 32, a systolic blood pressure of 85 and a Glasgow Coma Score of 10. His triage score can therefore be calculated as follows.

		Score
Respiratory rate	32	3
Systolic blood pressure	85	3
Glasgow Coma Score	10	3
Total		9

Using the Triage Revised Trauma Score, he therefore has a priority of T1.

Box 59.1 The CRAMS score

Circulation

2 Normal capillary refill or systolic BP more than 100 mmHg
1 Delayed capillary refill or systolic BP 85–99 mmHg
0 No capillary refill or systolic BP less than 85 mmHg

Respiration

2 Normal respiration
1 Laboured, shallow or rate above 20/min
0 Respiration absent

Abdomen thorax

2 Abdomen not tender
1 Abdomen tender
0 Abdomen rigid, flail chest or penetrating injury

Motor response

2 Normal (obeys commands)
1 Responds only to pain
0 Postures or no response

Speech

2 Normal speech (oriented)
1 Confused or inappropriate
0 Nil or unintelligible sounds

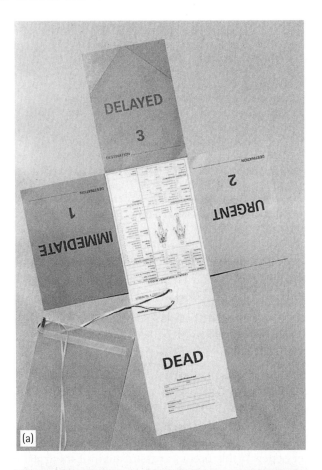

(a)

Table 59.6 Triage categories using the CRAMS score

Priority	CRAMS score	Mortality (%)
Immediate (red)	<6	15–100
Urgent (yellow)	7	3
Delayed (green)	8–10	0–0.5

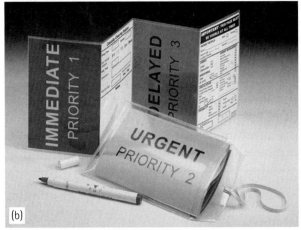

(b)

Figure 59.10 Triage cards. (a) Cruciform card; (b) concertina type

be heavily dependent on the triage status of the patients) does not go awry.

The best cards currently available are cruciform (i.e. in the shape of a cross – Figure 59.10a) or concertina shape (Figure 59.10b). Folding the corners of the cruciform card into the middle causes the card to become rectangular; the colour and markings that remain visible depend on the way in which the folds are made so the card can show any priority. If the priority changes it is simple to adjust the card so that it shows the appropriate colour and markings. This system elegantly overcomes the problems inherent to dynamic triage in that category changes are simple and clinical notes are secure since only one card is ever used for each patient. Additionally, there is no reason why the card initially placed on the patient during or immediately after the triage sieve cannot be used at all subsequent stages of triage.

The disadvantage of the cruciform card is that because the categories are so easily changed, the method is open to abuse by the patients and their relatives. The Mettag triage card is in widespread use in Europe (Figure 59.11). A disadvantage of this system is that patients can only deteriorate on the same card, as the category is indicated using a tear-off strip: any improvement in the patient's condition requires a new card.

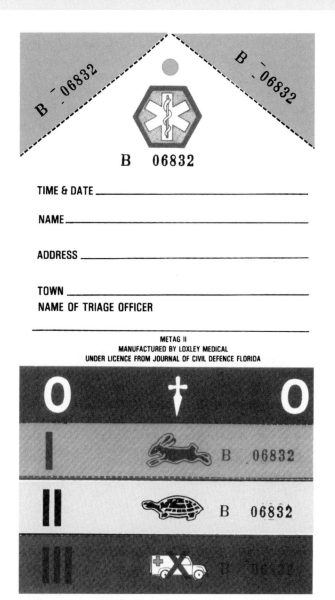

Figure 59.11 The Mettag triage label

determining treatment and transport priorities, the medical response will be suboptimal and patients will suffer.

Although triage is an unfamiliar process to most clinicians, dealing as it does with the management of groups of patients rather than concentrating on the detailed management of a single patient, it is straightforward as long as the algorithms are followed.

Triage is a dynamic process and a patient's triage category will change as his condition improves or deteriorates, with or without treatment. Similarly, it is inevitable that some patients will be assigned to an incorrect category at the initial triage stage: this will be corrected as the triage and treatment process progresses.

FURTHER READING

Advanced Life Support Group 2002 Major incident medical management and support. BMJ Books, London

CONCLUSION

In any system where patient numbers and injury severity mean that there will be a shortage of medical resources, triage is the key component in ensuring the most appropriate use of what is available. Without an effective way of

Chapter 60

The ambulance service at mass gatherings

INTRODUCTION

Mass gathering medicine is a new development in prehospital care and is only a modification of our routine work, frequently providing light relief, a training opportunity (particularly for contingency planning) and a wide range of new experiences.

A mass gathering is defined as a collection of 1 000 people or more and the emergencies that may occur depend on the people, the venue and the environment. Some mass gatherings, such as political marches, rallies and local derby sports matches, may give rise to outbreaks of violence, often

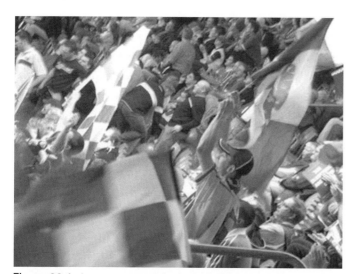

Figure 60.1 A recent mass gathering at a football match

exacerbated by alcohol. Peaceful gatherings, even if attracting crowds in their millions such as Papal masses, may be totally uneventful. However, in any mass gathering the individual members of the crowd are at risk from day-to-day minor and major medical crises, as well as accidents associated with both the venue and the sheer volume of the crowd.

CASUALTY ESTIMATES

Casualty figures reported at mass gatherings range from 0.11 per thousand to 9.0 per thousand. Surprisingly, the lower figure relates to a 1982 Rolling Stones concert with an audience of 92 000. A low figure (1.6 per thousand) was also reported for the estimated 3 500 000 people who attended the Los Angeles Olympic Games (despite the length of the event). The higher figures relate to the US air show and the US Open golf tournament; at first this was thought to be because it attracted an older population but this would not account for a New Zealand music festival reporting a casualty rate of 9 per thousand in 1973. Part of the difference may be due to the absence of a standard method of recording casualty statistics but weather conditions and other factors cause wide daily variations at similar events.

CASUALTY TYPES

Mass gatherings worldwide seem to produce medical statistics that are surprisingly similar: about 20–25% of the work is caused by preexisting disease (such as diabetes mellitus, bronchitis, epilepsy and ischaemic heart disease) and 20–30% is due to trauma such as sprains, strains and abrasions, burns and scalds, foreign bodies in the eye and the inevitable blisters at events that involve walking around all day. Environment-related illnesses are common – heat stroke and exhaustion in the warmer zones, hypothermia (especially associated with alcohol excess) in colder climates. The occasional collapse due to cardiac arrest, stroke or a drug-related incident is seen at many events. Minor complaints such as headache, allergic conjunctivitis, sore throats and non-specific maladies make up the rest. The voluntary aid societies keep statistics on the ailments they see, which is a useful guide when planning dressing and drug requirements.

Just as conditions seem to vary little from event to event, the same applies from year to year. If an event is expected to last several days, plans must be in place to replenish supplies.

PLANNING

Contingency planning for such events should always include major incident planning, working closely with venue owners, the organizers of the gathering, the police and local authorities. As a member of the ambulance service, one may well be aware of existing plans but familiarity with the local geography, evacuation routes and specific amendments to baseline plans for a specific event is mandatory. An empty stadium is easy to memorize but once filled to capacity, it offers a great challenge when trying to evacuate part of the crowd (or even a single casualty).

MASS GATHERINGS AND THE LAW

In the UK interest in mass gatherings has been spurred on by several football tragedies, notably the Bradford fire in 1985, and the report of the subsequent inquiry undertaken by Mr Justice Popplewell, and the Hillsborough stadium disaster in 1989 (Figure 60.2). The latter was seen by millions of people worldwide through the media and caused a public outcry. Lord Justice Taylor chaired the public inquiry and made many wide-reaching recommendations in his comprehensive report. Many measures to ensure safety were not medical and the Football Licensing Authority (which had first been set up under Section 8 of the Football Spectators Act 1989 as a direct result of the Heisel stadium tragedy, in order to oversee the introduction of the Football Membership Scheme) was asked to take the lead in ensuring the implementation of certain key Taylor Report recommendations concerning safety at football grounds. These included the operating of a licensing scheme for grounds at which designated football matches were played, advising the government on the introduction of all-seater stadia and keeping under review the discharge by local authorities of

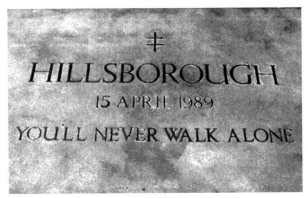

Figure 60.2 The Hillsborough disaster

their function under the Safety of Sports Grounds Act 1975. The Football Membership Scheme itself was shelved after the final Hillsborough report.

Until the Popplewell and Taylor Reports were published, the bible for mass gatherings was the HMSO publication known everywhere as the "Green Guide": *A guide to safety at sports grounds*, first produced in 1975 and regularly updated since, the latest edition being in 1997. This now incorporates the Taylor recommendations, which are seen as appropriate not only for football but all sports gatherings. For the wider health, safety and welfare issues involved in preparation for music and similar mass gatherings, the Green Guide should be read in association with the Purple Guide (*The event safety guide*, published by the Health and Safety Executive).

In the Taylor Report, overall responsibility for medical matters at football stadia was given to the ambulance service. After the report was published, Myles Gibson, honorary medical adviser to the Football Association, was asked to make recommendations on the implementation of the spirit and the letter of Lord Justice Taylor's recommendations concerning first aid, medical facilities and ambulances. He consulted with medical, ambulance and voluntary aid society colleagues and the recommendations were interpreted as follows.

Recommendation 64

"There should be at each sports ground at each match at least one first aider per 1000 spectators."

The club should have responsibility for securing such attendance. As first aiders are trained to work in pairs and have rest needs too, a minimum of three first aiders at any match is required. A first aider should be defined as a person who holds the standard certificate of the voluntary aid societies. Local knowledge may decree that on occasions such as local derbies, more first aiders may be needed.

Recommendation 65

"There should be at each designated sports ground one or more first aid rooms. The number of such rooms and the

equipment to be maintained within them should be specified by the local authority and subject to minimum standards."

To provide a guide to the equipment needed, the Gibson Report looked at the list of items agreed by the Scottish Football Association (predominantly the dressings needed to equip a first aid room) and added to this further equipment needed for resuscitation as well as a list of emergency drugs, including those to be carried by the crowd doctor. Equipment for cardiopulmonary resuscitation is mandatory.

Recommendation 66a

"At every match where the number of spectators is expected to exceed 2000, the club should employ a medical practitioner to be present and available to deal with any medical exigencies at the ground. He should be trained and competent in advanced first aid. He should be present at the ground at least an hour before kick off and should remain until half an hour after the end of the match. His whereabouts should be known to those in the police control room and he should be immediately contactable."

Recommendation 66b

"At any match where the number of spectators is not expected to exceed 2000, the club should make arrangements to enable a medical practitioner to be summoned immediately to deal with any medical emergency at the ground. The arrangements made should be known to those in the police control room."

Although the requirement is for the club and police to be aware of the doctor's whereabouts, it is more important that the ambulance service knows too and works closely with the doctor, maintaining contact (preferably through the ambulance radio network) and cooperating on the ambulance plans for the match, including any exercises.

Since these recommendations came out, more than 700 doctors have gone through a one-day introductory course for football crowd doctors, some more than once, and doctors from other mass gathering events have joined them. A more detailed refresher course is also held and doctors are expected to attend every 3 years. This may not produce a cadre of doctors highly skilled in resuscitation techniques but they are competent and aware of the role of the ambulance service and their place in the medical response. Doctors providing cover at the Premier Division football events are required to have attended both days of this course. More and more doctors are taking the Diploma in Immediate Medical Care under the aegis of the Royal College of Surgeons of Edinburgh. Such doctors have to demonstrate their skills in many medical and surgical emergencies and major incident management. Many are already known to their local ambulance service as members of the

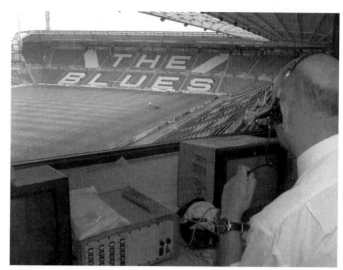

Figure 60.3 A Premier League football ground control centre

British Association for Immediate Care (BASICS), having worked together at the roadside. It is likely that the Football Association will increase its requirements for crowd doctors, insisting they hold this diploma in future.

For longer events, doctors often make arrangements with a local pharmacy for drug resupply rather than carrying very large stocks.

Recommendation 67

"At least one fully equipped ambulance from or approved by the appropriate ambulance authority should be in attendance at all matches with an expected crowd of 5000 or more."

Recommendation 67 allows a busy ambulance service to delegate attendance to an appropriate private or voluntary ambulance service, but the responsibility remains with the statutory ambulance service. It is usually when this service deems that more than one ambulance is required that other non-service vehicles are used. The vehicle should be equipped to paramedic standard and have at least one paramedic in the crew. In the event of a major incident this vehicle may initially be used as the control vehicle rather than for patient transport. However, many Premier and First Division football grounds have excellent multidisciplinary control rooms, equipped with adequate communications, including with ambulance control, where the silver control can be established.

Recommendation 68

"The number of ambulances to be in attendance for matches where larger crowds are expected should be

specified by the local authority after consultation with the ambulance service and should be made a requirement of the safety certificate."

It is important that services are aware of this and do not have arbitrary numbers dictated to them by the local authority through the safety certificate.

Recommendation 69

"The need for liaison between the various people in ensuring safety is encouraged by recommending a liaison meeting each season and before each match."

This seasonal meeting should include representatives from the club, preferably the club secretary and safety officer, a representative from the local authority, all the statutory services, the accident and emergency consultants from the hospitals designated to take casualties in the event of a major incident, and the club and crowd doctors. This is a vitally important meeting and must take place at a time when all senior people can attend, rather than sending deputies. This meeting sets the standards, deals with problems from the previous season and reviews any changes – structural, managerial or legislative. The future events in the season should accommodate both prematch and postmatch meetings where day-to-day strategy can be reviewed.

Recommendation

"A major incident equipment vehicle designed and equipped to deal with up to 50 casualties should be deployed in addition to other ambulance attendance at a match where a crowd in excess of 25 000 is expected."

Again, this is left to the discretion of the local ambulance service and many feel the major incident vehicle should be present at smaller gatherings where trouble may be expected.

CONCLUSION

Although this chapter has concentrated on sports grounds, particularly football, the lessons learned at such venues are providing guidance for other events. Courses relating to mass gatherings have been held at the Civil Emergencies Planning College at Easingwold and useful publications and resources are held at the college library. The college's publication on crowd-related disasters draws on experience gained from a wide range of disasters.

With these recommendations in place and the analysis of the morbidity and mortality rates of the many mass gathering events worldwide, mass gathering medicine is becoming a recognized and rewarding aspect of paramedic work.

FURTHER READING

Emergency Planning College 1992 Lessons learned from crowd-related disasters. Paper 4. Home Office Emergency Planning College, Easingwold

Football Licensing Authority 1994 Football club contingency planning: a guide to safety management and practices and appointment, training and duties of stewards at football grounds. FLA, London

HMSO 1975 Safety of Sports Grounds Act 1975. HMSO, London

HMSO 1997 A guide to safety at sports grounds, 5th edn (the Green Guide). HMSO, London

HSE 1999 The event safety guide: a guide to health, safety and welfare at music and similar events. HSE Books, Sudbury

Popplewell (initial) 1985 Report of the Committee of Enquiry into Crowd Safety and Control at Sports Grounds. HMSO, London

Sports Council/Football Stadia Development Committee (year) Stadium control rooms. Sports Council, London

Taylor (initial) 1990 The Hillsborough stadium disaster 15th April 1989. HMSO, London

Section

12

ADMINISTRATION, ETHICS AND THE LAW

Chapter 61

Record keeping in prehospital care

CHAPTER CONTENTS

INTRODUCTION

Record keeping is viewed as a major chore by both para-medics and doctors involved in prehospital care. The acknowledged stresses faced in the field by these individuals pale into insignificance compared with the sight of the standard A3 sheet, at the end of a difficult patient care episode.

"No-one ever looks at them", *"They throw them straight into the bin"*, *"I've already given them a complete verbal report"*, are all familiar complaints which are expressed while completing the prehospital record. The importance attached by para-medics to keeping a good and accurate record is often not high, usually because the value of the exercise is not apparent, and as a result the information generated is frequently incomplete and of questionable accuracy. However, the real value of accurate prehospital record keeping must not be underestimated.

WHY KEEP GOOD RECORDS?

The report form is a statement of one's professional attitude to practice. A well-documented and accurate patient record creates the immediate image of a competent and professional practitioner in the eyes of the reader. An incomplete and poorly completed record creates the opposite impression. The absence of any report form at all for the incident leaves one even more vulnerable, as it questions the very professional basis of one's clinical practice.

It is important to remember that the hospital copy is retained within the patient's hospital file and may well be referred to for information hours, days or weeks after admission by hospital medical and nursing staff. This is particularly the case since hospitals are notoriously bad at listening to, and recording, verbal handovers at the time of admission. On occasion, that report form will be the sole source of information regarding the circumstances and mechanism of injury as well as on-scene findings and interventions.

An accurately completed report form can be a very good ally when, for example, a solicitor's letter arrives 2 years after the incident threatening legal action because of an apparent omission of care. The incident itself may well have long faded from memory, but unearthing the completed report form can aid greatly in refuting allegations and refreshing one's memory of the event. In addition, the names of all professionals who have been involved in the care of a patient should be clearly recorded *in full*.

> Good notes – good defence
> Poor notes – poor defence
> No notes – no defence

If procedures have not been recorded, it will leave one vulnerable to the allegation that if it was not written down, it was not done. The form must therefore be viewed as a legal document and stored safely for future recall.

> If it was not written down, it was not done!

Because the report may act as a record for future recall of an incident, it is worth noting any peculiar aspects, especially in incidents likely to result in police or other legal action, such as fatal road accidents and assaults. In addition, if a patient (or his relatives or friends) is aggressive or unco-operative, this should be recorded. Unfortunately a signifi-cant number of complaints are made by those whose own behaviour leaves the most to be desired. There is no point in retrospective allegations of unacceptable behaviour if these were not recorded at the time.

The report form is an integral part of the clinical record and merits time and commitment to record accurately all relevant prehospital data.

AUDIT

Many prehospital care practices have never been subjected to scientific scrutiny. Similarly, the benefits of many proced-ures used in accident and emergency departments have yet to be scientifically proved. It is important for the advance-ment and validation of prehospital care to evaluate aspects of care in order to determine whether they result in any patient benefit.

Audit is the process used to assess the effectiveness of a particular clinical intervention and to compare the results with an established standard. Once that comparison has been made, suggestions for improvement can be implemented and the process reassessed in the wake of these changes to see if improvement has occurred (Figure 61.1).

This process, along with scientific research into areas of prehospital practice, is central to any scientific evaluation of prehospital care. It can be used to prove or disprove whether impressions of the effectiveness of practices in a system are correct. It also allows reassessment after changes in practice, to ensure that such changes bring about the intended improvements.

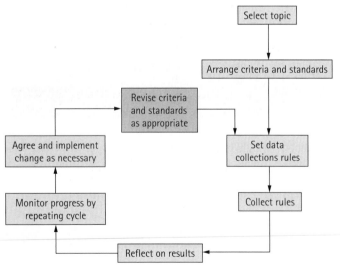

Figure 61.1 The audit loop

Audit and research are impossible without accurate, con-sistent and reliable prehospital data. Virtually all these data will originate from the patient report form and omissions and inaccuracies will minimize the validity of any research. This is not just a minor problem for those who try to analyse the inadequate data. Accurate and scientifically valid proof of the effectiveness of prehospital care is critical if service provision and funding for prehospital ambulance and med-ical care is to be successfully sought from increasingly cash-limited health authority purchasers. In effect, the security of paramedic jobs in the future may depend on careful record-ing of patient data and information now.

An example of a section of a patient data collection form, designed to collect data in the order that the paramedic clin-ically assesses the patient, is shown in Figure 61.2.

As an example, the UK Trauma Audit Research Network (TARN) has a data set for prehospital patient recordings. The use of data and evaluation of the prehospital compon-ent of the care of most of these patients have been frustrated since the outset of the study by the frequent omission from report forms of key data such as respiratory rate.

Trauma scoring as a method of field triage has a number of practical problems, mainly related to time, particularly in major trauma cases. The use of the primary survey as a basic field triage tool in trauma cases appears to work in practice, as any major "ABCD" problem merits a "critical" category and consideration for trauma unit admission.

However, retrospective gathering of trauma scoring data is the key to the effective assessment of the potential merits of prehospital care procedures. Recognition of training deficits within an ambulance service can also be highlighted by accurate and coordinated report form audit. Without this, training efforts may be wasted or misdirected.

Finally, patient safety depends on well-completed report forms. Verbal information about fluid volumes and drug administration given to the accident and emergency depart-ment doctor during the handover may not be passed on to doctors who care for the patient subsequently. Over-dosage of opiate drugs and overinfusion of intravenous fluids have occurred because of the lack of a written report at the handover of a patient, and omissions in the verbal reports.

CONCLUSION

The completion of paperwork is undoubtedly a burden for prehospital carers, but it is one of the most important tasks of the professional paramedic or doctor. The patient's well-being and the professional integrity of the paramedic or doctor may depend on the time and effort spent on com-pleting an accurate patient report form, and therefore few tasks in prehospital medicine can rate more highly than pre-cise record keeping.

BASIC OBSERVATIONS							INTERVENTIONS			
TIME ➤➤➤➤➤➤							OP Airway ☐ NP Airway ☐			
1	AIRWAY	Clear					Suction ☐ ET ☐ NT ☐			
		Obstructed					Attemps ....Success ☐			
2	**BREATHING RATE** ➤➤						Man C-sp immob ☐			
3	Breathing Qual.	Normal					C-sp collar ☐			
		Shallow					Red ☐			
		Deep					Spinal board ☐			
		Laboured					Traction splint			
4	Breath Sounds	Present					Mask ☐ B&M ☐ Assisted ☐			
	Left	Absent					Mechanical ☐			
		Clear					Oxygen ☐ .... %			
		Noisy								
5	Breath Sounds	Present					*Needle cricothyrotomy* ☐			
	Right	Absent					Cannula size........... | Time.............			
		Clear								
		Noisy					*Chest decompression* ☐			
6	**BREATHING RATE** ➤➤						Cannula size........... | Time.............			
7	Pulse	Strong					Left ☐	Right ☐		
		Weak					Site			
		Regular					*CANNULATION*			
		Irregular						No att	Site	✓ ✗
8	Pulse Site	Radial								☐ ☐
		Brachial								☐ ☐
		Femoral								☐ ☐
		Carotid					*INFUSION*			
9	Skin Condition	Normal					Fluid	Time	Finish	Total
		Pale								
		Perspiring								
		Flushed								
10	Capillary Refill	Normal								
		Delayed								
11	Blood Pressure ➤ ➤						*DRUGS*			
12	LOC	Alert					Name	Time	Dose	Batch #
		Voice								
		Pain								
		Unresponsive								
13	Pupils N=normal D=dilated R=reactive		L:	L:	L:	L:				
	c=constricted U/R=unreactive		R:	R:	R:	R:				
14	Oxygen Saturation ➤➤➤									
15	Peak Flow Reading ➤➤➤									
16	Blood Gluc (mmol) ➤➤➤									

Figure 61.2 A patient data collection form

Chapter 62

Communications and despatch

INTRODUCTION

Communications are the cornerstone of a successful emergency medical services operation. Accessibility of the service to the public is the first essential requirement and in this respect, the national 999 emergency telephone system is well known to the population as a whole.

THE 999 CALL

It is vital to have well-trained call-takers and an effective handling system for calls received by the ambulance control centre. Emergency calls must be readily identified on receipt in the control room and details passed directly into the ambulance computer-aided despatch (CAD) system. This permits rapid despatch of an emergency ambulance as soon as the despatcher knows the location of the incident. The call-taker will still be taking further details while the ambulance mobilizes and an update message to confirm location and clinical details is passed by the ambulance controller to the vehicle as it is en route to the emergency.

Additional resources such as paramedic or medical support may be despatched to the scene depending on initial information received. The initial information gathering by the call-taker has to be of the highest quality if appropriate care is to be provided for every emergency.

The new generation of computerized telephone exchanges can provide an enhanced service to emergency service controls, identifying the call-back number and subscriber details (such as address) on receipt of the call. This information can be put directly into the CAD system via an interface, which speeds up mobilization since the call-taker has only to confirm these details with the caller. Some CAD systems are able to hold useful information about the patient's condition and circumstances and may also hold registers of "at-risk" cases such as asthma and anaphylaxis.

Prearrival instructions to the caller about life-saving first-aid procedures should be a feature of every ambulance control centre's service to the public. There is evidence of the effectiveness of "telephone CPR" and the case for prolonging the period of ventricular fibrillation with early basic life support is now convincing.

The ambulance service must concentrate on reducing the time taken for well-trained and well-equipped crews to reach patients with life-threatening problems. If all life-threatening emergencies were attended within 8 minutes by a defibrillator-equipped ambulance crew and telephone-advised CPR were widely used, cardiac arrest survival in the UK could well improve significantly.

PRIORITY DESPATCH

Two systems are in use which provide an enhanced ability to judge the medical priority of incoming emergency calls to the ambulance control centre. These systems allow structured and thorough questioning of the caller, so that more medical detail can be obtained from the initial emergency call. This has a number of advantages. First, it allows better information to be passed to crews en route to emergency calls; this reduces stress and allows the crew to make decisions about the correct approach and selection of appropriate equipment prior to reaching the patient.

Second, a better judgement may be made as to the despatch priority for the ambulance. If it becomes apparent that the

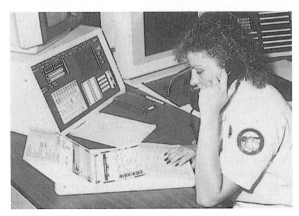

Figure 62.1 Using the AMPDS card set

call is not to a life-threatening emergency, the ambulance crew can be advised by radio to attend without using blue lights and siren, reducing the risk to both the public and the crew. In rural and quieter urban areas, blue light and siren progress makes little time difference in reaching the casualty but in traffic-choked inner cities the difference may be more significant. The despatch system must be both safe and accurate and the tendency of both systems is to err on the side of caution by sending an emergency response in situations where there is doubt. There will, however, be a reduction in unnecessary emergency responses with these systems.

In the UK, the emergency ambulance service is effectively a paramedic-based service. Another function of a medical priority despatch system is to differentiate between calls requiring a response from the ambulance service in the form of a paramedic ambulance rather than an alternative non-paramedic response. Medical triage at the time of the call will allow the screening of non-emergency calls and offer a more appropriate response such as linkage to a primary care cooperative or an NHS Direct nurse-led advice centre.

Finally, a major feature of these systems is the provision of prearrival instructions to emergency callers. This scripted advice extends from looking out for the ambulance and restraining the family dog to basic life support (BLS) instruction. Lives have undoubtedly been saved by advice on BLS and the relief of choking given over the telephone. Ambulance services in the USA have suffered lawsuits as a result of failing to provide prearrival instructions to callers.

There are two prioritized despatch systems which vary in principle. The Advanced Medical Priority Despatch System (AMPDS) is protocol driven and is designed for use by emergency medical despatchers without paramedic training. The second, the Criteria-Based Despatch System (CBDS), is designed as an advisory system for paramedic use in the control centre. There are extensive quality assurance procedures involved in the AMPDS, which have been refined over some 15 years of operation, and the majority of ambulance services in the UK now use the AMPDS (Figure 62.1).

Both systems are based on a set of cards or computer software stratified into individual "Chief Complaint" protocols of guidelines, each with its own specific questions. A base information set including age, sex, breathing status and conscious level precedes each condition-specific card. Computerization of the priority despatch codes into a database facilitates quality assurance, audit and planning.

These systems are an essential part of any modern control centre and the advantages of medical information gathering, better prepared crews, fewer unnecessary emergency responses and life-saving telephone instruction cannot be overstated.

RADIO AND PAGING SYSTEMS

The alert message must reach the ambulance without delay. Telephone contact with an ambulance station and turnout from the station may take up to 1–2 minutes, whereas direct radio alert to a vehicle at a standby location achieves mobilization in around 30 seconds.

Taking longer than 8 minutes to reach a cardiac arrest costs approximately 7–10% of lives per minute of delay. Saving just 90 seconds by more rapid mobilization will save lives.

Ambulance stations are usually in or near town centres. The majority of the population live in the outlying suburbs, where most emergencies occur. Strategic predeployment of ambulances around these population centres will often reduce attendance times.

Ambulances use very high frequency (VHF) radio systems, both fixed in the vehicle and as lower-powered portable handsets. These handsets may be VHF or ultra-high frequency (UHF) linked to a UHF repeater radio linked to the vehicle VHF set (Figure 62.2). Communication is greatly enhanced with the handsets, as crew-to-crew and crew-to-vehicle communication is possible in addition to contact with the control centre.

Many services use an automatic updating system, with status codes sent by radio to update the control centre on vehicle status, without the need for repeated speech updates. This allows a largely speech-free radio system and obviates the need to record times in the control centre. Ambulances can travel with muted radios until the control centre opens up the vehicle radio for a call. The disadvantage of this system is the absence of awareness of the operational situation in the service by crews; they are unable to offer help if nearer to an emergency than a tasked unit or to offer assistance in finding a location for a crew operating in an unfamiliar area.

Most ambulance services are in radio communication with local accident and emergency departments. This is a much better system than telephone relay of information by the control centre. Ambulance crews should have direct "talk-through" of their own priority messages with the receiving senior nurse or doctor in the accident and emergency department. Reluctance of hospital staff to use a radio and the siting of the sets in the reception area and their operation by reception staff are the only major problems in

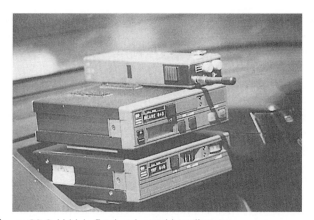

Figure 62.2 Vehicle fixed and portable radio sets

the use of this facility. Crews must present a brief but comprehensive alert message and ideally a proforma for these reports should be provided in consultation with the accident and emergency departments.

One system in use is ASHICE.

A	>	Age
S	>	Sex
H	>	History
I	>	Injuries/illness
C	>	Condition (ECS, TRTS, vital signs)
E	>	Estimated time of arrival

The scarcity of radio frequencies available to ambulance services is a major constraint in providing even more elaborate ambulance–hospital communications. Medical guidance for on-line advice would be far more practical if more radio frequencies were available.

The development of digital trunked radio systems for emergency service use will provide both higher speech quality and more efficient use of radio channels. Interlinking with more elaborate facilities via the CAD system will also be easier with a digital radio system. Mobile computer-based patient report forms are now in use and can be linked to the CAD via the vehicle radio. Direct entry of the call details into a laptop computer and download of patient data to the receiving accident and emergency department during transport of the patient are both feasible.

PAGING

Paging is often used as a duplicate or reserve alerting system for emergency ambulance crews. Alphanumeric paging offers rapid alerting with location and call details as a parallel alert to the radio; it allows a location confirmation if this is in doubt and allows updates to be passed by control without the need to use radio (Figure 62.3). Issuing personal pagers to all crew members allows operational messages to be passed at any time, for instance if extra personnel are needed for a major incident to cover shifts. Paging also

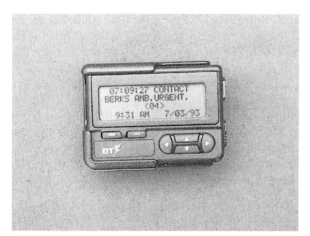

Figure 62.3 Alphanumeric pager

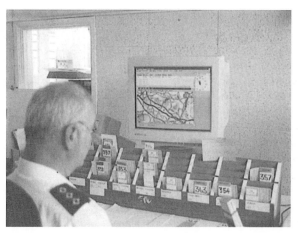

Figure 62.4 Automatic vehicle location system

provides a medium for sending discreet messages to crews, where open channel radio would allow the patient or relatives to be aware of the nature of the message.

These pagers can be linked through the CAD to an internal paging system or linked to a commercial paging agency. This facility, along with other communication services, also provides a basis for the ambulance service to fulfil the communication needs of other NHS agencies.

Cellular telephones may offer a useful facility for major incident management, if the access override system (ACCOLC) has been implemented to provide preferential access in these situations for the emergency services. Certain specialist functions can be performed using cellular telephones, including WAP messaging, fax and electrocardiograph transmissions, but variable performance and recurring costs may still inhibit more widespread use.

AUTOMATIC VEHICLE LOCATING SYSTEMS

A variety of automatic vehicle locating systems (AVLS) are commercially available and in use by most UK ambulance services. They are based either on triangulation of transmitted radio signals or on positioning derived from the global positioning satellite system (Figure 62.4).

These systems use vehicle locator transmitters and a mapping system to show the vehicle location on a visual display unit (VDU) screen. Additional data transmission is possible, including status reporting using keypads in the vehicle. These status and location reports can be integrated with the CAD system. Vehicle location, status and even speed can be displayed on screen and the system can further locate incidents on the mapping screen using six-figure map references incorporated in a gazetteer. This can use the CAD facilities to locate the incident and nearest vehicle on the mapping screen, enabling rapid deployment of the most appropriate ambulance.

CONCLUSION

Effective communication with the public, ambulance vehicles and staff and other emergency services is the key to a responsive ambulance service. Modern performance targets must reflect current medical practice and a knowledge of the needs of their patients, in particular those with a life-threatening emergency.

Operational performance must be geared to providing a rapid response (under 8 minutes in urban areas) to life-threatening emergencies. This is only possible with a rapidly accessible 999 system, medical priority despatch and high-quality radio and pager communications. It also requires the redesign of ambulance systems to enable ambulance numbers to be tailored to fluctuations in demand and vehicles to be located in areas of maximum call density. These changes will enable the service to fulfil its commitment to the public.

Chapter 63

Ethical issues

ETHICS AND MORALS

DEFINITIONS

A dictionary definition of *ethics* is *"a system of moral behaviour"*, something which is, with *ethical*, defined as *"that which is morally good"*. *Moral* is defined as *"of, or based on the difference between good and evil or right and wrong. Pure and honest in character and behaviour"*.

WHAT IS MORALITY?

It is necessary to be "moral" to be "ethical". The problem of the definitions provided is that they do not actually state what conduct constitutes these behaviours. Who defines what is good or evil, right or wrong? Essentially society does and the actions and responses of everyone around us set the standards for what is acceptable and what is not. A consensus is developed through an unwritten process of precedent set over many generations, passed on through the teaching and example of parents, schools and, where appropriate, religious institutions.

An important consideration is the concept that society is a product of culture; because cultures vary in different parts of the world, it is not surprising that each culture's perception of what is moral and ethical will be different. As a paramedic, one is privileged to be involved in working intimately with people from many different ethnic communities and it is important to be aware that there may be differences in their moral and ethical beliefs. These must be respected and individuals should not necessarily be judged by the standards that one adopts for oneself. It should be remembered that each society generates its own perceptions and rules of good and evil, right and wrong and that none of these necessarily represents the correct or only view. In some cultures the relationship between men and women and the individual roles of each sex are seen as being very different from that generally accepted by Western society. When behavioural patterns are encountered which are different from those that arise from one's own society's norm, it may seem that one is encountering prejudice or sexism. In reality, some cultures do not share what is after all a Western concept and should not therefore be judged adversely if they do not subscribe to "conventional" culturally based beliefs.

On the other hand, it is our own ethical and moral values that we should use to measure our personal behaviour. They are what form our conscience and provide us with guidance as to what is right and wrong in our own actions. Generally, if one listens to one's conscience, one feels comfortable about what one does but if it is ignored and the nagging voice of doubt or self-criticism is acted against, second thoughts are likely to result. If it feels wrong, then it probably is!

ETHICAL DILEMMAS

The most fundamental ethical dilemmas arise from a conflict between conscience and ego. This occurs when one "knows" something is wrong but the desire for personal gain suggests that one should break one's own internal rule system. What happens most commonly under circumstances such as this is that we rationalize "good" reasons for deviating from our normal code of moral conduct. For example, it is not unusual to be offered "tips" by grateful patients. Unfortunately this generosity is most often displayed by those least able to afford it, such as the elderly whose only income is a small pension.

The argument most often voiced for accepting tips is that patients only offer what they can afford and would be offended if refused. In reality this is unlikely to be true. The offering of tips is probably an unconscious response to the pressure of another norm: that of providing gratuities to those in "service" occupations, who were traditionally poorly paid. There are many logical reasons as to why acceptance of money could be judged by society at large as unethical.

- Ambulance paramedics earn far more than most pensioners.
- Patients have already paid for their use of the ambulance service (and hence the wages of its employees) via their National Insurance contributions and by tipping they are in effect paying again.
- Ambulance paramedics have the controlling stake in their relationship with subsequently vulnerable patients and should not abuse this.
- Employing ambulance trusts typically have rules stating that staff should not accept gratuities.
- Patients who give gifts may feel that they subsequently have the right to preferential treatment and if this is not forthcoming, can become upset or angry. This type of manipulative behaviour can be very difficult for ambulance staff to cope with and may unfairly prejudice the interests of other patients who are unable or unwilling to give tips.

Nurses and fire-fighters are rarely offered gifts of money in gratitude for their services, nor do they expect them. The reasons for this difference are likely to be complex but may possibly centre around the view of the ambulance professional as a "driver" (particularly common among the elderly), which is the very image the modern ambulance service has tried to avoid.

Other ethical dilemmas are more complex and occur when a society's unwritten guidelines for personal conduct are unclear or at conflict with each other.

CASE HISTORY 1

You attend a road accident involving a car that has hit a bridge. The passengers consist of a family of three: father (who was driving), mother and 6-year-old daughter. On arrival everyone is out of the car. You take care of the father. During your examination you discover a needle and syringe in his clothing. You challenge him and he admits that he is a heroin addict and had "*shot up*" prior to getting in the car.

Should you tell the police? The driver has clearly broken the law and by his actions endangered the life of his family and other road users. The information you have received has come to you as part of your therapeutic relationship: are you bound by the rules of confidentiality?

Discussion

There is probably no right or wrong answer to this or other similar dilemmas. Opinion will be divided depending on an individual's life experiences and cultural background and society's current standards of behaviour. Perhaps the best approach is to focus, as a caregiver, entirely on the patient, addressing his immediate needs and maintaining confidentiality. It is not appropriate for paramedics to stand in judgement on others and we must therefore avoid imposing our standards of behaviour and world view of what is right or wrong. However, if the information one receives indicates that future harm may be caused by the behaviour of the patient and, furthermore, that such harm may be prevented by timely action on your part, it may well be appropriate to inform the doctor in charge of the patient's case, who can then consider what action is appropriate.

FIELD TRIALS

Paramedics are occasionally asked to participate in the field trials of new drugs (or new applications of drugs in the field) and medical devices. These trials must be approved by both the Trust's Research Governance Committee and a local or multicentre research ethics committee. The role of an ethics committee is primarily to act as the patients' advocate. Its members must ensure that, where possible, the consent of each patient to participate in the study is gained or, if this is not possible, that consent is given by the patient's immediate relatives.

"Consent" requires that patients fully understand:

- that they are being invited to participate in a study
- that they have the right to refuse to take part
- the purpose of the study
- the potential beneficial effects (if known) of the drug or device
- any potential risks
- any side-effects that have occurred in previous usage of the drug or device.

The ethics committee must also ensure that patients are given no inducement to participate in the study. Inducements may include financial reward, gifts or a promise of speedier treatment. The committee must ensure that the study is reasonable in its design and that in their best judgement is likely to produce a valid result. It is a primary responsibility to ensure that the risk involved for consenting patients is minimal.

The membership of ethics committees will typically consist of physicians, nurses, scientists of appropriate background and representatives of the community at large. It is generally accepted that the community representatives should outnumber the medically trained and that the chairperson of the group should be drawn from their ranks. Where possible patients should be included in the committee. For a study in which ambulance personnel are participating the membership of a paramedic would be invaluable, although this individual should probably be drawn from the ranks of a service not directly involved in the trial. Ethics committee members also have the potential to contribute positively to the development of ambulance service policy in other matters discussed later in this chapter. The Medicines for Human Use (Clinical Trials) Regulations 2004 has now made it illegal for any clinical trial to be commenced or conducted without prior authorization from the Medicines and Healthcare Products Regulatory Agency (MHRA) and obtaining a favourable opinion from an ethics committee. The Regulations also establish a "cascade" system by which a decision can be made on behalf of an incapacitated adult whether to consent or refuse on their behalf to their participation in a trial. In the first instance, informed consent is sought from a person whose relationship to the patient is suitable for them to act as a legal representative. If no-one is able to take this responsibility, consent may be given by the doctor primarily responsible for the care of the patient, unless he is involved in the conduct of the trial. In this case, or if they are unable to give consent, the health care provider may nominate a person not involved in the conduct of the trial to decide consent or refusal.

The process for approval of studies is necessarily bureaucratic in order to protect the interest of patients. It would be highly unethical for ambulance paramedics to introduce new equipment or drug regimens on an experimental basis without this type of approval and would almost certainly result in a breach of both protocol and their contract of employment.

MAKING ASSUMPTIONS

Circumstances often tempt paramedics to judge the integrity of certain types of patients or the validity of their complaint. We hate to see our service "abused" and often justify our attitude with a stated desire to reserve resources for those patients "who truly need them". Unfortunately, attempting to filter out the so-called "abusers" without careful checks and balances (such as physically examining the patient) will also result in inadvertently and inevitably filtering out those who demonstrably need emergency medical aid. It is a common feature of emergency services all over the world that they spend much of their time responding in emergency mode to what turn out to be non-emergency calls. Nevertheless, it is undoubtedly better to overrespond than to underrespond.

It would be unreasonable to expect ambulance personnel to be entirely free from personal prejudices and preconceptions; however, it is essential to prevent these attitudes affecting clinical practice. All personnel should identify their own prejudices clearly and make a consistent and disciplined effort to avoid being influenced by them. For example, the common distaste for individuals who abuse alcohol and who make a public nuisance of themselves has led to many problems. Patients have died in police cells from airway obstruction or alcoholic poisoning because ambulance staff did not

wish to burden themselves or hospital staff with their treatment. Even in hospital, this prejudice can lead to inappropriate care (or lack of care) for patients who appear to be drunk, but are actually suffering from medical or traumatic conditions.

In order to protect oneself and one's patients from the results of such human preconceptions and prejudices, it is necessary to be disciplined regarding never judging the integrity of the patient, relatives, bystanders or other professional caregivers.

CASE HISTORY 2

You respond following a 999 call to a man who is unable to talk. On arrival you are met by a colleague of the patient. The colleague appears friendly and sympathetic and tells you that the patient is a malingerer with a poor attendance record and a multitude of complaints. "Now he's pretending he can't talk!"

The patient indicates by vigorous and theatrical hand signals that he is unable to utter a sound. He appears unconvincing and when you give him a piece of paper and a pen, attempts to explain that he is unable to write either. You are convinced he is a fraud, but take him to hospital anyway.

Two months later you receive a letter of grateful thanks from the same patient who tells you that he has just been discharged from hospital following a stroke which affected the speech centre of the brain, resulting in expressive dysphasia – inability to talk. Interestingly, this area of the brain also controls other forms of expression such as writing skills.

LIVING WILLS

The legal status of "living wills" in the UK is vague and needs clarification and these documents are therefore currently best viewed on an ethical basis. Living wills (also known as "advance directives") are documents in which people state their wishes for restricted medical care should they become seriously ill in the future. It is a method of withholding consent to treatment in the event that any future illness incapacitates them to the extent that they cannot express their wishes.

The legal issues associated with "living wills" have been the subject of much discussion. A precedent was set regarding the validity of advance directives by a ruling by the House of Lords in the Tony Bland case. This stated that it would be unlawful to give treatment against the previously expressed wishes of the patient. Consequently, although no statutory legislation exists, this precedent implies that advance directives will have force in common law. As a result, if a caregiver fails to follow the clear instructions of a patient regarding limitation of treatment, even if the instructions are given in advance, that patient will have a right of action for trespass against the person. Additionally, the Law Commission published a consultation paper in March 1995 that included draft legislation regarding "living wills". Some or all of its recommendations may eventually find their way into law, conferring statutory rights on patients enacting advance directives and providing further guidance for healthcare workers.

The circumstances in which an advance directive will have the greatest impact for paramedics are where an individual with a "living will" suffers a cardiac arrest out of hospital. Ethically, it would probably be generally agreed that the wishes of the victim should be honoured; it is not a pleasant thought that we as citizens potentially have no control over our destiny, even in death. On the other hand, as the legal status of these directives is so vague, there may not be incontrovertible evidence available in an emergency that such a document is genuine or does indeed represent the patient's current wishes. There is a potential for unscrupulous or even well-meaning relatives to produce "fake" documentation. Withholding resuscitation attempts under these circumstances may not represent the patient's wishes and is unlikely to be in their best interest.

There is no universal answer to the problem of how paramedics should respond when presented with a "living will". The most important step is for each service to establish a clear written policy on how they would wish their staff to act. This should be formulated by either the local paramedic steering group or the ethics committee and in any event, must have medical as well as managerial approval. The British Medical Association has produced guidelines for doctors that will form a useful reference point. Any ambulance service policy would also need to encompass the delivery of telephone cardiopulmonary resuscitation (CPR) instructions, as provision of this type of aid is becoming increasingly common in ambulance controls.

The state of Florida in the USA has issued legislation to mandate how "living wills" should be enacted, verified and responded to. It recognizes the right of individuals to determine their fate and the medical care they receive and provides a standard form for documenting their wishes in this regard. This has to be signed by the person and a physician, who must confirm that the patient is of sound mind at the time the document is enacted. Medical staff are required to honour "living wills", with the strict provision that they must see the signed original form and evidence that this relates to the patient concerned. Despite this, telephone CPR instructions are normally given prior to the arrival of medical care at the incident, as despatchers are of course unable to see these documents; however, relatives are not obliged to follow these instructions. Once reasonable proof of the veracity of a document has been provided to personnel at the scene, failure to comply with the patient's wishes as set down in the document is viewed as assault.

There is a need for similar legislation in this country, not only to protect patients' interests and wishes but also to define the role and actions of responders and to protect them after the event. Until this has been enacted the most important action for individual ambulance services is to establish a written policy.

"DO NOT RESUSCITATE" ORDERS

"Do not resuscitate" orders take the form of written and signed instructions from the physician responsible for the care of the patient concerned. They are developed after discussion with, and the consent of, the patient (where possible), relatives and other healthcare professionals associated with the individual affected. With the advent of registration paramedics are now responsible for their own actions and may be called to justify them where necessary. The paramedic therefore has a degree of discretion within which to act, dependent upon the situation. Clearly the ethical position is that the wishes of the patient, family and their doctor responsible for ongoing care should be followed but there may be circumstances which are deemed inappropriate to the order; for example, a patient who has a simple blocked airway after choking on food should not be left untreated simply because of a "do not resuscitate" order relating to an ongoing terminal condition.

If possible, "do not resuscitate" orders should be confirmed with the doctor face to face and clarification sought as necessary. "Do not resuscitate" orders must always be in writing in order to protect the interests of caregivers other than the physician making the order. During interhospital transfers such documentation should accompany the patient as a part of their medical notes. If there is any doubt about the situation in which one finds oneself, basic life support should be commenced and radio or telephone guidance requested from the local hospital.

REGISTRATION

Registration is covered in more detail in Chapter 64 but it is worth noting here the reliance upon ethics in all medical professions covered by state registration. Whilst there will always be some procedures which are beyond the remit of paramedics, the decision-making process within the range of skills available is now considered much more of an individual responsibility. Paramedics may be called before the Health Professions Council to justify their actions or lack of action in a particular situation. A commitment to acting in the best interests of the patient, to prevent death or deterioration and to promote recovery, is the ethical basis of the profession. It is vital always to act in the way one considers to be, and can justify as being, in the best interest of the patient at the time (but always within one's scope of practice). If this principle is followed any criticism or complaint can be successfully countered.

Chapter 64

Legal issues

CHAPTER CONTENTS

INTRODUCTION

In the UK paramedical staff are fortunate that litigation has historically been relatively rare. However, litigation is now on the increase and far more responsibility is placed on ambulance trusts for the financial liability resulting from successful actions against them than was the case in the past.

While it is generally true that an employer is legally liable for the actions of its employees, it would be unwise for an individual paramedic to feel immune from legal action. Civil law allows anyone to sue anyone else, whether their claim is justified or not. Regardless of whether a case is successfully defended or whether an individual practitioner or their employer is liable, the experience of having one's actions questioned and dissected in court is never pleasant. This chapter aims to identify those areas where one can plan one's conduct in order to lessen the chances of such an experience.

THE STATUS OF THE PARAMEDIC

In September 2000 the professional status of the paramedic has been formally recognized in the United Kingdom through the Paramedics Board of the Council for Professions Supplementary to Medicines, set up under the Professions Supplementary to Medicine Act 1960. This important change,

which applies only to paramedics, not technicians, has put much greater responsibility on individual paramedics to maintain ongoing professional education and standards of discipline. In 2001, the responsibility for the registration of paramedics moved to the Health Professions Council (HPC). Legislation has now made it illegal for someone to use the title "paramedic" (or any title containing this word) unless they hold valid registration with the HPC. Anyone who wishes to work as a paramedic in the National Health Service must be state registered.

A complaints procedure exists which allows for a paramedic to be removed from the register if he or she is found guilty of "infamous conduct". The definition of infamous conduct is itself vague and the HPC explicitly retains the right to find someone guilty of infamous conduct at their discretion, even where the offence is not of the same nature as any of the examples which they give for guidance. It follows that once closure of title has occurred the loss of registration will lead to an inability to gain employment as a paramedic anywhere within the public sector.

The November 1992 amendment to the 1983 Medicines Order provides the legislative authority for the administration of a limited list of prescription-only medications (POMs) by paramedics and also addresses the issue of invasive techniques such as intubation and venepuncture. These skills are restricted to those holding a certificate of proficiency in ambulance paramedic skills issued by the Secretary of State (formerly through the NHS Training Directorate (NHSTD), now the Institute for Health Care Development (IHCD)). Since practitioners holding such a certificate are now those eligible for state registration it could be assumed that this legislation now applies only to those holding registration. Since October 2000 the list of licensed medications has been further expanded to include such drugs as benzyl penicillin and morphine sulphate and the intention is to regularly review the list in order to ensure that it is kept up to date and appropriate. Furthermore, after recent media criticism of varying regional practice, an integrated national paramedic guidelines manual, utilizing a best evidence base, was introduced in 2002. The manual has been produced under the supervision of the Joint Royal Colleges Ambulance Liaison Committee (JRCALC). Regional needs for additional drugs can still be met using a Patient Group Directive signed by a Trust's Chief Executive, Medical Director and a senior pharmacist, but there will be considerable political pressure to ensure that this is not used in a way that again promotes regional differences.

"Bogus" paramedics are an increasingly common problem despite state registration. In the event of an unrecognized healthcare professional attending the scene of an accident, it is essential to ask them to identify themselves: doctors who are members of BASICS (the British Association for Immediate Care) or a valid immediate-care scheme will carry identification. If necessary, individuals who are unable to prove a genuine reason for attendance should be escorted from the scene by the police.

CONSENT

Patient consent is required before providing any form of treatment to the victim of a medical illness or trauma incident. Consent may take one of three forms according to the circumstances of the incident:

- express
- implied
- presumed.

Express consent is where a patient grants specific permission for a treatment to be carried out. *Implied* consent is where patients, by their actions, present themselves for treatment but without specific verbal or written authorization. *Presumed* consent can be used, for example in the unconscious patient, where the patient is not able to give consent but it could be presumed that if they were able to give consent, they would do so in the given circumstances. The measure of whether or not this is a reasonable implication is to ask if an ordinary person would, given the opportunity, consent to the treatment being provided under the same or similar circumstances. Obviously, presumed consent must be used with caution and limited to appropriate circumstances.

What is more, any consent should be *informed consent*, which implies that the patient has been informed of the foreseeable benefits and possible side-effects of the treatment

concerned and understands their right to refuse treatment and the consequences of so doing. Failure to obtain consent or, more explicitly, providing treatment against a patient's will is, in legal terms, an assault and such an action brings with it the risk of prosecution. As a minimum the patient has the right of action for "trespass against the person". Even threatening to provide treatment against a patient's will constitutes the tort of assault at common law.

It is not always possible or practical to obtain consent in emergencies where time is crucial, even if the patient is conscious or relatives are present. In a situation where seconds count, and provided one's actions are reasonable and justifiable, it is likely that any treatment carried out to save life would be considered to be associated with implied consent or under the common law principle of necessity. However, explanations can help prevent distress for relatives and avoid serious misunderstanding.

It is vital to ensure that patients are fully aware of the possible consequences if they reject treatment. Ideally, written evidence should be recorded that this is the case. It is helpful to include a section on the patient report form to allow documentation of this. Patients should be asked to sign a statement to the effect that they have refused treatment and that the ambulance personnel have informed them of the possible consequences of their action. The patient's signature should be witnessed by someone other than the ambulance personnel, who can confirm the veracity of this statement. In the event that the patient refuses to sign, two witnesses should be asked to provide their signature. Ambulance control should be informed of the incident and any further information carefully documented on the patient report form. This procedure is not designed to threaten patients or to attempt to force them to change their minds. Technically, healthcare staff must demonstrate that the patient has given informed consent to refuse treatment and this process may help provide that evidence when necessary.

Refusing treatment should not be confused with the situation where the paramedic either expressly tells the patient or even simply implies that hospital is not necessary for the presenting condition. One of the most common causes of legal action against ambulance services relates to patients who have been left at home and are subsequently found to have a serious condition. Any patient who wishes to be taken to hospital should be transported as there is, as yet, no clearly defined policy which allows an ambulance service to refuse to convey a patient. If a patient is properly examined and there appear to be no grounds for attending hospital, the patient must be fully in agreement with the decision to stay at home. The documentation must be comprehensive so as to demonstrate that the assessment on which the decision was made was thorough and that the decision was reasonable in the presenting circumstances. It is important to leave the patient with appropriate advice on things to look out for which might suggest that their condition is worsening together with advice regarding what to do in such an eventuality.

Difficult situations arise with patients who refuse treatment but are not competent to do so. Clearly the hypoglycaemic diabetic who is violently resisting treatment needs to be treated anyway and will invariably be grateful afterwards. Because hypoglycaemia carries a real risk of death if it is left untreated and because the mental state of the patient is such that any refusal is not informed, then necessity can apply to such a case.

The head-injured intoxicated patient is always a complicated issue. The majority of these patients have no significant injury and their refusal is based on the effects of alcohol. As such, necessity could not apply to treating them against their will. However, if later it transpires that they have a serious underlying injury, they may claim that their refusal was as a result of the head injury and not the alcohol. There is no simple answer to such a case. Documentation must be very thorough and an independent witness should be sought to sign the case report form. In the event of their refusing treatment, every effort should be made either to refer the matter to the patient's GP or to leave the patient in the care of an appropriate sober adult with comprehensive advice, which again must be fully documented. This may not always be possible where the patient is alone in a public place and in such a case, where there are no grounds for the police to become involved, comprehensive documentation together with a recorded radio or telephone message to ambulance control must suffice as protection. It is much harder to try to justify one's actions as correct at a later date if the opportunity to record them as such at the time of the incident was not taken.

The rights of the child are increasingly important within society and this is reflected in the law. A minor, that is someone under 16 years of age, may consent to or refuse treatment without reference to an adult where they are of sufficient maturity to understand the full implications of what is happening to them. In extremis, a child can ask for the official solicitor to represent their views but this is clearly inappropriate to the emergency setting. Where treatment is absolutely necessary to save life or prevent permanent disability, the minimum treatment should be carried out under presumed consent or necessity with the rights and wrongs being argued at a later stage. A child may consent to treatment against the wishes of their parents, but *may not* refuse treatment of a serious or life-threatening illness if the parents consent.

MEDICAL ERRORS AND NEGLIGENCE CLAIMS

The test for negligence is the same in the medical and paramedical field as it is in any other profession. Defined in the case of *Bolam v. Friern Hospital Management Committee* (1957):

> The standard is that of the ordinary man exercising and professing to have that special skill ...

or, put more simply:

> The failure to exercise that degree of care which a person of ordinary prudence with the same or similar training would exercise in the same or similar circumstances.

What this means for paramedics is that in the event of a negligence claim, their performance or actions would be judged against that of their peers, who are other similarly qualified paramedics. Comparison is not made against the care a physician might be expected to provide. Care would, however, be expected to exceed that provided by a first-aider or member of the public (provided appropriate equipment was available).

Negligence claims can arise as a result of a perceived act of commission or one of omission. Negligence can be very difficult to prove; "proof" requires evidence that the following four components are all present:

- duty to act
- breach of duty
- damage
- causation.

DUTY TO ACT

Evidence is required that an individual was reasonably required to act in the situation found. For instance, if one reports to work as a paramedic for the ambulance service and responds to emergency calls then one has a duty to provide care to patients. Similarly the ambulance service as an organization may accept a duty of care from the moment they answer a 999 call before any individual paramedic is involved in patient care.

BREACH OF DUTY

Breach of duty is failure to act appropriately where one has a duty to do so. If, in responding to a patient with severe external haemorrhage, no attempt is made to control the bleeding, breach of duty as a paramedic has occurred. Similarly, if a tourniquet is applied to a patient with a minor haemorrhage and they lose their arm as a result of the lack of a blood supply, breach of duty has taken place. If, however, a body of peers, namely other paramedics, would reasonably have dealt with the same situation in the same way then there is no breach of duty.

DAMAGE

For a case of negligence to succeed, it is necessary to demonstrate that damage or harm occurred to the individual. This may occur in more than one way. There may be a new injury (such as dropping a patient through not using appropriate lifting aids), a worsened condition, an unimproved condition (where the patient has been in distress longer than was necessary) or the loss of opportunity. The loss of opportunity is becoming more widely known about through initiatives such as thrombolysis within one hour of onset of chest pain. If a crew were to attend a patient with chest pain and remain on scene for 40 minutes without a good explanation, this might contribute to the failure to thrombolyse the patient within the hour. Were the subsequent thrombolysis to fail, it could be argued that the delay by the crew caused the loss of opportunity for successful thrombolysis, leading to a greater impairment of long-term myocardial function.

CAUSATION

Causation is the requirement to demonstrate that the damage or harm resulted from the breach of duty. This rests on the plaintiff to prove and can often be difficult to establish. It is often difficult to prove, on the balance of probabilities, that the damage was the result of an act or omission by the paramedic rather than a consequence of the patient's initial illness or injury which, as they have called a 999 ambulance, should have been serious in the first place.

It should be remembered that to prove negligence it is necessary to provide evidence that all four of the above elements were in place. Generally a negligence claim can be brought up to 3 years after the event. In the case of children this is 3 years from their 18th birthday – up to 21 years if the case involves a newborn. This shows why it is so important that paramedics fully document all their observations and treatments, both positive and negative, at the time of the incident.

CONFIDENTIALITY

The ethical obligation to maintain confidentiality amongst doctors has seemingly progressed to become a legal duty. The General Medical Council rules confirm that confidentiality is a fundamental ethical obligation and the case of *E v. Egdell* has gone further by stating that the GMC rules "accurately state the general rule as the law now stands." This does not apply directly to paramedics who are bound by no such ethical oath but there are important reasons for maintaining confidentiality. First, confidentiality is a general rule of all professions where a practitioner has a privileged relationship with a client. Second, it is a generally accepted standard and expectation amongst the population at large that healthcare personnel do not discuss confidential matters outside their own profession, and only within it for educational purposes and (wherever possible) with the patient's consent. It is reasonable, therefore, to assume that a breach of confidentiality will be considered "unethical" by the public. Third, such a breach would prejudice the relationship with the person concerned, who would be unlikely to trust or consent to treatment by that practitioner in the future. Finally, most ambulance services have rules that define conduct and prohibit discussion of confidential patient-related matters. If any such rule is broken it could be judged as a major breach of contract and dismissal may

follow. Indeed, a wise employer must consider this level of action: if they fail to do so and the breach of confidentiality is repeated, the employer could be liable for a negligence suit.

Over the course of time the legal position may well change. The HPC, responsible for the state registration of paramedics, includes breach of confidentiality as an example of infamous conduct which could result in paramedics losing their registration and thus their ability to practise. It may be that once this rule has been in force for some time, it will progress to having the backing of the legal system as a matter of law rather than ethics.

It is not always as easy to maintain confidentiality as one would imagine. Inadvertent slips are unfortunately all too easy, for example when relaying patient information to a nurse or physician within earshot of other patients or their relatives. A further risk occurs with radio and telephone transmissions. It is easy and cheap for members of the public to buy a scanner that will allow monitoring of ambulance frequency radio transmissions. Inevitably, much patient information passes via these media with a subsequent risk of loss of privacy. Many services, in addition to providing the address of incidents, will pass details of the patient's medical condition over the radio and sometimes even the patient's name. It is worthwhile considering if a name is of any real value to responders prior to their arrival at the scene and if any such value outweighs the patient's right to privacy.

A number of strategies can be employed to reduce the risk of loss of confidentiality. First, where possible, call details should be passed via telephone landline which, while not entirely secure, is far less prone to amateur interception.

One method of increasing the privacy of data transferred from the ambulance control to responders is to send it as text to a mobile data terminal. Such devices are now becoming increasingly common in UK ambulance services. Another advantage of this technology is that it reduces transcription errors when crews take down details of incident locations.

The next technological leap in communications will be the introduction of digital technology. Digital mobile phones and their associated networks have been available in the UK since the end of 1994 and a working group led by the Home Office is investigating the potential application of digital (800 MHz) trunked radio systems for the ambulance service. Digital communications technologies have a far higher level of security than conventional analogue systems, as they encode voice data and select from a large number of available frequencies on a random basis before effecting each transmission. While it is theoretically possible to monitor calls sent in this way, the equipment required would be prohibitively expensive and extremely complex. Another advantage with these systems is that portable and mobile devices can be remotely turned off from the control centre, thus providing security in the event of their theft.

One area of constant concern to paramedics is the threat of infection with human immunodeficiency virus (HIV). This very real fear has, on occasion, led to what was assumed to be a "justified" breach of confidentiality. The rationale where confirmation that a patient has acquired immune deficiency syndrome (AIDS) has been transmitted over the radio is that it allows ambulance staff to "protect" themselves or to "take precautions". In reality this is no justification at all. All services should by now have policies in place that require paramedics to take universal precautions against direct contact with any body fluids from any patient. This implies that whenever a member of staff is exposed to the risk of HIV infection they will already be protected. It also implies that, logically, there will be no additional necessary precautions that they can take. Consequently the knowledge that any specific patient has HIV should have no effect on the handling of that particular person and the information is therefore unnecessary to protect crews' safety.

RESTRAINT OR ASSAULT

Ambulance personnel have no legal right to restrain a patient over and above that of the ordinary citizen, even if the patient is being admitted under a relevant section of the Mental Health Act on the orders of a doctor. As a result, any attempt to restrain a patient under any circumstances is a criminal assault. The only exception to this rule is the right to make a citizen's arrest and this is only lawful if it is known beyond doubt that a criminal act has taken place. Being mentally ill is not a criminal act, nor is refusing treatment for any other reason. Therefore should restraint or forced transportation be necessary for any reason, the assistance of the police should be requested. In addition to assisting with the enforcement of a section of the Mental Health Act, police officers may also order on their own initiative that a person should be removed to a place of safety if they are a risk to themselves or others. They are naturally somewhat reluctant to apply this power to confused aged persons who are refusing to go to hospital for treatment for their fractured neck of femur, but who have not injured themselves as the result of a criminal act. However, with a little tact and diplomacy, the police can usually be persuaded to do so.

In the event of an assault, one has a legal right to defend oneself but the power to do so does not extend beyond that granted to a member of the general public. In effect, this means that it is only permissible to use "reasonable force" to prevent harm being inflicted.

PRONOUNCING DEATH

In law the ability to certify death is confined to registered medical practitioners. This should not be confused with the pronouncement that death has occurred. Paramedics and technicians are not legally entitled to "certify" patients dead, nor are other medically unqualified persons. However, this

Table 64.1 Findings defining "obvious" death

Finding	Caution
Decomposition	Requires clear definition
Rigor mortis	Beware of muscle rigidity as a result of parkinsonism or hypothermia
Dependent lividity (postmortem staining)	Can be an uncertain finding
Decapitation	
Total incineration	Death is not always immediate in these circumstances
Gross mutilation through trauma	Requires clear definition and some experience to determine
Submersion confirmed as being greater than 24 hours	A very rare event (if a submersed body is visible for 24 hours, why has no-one taken action during that time?)

Box 64.1

- History   Patient in a lifeless condition for at least 10 minutes with no bystander CPR
- Vital signs No carotid or femoral pulses
              No spontaneous respirations
              Fixed and dilated pupils
              30-second trace of continuous asystole

does not impose a requirement on them to start treatment when, according to the definition of a medically approved and established policy, the patient has a non-salvageable condition.

There will be some circumstances where it is not appropriate for the paramedic to attempt resuscitation. It has long been the case that resuscitation should not be attempted where a patient is "obviously deceased". Examples of the "obviously deceased" are included in Table 64.1.

Many ambulance services are now introducing guidelines to allow paramedics to identify "irreversible death" and thus not commence resuscitation in much wider circumstances than those detailed for obvious death. An example of irreversible death is given in Box 64.1.

Whatever local policy is established, any pronouncement of death by a paramedic must be unquestionable. If errors occur they must be in the direction of patient safety, to maximize the potential for survival. If in doubt, the best advice is to resuscitate and let a doctor at the receiving hospital make the decision to stop.

STOPPING RESUSCITATION

Research in both the USA and the UK has demonstrated that few patients receiving full advanced cardiac life support in the field who did not develop a perfusing rhythm prior to transportation responded to hospital treatment, and none survived to discharge. This suggests that provided adequate and comparable treatment regimens are given by paramedics for the victims of medical cardiac arrest (as opposed to trauma-related death), failure to respond in the field implies irreversible death.

Subsequent removal of non-responsive patients to hospital is potentially hazardous as it requires rapid transportation with the use of lights and sirens and with unrestrained staff providing treatment in the patient compartment. It prolongs the period for which an ambulance is unavailable and inappropriately ties up medical and other resources at the receiving hospital. The whole process of transportation of the patient may be distressing for relatives as it may raise their expectations unfairly and could be perceived as depriving the victim of their dignity.

There is no legal bar to paramedics stopping resuscitation in the field and some services are now introducing appropriate policies which have medical approval, authorizing paramedics to abandon resuscitation attempts after a particular point in their protocol has been reached. This point has to be defined by the local paramedic steering group but is most often applied to cases of persistent asystole where the relevant advanced life support protocol loop has been applied at least three times without response.

If resuscitation is stopped in the field it will be necessary to inform the patient's general practitioner (or, rarely, the police surgeon if the former cannot be identified) and the police, who will act for the coroner's officer.

In modern times the technology available to paramedics to confirm death is often greater than that which the attending physician can bring. Electrocardiographs with time stamps on their printouts and end-tidal carbon dioxide monitors can provide reliable evidence, although this is not always acceptable to the physician.

RESPONDING TO EMERGENCY CALLS

Drivers of ambulances are able to claim exemption from certain specific sections of the Road Traffic Act when responding to an emergency call or, if appropriate, when transporting a seriously ill patient to a hospital. More accurately, these exemptions are considered to be applicable when observance of the referenced sections of the Act *"would be likely to hinder the use of the vehicle for the purpose for which it is being used on that occasion"*. Theoretically this leaves space for interpretation as to what constitutes hindrance of the vehicle and for precisely what uses of the vehicle the exemptions would apply. For example, it may

---

Box 64.2 Exemptions from the Road Traffic Act

- Exceeding the statutory speed limit
- Treating red traffic lights as a "give way" sign rather than an instruction to stop and wait
- Passing on the offside of a refuge (including those with "keep left" or "keep right" signs)
- Turning right at junctions where this is normally banned or restricted to buses
- Using bus lanes during their times of restricted operation
- Stopping and parking on clearways
- Stopping and parking in a pedestrian crossing controlled area or on the crossing itself
- Parking at or near to double white lines
- Using white lights (e.g. floodlights) other than reversing lamps and showing these to the rear of the vehicle while stationary
- Using audible warning devices at night when necessary
- You may leave the engine running when the vehicle is stationary

---

Box 64.3 Actions which are not permissible under the Road Traffic Act

- Parking dangerously
- Driving without reasonable consideration for other road users
- Ignoring one-way signs
- Ignoring stop signs
- Driving against the flow of traffic at a roundabout
- Crossing double white lines (other than as described in the Highway Code).

---

well be considered in a court of law that exceeding the statutory speed limit while transporting someone with a twisted ankle to a hospital does not warrant the application of the relevant exemption.

Box 64.2 details the specific exemptions that drivers of ambulance vehicles engaged in true emergency duties may reasonably expect to be able to claim.

All these exemptions must only be claimed when it is safe to do so. Should an accident occur, either involving or caused by the ambulance service vehicle, it may subsequently be considered to be the fault of the driver if his or her action was not deemed to be safe. For example, if a collision occurs whilst exceeding the speed limit, it is perfectly possible that the driver could be charged with dangerous driving.

If a collision happened while proceeding through a red traffic light, a subsequent charge might relate to failing to observe a "give way" sign or driving without due care and attention. Similarly, if an accident resulted from passage through a red traffic light without any direct involvement of the ambulance vehicle, one could still be liable (e.g. if a car runs into the back of another vehicle which has stopped to allow an ambulance to progress through a red traffic light, even if the ambulance is not struck, the action of proceeding through the light could legitimately be considered to be the cause of the accident). The policy of the police is to refer all such cases to the Director of Public Prosecutions.

Interestingly the exemptions listed above are defined as applying to vehicles "used for ambulance service purposes", and are therefore not restricted to ambulances.

Box 64.3 lists the most important non-exemptions. It is essential that all ambulance crew are aware of these.

It is essential to use good defensive driving practices at all times; exemptions should be claimed only when responding to emergency calls or when transporting to hospital the very, very small percentage of patients whose condition suggests that a few seconds or minutes saved will positively affect outcome.

ACCIDENTS WHILE DRIVING

Ambulance personnel have the same duties as the general public under the Road Traffic Act if involved in an accident, regardless of whether they are responding to an emergency call or not. This Act requires that the driver stops and provides to persons having reasonable grounds for requesting it the following information:

- name and address
- name and address of the owner of the vehicle
- registration number of the vehicle
- insurance certificate.

If this information cannot be provided because the relevant person is not present or would be unable to understand this information, the accident must be reported to a police officer as soon as possible and within 24 hours. It should be noted that "*I was responding to an emergency call*" is never an acceptable reason for not stopping and providing the required information.

In the event that an injury occurs to a person other than the driver of the vehicle, this should be reported to the police as soon as practicable and in any case within 24 hours of the accident occurring, although prudence suggests that immediate police attendance at the scene should be requested.

All ambulance services have policies setting out their expectations of their employees should they be involved in a road traffic accident. These steps should be followed precisely and will almost certainly include the requirement that an NHS Traffic Accident Report form is completed. It is most unwise to say anything that might indicate acceptance of liability for an accident and to do so would almost certainly be in breach of the policy of one's ambulance service.

BREAKING AND ENTERING

Unlike the police and fire services, ambulance personnel have no legal rights to force entry into private property, even if they suspect that an individual's life is at risk.

However, in practice, it seems unlikely that anyone would press charges in the event of such a suspicion proving correct. A prudent paramedic would ensure that there was sound evidence that a patient was indeed at risk before using force to make an entry. In all other instances the assistance of the police should be requested and their arrival awaited before forcing an entry.

DRUG SECURITY

Since October 2000, the use of morphine sulphate by paramedics has been approved. Morphine sulphate is a controlled drug and drugs so classified must, by law, be kept in a locked container within a locked cabinet fixed to an immovable surface. While it could be argued that an ambulance is anything but an immovable surface, it does apparently suffice for legal purposes.

Common sense and safety precautions suggest that all drugs carried by ambulance personnel should be afforded some form of security. Although there is no legal requirement to keep non-controlled prescription-only drugs locked up, there have been many instances of the theft of these substances from ambulances. These drugs can be dangerous if administered inappropriately and it could be argued that there is a moral requirement to minimize the chances of such thefts occurring.

Some modern ambulances are now being fitted with remote control central locking devices to facilitate both security and easy access. Failure to secure drugs could potentially result in a charge of negligence if a child gained access to them and was harmed as a result and the prevention of theft will at least help to ensure the ability to treat patients when drug therapy is indicated.

THE HEALTH AND SAFETY AT WORK ACT

The Health and Safety at Work Act establishes a duty on an employer to take all reasonable precautions to ensure the safety of employees and to minimize risks to them resulting from their employment. Resulting activity should include a formal assessment of potential risks, the development of policy and procedures offering guidance in reducing risk and coping with hazards, and the provision of safety equipment and relevant healthcare designed to offer protection from identifiable or predictable risks.

The Act also places a statutory duty on employees to minimize risk to themselves. Failure to follow policy, to use safety equipment provided or to identify hazards to one's employer will place an employee in breach of this duty. For example, failing to follow a written policy that requires the wearing of gloves provided by the employer whenever there is a risk of contact with body fluids is technically a breach of the law and there would certainly be no redress were the employee to contract an infectious disease as a result of the omission.

CONCLUSION

There are some surprising inadequacies and oversights in the legislation regarding certain areas of paramedic practice. However, where such guidance is either vague or not available, it is important to apply sound ethical practices by following the example set by colleagues in the medical profession. Reference should always be made to the employer's policies and if these appear be inadequate or missing, a request should be made for written directions which will provide appropriate guidance whilst carrying out the challenging duties of a paramedic.

Chapter 65

Clinical governance and audit in prehospital care

CHAPTER CONTENTS

INTRODUCTION

The prehospital component of patient care, particularly of those patients with serious injury or illness, has only become a point of focus and interest in recent years. In the United Kingdom organized local authority ambulance services began in the wake of World War II with the provision of basic first aid and the development of urgent transfer of the sick and injured to the nearest hospital.

Ambulance services were transferred to the National Health Service in 1974 and these NHS ambulance services have, since then, provided the backbone of prehospital care for the acutely ill or injured patient. Medical support to the ambulance service, when required, has been provided by doctors with prehospital care training or by hospital-based medical teams.

From 1966 onwards, the ambulance service provided advanced levels of first aid in the form of ambulance aid training, until the 1970s when the gradual introduction of paramedic training resulted in an upgrading of the skill levels of some ambulance technicians.

TRAINING OF AMBULANCE PARAMEDICS

Paramedic training has traditionally been orientated around the acquisition of resuscitation skills with teaching of the necessary underpinning knowledge. These skills include achieving competence in endotracheal intubation, intravenous cannulation, defibrillation and the administration of a number of drugs.

More recently, the paramedic course has been extended and it now includes elements of improved trauma, obstetric, and paediatric care. Many services had recognized the increasing limitations of the original paramedic course and implemented additional training outside the basic paramedic curriculum, including the Pre-Hospital Trauma Life Support (PHTLS) course and the Pre-Hospital Paediatric Life Support (PHPLS) course.

Comprehensive clinical protocols have rarely been available and have, in the main, been derived from the procedures taught in the original paramedic course, augmented by specifically local protocols. This has lead to varying levels of practice and capability across the UK, as services have had to respond to many changing demands.

Much of the preparation for practice of the current generation of ambulance paramedics and technicians has therefore been based on fairly rigid training programmes, in comparison with the path taken by other groups of healthcare professionals. In other courses, a variety of higher education pathways are offered alongside specific patient-orientated teaching. The less flexible methodology of training paramedics has resulted in a very real barrier to the easy and safe extension of current paramedic practice.

This narrower training approach focused on skill acquisition breeds an inevitable dependency on rigid procedures and guidelines and lessens the tendency for informed decision making in clinical situations. The limited training period and curriculum further aggravates easy augmentation of paramedic practice by producing varying levels of understanding of some of the important areas that support safe practice. Examples include pharmacology, the pathophysiology of key conditions and, vitally important, the ability to assess and examine patients consistently.

THE NATIONAL PICTURE – AN EMPHASIS ON CLINICAL QUALITY

The government indicated an intention to focus on clinical practice and quality by the publication of *The new NHS: modern, dependable* in 1997. Some services, often led by their medical director, have led the way by developing comprehensive clinical protocols and procedures, implementing clinical audit when supported by their commissioning health authorities, and beginning to tackle clinical quality issues by implementing key strands of clinical governance.

Although the introduction of formal medical direction of ambulance services has been slow to develop, the original isolated band of medical directors in the mid-1990s has now grown to a level where most ambulance services now have some level of dedicated medical direction.

In the wake of *The new NHS: modern, dependable*, the National Service Framework for Coronary Heart Disease has been published by the Department of Health. This is one of the first evidence-based documents in which the treatment standards for patients with coronary heart disease are laid down for implementation by NHS organizations and practitioners. There are two specific standards which apply to ambulance services relating to patients presenting with suspected acute myocardial infarction. The first requires the provision of a defibrillator by the patient's side within 8 minutes of a 999 call. The second requires prompt thrombolytic treatment for patients suffering from acute myocardial infarction, within 60 minutes of a call. These standards are also reflected in the more recent publication of the *NHS Plan* and will require significant improvements in both ambulance response times and prehospital cardiac care. In urban areas, thrombolysis will in the main be provided by hospitals but in more rural areas, dependence on a hospital-based thrombolysis administration service will result in failure to achieve the 60-minute standard for patients. Paramedics, sometimes working closely with interested general practitioners, will be providing thrombolytic drug treatment in these areas and will therefore need to undertake 12-lead electrocardiograms and administer thrombolytic drugs to patients in the prehospital environment.

Ambulance paramedics will therefore be providing more interventions, with inherent risks to patients, as part of achieving the standards laid down in the CHD NSF. It is therefore in this context that the ever more important role of clinical audit and clinical governance should be considered.

CLINICAL AUDIT

BACKGROUND

Clinical audit is an essential component of clinical governance as outlined below. It was defined in the White Paper *Working for patients* as:

"the systematic, critical analysis of the quality of medical care, including the procedures used for diagnosis and treatment, the use of resources, and the resulting outcome and quality of life for the patient."

It has also been defined as:

"a method used by health professionals to assess, evaluate and improve the care of patients in a systematic way."

Clinical audit was being introduced into hospital practice and primary care in the early 1990s as a quality improvement tool, to enable variations in practice to be identified, evaluated and either promoted, if shown to be compliant with recognized standards, or discouraged if not. It needed careful and considered introduction as it inevitably consumed practitioner time and could result in challenges to individual clinicians' methods and practice. It also had implications for the overall system of care and for those practising within it.

During the early to mid-1990s many areas of hospital medicine and primary care practice were becoming proficient at the tasks of data collection and comparison of results against an established or agreed standard. Many audits, however, failed to follow the full audit cycle (Figure 65.1). Changes in clinical practice have not always resulted despite evidence supporting the need for change arising from systematic audit analysis.

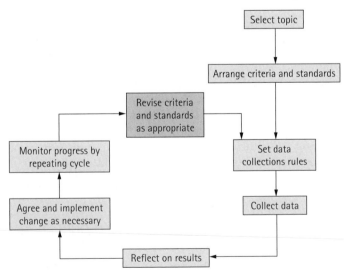

Figure 65.1 The audit cycle

Resistance to change was often a major stumbling block, notably where the audit process was neither led nor "owned" by the clinicians involved. Clinical audit did, however, fundamentally shift the emphasis away from attempts solely aimed at monitoring practice to those aimed at evolving and improving practice in the light of more objective assessment of its effectiveness.

To succeed, therefore, the commitment of those practitioners involved in the process was essential since lack of willingness, firstly to expose one's practice (and all the inherent beliefs held about its effectiveness) and secondly to be open to evolving it in the light of analysis, would rapidly see the value of clinical audit decline.

CLINICAL AUDIT IN AMBULANCE SERVICES

In the early days of the introduction of clinical audit to ambulance services, the process was introduced to varying levels of development and sophistication. The level of development was often more dependent on commitment and funding by commissioning health authorities and their public health physicians than any variation in the level of enthusiasm shown by individual ambulance services.

For many years, paramedics were required to participate in an activity audit, run nationally by the paramedic award's accrediting body, now the Institute of Health Care and Development (IHCD). This audit collected data on the number of occasions "advanced skills" were used. This information was subsequently used as part of the paramedic's recertification process and collated into a national annual report.

It was, however, never used to attempt to relate paramedic practice to appropriateness or to assess the outcome or effectiveness of their patient interventions.

More recently, as confidence and expertise have grown, services have expanded the range of audits which are undertaken. These now vary from the simple audit of compliance with guidelines and clinical procedures, such as the management of hypoglycaemia and use of nebulization in patients with acute asthma, to complex interservice analyses of patient outcome from different cardiac arrest rhythms.

Following professional registration of paramedics during 2000, involvement in clinical audit and some element of self-appraisal is now essential at individual paramedic level and this will inevitably boost the more general interest in clinical audit as a part of self-assessment.

CLINICAL AUDIT IN PERFORMANCE MONITORING

The evolution of more sophisticated audit processes will allow ambulance services to develop clinical performance comparison tools. These will replace current simple performance comparators which act as a proxy for clinical quality, such as response times to emergency calls. Comparator audits, such as survival from ventricular fibrillation (VF), can form a useful clinically based outcome measure for comparison of similar ambulance services. There is compelling evidence that survival from VF is critically dependent on a small number of key factors, such as the early provision of basic life support and the time delay from collapse to providing defibrillatory shocks.

Analysis of survival rates from VF arrests in an ambulance service operational area, therefore, tests the effectiveness of a number of separate elements of service provision, both independently and as a whole during a call. These include the level of basic life support capability in the communities served, the provision of effective telephone resuscitation advice to 999 callers, ambulance or first responder response times to reach the patient and the clinical performance of the responders on arrival. These are all tested as part of the chain of survival necessary to produce a successful patient outcome.

There is already recognition that outcome from VF may provide a good evaluation of ambulance system performance and implementing this in the UK is entirely feasible, although it demands committed, open and collaborative working with ambulance and hospital trusts.

In addition, many ambulance services are developing clinical performance indicators or audited standards of care with their commissioning health authorities. This again is intended to facilitate a move away from simplistic monitoring of response times as a surrogate for clinical quality.

Further development of more sophisticated system-wide and interdisciplinary audits involving ambulance services, medically staffed immediate care schemes and accident and emergency and coronary care units is an inevitable consequence of the monitoring of standards of care and performance against targets laid down in National Service Frameworks.

Alongside the ambulance service, many progressive immediate care schemes, committed to work with ambulance services to provide improved patient care, have initiated their own practitioner audit programmes and clinical governance procedures. Prehospital care providers can also establish audit links with those hospital A&E departments which contribute to the Trauma Audit and Research Network (TARN). This national audit system, which arose from the Major Trauma Outcome Study (MTOS), collates audit data to confidentially assess the performance of the hospital and some of the elements of the prehospital care of patients with major injury. It also provides comparison of the individual hospital's performance with other anonymous hospitals which also contribute to TARN.

Finally, assessing the satisfaction of patients with the service provided is a key part of auditing the performance of prehospital care organizations. Patient satisfaction studies provide nuggets of information about the patient's perception of their care and repeatedly demonstrate that the attitude of the attending crew or doctor weighs as heavily as the actual care administered.

CLINICAL GOVERNANCE

BACKGROUND

An intent to see defined improvements in the quality and safety of patient care was a key element in the government's White Paper *A new NHS. Modern, dependable* in 1997. It introduced a new responsibility of NHS trust chief executives for clinical governance, alongside others already in place for ensuring corporate governance and other statutory responsibilities. All NHS trust boards, including ambulance service trusts, have now established formal subcommittees to monitor and promote clinical governance, alongside the general management of risk.

Clinical governance was defined in the White Paper as:

"A framework through which NHS organizations are accountable for continuously improving the quality of their services and safeguarding high standards of care by creating an environment in which excellence in clinical care will flourish."

This rather long definition essentially introduces the duty to ensure quality of patient care in NHS organizations. As mentioned above, ultimate responsibility for assuring the quality of services rests with NHS trust chief executives. However, this is only part of a process designed to engage all those responsible for the provision of healthcare and to ensure they practise proficient and safe patient care.

Individual responsibility for aspects of clinical governance therefore rests with all practitioners and carers in the NHS. All healthcare professionals, including paramedics, must demonstrate individual commitment to continuing education and involvement in clinical audit and the identification of clinical risk.

Clinical governance incorporates several interrelated strands, namely staff training and education, a commitment to lifelong learning and the identification and management of clinical risk. It also includes implementing clinical audit, the establishment of suitable arrangements for accountability for managing clinical risk and the need to steadily improve clinical quality and effectiveness.

CLINICAL GOVERNANCE IN AMBULANCE SERVICES

Ambulance trusts have established accountability arrangements for clinical governance since its launch in 1997. Clinical audit has been implemented in the majority of services. This brings with it the first essential requirement, which is to implement a foolproof system for collecting and storing accurate clinical data, either on paper or electronically, about every patient contact.

Collection, access and safe storage of all patient records must be assured, followed by the introduction of effective audit processes and their reporting and feedback to staff and managers. Issues of access to patient information and its security must also be addressed.

Current clinical guidelines and standards of practice must be implemented. Problems have existed in ambulance services for years in agreeing common national guidelines for patient care. However, a standard set of clinical guidelines is now available to all ambulance services in the UK. These have been compiled under the supervision of the Joint Royal Colleges Ambulance Liaison Committee.

These guidelines were initially based largely on expert consensus regarding best practice but are being developed to provide guidelines supported by an increasing evidence base. Mechanisms are in place to achieve this and progressive review of these guidelines should place UK ambulance services in a strong position as one of few worldwide with national standards of clinical practice.

Clinical risk identification and reporting of events or "near misses" must be universally adopted. This will simply not happen whilst clinical errors are treated as episodes of misconduct and a different policy of organizational and individual learning must be implemented to deal with clinical errors and omissions.

Progress has been made in creating organizations with the "no blame" culture necessary to encourage openness about clinical errors and near misses and to allow system and practitioner deficits to be addressed and rectified. For many ambulance services, however, full implementation of these changes will remain a long-term objective.

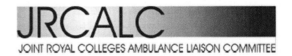

JOINT ROYAL COLLEGES AMBULANCE LIAISON COMMITTEE

Clinical Practice Guidelines 2004

For Use in U.K. Ambulance Services
(Version 3.0)

Also available online at:
www.nelh.nhs.uk/emergency

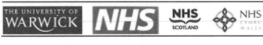

Edited by Ian Todd, University of Warwick
© University of Warwick and JRCALC 2004

Version 3.0   Issued April 2004   For review April 2006

Figure 65.2 The new ambulance service clinical guidelines

IMPROVING CLINICAL PERFORMANCE

Improving clinical performance requires a well-educated and trained workforce who remain current in their knowledge and competencies. Individual lifelong learning is therefore essential, as is the provision of appropriate training and education to undertake the tasks with which paramedics are faced.

Environment is key to effective practice and ambulance services have a lot of control over the clinical environment of the ambulance vehicle, if little over the external environment where much patient care occurs. Well-designed clinical compartments, safe and effective equipment and a focused identification of health and safety risks when designing vehicles and purchasing equipment are all requirements of an effective safety-conscious service.

Clinical audit supports the drive to improve patient care and, when implemented, offers a largely "paper-based" evaluation of the standard of clinical practice and compliance with accepted guidelines. It does, however, have obvious weaknesses in terms of consistent practitioner compliance, its retrospective nature and the limitations in visualizing the actual effectiveness of practitioners' "hands–on" management of the patient.

One can therefore be encouraged when paper-based audits report excellent performance. However, in reality this in no way guarantees actual standards of field performance and to believe that it does is perhaps a little naive.

Audit results can only really be validated by assessment in the field of actual clinical performance delivery. This is a vital part of providing high-quality care as well as patient satisfaction.

Field observation must not be seen as a "policing with a clipboard" exercise, which may be perceived by many staff as checking and spying. It must be a process of clinical support, committed to commendation and reinforcement of good practice but combining this with rapid but fair and respectful addressing of poor practice. Where poor practice is identified, most organizational cultures react in a way that results in other practitioners watching anxiously to see how poor performance is approached and managed.

Identification of poor practice must be followed up by active coaching and intensive support of individuals, not punishment, as we must surely believe that few practitioners arrive for duty in the morning with a wish to do a poor day's work and fail their patients. The process must give time and opportunity for improvement and provide long-term support where necessary. Rarely do practitioners need

removing from their field of practice, but this must be addressed if sufficient improvement cannot be made.

The field observers need to have peer credibility, practise to the highest standards and be actively supported by the organization's management structure.

CONCLUSION

By combining effective patient documentation with clinical audits owned by and seen as relevant by practitioners in the service, and field observation, a good baseline can be established for clinical performance in a service. Policy changes, such as education or treatment initiatives, can thereafter be monitored for impact with some confidence.

By implementing appropriate training and education initiatives which stretch individuals, promptly identifying episodes of deficient practice by auditing or observing practice and changing from a pure training approach towards an educational approach to developing staff, the original baseline of patient care and safety can be expanded and improved.

From an organizational responsibility perspective, many clinical errors are more to do with deficits in the system in which practitioners operate than in the individual practitioner. Managers must be prepared to act speedily and effectively to correct deficits in the system identified by investigating untoward clinical incidents. To fail to do this and leave risks unaddressed will jeopordize the whole credibility of the organization's efforts to implement effective clinical governance and we cannot expect clinicians to "get their act together" if the leaders of the organization are seen to shirk their own responsibilities.

FURTHER READING

Advanced Life Support Group 1997 Prehospital paediatric life support, 2nd edn. BMJ Books, London

Department of Health 1997 The new NHS. Modern, dependable. Department of Health, London

Irvine D, Irvine S 1991 Making sense of audit. Radcliffe Medical Press, Oxford

Prehospital Trauma Life Support Committee of the National Association of Emergency Medical Technicians and the Committee on Trauma of the American College of Surgeons 1999 Prehospital trauma life support, 4th edn

APPENDICES

Appendix A

Glossary

a- Prefix meaning without or absent.

ab- Prefix meaning away from (e.g. abduct).

abdomen The portion of the body between the thorax and the pelvis containing the majority of the organs of digestion as well as the liver and spleen.

abduct To move away from the midline.

aberrant Deviating from the normal path or site.

ABO blood groups One of a number of classifications of blood types based on the presence of the protein groups A or B on the red corpuscles. Groups are divided into A (the presence of group A proteins), B (the presence of group B proteins), AB (both A and B present) or O (no antigens present). Normally blood requires crossmatching into at least a similar blood group between patient and donor before transfusion, though in a desperate emergency blood from group O may be given to any patient.

abortion The termination of a pregnancy before the fetus is viable. This may be a pathological process, related to disease of the fetus or disease of the mother, or a deliberate attempt to terminate a pregnancy.

abruptio placentae Separation of the placenta from the uterine wall prior to the commencement of labour, normally associated with massive haemorrhage. It more frequently occurs during the third trimester.

absolute refractory period Period of time when cardiac muscle cells or neurones are completely refractory to depolarization however large the depolarizing stimulus is.

acetabulum The socket of the hip joint in the pelvic bone.

Achilles tendon The major tendon of the gastrocnemius muscle running down from the midcalf to insert in the heel on the calcaneal bone; it can be easily felt posteriorly at the ankle.

acidosis The condition of an excess concentration of hydrogen ions in the body. This may be as a result of either a metabolic problem or a respiratory problem. Treatment relies on treating the cause to correct the imbalance. This is the opposite of alkalosis.

acoustic Related to hearing and the ear.

acromion The tip of the scapula articulating with the clavicle.

activated charcoal A compound used in the treatment of acute poisoning where it is given orally to prevent further absorption of ingested poisons from the gut.

acute abdomen The condition of acute onset of severe pain within the abdominal cavity. It may indicate a condition that requires urgent surgery and therefore normally requires rapid assessment by a doctor.

acute confusional state Confusion caused by interference with the normal brain activity by drugs or metabolic insults.

acute epiglottitis Rapid progressive bacterial infection of the upper airway in young children. One of the key features is a markedly swollen and infected epiglottis which may actually cause sudden airway obstruction and respiratory arrest.

acute hypoxia Sudden fall in oxygen concentration within the bloodstream. It may be caused by airway obstruction, lung failure or cardiac failure. Signs may be subtle, such as confusion, or more obvious, such as acute loss of consciousness.

ad- Prefix meaning towards (e.g. adduct).

addiction Condition characterized by physical and psychological dependence on a substance.

adduct To move towards the midline.

adeno- Relating to a gland.

ADH (antidiuretic hormone) Hormone secreted by the posterior pituitary which has a water-retaining effect on the kidney. It affects the permeability of parts of the kidney leading to water being removed from the urine, concentrating the urine and reducing its volume.

adhesion A fold of scar tissue which causes abnormal tethering of tissue. Most problematic within the abdominal cavity, where it may cause obstruction of the bowel.

adipose Pertaining to fatty tissue.

adrenal glands Two glands each lying superior to the two kidneys in contact with their upper surfaces. Anatomically they are divided into two distinct regions: the medulla and the cortex. They are responsible for secreting a variety of compounds such as adrenaline and noradrenaline (from the adrenal medulla) and cortisol and androgens (from the adrenal cortex).

advanced life support (ALS) The combination of basic life support (BLS) with advanced and invasive techniques including drug therapy and defibrillation.

afebrile Without fever (i.e. normal physiological temperature).

afterbirth Placenta.

afterload The resistance against which the ventricle has to pump.

agitation Restlessness and anxiety; may be pathological, as part of a psychiatric illness.

agonal rhythm The terminal dysrhythmia recorded before death, normally consisting of broad-based bradycardic tracing with no cardiac output.

AIDS Acquired immune deficiency syndrome. A disease characterized by a deficiency in the cell-mediated part of the immune system. It is caused by the human immune deficiency virus (HIV) which is transmitted either through exposure to contaminated blood or blood products or via sexual contact. There is an increased risk of infection in these patients, particularly recurrent infection. Certain cancers such as Kaposi's sarcoma and non-Hodgkin's lymphoma are more common in these patients.

air embolism The presence of pockets of air within the cardiovascular system. If the volume is large enough this results in the obstruction of normal flow of blood.

air hunger Dyspnoea: shortness of breath and rapid, laboured breathing.

airway The passage allowing free movement of air into and out of the lungs. The term is also used to describe clinical devices for maintenance of a patent airway; these may range from simple devices such as Guedel airways to endotracheal tubes.

alcoholic (1) One who has a physical and psychological dependence on alcohol. (2) Mixed or diluted with alcohol.

aldosterone A mineralocorticoid secreted by the adrenal glands that are responsible for the reabsorption of sodium ions from the urine, sweat and gastric juice. In the kidneys this is accomplished by the exchange of sodium ions for potassium; the latter is then excreted instead.

aliquot A small quantity or volume of a substance.

alkalosis The condition of a decrease in the body's concentration of hydrogen ions or an increase in bicarbonate ions. Like acidosis, this may be caused by respiratory (hyperventilation) or metabolic causes (the ingestion of excess bicarbonate or loss of excess gastric acid following vomiting).

allergy Abnormal sensitivity to normally harmless antigens. In the severest form this may result in an anaphylactic reaction.

alveolus (Latin, a small hollow) The small sac-like terminations of lung tissue at which level gas exchange takes place.

ambulatory Able to walk. Often refers to patients who are not hospitalized, e.g. day-case surgery is often referred to as "ambulatory" surgery.

amnesia Loss of memory induced by severe physical or emotional trauma.

amniotic fluid The fluid surrounding and cushioning the fetus within the mother's womb.

amputation The loss of a digit, limb or appendage, either deliberately (surgically) or as a result of trauma, vascular disease or infection.

anaemia An abnormally low haemoglobin concentration in the blood.

anaesthesia (Greek, absence of feeling) A loss of normal sensation, particularly pain. This may be as a result of disease or induced deliberately. Anaesthesia may be local (by injecting local anaesthetic drugs around an area), regional (by blocking a nerve or nerves supplying a region) or general, which normally involves reducing a patient to a state of unconsciousness.

analgesic A pain-relieving drug.

anaphylactic reaction An extreme reaction to an allergen characterized by release of histamine from cells of the immune system and resulting in generalized itching, angiooedema, collapse, tachycardia, bronchospasm and (in the worst cases) death.

anastomosis The surgical joining of two tubular structures.

aneurysm A saccular swelling of a blood vessel.

angina (Latin, choking distress) A term primarily used to describe chest pain of myocardial origin relating to insufficient coronary blood flow. This may be stable, occurring only in episodes of excitement or exercise, or may be unstable, preceding a myocardial infarction.

angio- Relating to blood vessels.

angle of Louis The prominence of the sternum opposite the second intercostal rib space.

antecubital The anatomical area at the front of the elbow (e.g. antecubital fossa).

antepartum Referring to the period before delivery.

anterior In front of or at the forward limits of the body (see Figure 1).

antiarrhythmic A drug that may be used either to control a cardiac dysrhythmia or to prevent it occurring.

antibiotic A drug with antibacterial actions.

anticoagulant A drug that delays or prevents the normal clotting of blood.

anticonvulsant Drug with antiepileptic activity used to stop fits or to prevent their occurrence.

antihypertensive agent A drug designed to lower a raised blood pressure.

aorta The main arterial supply to the body. It commences at the outflow of the left ventricle as the ascending aorta and arches within the chest cavity (aortic arch) to give off the main vascular supply to the head. It then descends through the thorax (thoracic aorta) and into the abdomen (abdominal aorta) to supply the intestines before splitting into two terminal branches (the common iliac arteries).

Apgar score An assessment of the newborn infant based on five factors (irritability, heart rate, respiratory effort, colour and muscle tone), each of which is scored between 0 and 2 at 1 minute and at 5 minutes after delivery.

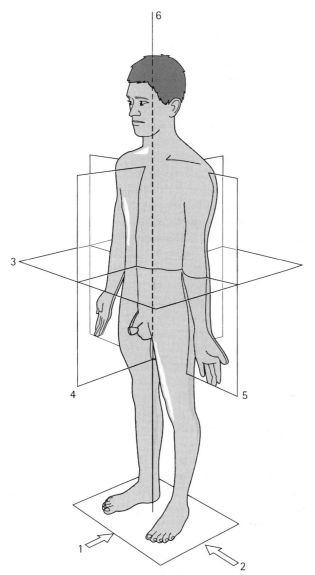

Figure 1 Anatomical position: 1, anterior aspect; 2, lateral aspect; 3, transverse plane; 4, sagittal plane; 5, coronal plane; 6, median line

aphasia A feature of a disease resulting in problems with speaking and understanding speech.

apnoea Absence of breathing.

appendicitis Inflammation of the appendix; normally requires surgical removal of the appendix.

appendix A small blind-ending sac at the junction of the ileum with the caecum. It may become inflamed, giving rise to the condition of appendicitis, and may go on to perforate, leading to peritonitis.

ARDS Acute (or adult) respiratory distress syndrome. A sudden onset of respiratory failure often associated with the critically ill patient and may frequently require ventilatory support.

arrhythmia *see* Dysrhythmia.

arterio- Relating to an artery or arteries.

artery Blood vessel supplying tissues with oxygenated blood.

arthritis Inflammation of one or more joints.

arthro- Pertaining to the joints.

articulation The junction between ends of bones or cartilage which form joints.

artificial respiration The artificial maintenance of respiration when normal breathing has ceased. This may be from basic respiration as mouth-to-mouth respiration up to respiration via an endotracheal tube and ventilator.

ascites The abnormal collection of fluid within the peritoneal cavity which may lead to problems with fluid balance. It is a complication associated with malignancy, cirrhosis and cardiac failure.

assisted ventilation The boosting of tidal volume in a spontaneously breathing patient.

asthma A disease characterized by episodes of narrowing of the small airways (bronchospasm) resulting in difficulty with breathing, wheeze and mucus plugging of the small airways. In its severest form it may be fatal without rapid medical aid.

asystole Complete absence of a heart beat and a straight-line ECG.

ataxia The inability to coordinate muscles.

atheroma The deposition of fatty material within the walls of the arteries, leading to narrowing and the conditions of stroke, coronary artery disease or peripheral vascular disease, depending on the area affected.

atlas The first cervical vertebra supporting the head (after Atlas, the Greek god who held up the World).

atrial depolarization The process of electrical depolarization and contraction of the atria.

atrial fibrillation The rapid and disorganized contraction of the atrium. In response the ventricles capture only some of the beats but this still results in an increase in the cardiac rate of up to 150 beats/min. These contractions are irregularly irregular in their timing and also in their pumping ability.

atrial flutter A state of rapid but organized and regular contraction of the atria, resulting in a subsequent increase in the cardiac rate, often associated with varying degrees of block between the atrial rate and the ventricular rate.

atrioventricular block Hindering or prevention of the passage of impulses from the atrium to the ventricle.

atrioventricular dissociation Complete lack of coordination of the electrical activity between the atria and the ventricles.

auditory Pertaining to hearing.

auscultation Listening and interpreting sounds as heard through the stethoscope.

avulsion Injury that tears tissue away from its anatomical connections, e.g. a finger may be avulsed from the hand.

axilla The armpit.

bacteraemia The presence of bacteria within the bloodstream (*see also* Septic shock).

baroreceptor Specialist receptor within the aortic arch and carotid sinus detecting the changes in pressure within the vascular system.

barotrauma Injury as a result of pressure change across a body or organ, such as may occur with rapid ascents following diving, etc.

basic life support   The maintenance of airway, breathing and circulation without any equipment.

Battle's sign   Bruising behind the ear over the mastoid region due to a basilar skull fracture.

Beck's triad   The three principal physical signs of cardiac tamponade: muffled heart sounds, hypotension and neck vein distension.

bends   The formation of bubbles of nitrogen within the bloodstream as a result of rapid decompression.

benign neoplasm   A tumour with limited potential to grow. It does not invade local tissues or metastasize and is frequently surrounded by a capsule. Its dangers lie in its site of expansion and the damage which may result from any pressure it exerts.

benign prostatic hypertrophy   An expansion of the prostate seen characteristically in elderly men and a common cause of acute retention of urine. It may be preceded by a history of frequency of passage of urine, nocturia and poor stream.

bi-   Prefix meaning two.

biceps   (Latin, two heads) One of the main muscles in the upper arm responsible for flexion of the elbow.

bifurcate   To split in two.

bigeminy   An abnormal cardiac rhythm with two rapid beats followed by a longer pause. Caused by every other beat being premature.

bile duct   The terminal part of the biliary tree, which leads from the junction of the cystic duct (which drains the gallbladder) and the common hepatic duct (draining bile from the liver) through to open in common with the pancreatic duct into the duodenum.

bilirubin   A yellow pigment excreted by the liver and giving rise to the yellow colour of the skin in jaundice, when it is inadequately excreted by the liver.

biopsy   The surgical removal of a small piece of tissue for histological (microscopic) analysis.

blood glucose   The concentration of glucose within the blood. In diabetic patients who lack adequate insulin secretion the blood glucose level would be expected to be raised (hyperglycaemia) owing to lack of control. It may become dangerously low (hypoglycaemia) as a result of excessive amounts of insulin relative to the oral intake of food.

blood pressure   The pressure exerted by the circulating blood on the arteries as it is pumped around the circulation.

bone marrow   The contents filling the cancellous bone, responsible for the maturation and production of red blood cells.

bounding pulse   A peripheral pulse which when palpated seems to be of excessive volume.

brachio-   Relating to the arm.

bradycardia   An unusually slow pulse rate, generally understood to be less than 60 beats/min, though this may be normal in a fit young individual.

breech birth   Delivery where the presenting part is a foot or the buttocks.

bronchiectasis   A pathological dilation of the small airways, forming chambers within which infection may pool and multiply.

bronchitis   Infection or inflammation of the bronchi.

bronchopneumonia   Acute infection of the lungs, particularly the bronchioles. Patients are severely ill with fever and rigors; the condition may result in pleural effusions and empyema as complications.

bronchospasm   Severe constriction of the bronchial tree.

bronchus   (plural bronchi) The division of the trachea leading down to the alveoli; the two first divisions after the trachea are known as the right and left main bronchi.

bulla   A large fluid-filled blister or thin-walled, air-containing space within the lung.

bundle branch block   Disturbance in electrical conduction through either the right or left bundle branch of the heart's conducting system.

burn   An injury caused by extremes of temperature – hot or cold. Classified as full thickness or partial thickness, depending on the depth of tissue damage. Other causes of burns include chemicals and electricity.

bursa   A synovial-lined cavity whose function is to enable the passage of tendons, muscle and soft tissues over bony points to be smoothed and effectively lubricated. The most common and well known are the infrapatellar and prepatellar bursae which may become inflamed in the conditions of clergyman's knee and housemaid's knee respectively.

caecum   The first segment of the colon at the site of the junction of the ileum and the appendix.

caesarean section   The delivery of a baby through an abdominal incision into the uterus.

calcaneus   The heel bone.

caput medusae   The pattern of veins on the abdomen seen in such conditions as advanced cirrhosis.

carbon dioxide retention   An increase in the concentration of carbon dioxide within the bloodstream, often secondary to respiratory failure. Care must be taken in treating these patients with oxygen as this can precipitate a sudden respiratory arrest if this condition is chronic.

carbon monoxide   A colourless, odourless gas. It has the ability to combine with haemoglobin in an almost irreversible manner, displacing oxygen and causing anoxia of the tissues.

carboxyhaemoglobin   The product of combination between carbon monoxide and haemoglobin.

carcinoma   A malignant neoplasm which has the ability to grow and metastasize and eventually kill.

cardiac arrest   Sudden stop to effective circulation. It may be caused by a variety of arrhythmias, including electromechanical dissociation, asystole and ventricular fibrillation.

cardiac output   The volume of blood pumped out by the heart in 1 minute. It is derived from the stroke volume (the amount of blood pumped per heart beat) multiplied by heart rate.

cardiac tamponade A collection of fluid within the pericardial sac that leads to a reduction in the output of the heart.

cardio- Relating to the heart.

cardiogenic shock Normally due to the effects of a myocardial infarction where sufficient ventricular damage has taken place such that the heart cannot maintain an adequate perfusion of tissues.

cardiogram *see* ECG.

cardiomyopathy A pathological condition of the muscles of the heart. It may take the form of the heart cells becoming weak and unable to pump properly or they may multiply in number, obstructing the outflow of the heart.

cardioversion The use of an electrical shock synchronized to the heart's rhythm to change an abnormal heart rhythm.

carotid arteries (from Greek *karos*, heavy sleep) The two major arteries that can be felt in the neck giving arterial supply to the face and brain.

carotid sinus massage The use of pressure over the carotid sinus to stimulate a vagal mediated reflex that slows the heart. It also can be used to try to convert certain supraventricular tachyarrhythmias into normal sinus rhythm.

carpo- Relating to the wrist.

cartilage (Latin, gristle) A supporting tissue found in a number of anatomical sites, e.g. joints, trachea and ear. It varies in its make-up depending on its anatomical site, e.g. fibrocartilage or articular cartilage. In the joints articular cartilage provides the smooth gliding surface to allow smooth movement between joints.

cataract An opacity of the lens of the eye. A common condition in the elderly.

catheter Any flexible tube that may be placed within a body cavity to drain or instil fluids, e.g. urinary catheter for draining the bladder.

cephalo- Relating to the head.

cerebellum The part of the brain responsible for coordination of voluntary motor activity; it resides within the posteroinferior portion of the cranial cavity.

cerebral haemorrhage Bleeding into the cerebrum – a form of stroke or cerebrovascular accident (CVA).

cerebral oedema An increase in the fluid around the cells in brain tissue with resultant swelling. A number of causes include head injury (the most common). It may present with signs of raised intracranial pressure owing to the closed nature of the skull.

cerebral perfusion pressure A measure of the circulatory pressure to the brain. It can be calculated as the mean arterial pressure minus the intracranial pressure.

cerebro- Relating to the brain.

chest lead One of six conducting leads placed on a patient's chest in predetermined positions during 12-lead electrocardiography.

chest pain A physical complaint, symptomatic of many differing disorders, some extremely serious such as myocardial infarction, others less dangerous such as hiatus hernia or indigestion. It should be taken seriously until investigated thoroughly.

Cheyne–Stokes respiration An abnormal pattern of breathing characterized by slow, shallow breaths, building to deep, rapid breathing and finally dying away to a period of apnoea lasting up to 20 seconds before the next cycle begins.

cholecystectomy The surgical removal of the gallbladder, often performed by "keyhole" or laparoscopic surgery.

cholecystitis Inflammation of the gallbladder (may present as an acute abdomen).

chondro- Relating to cartilage.

chronic bronchitis A common respiratory disease, with increased sputum production for at least 3 months of the year for 2 years.

chronic obstructive pulmonary disease (COPD) A blanket term for the three chronic diseases (chronic bronchitis, emphysema and asthma) that may cause obstructive problems with the airways. Formely known as Chronic Obstructive Airways Disease (COAD)

circum- Prefix meaning surrounding, around.

claudication Pain felt in a limb or muscle group (particularly the calves) on exercising the muscle group. Caused by poor arterial circulation to the muscle, leading to ischaemic pain when the muscle action outstrips the blood supply to it.

clavicle The supporting bone articulating between the scapula and the sternum.

coagulation factors Thirteen named factors circulating in the bloodstream, which are responsible for the successful and efficient clotting of blood.

coagulopathy An abnormal condition characterized by a decreased ability of the blood to clot. In trauma this may be caused by continual bleeding and an inadequate replacement of coagulation factors after large blood loss.

coccyx The small bone at the base of the spine joined to the sacrum.

colic A pain, originating from a tubular structure, that characteristically comes in waves; it may be caused by obstruction or spasm of the muscular coat of the structure. Typical organs that may produce colic include the gut and the ureter.

colitis Inflammation of the colon (large bowel).

collateral Running alongside (e.g. collateral ligament).

colloid A solution used to increase circulating volume by intravenous transfusion, which contains proteins and large molecules, e.g. hetastarches, dextrans or albumin.

colon The large bowel reaching from the caecum to the rectum. Divided into four parts: the ascending, transverse, descending and sigmoid colon.

colostomy The surgical creation of an opening of the large bowel on the abdominal wall after resection or decompression of the bowel.

coma Deep unconsciousness with no response to vocal or painful stimuli or spontaneous eye movement. Causes are many and include trauma, infection and metabolic states.

compensatory pause A longer than normal interval between heart beats. Often associated with premature ventricular contractions.

complete heart block A block anywhere between the atria and the ventricles to electrical conduction. Thus the ventricles are driven by an ectopic pacemaker at some level below the block, at a slower than normal rate.

concussion The injury (used with regard to head injury) following a violent jar or shock.

condyle A rounded projection at the end of a bone (e.g. femoral condyle at the distal femur).

congenital Any condition acquired before or present at birth.

congestive heart failure (CHF) Also known as congestive cardiac failure. Pathological condition most frequently related to a myocardial infarction or to ischaemic cardiac disease where the heart does not pump efficiently enough to clear fluid around the circulation. It is characterized by peripheral oedema and shortness of breath; the symptoms that predominate depend on whether the right or left side of the heart is most affected.

conjunctiva The membrane that lines the eyelids and the sclera of the eye.

contaminated Infected with bacteria (or viral or fungal organisms); this may apply to a wound or to any substance or area.

contra- Prefix meaning against.

contracoup The head injury sustained on the opposite side of the head to the site of the blow. It results from the movement of the soft brain against the inside of the cranium on the opposite side.

contralateral On the opposite side.

contusion The result of a blow to the body which fails to break the skin but produces swelling, bruising and pain.

coracoid A bony projection from the scapula that can be felt below the clavicle.

cornea The transparent covering over the anterior part of the eye.

coronary (1) Referring to the heart or to its encircling vessels, e.g. coronary vessels. (2) Alternative term for myocardial infarction, as in coronary thrombosis.

coronary artery bypass The surgical reconstruction of the coronary arteries with vein or graft in order to bypass areas of narrowing.

coronary artery disease A common affliction, particularly of the Western world. The coronary arteries become narrowed owing to the deposition of atheroma within their walls. This results in symptoms of angina or may lead to thrombosis and further narrowing of the artery which may clot off completely, producing a myocardial infarction.

coronary care unit Hospital unit equipped and staffed to deal with the acute problems associated with coronary disease, particularly relating to myocardial infarctions.

cor pulmonale Heart disease arising secondarily to lung disease.

corpuscle (Latin, a small body) One of the cells suspended within the bloodstream, e.g. white or red corpuscles.

costo- Relating to the ribs.

coup injury Head injury occurring on the side of the blow.

CPR Cardiopulmonary resuscitation: the provision of cardiac massage and artificial ventilation during attempts to resuscitate patients in a state of cardiac arrest.

cranio- Relating to the skull.

cranium The bony framework of the skull.

cricoid (Greek, ring-like) The last complete ring of cartilage in the upper airway before the horseshoe-like cartilages of the trachea.

cricothyrotomy Puncturing of the cricothyroid membrane in order to create an emergency airway. This may be done using a thick needle or a formal surgical incision may be made.

cruciate Crossed (e.g. the posterior and anterior cruciate ligaments which stabilize the knee and cross each other).

crush syndrome The life-threatening condition seen after massive crush injury to the body which results in haemodynamic instability and potential renal impairment.

crystalloid Solution used for intravenous fluid replacement, containing only electrolytes and water.

CSF Cerebrospinal fluid: the fluid surrounding the brain and spinal cord.

cubital Relating to the elbow (e.g. antecubital fossa).

cutaneous Pertaining to the skin.

cyanosis The blue colour seen at the periphery or centrally caused by the inadequate oxygenation of blood, which thus contains too much deoxyhaemoglobin which has a bluish colour.

cyst- Relating to the bladder.

dead space The area of the lung that is in contact with oxygen but is not being perfused with blood; also applied to the volume of air that is contained within the trachea and the bronchi which never reaches the gas exchange surface.

death The absence of palpable heart beat and spontaneous respiration.

decerebrate A condition of profound brain dysfunction associated with a classical posture of extension of both arms and legs and internal rotation of the arms.

decorticate Similar to decerebrate; a severe brain dysfunction but owing to the difference in area affected, the posture is different with flexion of the upper limbs and extension of the legs.

deep vein thrombosis The development of a blood clot within the deep venous system (normally within the lower limb). It may be detected clinically by swelling of the calf and accompanying tenderness. It may be complicated by fragments of the clot breaking off and travelling to the lungs as pulmonary emboli.

defibrillate To use an electric shock to convert an abnormal rhythm of the heart (fibrillation) to a normal rhythm.

definitive care In-hospital management of the trauma victim, usually surgical.

dehiscence A separation. Used to describe a healing surgical wound breaking apart (wound dehiscence).

delirium tremens (DTs) The stage of agitation and hallucination sometimes experienced in uncontrolled withdrawal from alcohol.

deltoid   A muscle clothing the shoulder and linking scapula and clavicle to the humerus.

dementia   A deterioration in mental function, frequently associated with old age although it may occur in younger age groups as a result of pathological processes.

dermato-   Relating to the skin.

dermatome   An area of skin supplied by sensation by one particular spinal root.

dermis   The skin.

dextrose   A sugar used in intravenous nutrition and in some crystalloid solutions.

dia-   Prefix meaning through.

diabetes mellitus   The disorder of metabolism clinically due to inadequate secretion of insulin by the pancreas. A variety of classifications exist. Treatment may range from a diabetic diet through tablet therapy to insulin therapy.

diabetic coma   The lapsing into unconsciousness by a diabetic patient. Though occasionally this is due to an excess of sugar in the bloodstream (hyperglycaemia), it is much more frequently a result of low blood glucose levels (hypoglycaemia).

diabetic ketoacidosis   The condition where by dehydration high blood glucose levels and an increased quantity of fat breakdown lead to the state of extreme illness which may slide into coma and eventual death if untreated.

dialysis   *see* Haemodialysis.

diaphragm   The musculotendinous sheet that separates the thoracic cavity from the abdominal cavity.

diastole   The period of time during the cardiac cycle when the heart is relaxed and blood enters the atria or ventricles.

diastolic blood pressure   The systemic blood pressure during diastole. It rises slightly in the early phases of hypovolaemic shock.

digit   A finger or toe.

digitalis toxicity   The condition associated with overdosage of digoxin.

dilatation and curettage (D&C)   The scraping of the endometrium of the uterus after dilating the cervix. This may be performed to correct heavy periods or to remove the products of conception.

diplopia   Double vision.

dislocation   The displacement of any joint from its normal anatomical site and relationship with the surrounding tissues and bones.

distal   Further away along the body or a limb from a reference point.

diuresis   The excretion of a quantity of urine; normally used to describe the response to a drug or fluid load.

diuretic   A drug used to aid the excretion of urine; particularly useful in conditions of fluid overload such as heart failure.

diverticulitis   Inflammation of a diverticulum. This may lead to abdominal pain and may even perforate, leading to peritonitis.

diverticulum   A small outpouching through the muscular wall of a tubular organ, most commonly referring to those found in the colon (e.g. diverticular disease).

dorso-   Relating to the back or posterior aspect of the body or limb.

dorsum   A structure on the back of a body or limb (e.g. the dorsum of the hand).

duodenal ulcer   The common type of peptic ulcer.

duodenum   The first segment of small bowel linking the stomach to the jejunum. Contains the entry of the common bile duct and the pancreatic duct.

dura mater   One of the three layers of membrane that surround the brain and spinal cord. In the head this layer is fused to the cranial vault and is indistinguishable from the periosteum. Bleeding between the dura and the bone following head injury may lead to an extradural haematoma which may have potentially fatal results.

dys-   Prefix meaning painful or abnormal.

dysmenorrhoea   Pain that accompanies menstruation.

dyspepsia   Epigastric discomfort associated with eating, heartburn and bloating.

dysphagia   Difficulty in swallowing or painful swallowing.

dyspnoea   Shortness of breath whether as a result of disease or excessive exercise.

dysrhythmia   An abnormal cardiac rhythm: may be a tachydysrhythmia or a bradydysrhythmia.

dysuria   Pain on passing urine.

ECG   *see* Electrocardiogram.

eclampsia   The onset of fits associated with pregnancy; these may occur before or after delivery.

-ectasis   Dilation of a tubular structure or sac.

ecto-   Prefix meaning on the outside.

ectopic   The development of tissue away from its normal site – particularly ectopic pregnancy, when fetal growth begins in an abnormal site such as the fallopian tube. Other tissues such as bone may form in ectopic sites.

electrocardiogram (ECG)   A trace of the electrical activity of the heart normally taken as 12 differing views of the heart. Used to diagnose abnormalities of the heart such as arrhythmias and previous myocardial infarction.

electromechanical dissociation (EMD)   The state of cardiac arrest where electrical activity is maintained but no cardiac output results. Common causes include pulmonary embolus, cardiac tamponade, tension pneumothorax and hypovolaemia. Also known as Pulseless Electrical Activity (PEA).

embolism   The passage through the blood vessels of a substance (e.g. clot, amniotic fluid, plastic particles) not normally found within the bloodstream. Finally the embolus impacts within the vascular tree.

embryo   The human fetus from conception to 8 weeks gestation.

emphysema   A chronic disease where there is destruction of the parenchyma of the lung and distension of other parts of the lung. Alternatively described as chronic obstructive pulmonary disease.

encephalitis   An inflammation of the brain.

endo-   Prefix meaning innermost.

endocrine   Relating to glands or cells that release their secretions into the bloodstream or lymph rather than into the digestive tract or onto the skin.

endometrium   The lining of the uterus into which the fetus implants.

endothelium   The lining epithelial cells of the serous cavities, lymphatic vessels and blood vessels.

endotracheal tube   A large-bore tube used to secure an airway or to administer positive pressure ventilation. Apart from those used in small children, all tubes have an inflatable cuff at one end to secure the tube within the trachea.

epidemic   The occurrence of a disease in a large number of people over a large area.

epidermis   The superficial layers of the skin: the outer cornified layer and a deeper living layer.

epiglottis   Protective structure that overhangs the larynx and hinges backwards during swallowing to prevent food entering the larynx.

epiglottitis   A childhood disease characterized by swelling and inflammation of the epiglottis. A sudden obstruction of the upper airway may occur without warning, resulting in respiratory arrest.

epiphysis   The proximal or distal part of a long bone that is separated from the shaft by the epiphyseal plate that allows growth of that bone.

epistaxis   A nose bleed.

erythrocyte   A red blood cell.

exercise ECG   An ECG which is performed while the patient exercises in an attempt to disclose latent ischaemia.

exo-   Prefix meaning outermost.

exsanguinate   To bleed to death.

extension   Movement between two bones, generally in a direction to increase the angle between them.

external chest compressions   The application of rhythmical mechanical compression of the chest wall, compressing the ventricles and maintaining a cardiac output during a state of cardiac arrest.

extradural   Literally, outside the dura; particularly refers to the cerebral bleed associated with a temporal fracture where the middle meningeal artery bleeds into the extradural space, compressing the cerebral substance.

extrasystole   A cardiac contraction that is outside the timing of the normal cycle.

fascia   (Latin, a band or sash) Fibrous connective tissue found in a variety of sites in the body, often wrapped around structures such as muscle or as a lining below fat and skin.

femur   The thigh bone.

fever   An increase in body temperature above the normal value of 37°C.

fibrillation   Disordered uncoordinated activity, either electrical (of the heart) or muscular.

fibula   The small outer (lateral) bone of the lower leg.

FiO₂   The concentration of oxygen that a patient is receiving normally expressed as a fraction or percentage, e.g. FiO_2 0.56 or 56%.

fistula   An abnormal connection between two organs: this may take the form of a bowel-to-bowel fistula, a join between two blood vessels (arteriovenous fistula) or a connection between an organ and its surroundings (bronchopleural fistula).

flail chest   A chest cavity that as a result of trauma has two rows of multiple rib fractures leading to paradoxical movement of the chest wall.

flexion   Movement between two bones, generally in a direction to decrease the angle between them.

flutter waves   Regular sawtooth waves on the ECG diagnostic of atrial flutter.

Foley catheter   A rubber or Silastic catheter that is inserted into the bladder via the urethra and is left in situ to drain urine. It has a small balloon on the end which is inflated once the catheter is in the correct site in order to prevent the catheter falling out.

fontanelle   A space between certain of the cranial bones in the newborn, covered by tough membranes.

foramen   A small space or opening.

fracture   An injury to the bone at which the continuity of the bone is broken. There are a variety of classifications, but one important feature of note is whether the skin has been broken over the fracture site (compound or open fracture) or not (simple or closed).

frostbite   The damage to tissues caused by subjection to freezing temperatures.

gag reflex   The reflex occurring in response to irritation of the pharynx.

galea   The fibrous fascial layer that connects the frontalis muscles on the forehead to the occipital muscles of the posterior aspect of the head (the scalp).

gallbladder   A small sac linked to the bile duct and to the hepatic ducts of the liver whose role is to concentrate bile from the liver, store it and, when required, release it into the common bile duct, whence it flows into the duodenum to aid in digestion.

gallop rhythm   A description of an abnormal heart rhythm where there is an extra heart sound (either a third or fourth sound).

ganglion   (1) In anatomical terms, a group of nerve cells outside the central nervous system. (2) In pathological terms, a small cystic swelling associated with a tendon.

gangrene   Death of tissue, often due to inadequate blood supply as the main cause, though a variety of other conditions such as cold injury may also cause gangrenous changes. Often divided into wet or dry gangrene: typically, wet gangrene follows major tissue damage such as crush injury.

gas gangrene   Infection of tissues with a particular genus of bacterium (*Clostridium*), characterized by aggressive infection accompanied by bubbles of gas formation within the tissues. If untreated, it may rapidly become fatal.

gastric   Pertaining to the stomach.

gastric ulcer   Ulceration of the lining of the stomach which may present with pain and indigestion responsive to milk or antacids. It may also present as a perforation of the stomach wall or with an acute bleed and vomiting blood.

gastrocnemius   The most superficial muscle of the posterior aspect of the calf.

gastrointestinal bleed   Any bleeding that originates from the gastrointestinal (GI) tract. It may frequently be due to upper GI causes such as peptic ulcers or oesophageal varices or lower GI causes such as bleeding from diverticuli or bleeding due to cancer.

gastrointestinal obstruction   Any obstruction of the GI tract. Causes may be manifold. Symptoms are predominantly colic pain, decrease in bowel opening and vomiting.

geriatrics   The section of medicine that specializes in the care and medicine of the elderly.

gestation   Pregnancy.

glands   Collections of tissues or an organ which produces substances to excrete or secrete that are not primarily related to their normal metabolism.

Glasgow Coma Scale   A swift method for assessing and monitoring the conscious level of a patient. It is based on the verbal response, the motor response and eye opening.

glenoid   The socket part of the scapula against which the humeral head articulates.

glomerulus   (Latin, a small ball) The first part of the nephron where small blood vessels allow filtering of plasma to start the production of urine.

glosso-   Relating to the tongue.

glucose   A simple sugar, important as an energy source, whose metabolism is disturbed in diabetes.

goitre   An abnormal swelling of the thyroid gland. This may represent an overactive or an underactive gland or a growth (malignant or benign) within the gland.

graft   A portion of tissue or complete organ taken from one site in a body and placed in another site or into a different patient to correct a deficiency or absence of tissue.

grand mal seizure   Generalized motor seizure, a form of epilepsy.

gravidity   The number of pregnancies that a woman has had.

greenstick fracture   An incomplete fracture, usually in children, where the bone cortex is bent and deformed rather than disrupted.

guarding   The contraction of the abdominal muscles to protect a painful area from the pressure of an examining hand.

gynae-   Referring to woman or female reproductive organs.

haematemesis   The vomiting of bright red blood, normally signifying rapid upper gastrointestinal blood loss such as an ulcer or oesophageal varices.

haemato-   Relating to blood.

haematoma   A collection of blood within the tissues; this may be as a direct result of trauma or of surgery.

haematuria   Passage of blood in the urine.

haemodialysis   The procedure necessary in patients with renal failure to remove the toxic products of metabolism from the bloodstream. Blood is taken through a large-bore cannula from an arteriovenous fistula or from a central line and passed through a dialysis filter to remove the toxins before being returned to the body.

haemoglobin   The red pigment found in red blood cells that is responsible for the carriage of oxygen around the body.

haemoptysis   The coughing up of blood in the sputum.

haemorrhage   The loss of blood – a term normally referring to rapid loss of a large quantity of blood either internally or externally.

haemorrhoids (piles)   An abnormal dilation (or varicosity) of the lower rectal veins: may present with rectal bleeding or protrude through the anal rim and become thrombosed.

haemothorax   The filling of a pleural cavity with blood, usually after trauma to the chest or following thoracic surgery.

hallux   The great toe.

head tilt   The act of hyperextending the head to open the airway.

heart block   Illness where the passage of electrical impulses from the atria to the ventricles is delayed or prevented. Varying forms exist: first-degree block is characterized by a prolonged PR interval; second-degree block is where a variable percentage of the P waves are not followed by a QRS complex; third-degree block is a complete failure of impulses to reach the ventricle from the atria when an ectopic focus takes over (*see* Complete heart block).

heart failure   *see* Congestive heart failure.

heat cramps   Muscular cramps resulting from dehydration and salt loss following exercise.

heat exhaustion   A state of nausea, muscle cramps and eventual loss of consciousness due to excessive exertion in hot conditions, resulting in loss of fluid and electrolytes.

heat stroke   A disturbance of the ability to thermoregulate, resulting in extreme fever and dry skin, eventually progressing to coma.

hemi-   Prefix meaning half.

hemiplegia (half paralysis)   Paralysis of one half of the body; this may be as a result of congenital illness such as cerebral palsy or due to such causes as stroke.

hepatic, hepato-   Pertaining to the liver.

hepatitis   An inflammation of the liver which normally results in jaundice, abdominal discomfort and loss of appetite. There are many potential causes including infections (such as hepatitis B, hepatitis A), parasitic infections, drugs and alcohol.

hernia   The abnormal protrusion of an organ through the muscular wall surrounding it; may be congenital or acquired later in life. If in the abdomen, may present with obstruction due to incarceration or strangulation of the bowel by the margins of the hernial sac.

hormone   A chemical produced within the body that regulates cell activities, often at a distant site.

humerus   The long bone of the upper arm and shoulder.

hyaline   Glassy and smooth (e.g. hyaline cartilage).

hyper-   Prefix meaning increased.

hypercapnia (hypercarbia)   A high level of carbon dioxide in the blood.

hyperglycaemia   A higher than normal concentration of glucose in the bloodstream.

hyperkalaemia   A high level of potassium in the blood, normally as a result of administration of drugs affecting the excretion of potassium or the failure of the kidney to adequately excrete potassium. In excess this may result in cardiac dysrhythmias.

hyperlipidaemia   An excess of lipids within the blood.

hyperpyrexia   An extremely elevated body temperature. Malignant hyperpyrexia, a condition of rapidly rising temperature, is a complication of general anaesthesia.

hypertension   Disorder of blood pressure control that results in an elevated blood pressure.

hyperventilation   A rate and volume of breathing above that normally required for adequate gas exchange. The removal of carbon dioxide from the bloodstream as a result of this may cause dizzy spells, numbness of the periphery and chest pains.

hypervolaemia   A larger than required circulating volume, generally the result of overtransfusion, though overdrinking (particularly in the presence of reduced renal function) may also give rise to it.

hypo-   Prefix meaning low or inadequate.

hypoglycaemia   An abnormally low blood glucose level. In extremes it may cause faintness, then unconsciousness and coma.

hypokalaemia   Low or adequate levels of potassium in the blood. In extreme cases this may lead to flaccid muscles and an abnormal ECG.

hyponatraemia   A low or inadequate concentration of sodium in the blood.

hypotension   A low blood pressure which is inadequate for perfusion of the vital organs. This may be as a result of abnormalities of the heart, side-effects of drugs in excess or loss of circulating fluid.

hypothermia   A pathologically low body temperature (normally defined as below 35°C), most frequently due to exposure to cold conditions.

hypovolaemia   A state of low blood volume. *See also* Hypovolaemic shock.

hypovolaemic shock   The state of inadequate perfusion (and therefore oxygenation of the tissues) due to a fall in the circulating volume (usually due to blood loss) and a subsequent fall in blood pressure. Excessive loss of body fluids due to other causes (e.g. diarrhoea) can also occasionally cause this.

hypoxaemia   Low level of oxygen in the blood.

hypoxia   A fall in the concentration of oxygen in cells. This may result from inadequate oxygenation due to a decrease in the atmospheric oxygen, inadequate respiration (due to a reduction in the respiratory drive, an obstruction of the respiratory tract or lung injury) or inadequate circulation (e.g. shock).

hystero-   Relating to the uterus.

idiopathic   Of unknown cause.

ileostomy   The surgical creation of a connection between the ileum and the abdominal wall.

ileum   The terminal part of the small bowel linking the jejunum to the caecum.

iliac   Referring to structures around the inguinal and pelvic region or the ilium, e.g. the iliac vessels.

ilium   Upper portion of the hip bone.

incisor   A cutting tooth.

incomplete abortion   A spontaneous abortion that does not result in the complete expulsion of the products of conception and may result in haemorrhage from the vagina, needing surgical intervention.

incontinence   The inability to control the excretion of urine or faeces. This may be due to congenital problems or to problems ranging from damage to the nerve supply of the bladder or bowels to direct damage to the organs themselves.

inevitable abortion   A spontaneous abortion which is imminent and cannot be avoided. Bleeding, abdominal pain and cervical dilation are major features.

infant   Child of less than 1 year old.

infarct   An area of cell death that results from the interruption of the blood supply. Examples include myocardial infarction and some types of stroke.

infra-   Prefix meaning below or beneath.

infusion   The introduction of a drug or fluid directly into the venous system.

inguinal   Pertaining to the groin (e.g. inguinal hernia, a hernia that passes through the inguinal region of the body).

inotropic   Affecting the force of cardiac contraction.

insulin   A hormone secreted by the B cells of the pancreas which is responsible for the lowering of blood glucose levels.

inter-   Prefix meaning between.

intermittent positive pressure ventilation   Ventilation of a patient who is not breathing, using a positive pressure system.

intestinal obstruction   *see* Gastrointestinal obstruction.

intra-   Prefix meaning within.

intravenous   Into a vein (administration of fluid or drugs).

intraventricular block   The slowing or stopping of the cardiac excitatory impulse within the ventricles; it can be seen on an ECG and identified as a left or right bundle branch block.

intubation   The passage of an endotracheal tube through the mouth or nose to secure an airway to the trachea or allow the passage of an anaesthetic agent.

ion   An atom or molecule in its charged state, e.g. chlorine naturally exists as a negatively charged chloride ion (Cl^-), ammonia exists as the ammonia ion (NH_4^+).

ipsi-   Prefix meaning the same (e.g. ipsilateral, on the same side).

ischaemia   Pain within an organ or tissue caused by a lack of blood supply, e.g. angina, which is due to a decrease in the supply of blood to regions of the heart.

isotonic   In medical terms, having the same osmotic pressure as extracellular fluid.

jaundice   A yellow colour first noted in the mucous membranes and sclera, caused by excess circulating bilirubin.

jaw thrust   A manoeuvre to open the airway by pushing the mandible forward, normally with the fingers behind the angle of the mandible.

jejunum   The intermediate portion of the small bowel linking the duodenum to the ileum.

joint   A junction between two bones. This may be classified in a number of ways, for example by its structure (e.g. a ball and socket joint such as the hip) or by its type (e.g. fibrous, cartilaginous or synovial).

jugular   Pertaining to the neck (e.g. jugular vein, the major vein running on the right and left of the neck alongside the carotid artery draining blood from the face and head).

jugular veins   The veins lying either side of the neck that return blood to the heart. They may become full and visible when central venous pressure increases, as in cardiac failure.

junctional rhythm   A cardiac rhythm initiated by the atrioventricular node.

junctional tachycardia   An automatic rhythm of greater than 100 beats/min that is controlled from the atrioventricular node.

ketoacidosis   A complication of diabetes mellitus where excessive blood ketone levels (products of uncontrolled metabolism) create a metabolic acidosis which can result in nausea, vomiting, dehydration and eventually coma and death.

lactic acid   One of the waste products of protein and carbohydrate metabolism. It may accumulate in certain conditions to cause a metabolic acidosis which may lead to a loss of consciousness: this may be one of the causes of coma in diabetic patients.

landmark position   The correct position of the hands during CPR.

laparotomy   The surgical exploration of the abdominal cavity.

laryngo-   Relating to the larynx.

laryngoscope   A tool for examining the larynx or for aid in viewing the larynx to assist the passage of an endotracheal tube.

larynx   The upper part of the windpipe.

lateral   A position on the body further from the midline relative to another point.

latissimus dorsi   A large muscle running from the iliac crest posteriorly over the back to insert in the upper arm.

lavage   To wash out (e.g. gastric lavage to remove contents of the stomach).

left heart failure   Limited function of the left ventricle leading to back pressure in the pulmonary artery and veins, pulmonary oedema and breathlessness. Often accompanied by some degree of right heart failure. *See also* Congestive heart failure.

leuco-   Prefix meaning white.

leucocyte   A white blood cell. May be further differentiated into types such as neutrophil, eosinophil, etc., according to histological appearance and function.

leukaemia   A malignancy of the bone marrow cells characterized by the replacement of the marrow with immature white cells which are released into the circulation.

ligament   A band of connective tissue connecting bones and cartilages together and stabilizing these structures.

ligate   To tie off.

lipid   The fat of the body. This term includes the structural fats in the membrane of cells through to the layers of adipose tissue.

lipo-   Relating to fat.

lobar pneumonia   Bacterial infection of one of the five lung lobes. It passes through a series of stages eventually ending with consolidation of that lobe.

log roll   Manoeuvre to move a patient to expose the back but maintaining in-line stability of the whole spine.

longitudinal   Along the long axis of the body.

lumbar   (Latin *lumbus*, the loin) General term referring to the lower back between the thorax and the pelvis, e.g. lumbar spine.

lunate bone   One of the small bones in the wrist.

lymph   (Latin *lympha*, clear water) Fluid produced by the seepage of plasma through the intercellular spaces and drained into the lymphatic vessels.

lymph nodes   Small round or oval structures responsible for production of cells of the immune system and for filtering lymphatic fluid.

lymphatics   The series of hollow tubes responsible for draining lymph from the periphery back into the circulation.

macro-   Prefix meaning large.

malignant neoplasm   A tumour with the characteristics of growth, metastasis and invasion.

malleolus   (Latin, a little hammer) Rounded, bony protuberances found on the inner (medial) and outer (lateral) aspect of the ankles.

Mallory–Weiss tear   A partial-thickness tear of the oesophageal lining following an attempt at stopping vomiting by keeping the glottis closed, leading to a raised intra-oesophageal pressure that tears the oesophagus.

mammo-   Relating to the breast.

mandible   The lower bone of the jaw.

mean arterial pressure (MAP)   The mean of the systolic and diastolic blood pressure.

medial   Towards the midline.

median   In the midline of the body.

mediastinum   (Latin, a middle partition) The middle cavity of the thorax within which the heart, the trachea (and its bifurcation), the great vessels and the oesophagus are contained.

medulla   The marrow cavity of long bones, a useful site for gaining emergency vascular access in children using an interosseous needle.

meninges   The membranes surrounding the brain substance, which become inflamed in meningitis. They comprise the pia mater, dura mater and arachnoid.

meningitis   Any infection or inflammation of the lining membranes of the brain. The condition presents with headache, photophobia, neck stiffness and vomiting.

meniscus   (Greek, a crescent) The half moon-shaped cartilage found within the knee joint; may be damaged by sporting accidents.

mesentery   The fold of peritoneum that surrounds parts of the large and small bowel, tethering them to the posterior abdominal wall but allowing considerable mobility. May be torn by sudden deceleration injuries and result in intraabdominal bleeding.

metabolite   The product of any form of chemical reaction or process within the body. This may refer to the production of carbon dioxide (a metabolite of respiration) or to the breakdown of drugs.

metaphysis   The junction between diaphysis and epiphysis.

metastasis   The product of a malignant tumour seeded to a site distant from the original tumour, where it multiplies.

micro-   Prefix meaning small.

micturate   Urinate.

midclavicular line   The imaginary line that runs vertically downwards from the midpoint of the clavicle.

migraine   A severe headache caused by vascular spasm. It may be heralded by visual disturbance and a prodromal feeling, and may be accompanied by vomiting and nausea.

military antishock trousers (MAST)   A garment for application to the legs and abdomen that may be inflated to provide autotransfusion from the lower extremities and some degree of tamponade in cases of hypovolaemic shock.

minute volume   Volume of air expired (or inspired) in 1 minute.

missed abortion   A condition where the fetus dies but is not actually expelled for 2 or more months.

mitral valve   One of the four heart valves. As such it can be afflicted by the same disease processes as the other valves and become excessively tight (stenosis) or not close properly (incompetence), each condition being accompanied by its own characteristic sounds at varying times of the heart cycle.

mono-   Prefix meaning single.

morbidity   Illness or features of a disease.

mortality   Death.

mouth-to-mouth resuscitation   A procedure to supplement inadequate ventilation or absent breathing in a patient by exhaling air into the patient's lungs via a mouth-to-mouth seal.

multigravida   Woman who has had at least two pregnancies.

multipara   Woman who has had at least two deliveries.

murmur   Sound heard with a stethoscope over the heart, indicating that one of the valves is leaking or narrowed.

myelo-   Relating to the spinal cord.

myo-   Relating to muscle.

myocardial infarction   The blockage of a coronary artery by a thrombosis, leading to death of some of the tissue beyond. Also known as a heart attack or coronary artery thrombosis.

myocardium   The muscle that is unique to the heart; it contracts to pump the circulating blood.

myoglobin   Protein contained within the muscle structure. Its release into the circulation following a crush injury may result in renal failure.

myotome   A group of muscles supplied by one spinal segment.

narcotic   A drug that has pain-relieving properties and causes sleep.

nasal airway (nasopharyngeal airway)   A flexible piece of tubing designed to pass through the nose into the pharynx to maintain an airway.

nausea   The sensation often preceding vomiting.

navicular   A small bone in the forefoot, the equivalent of the scaphoid in the hand.

nebulize   To break up a drug or liquid into fine droplets in order for it to be inhaled and absorbed. Particularly useful for treating conditions of the lung such as asthma.

necrosis   The death of tissue, often due to ischaemia.

neonate   A young child between birth and 28 days old.

neoplasm   The benign or malignant new growth of tissue.

nephron   (Greek, the kidney) The basic unit of the kidney comprising the glomerulus and the renal tubule.

neurogenic shock   The condition of low blood pressure due to an injury to the spinal cord resulting in widespread dilation of blood vessels.

neurone   The basic nerve cell of the central and peripheral nervous system. Comprises the cell nucleus and one or more processes which extend and link with other neurones via synapses.

neutropenia   The state of an abnormally low number of circulating neutrophils in the bloodstream; if low enough may result in immunosuppression.

nocturia   The need to get up at night to pass urine.

normal sinus rhythm   The state of normal conduction of the electrical impulses in the heart with progression of depolarization from atria down to ventricle.

nucleus   The central part of the cell responsible for storage of DNA and regulation of the cell's activity. Also applied as a collective term to groups of nerve cells in the central nervous system with a common and integrated role.

nystagmus   Involuntary oscillations of the eye. This may be as a result of neurologic ear or eye disease. The oscillations may be in a vertical, horizontal or circular plane or may be a combination. They may be accompanied by other features of the disease such as nausea or vomiting.

oculogyric crisis   A state where the eyes are held in one position of gaze, often upwards, due most frequently to drug side-effects.

oculomotor nerve   The third cranial nerve.

oedema   The abnormal collection of fluid around tissue and cells or within tissue spaces.

oesophagus   The muscular structure that carries food from the oropharynx to the stomach, linking the two structures.

olecranon   The bony protuberance on the posterior aspect of the elbow formed by the proximal end of the ulna.

oliguria   A reduced output of urine resulting in a failure to detoxify the blood.

omentum   A large fatty sheet derived from a fold of peritoneum within the abdomen. It may have a role in limiting the spread of inflammation within the peritoneal cavity in such illnesses as appendicitis.

oncology   The branch of medicine specializing in the study of tumours and their treatment.

oophoro-   Relating to the ovary.

open fracture   *see* Fracture.

open pneumothorax   The collapse of a lung with entry of air into the pleural space and direct communication of the pleural space with the external environment. Also known as "sucking" chest wound.

ophthalmo-   Relating to the eye.

ophthalmoplegia   Paralysis of the oculomotor nerves. This may affect just one particular muscle (and thus lead to an inability to look in one direction), such as following a nerve injury, or be more widespread and affecting all eye muscles, leading to an inability to move the globe at all (for example, in some neuromuscular conditions such as myasthenia gravis).

-opia   Suffix meaning vision or visual.

opiates   Morphine and related drugs which may be used for pain relief. They have a tendency to cause respiratory depression and nausea. They may be administered subcutaneously, intramuscularly or intravenously.

oral airway   A plastic or rubber device such as the Guedel airway designed to maintain an open airway in the unconscious or anaesthetized patient. Also known as an oropharyngeal airway.

orthopnoea   Severe dyspnoea that occurs when lying flat but which may be relieved by sitting upright. Often a sign of left heart failure.

orthostatic hypotension   A fall in the blood pressure that occurs when changing from a supine to a standing position.

osteo-   Relating to bone or bony.

osteo-arthritis   Arthritis of any joint in which degeneration of the joint takes place. There is loss of the cartilage and the articulation of the bone on bone causes thickening and hardening of the bone (sclerosis).

osteomyelitis   Any bacterial infection of the bone, usually as a result of trauma, surgery or extension of local infection, or carried to that site by the bloodstream.

osteoporosis   The thinning of bone mass seen in the elderly or immobile, also caused by certain drugs such as steroids. Common complications of this are fractures as a result of very little stress or force.

oximeter   A device that measures the saturation of the bloodstream with oxygen by attaching a light-transmitting and -receiving probe to the skin.

oxygen   A colourless and odourless gas which is vital for cellular metabolism. In conditions of shock and respiratory deficiency its supplementation forms an important part of the therapy.

oxygen mask   A device which is strapped to the face and used for administering supplementary oxygen.

pacemaker   The sinoatrial node or other collection of specialized cells within the heart which is responsible for the initiation and maintenance of the heart rhythm. Also an artificial device which is implanted under the skin and linked to the heart in order to maintain a heart rhythm in cardiac disease. It may be set to fire only when the heart fails to initiate a beat or set to drive the heart rhythm permanently.

packed cells   The red cells from a bag of donor blood separated from the plasma (which is used for other purposes) so that the transfusion with packed cells is of a smaller volume.

paediatrics   The branch of medicine specializing in the care and study of sick children.

pain   A sensation mediated by sensory nerve endings that is representative of tissue damage and inflammation.

palate   The dividing tissue forming the roof of the mouth separating the oral and nasal cavities. It is split into the hard (bony) palate anteriorly and soft palate posteriorly.

palpation   To examine a patient by feeling for differences in tissues.

palpitation   A sensation of racing of the heart, often associated with emotional excitement or a premature ventricular contraction.

pancreas   A large, glandular structure lying across the posterior midline of the abdomen which provides enzymes (exocrine secretions) for digestion of food; these enzymes are secreted into the pancreatic duct which drains into the duodenum. The pancreas also produces insulin and glucagon which are secreted into the bloodstream (endocrine secretions) for regulation of the blood glucose level. It may become inflamed either acutely or chronically (pancreatitis).

pancreatitis   Inflammation of the pancreas; may be acute or chronic and may be caused by damage to the biliary tree, drugs, alcohol and certain infections. There may be severe pain and jaundice and if chronic, the decrease in enzymes produced by the pancreas may lead to malabsorption.

paracentesis   The insertion of a needle or drainage tube to drain fluid or blood from the abdominal cavity.

paradoxical breathing   Generally associated with traumatic damage to the chest, resulting in instability of the chest wall such that on inspiration the chest wall collapses in and the lung fails to expand.

paraesthesia   The sensation of "pins and needles" or tingling in the extremities.

paralysis   An abnormal loss of muscle function due to a variety of conditions.

paralytic ileus A lack of peristalsis in the gastrointestinal tract occurring because of a whole variety of conditions including local trauma, operations on the gut or painful conditions in the thorax or retroperitoneal space. There is retention of secretions in the bowel and therefore abdominal distension but there are no bowel sounds.

parasuicide A deliberate act of self-harm but without the intention of committing suicide, the act of parasuicide is associated with a high probability of suicide owing to the acts often performed during the parasuicide attempt.

parity The obstetric way of classifying a woman by the number of live births or stillbirths after 28 weeks.

Parkinson's disease A chronic neurological disease characterized by tremor, a mask-like face and rigidity of movement.

paronychia An infection of the skin of the nail fold.

parotid The largest of the salivary glands, lying between the posterior aspect of the mandible and the external ear canal.

patella The bone forming the kneecap; it is a sesamoid bone (i.e. it forms within a tendon).

patent The condition of a tabular structure being open and not blocked.

pathological fracture The fracture of a bone secondary to the bone being weakened by disease.

Pco$_2$ The concentration of carbon dioxide within the bloodstream.

pectoral (Latin *pectus,* the breast) Relating to the breast – usually the muscles (e.g. pectoralis major).

pelvic inflammatory disease (PID) An inflammatory condition of female pelvic organs, often a bacterial infection. There may be an offensive vaginal discharge, abdominal pain over the uterus or fallopian tube and signs of bacterial infection such as fever.

pelvis The lowest region of the trunk of the body, generally understood to be surrounded by the pelvic bones as its boundary (anterior, posterior and lateral). It contains female reproductive organs, bladder, coils of small bowel and the lower reaches of the colon and the rectum.

peptic ulcer Any ulceration, normally of the stomach or small intestine, which has as a major part of its causation acid damage to the bowel mucosa. Ulcers may be aided in their formation by mucosal damage due to a variety of factors including certain drugs and bacterial infections.

perfusion The passage of blood through a tissue at a rate adequate to supply it with the necessary nutrients and remove toxic metabolites.

peri- Prefix meaning around.

pericardial tamponade A collection of blood within the pericardial sac which prevents effective contraction of the heart. A cause of EMD cardiac arrest.

pericardiocentesis The aspiration of fluid or blood from a pericardial effusion.

pericardium The fibrous sac that surrounds the heart. Fluid collecting within this sac but outside the heart as a result of either inflammation of the sac or trauma may lead to pressure on the heart and reduction in cardiac output and in severest cases an EMD arrest.

perineum The area between the anal opening and the urethra perforated by the vaginal opening in the female.

peripheral vascular disease The development of vascular damage due to calcification and fat deposition within the arterial walls in any part of the arterial supply, excluding the heart's arteries. It may result in local effects to the tissues supplied by the vessels that may be noted on the use of the limb (e.g. claudication) or may present with acute loss of blood supply and gangrene.

peritoneal dialysis The removal of toxic metabolites from the body by fluid washed in and out of the peritoneal cavity.

peritoneum The lining membrane of the abdominal cavity, enfolding all the abdominal cavity. Organs in the abdomen may be within the peritoneal cavity or retroperitoneal (behind the peritoneal cavity): examples of the latter are the kidneys and pancreas.

peritonitis Inflammation of the abdominal cavity due to bacterial, chemical or other causes. Most, common causes include appendicitis, perforation of an ulcer or perforation of a large bowel diverticulum.

petit mal Momentary loss of concentration and awareness but with no motor symptoms. This form of epilepsy is seen in children.

pH The measure of acid and base balance within the body. It is a measure of the concentration of the hydrogen ions present in the blood (the log of the reciprocal of the hydrogen ion concentration). Normal body pH is 7.4. In cases of acidosis (metabolic or respiratory) the pH falls. In alkalotic conditions (metabolic or respiratory alkalosis) the pH rises.

pharynx The throat. It is divided into the nasal cavity (nasopharynx), the oral cavity (oropharynx) and the larynx (laryngopharynx).

phlebitis Inflammation of the veins, often accompanied by a clot within that segment of vein (thrombophlebitis). This may affect the superficial veins or the deep veins (deep venous thrombosis, DVT).

phlebo- Relating to veins.

phrenic nerve The nerve supplying the diaphragm (motor and sensory).

pituitary gland A small gland attached to the hypothalamus in the brain. It secretes a number of hormones vital to normal functioning including adrenocorticotrophic hormone, thyroid-stimulating hormone and follicle-stimulating hormone.

placenta The fetal organ through which the fetus absorbs nutrients and oxygen from the mother and excretes its waste products.

placenta praevia An abnormal position of the placenta such that it occludes the exit of the uterus. If labour commences it may cause a dramatic and exsanguinating haemorrhage.

plantar Relating to the sole of the foot.

plasma   The watery solution of salts and proteins that suspends the cellular components of the blood.

plasma expander   A substance given intravenously that is used to expand the plasma volume or increase the oncotic pressure.

pleura   The lining tissue that coats the inside of the thoracic cavity, the mediastinal contents and the lungs, allowing movement of the lungs relative to the thoracic cavity.

pleuritic pain   Chest pain worse on coughing or deep breathing, indicative of pleural inflammation.

pneumatic antishock garment *see* Military antishock trousers (MAST).

pneumonia   Acute infection of the lungs: often refers to bacterial infection although pneumonia may well be due to viral or other organisms.

pneumonitis   Acute inflammation of the lungs: may be due to viral infection, hypersensitivity to dust or allergens, or chemical contamination of the lung.

pneumothorax   A collection of air within the pleural space leading to collapse of the lung. This may be caused by a spontaneous leak from the lung or from perforation of the thoracic wall, e.g. in stabbing. When a leak exists with a "one-way valve" effect the pressure of the pneumothorax may increase, leading to distortion of the mediastinum, decreased venous return and collapse: this is known as a tension pneumothorax.

Po$_2$ The concentration of oxygen within the bloodstream.

podo-   Relating to the foot.

poisoning   The absorption in some manner of a substance that has toxic effects on the body.

polydipsia   Excessive drinking; this may indicate a variety of pathologies including diabetes mellitus.

polymorphonuclear leucocyte   A white blood cell with a lobulated nucleus.

popliteal fossa   The fossa found at the back of the knee through which in its depths the major vascular and nervous tissues run to the calf and foot.

portal hypertension   An increase in the venous pressure within the portal vein, resulting in spleen enlargement and oesophageal varices, among other effects.

postero-   Prefix meaning back.

postictal   Relating to the state seen after a grand mal seizure.

pre-   Prefix meaning in front of.

precordium   The area over the front of the heart. In some resuscitation protocols the area that should be hit in a precordial thump.

preeclampsia   An abnormal condition associated with pregnancy of hypertension and limb swelling, preceding eclampsia.

preload   The pressure that causes ventricular filling.

premature   Description of an infant born before 37 weeks of gestation.

presenting part   The first part of the baby to be delivered.

priapism   Persistent penile erection which may be secondary to spinal cord injury.

pro-   Prefix meaning before.

proctitis   An inflammation of the rectum and anus; may be due to local trauma, drug administration or a variety of disease processes, and may be acute or chronic.

procto-   Pertaining to the rectum or rectal.

proprioception   The perception of the position in space of the body and limbs.

prostate   A small gland in the male urogenital tract responsible for the addition of certain key secretions to semen. In elderly men it may enlarge as a result of either benign or malignant change, causing a decrease in urinary stream and eventual urinary retention.

prostatectomy   The surgical removal or partial removal of the prostate gland. This may be by either an open approach through the abdominal wall or an endoscopic approach via the urethra.

proteinuria   The presence of unusually high quantities of protein in the urine; this may signify renal tract disease or renal involvement secondary to some other disease, for example diabetes mellitus.

proximal   Usually referring to a point on a limb which is closer to the trunk than another point, e.g. the elbow is more proximal than the fingers.

psychiatrist   A doctor who specializes in psychiatry.

psychiatry   The study and treatment of mental illness.

psychosis   An extreme form of behavioural disturbance, whether organic or mental in origin, normally requiring hospitalization for its treatment and characterized by severe changes in the behaviour of an individual.

PTCA   Percutaneous transluminal coronary angioplasty: an effective form of treating coronary artery disease where a small catheter is inserted through a small opening in a major artery and threaded into the coronary arteries. At the site of narrowings in the artery a small balloon can be inflated to stretch the constriction, allowing greater blood flow to the tissues of the heart.

pubis   One of the three paired bones (including the ischium and ilium) that constitute the pelvis.

puerperium   The period during which the reproductive organs return to their pre-pregnant condition – usually regarded as an interval of 6 weeks after delivery.

pulmo-   Relating to the lung.

pulmonary   Pertaining to the lungs and respiratory system.

pulmonary embolism (PE)   The obstruction of a pulmonary artery, most commonly by a blood clot, though fat, air or amniotic fluid may also cause obstruction. It may present with chest pain, shortness of breath, cyanosis, tachycardia and shock.

pulmonary oedema   The accumulation of excess fluid, firstly within the interstitial tissues of the lung and in severe cases within the actual alveoli of the lungs. Most commonly caused by congestive cardiac failure, though also associated with other acute conditions such as following acute head injury, near drowning and following inhalation injuries.

pulmonary vein   One of two blood vessels that transmit oxygenated blood from the lungs back to the left side of the heart.

pulse The expansion and contraction of an artery as a result of the intermittent flow of arterial blood; can be detected by palpation or other means.

pulse pressure The difference between the systolic and diastolic blood pressure. A reduction in the pulse pressure as a result of an increase in the diastolic pressure may be one of the first and subtle signs of shock.

pus A thick, creamy liquid of varying colour, a result of tissue or bacterial necrosis. Its main constituent is the polymorphonuclear white cell.

P wave The upward deflection on an ECG preceding the QRS complex and representing atrial depolarization.

pyloric stenosis Obstruction of the outflow tract of the stomach, resulting in a reduction of flow of food to the small bowel. This presents with vomiting which may be enough to cause systemic alkalosis.

pyrexia *see* Fever.

QRS The complex of electrical activity seen on an ECG that represents ventricular depolarization.

quadri- Prefix meaning four.

quadriceps The group of four muscles that comprise the front (anterior) part of the thigh.

quadriplegia The condition of paralysis of all four limbs, normally below the level of a spinal cord injury.

radial pulse The pulse of the radial artery which can be felt in the wrist; because of the ease with which it can be felt, it is the most frequently palpated.

radiograph An X-ray image.

radiotherapy The branch of medicine concerned with the treatment of disease using ionizing radiation.

rebound tenderness The pain felt on sudden release of a hand palpating the abdomen. It is seen in conditions of inflammation of the peritoneum.

rectum The terminal portion of the large bowel where faeces are stored prior to evacuation.

reduction Surgical term used to describe the manipulation of tissues back into their original position after they have been moved abnormally. Particularly refers to fractured bones being brought back into alignment.

referred pain Pain felt at one site but caused by disease or illness at another anatomical site, e.g. hip disease may present with knee pain.

regional anaesthesia Loss of feeling in an area of the body by injection of local anaesthetic solution around the sensory nerves supplying that area.

renal failure Failure of the kidneys to perform their normal function of waste product filtration, concentration and excretion. This may be a manifestation of disease affecting only the kidney or may reflect the kidneys' involvement by other disease.

reno- Relating to the kidney.

reservoir bag A component in anaesthetic or resuscitative apparatus that is used as a store for ventilatory gases between ventilatory cycles.

respiration (1) The process of inhaling oxygen-rich atmospheric air and exhaling carbon dioxide-enriched air. This may be affected pathologically by central factors such as in Cheyne–Stokes respiration or by the degree of acidosis or alkalosis within the bloodstream. (2) At a cellular level, the process of cellular exchange of oxygen as a fuel, metabolizing it into carbon dioxide and excreting it.

respiratory acidosis The condition of increased carbon dioxide and carbonic acid (thus an increased hydrogen ion concentration) due to failure of excretion of carbon dioxide by the lungs. This may be due to suppression of the respiratory centre in the brain (head injury, drugs, etc.) or lung disease.

respiratory alkalosis A condition characterized by a decrease in the concentration of carbon dioxide in the bloodstream. Like respiratory acidosis, it may be caused by lung disease, through hyperventilation and excess excretion of carbon dioxide (e.g. asthma or pneumonia). Other causes may include drugs and a variety of medical conditions.

respiratory arrest A sudden cessation of respiration which, if not corrected by artificial respiration, may progress to cardiorespiratory arrest.

respiratory centre A group of neurones in the brain that control the rate of respiration in response to the circulating levels of oxygen, carbon dioxide and hydrogen ions.

respiratory rate The number of breaths taken per minute. Normally this is between 12 and 15. Slower rates may be due to drugs or head injury. Higher rates may be due to a range of acute medical conditions, pain or anxiety.

respiratory tract infection Any infection (bacterial, viral or with any other organism) that is harboured within the upper or lower respiratory tract.

retained placenta The retention of all or part of the placenta following delivery.

retina The light-absorbing surface within the eyeball.

retinopathy The degeneration of the retina, seen particularly in diabetic patients, which may be complicated by the occurrence of haemorrhage and visual loss.

retro- Prefix meaning behind.

retrograde A movement in the opposite direction to that considered normal.

retroperitoneum The potential space lying behind the peritoneum in which the retroperitoneal organs may be found (e.g. the pancreas and kidneys).

Reyes' syndrome An acute condition characterized by disturbed liver and brain function. Viral illness and aspirin have been implicated as causative agents.

rheumatoid arthritis A chronic and destructive inflammatory disease particularly characterized by swelling of the synovium of the joints and joint swelling. It may have an autoimmune element to it.

rhino- Relating to the nose.

rhinorrhoea The passage of cerebrospinal fluid from the nose following a head injury.

right heart failure A condition characterized by impairment of the right ventricle and a subsequent increase in the systemic veins and capillaries.

rule of nines   An approximate formula that may be used to calculate the surface area of a body affected by thermal injury: 9% is allocated to each arm and the head; 18% (2×9) to each leg and the front and back of the trunk; and 1% to the perineum.

sacrum   The penultimate segment of the lower spine. It lies between the two hip bones, articulating with them via the sacroiliac joints.

sagittal   Anatomical term describing the plane that runs from the front to the back of a body.

salpinx   (Greek, a tube) Any tube, though normally used to describe the tubes leading between the ovary and the womb in a female.

scaphoid bone   One of the small bones of the wrist. May be broken and then fail to unite properly, leading to chronic disability; this is related to the blood supply of the bone which enters from the far end and may be disrupted by the fracture.

scapula   The bone forming the shoulder blade.

sciatica   The presence of leg pain often with back pain due to a prolapse of an intervertebral disc which through either direct pressure or other mechanisms leads to irritation of the nerve roots to the lower limbs.

segmental fracture   A fracture where the bone breaks into more than one large fragment.

semi-   Prefix meaning half.

septic arthritis   The bacterial infection of a joint, normally by haematogenous spread or direct contamination of the joint, presenting with acute pain, swollen joint and fever as the main constituents.

septic shock   A form of shock secondary to the release of toxins from certain bacteria when they infect a patient. These cause decrease in the vascular resistance and a drop in blood pressure. Fever, an increased respiratory rate and confusion may also be features.

serum   The thin clear fluid that is left behind after blood has clotted or after plasma has been allowed to form a clot.

shock   Reduced perfusion of tissues inadequate to maintain their metabolic rate and oxygenation. It may have many causes, which fall into five main groups: septic, cardiogenic, spinal, hypovolaemic and anaphylactic.

sickle cell anaemia   A severe, chronic inherited condition, characterized by low haemoglobin levels as a result of an abnormal haemoglobin (Hb-S) within the red cell. The abnormality predisposes to fragile red blood cells which break down or distort, blocking capillary flow and leading to painful infarcted areas. This occurs sporadically and such blockages are known as crises.

sick sinus syndrome   The presentation of a variety of cardiac diseases with a combination of varying cardiac arrhythmias, all of which contain some kind of bradycardia (this may be alternated with tachycardia or atrioventricular block).

sigmoid   S-shaped; applies to any S-shaped bodily curve, in particular the terminal part of the colon before it joins the rectum.

sigmoidoscopy   The inspection of the rectum and sigmoid colon with a sigmoidoscope.

sinus arrhythmia   The slight variation in pulse rate caused by breathing changing the resting parasympathetic tone.

sinus bradycardia   Sinus rhythm less than 60 beats per minute.

sinus tachycardia   Sinus rhythm greater than 100 beats per minute.

skin traction   A method for attaching bandage or material (either adhesive or non-adhesive) to the skin of a limb in order to apply a corrective force reducing a fracture or orthopaedic deformity.

sphincter   (Greek, a tight binder) A controlling band of muscle surrounding a hollow, tubular structure such as the gut or urinary tract.

sphygmomanometer   A device for measuring the arterial blood pressure.

spinal cord injury   Traumatic damage of the spinal cord. The results depend on the level of the cord at which the injury occurs and the severity of the cord damage. Cord damage below C5 and above T1 is associated with quadriplegia, while damage below T1 produces paraplegia. The effects depend on the severity of the damage and may range from temporary to permanent. Transection of the cord is associated with spinal shock characterized by warm peripheries, low blood pressure and absence of sensation and movement below the level of the injury.

spine   The collective term for the group of bones which articulate together to form the backbone.

splanchnic   (Greek *splanchnos*, an entrail) Relating to the viscera.

spleen   A vascular organ in the upper left quadrant of the abdomen. Its role is primarily producing cells for the lymphoreticular system. Traumatic damage may result in severe haemorrhage owing to its vascular nature.

spleno-   Relating to the spleen.

splint   Any device that may be used to immobilize an injured part of the body.

spondylo-   Relating to the vertebrae.

spontaneous abortion   The expulsion of the fetus and placenta before the 24th week of gestation.

sputum   The products coughed up from the lung. These may be expectorated into a specimen container to gather a sputum sample.

Staphylococcus aureus   A natural bacterial inhabitant of the skin which may infect open wounds or may cause infection of internal organs if it enters the bloodstream.

status asthmaticus   A particularly severe and prolonged asthma attack.

status epilepticus   A prolonged and continuous epileptic fit with no regaining of consciousness between the seizures.

stenosis   An abnormal narrowing of a tubular structure. This term may be used in relation to the gut, blood vessels or bony canals such as the spinal column.

sternum   The breastbone.

stillbirth The delivery after the 24th week of gestation of a baby showing no spontaneous signs of life at delivery.

stoma Literally, a pore or orifice on the surface. Generally refers to the artificial surgical creation of a communication between an internal organ and the skin.

strangulation The constriction of a tubular structure within the body, preventing effective function.

stroke A sudden onset of neurological deficit corresponding to an area supplied by a cerebral vessel, normally caused by obstruction of the vessel and loss of blood supply.

sub- Prefix meaning under.

subacute bacterial endocarditis A chronic bacterial infection of the heart valves presenting with fever and heart murmur.

subarachnoid haemorrhage The presence of blood within the subarachnoid space. This may be due to the rupture of a small aneurysm of the arteries of the brain with resultant leakage of blood into the space.

subcutaneous emphysema The presence of free gas within the subcutaneous tissues. The gas originates from airway or alveolar damage and tracks through the soft tissues to the subcutaneous plane.

supination The movement of a limb or body towards the supine position, i.e. flat on the back with hands in a palms upward position.

supra- Prefix meaning above.

suprarenal Above the kidney.

supraventricular tachycardia An abnormal tachycardia that can be identified as originating from a focus above the ventricles, but more precise identification of the focus of origin may not be possible.

sural Relating to the calf or leg. The sural nerve supplies part of the lower limb with sensation.

surgical emphysema The presence of gas in the subcutaneous or deep tissues of the body that has been forced there due to a leak of air from the lungs (rarely the gut). It may indicate the presence of a penetrating neck wound or a pneumothorax, for example.

suture A material used to join surgical wounds or damaged tissues.

syndrome A collection of symptoms or clinical signs that are recognized to exist together in certain disease states.

synovial Relating to synovia, the fluid secreted by the synovial membranes which lubricates joints and tendon sheaths.

systole The part of the cardiac cycle in which the heart contracts and blood is expelled into the aorta.

tachycardia An abnormally fast pulse rate, generally defined as a pulse rate above 100 beats per minute.

talus (Latin, ankle) The small bone that fits into the mortice formed by the tibia and fibula at the ankle joint.

tendon The connective tissue that joints muscle to bone.

tension pneumothorax *see* Pneumothorax.

term Pregnancy from 37 weeks up to 42 weeks.

tetanus A potentially fatal infection affecting the central nervous system, caused by the release of a toxin from the bacterium *Clostridium tetani*. The bacterium is a common inhabitant of the soil and a normal commensal of the gastrointestinal tract of cows and horses, and infects wounds that contain dead tissue. The disease consists of fever, headache and muscular spasm, eventually affecting all the muscles of the body.

tetanus immunoglobulin An effective injectable antibody originating from humans immune to the tetanus toxin and used in the treatment of tetanus and protection following possible exposure.

tetanus toxoid The material used for conferring active immunity to tetanus by production of an antigenic response within the body.

tetany A state of cramps, muscular twitching and (at its worst) convulsions. It is due to an abnormality of calcium metabolism.

thenar Relating to the palm of the hand. The *hypothenar* eminence is the small group of muscles over the little finger side of the palm and the *thenar* eminence is the group of muscles at the base of the thumb.

thermoregulation The natural physiological ability to maintain heat production and loss.

thoraco- Relating to the chest.

thoracostomy The formation of a hole in the thoracic wall to enable the passage of a chest drain. In the emergency setting this may be performed by the insertion of a needle (needle thoracocentesis).

thoracotomy The surgical incision and opening of the thoracic cavity.

thorax, thoracic cage The upper body cavity containing the principal organs of respiration and circulation. Bounded by the sternum at the front, the thoracic vertebrae at the back and the ribs around the sides.

thready pulse A pulse that is weak or difficult to feel; may be related to a small pulse volume secondary to shock.

threatened abortion Uterine bleeding and abdominal cramps suggestive of a miscarriage occurring before 24 weeks of gestation.

thrill A palpable disturbance indicating underlying disease of either blood vessel or heart.

thrombocytopenia An abnormally low level of platelets circulating in the blood. This may present as a tendency to bleed, particularly from small cuts or into the subcutaneous tissues.

thromboembolism The blockage of a blood vessel by an embolus which has been carried within the vessel from upstream. This may result in an ischaemic periphery in the region normally supplied by the vessel or, in the event of a pulmonary embolus, chest pain, cough and tachycardia.

thrombolytic The dissolving of a thrombus; the term is normally used to refer to drugs that cause breakdown of an established clot.

thrombophlebitis The inflammation of a vein, often accompanied by formation of clot within the vein wall. In deep venous thrombi this may be indicated by calf pain and swelling.

thrombus The collective constituents of a blood clot (fibrin, red blood cells, white blood cells, clotting factors, etc.)

adherent to a blood vessel wall; thus it is possible to have an arterial or a venous thrombosis.

thrush Candidal infection of tissues, usually the mouth, vulva or gastrointestinal tract.

thyroid (Greek *thyroeides*, like a shield) The small gland found in the neck, consisting of two lobes joined in the middle (the isthmus), responsible for secreting a mixture of hormones which control and influence the metabolic rate and growth. It may be overactive or underactive in disease states.

thyroid function test Biochemical tests used to assess the activity of the thyroid gland.

tibia The main weight-bearing bone of the lower limb below the knee joint.

tidal volume The volume of air breathed in and out during normal respiration.

tinnitus Ringing heard in one or both ears; it may be associated with acoustic trauma or as a feature of disease such as Ménière's disease.

tonsil A small quantity of lymphoid tissue found in the oropharynx, inflamed in the condition of tonsillitis.

torsades des pointes (twisting of points) A form of ventricular tachycardia.

torsion fracture A spinal fracture, usually the result of a twisting injury.

total joint replacement Surgical treatment of severe arthritis of joints such as the hip, knee, elbow and shoulder.

total peripheral resistance The overall peripheral resistance to blood flow caused by the constricting effects of the peripheral vessels.

toxicity The results of exposure to a toxin which in smaller quantities gives rise to no such effects.

toxin A substance which may act as a poison.

trachea The main air passage connecting the lungs to the oropharynx and nasopharynx.

tracheostomy The surgical creation of an artificial airway by incising the trachea. This may be performed to aid long-term ventilation on an intensive care unit or as an emergency to circumvent an airway problem.

traction The placement of a limb or body part under tension; often used in orthopaedics to correct deformity, realign broken bones and as a temporary method of pain relief at a fracture site.

trans- Prefix meaning across or over.

transfusion The replacement of lost blood with stored blood. This is most commonly from an unrelated donor and as such the blood requires crossmatching prior to transfusion. Occasionally in routine surgery the blood may be given by the patient in advance of the operation and stored until the procedure.

transfusion reaction The response of the body to a transfusion of unmatched and incompatible blood. Fever, bronchoconstriction and renal failure may result. At its worst profound shock may develop.

transient ischaemic attack The occlusion or partial occlusion of a cerebral vessel, with symptoms related to the area supplied by that vessel (often called a "mini-stroke"); symptoms resolve within 24 hours or else they are classed as a stroke. Often the eyes are affected, with disturbance of vision.

transplant The movement of tissue from one anatomical site to another or from one individual (donor) to another individual (recipient). In the case of the movement from one individual to another they require to be as closely matched as possible with regard to blood groups and immunological typing.

transverse At right angles to the long axis of the body (this plane is also at right angles to the coronal and sagittal planes).

transverse lie An abnormal presentation of the fetus within the uterus.

tri- Prefix meaning three.

triage The classification and sorting of casualties into groups based on the severity of injury and chance of survival. Successful triage aims to do the most for the most, even if resources are limited.

triceps The large muscle on the posterior aspect of the upper arm whose main action is to straighten the arm at the elbow.

trimester One of the three periods into which pregnancy is divided.

truss A belt or device used to prevent the passage of abdominal contents into a hernia.

tubal pregnancy An ectopic pregnancy where the embryo implants into the uterine tube; this may be predisposed to by previous uterine infection or injury.

tuberculosis (TB) A chronic disease caused by infection with the bacterium *Mycobacterium tuberculosis*. Histologically this is characterized by granulomatous areas in the tissues. Primarily the lung is affected, though infection may spread from the lung to other tissues.

tumour A swelling or enlargement of tissues, which may be a result of local inflammation or a new growth. The latter may be a benign or malignant neoplasm.

ulcerative colitis Chronic inflammatory disease of the large bowel: a relapsing and remitting disorder. During attacks there is diarrhoea with blood, pus and mucus. There is a higher than average risk of developing carcinoma of the large bowel in the long term.

ulna The long bone of the forearm that runs on the inner aspect of the forearm from the elbow to the wrist. At the elbow it forms the olecranon.

ultrasound High-frequency sound waves (>20 000 Hz). There are numerous applications in medicine, from imaging to physiotherapy treatment.

umbilical cord The flexible link between the fetus and the maternal circulation (via the placenta).

umbilicus (Latin, the navel) The site of the junction of the umbilical cord in the newborn with the abdominal wall.

unconsciousness The inability to sense and respond to external stimuli, due to a variety of causes.

undisplaced fracture A fracture which although completely across the cortices has failed to displace away from the anatomical position of the bone.

uni- Prefix meaning one.

universal donor The blood group O Rh negative which can be given to almost any individual in the event of an emergency, with minimal risk of a transfusion reaction.

ureter The muscular tubes responsible for passage of urine from each kidney into the bladder. They originate from the continuation of the renal pelvis and terminate by passing obliquely through the bladder wall, forming a one-way valve into the bladder.

urethra The terminal passage from the bladder for voiding of urine. In females it is a short tube that lies anterior to the vagina; in males it is about 20 cm long and passes through the middle of the prostate before running the length of the penis to the external meatus.

urinary retention The inability to pass urine; in the male, it may well be preceded by the symptoms of frequency, poor stream, nocturia and dribbling.

urology The branch of medicine concerned with the study, treatment and surgery of disorders of the urinary tract.

vaccination The injection of organisms attenuated so that they cannot cause disease but are capable of stimulating a reaction and active immunity.

vagus A nerve lying next to the carotid artery on either side of the neck. Its sensory fibres are wide ranging and supply sensation to the thoracic viscera and motor supply to the gut from the soft palate to the splenic flexure of the colon.

valgus The abnormal deformity of a joint away from the midline.

Valsalva manoeuvre Breathing out against a closed glottis to increase intrathoracic pressure. This may be used as a method for testing the physiological mechanisms that control the blood pressure.

valvular heart disease Congenital or acquired disease of heart valves; may take the form of stenosis of the valve or incompetence. Features may include cardiac failure, arrhythmia and more chronic features such as weight loss and anorexia.

varicose veins Abnormally tortuous and dilated veins. Although occurring in other anatomical locations, they are most common in the legs.

varus The abnormal deformity of a joint towards the midline.

vascular insufficiency The inadequate flow of blood through a periphery owing to stenosis of the vessels by arteriosclerosis. Symptoms may consist of pain on use of the limb (e.g. intermittent claudication) and in severe disease the skin may have reduced capillary return and be pale.

vaso- Relating to a vessel.

vasoconstriction The narrowing of the blood vessels, particularly the arterioles and veins. This may be accomplished by a variety of stimuli and is useful in the response to shock or to control blood pressure.

vasodilation The widening of the various small vessels (*see* Vasoconstriction) brought about by relaxation of the smooth muscle in the walls of the vessels.

vasovagal attack Loss of consciousness due to a sudden decrease in blood pressure following bradycardia, decrease in cardiac output and vasodilation, causing cerebral ischaemia. This may be triggered by a variety of stimuli, including pain or fright.

ventilation The process of exchanging gases from within the lung to the atmosphere.

ventilator A device that may be used either to provide ventilatory support or to perform complete ventilation.

ventricular fibrillation A cardiac dysrhythmia with rapid and disorganized depolarization of the whole ventricle resulting in no effective organized electrical signal and no cardiac output. Unless CPR and subsequent defibrillation take place, death occurs.

ventricular tachycardia A cardiac dysrhythmia originating normally from the Purkinje fibres of the ventricle.

Venturi mask A mask that is designed to mix atmospheric air with oxygen to create fixed oxygen concentrations.

vertebra One of the constituent bones of the spinal column. It may be a cervical, thoracic, lumbar, sacral or coccygeal vertebra.

virus A microorganism smaller than a bacterium that may only replicate by infecting another organism. The key constituent is a core of DNA or RNA which provides the information necessary for replication.

visceral Relating to any internal organ in a body cavity. Though often referring to organs of the abdominal cavity, it can also refer to those of the thoracic cavity.

vital capacity The maximum amount of air that can be expelled slowly after full inspiration.

vital signs The pulse rate, blood pressure, respiratory rate and temperature.

volume expander Any form of intravenous fluid that stays within the intravascular space, expanding it (normally refers to colloid, though blood is also classified as a volume expander).

volvulus A twist of the bowel upon itself causing intestinal obstruction.

Weil's disease (leptospirosis) An infectious disease caused by the organism *Leptospira icterohaemorrhagiae*. Most commonly caught from contaminated water, clinical features include jaundice, haemorrhages, kidney and liver failure.

wheeze A whistling sound produced by bronchoconstriction.

whiplash injury Forced flexion extension injury of the neck often seen following a road traffic accident.

xiphoid The lower part of the sternal bone, generally cartilaginous in nature. It may be used as an anatomical reference point to decide where to place the hands for CPR.

X-ray A form of electromagnetic radiation that penetrates soft tissues more than bone and therefore can be used in conjunction with an appropriate film to show structures of the body.

zygoma An extension of the temporal bone of the head which forms the prominence of the cheek.

Appendix B

Glossary of obstetric terms

abortion   The process by which the products of conception are expelled from the uterus via the birth canal before the 24th week of gestation.

abruptio placentae   (accidental haemorrhage) Bleeding from a normally situated placenta causing its complete or partial detachment after the 24th week of gestation. The diagnosis is confirmed by the demonstration of an old retroplacental clot after delivery.

accoucheur   Deliverer of babies, midwife (originally male).

antepartum haemorrhage   Bleeding from the birth canal in excess of 15 ml in the period from the 24th week of gestation to the birth of the baby.

Apgar score   A numerical scoring system usually applied at 1 minute and 5 minutes after birth to evaluate the condition of the baby, based on the heart rate, respiration, muscle tone, reflexes and colour.

blastocyst   A collection of cells produced by division of the fertilized ovum.

bradycardia   Fetal heart rate below 120 beats per minute.

Brandt–Andrews method   Method of delivery of the placenta from the uterus: controlled cord traction is applied with one hand while the contracted uterus is pushed upwards away from the placenta with the other hand on the mother's abdomen.

Braxton Hicks contractions   Spontaneous, painless uterine contractions described originally as a sign of pregnancy. Occur from the first trimester onward and probably promote uterine blood flow and transfer of oxygen to the fetus.

breech presentation:
Complete: the fetus is flexed and buttocks, genitalia and the feet present
Incomplete: (frank breech) the legs are extended and buttocks and genitalia present
Footling: one or both feet present; there is a 10% risk of cord prolapse

caesarean section   Surgical removal of the uterine contents by the abdominal route after fetal viability (24 weeks).

cord presentation   The cord is below the presenting part with the membranes intact.

cord prolapse   As for cord presentation, except that the membranes have ruptured and pressure on the umbilical cord vessels is more likely to occur.

corpus luteum   The yellowish body formed from the Graafian follicle after ovulation which produces oestrogen and progesterone.

crowning of the head   Visualization of the fetal head as birth becomes imminent. The widest diameter has passed the bony pelvic outlet and emerged from under the pubic arch.

delay in the second stage of labour   More than 1 hour in a nullipara or 30 minutes in a multipara.

delivery   The process of expulsion of the fetus at the time of birth.

dystocia   Difficult or abnormal labour due to cephalopelvic disproportion or a primary disorder of uterine action.

eclampsia   (Greek *eklampein*, to flash forth) A clinical state characterized by convulsions, not attributable to cerebral conditions such as epilepsy or cerebral haemorrhage, and usually superimposed on preceding severe preeclampsia.

ectopic pregnancy   Implantation of the fertilized ovum outside the uterine cavity. The most common site is the fallopian tube.

effacement of cervix   Thinning of the muscle of the cervix with shortening of the cervical canal prior to delivery.

embryo   The name given to the conceptus up to the 10th week of gestation (8th week post conception); after which the word fetus is used.

endometrium   The mucous membrane lining the uterus which responds to ovarian hormones during the menstrual cycle.

engagement   The fetal head is engaged when its maximum diameters have passed the pelvic inlet.

engorgement of breasts   Full, red, hard, sore breasts due to increased blood flow before milk secretion commences.

episiotomy   An incision of perineum and vagina that enlarges the introitus and lessens the curve of the birth canal.

ergometrine   The active oxytocic principle derived from ergot.

face   The area of fetal head below the root of the nose and the orbital ridges.

fertilization   The union of one sperm and the mature ovum; usually occurs in the outer half of the fallopian tube.

fourchette   The fold of skin formed by merging of the labia minora and labia majora posteriorly.

generalized oedema Excessive accumulation of fluid in the tissues demonstrated by the swelling of the legs, hands and face; one of the definitive signs of preeclampsia.

Graafian follicle A ripened primordial follicle with a proliferation of granulosa cells and an accumulation of fluid within it.

grand multipara Para 4 or more; a patient likely to have powerful uterine contractions – hence the risk of uterine rupture if there is cephalopelvic disproportion.

gravid Pregnant; a primigravida is a woman pregnant for the first time.

hyperemesis gravidarum Vomiting during pregnancy sufficient to warrant admission of the patient to hospital.

hypertension A blood pressure of 140/90 mmHg or above or a rise of 15–20 mmHg systolic and 10–15 mmHg diastolic. Essential hypertension is diagnosed when hypertension is known to be present before or during early pregnancy.

Implantation Penetration of the endometrium by the early fertilized ovum (blastocyst) which becomes completely surrounded by decidua. Occurs 6–8 days after ovulation.

introitus Entrance to the vagina.

inversion of the uterus Uterus turned inside out, usually due to pulling on the cord with the uterus relaxed.

labour The process by which the products of conception are expelled from the uterus via the birth canal after the 24th week of gestation.

left lateral position The preferred position for rest in bed in late pregnancy; when a patient turns from the supine position to her right side, cardiac output increases 10%; from supine to her left side, the increase is 20%.

lie of the fetus Relationship of the long axis of the fetus to the long axis of the uterus. Usually longitudinal, but can be transverse or oblique.

lightening Usually occurs after 36 weeks and is more common in nulliparas; the presenting part enters the pelvis and thus reduces the pressure on the diaphragm; the mother notices that it is easier to breathe. Lightening is not synonymous with engagement; often 3–4 cm of the head remains palpable abdominally.

lochia The discharge from the uterus during the puerperium; it is initially red (lochia rubra), then yellow (serosa) and finally white (alba).

Lovset manoeuvre Rotation and traction of the fetal trunk during breech birth to facilitate delivery of the arms and shoulders.

lower uterine segment The thin, expanded lower portion of the uterus which forms from the isthmus in the last trimester of pregnancy; it provides the usual method of approach to the baby in the operation of caesarean section.

manual removal of the placenta Removal of the placenta by means of a hand inside the uterus; it is performed when other methods fail.

maternal death Death occurring during pregnancy, childbirth or in the first year following birth or abortion, from any cause related to or aggravated by the pregnancy or its management. The maternal mortality rate ranges from 10 to 40 per 100 000 births in developed countries.

meconium Greenish-black, fetal faeces composed of cellular debris, bile, lanugo and vernix caseosa.

moulding Alteration in shape and diameters of the fetal head during labour. The fontanelles and sutures permit the force of contractions to compress the head against the bony pelvis and adapt its shape to that of the birth canal.

multigravida A woman who is pregnant for the second or subsequent time.

neonatal death A liveborn infant who dies within 28 days of birth.

normal labour A labour in which the fetus presents by the vertex, the occiput rotates anteriorly and the result is the birth of a living, mature fetus with no complications, the duration of labour ranging from 4–24 hours.

occiput The back of the fetal head behind the posterior fontanelle.

operculum The plug of mucus that occludes the cervical canal during pregnancy.

ovulation Extrusion of the ripened ovum from the Graafian follicle in the ovary to the peritoneal cavity (and then into the tube).

oxytocic An agent that hastens the birth of the fetus and/or placenta by stimulating contractions of the uterine muscle; by definition may accelerate first, second or third stages of labour.

parous Having delivered a viable (28 weeks or more) child. A nullipara is a woman who has never reached 28 weeks in a previous pregnancy, although she may have been pregnant more than once (multigravida).

perineal body A triangular wedge of tissue based on the perineum, separating the lower third of the posterior vaginal wall from the anal canal.

period of gestation The number of completed weeks from the first day of the last menstrual period to the date in question.

placenta The organ of communication (nutrition and products of metabolism) between the fetus and the mother. Forms from the chorion frondosum with a maternal decidual contribution.

positive signs of pregnancy Signs that are infallible: fetal heart sounds, palpable fetal parts or movements, X-ray and tests for the presence of chorionic gonadotrophic hormone in the urine or blood.

postpartum haemorrhage:
Primary: blood loss in excess of 500 ml from the birth canal during the third stage, and for 24 hours afterwards
Secondary: bleeding occurring in the interval from 24 hours after delivery until the end of the puerperium

precipitate labour Labour of less than 4 hours duration.

preeclampsia Diagnosed when any two of the following signs are present: hypertension (140/90 mmHg or above), generalized oedema and proteinuria not due to infection or contamination of the urine. Also called proteinuria-hypertension syndrome of pregnancy.

premature infant   One born before 37 completed weeks of gestation, i.e. 259 days (previously, one weighing less than 2500 g). The incidence of prematurity is 8% and it accounts for 80% of all neonatal deaths.

premature rupture of the membranes   Spontaneous rupture of the membranes before the onset of contractions; usually the membranes rupture at the end of the first stage of labour (this flushes the vagina with sterile fluid before the fetus is born).

presenting part   The part of the fetus felt on vaginal examination.

prolapsed cord   An obstetric emergency where the umbilical cord is delivered before any part of the baby.

proliferative phase of menstrual cycle   The interval after menstruation and up to ovulation during which growth of the endometrium is stimulated by oestrogen from the developing Graafian follicle.

prolonged labour   Labour of more than 24 hours duration.

puerperal infection   An infection of the genital tract arising as a complication of childbirth.

puerperium   The period during which the reproductive organs return to their pre-pregnant condition, usually regarded as an interval of 6 weeks after delivery.

quickening   When the patient becomes aware of fetal movements; add 5 calendar months (22 weeks) to calculate the due date.

respiratory distress syndrome in the newborn   Diagnosed in any infant who develops a respiratory rate above 60 per minute, has difficulties in breathing as shown by retraction of the sternum and lower costal margin, has an expiratory grunt and central cyanosis. The incidence is about 3% of neonates and the mortality is about 20%.

restitution   When the fetal head is born, it is free to undo any neck twisting caused by rotation during delivery.

retraction   The quality of uterine muscle whereby permanent shortening occurs after contractions in labour. The uterine fundus thickens and pulls up the dilating cervix like a hood over the presenting part.

rotation of the head:
   Internal: the occiput rotates to the anterior position, rarely (1–2%) posterior
   External: the head rotates after it is born because the shoulders are turning into the anteroposterior diameter of the pelvic outlet

secondary powers in labour   Voluntary muscles of the abdominal wall and diaphragm which, by their contraction, increase intraabdominal pressure in the second stage of labour. Intrauterine pressure rises to 110 mmHg with the combined effect of primary uterine action (35–66 mmHg) and secondary powers (50 mmHg).

secretory phase of menstrual cycle   The interval between ovulation and the succeeding menstrual period during which oestrogen and progesterone from the corpus luteum stimulate growth of the endometrium and glycogen secretion of the glands.

shoulder dystocia   (impacted shoulders) Obstruction to the passage of the shoulders through the bony pelvis, the head having been delivered – the neck fails to appear and the baby's chin burrows into the mother's perineum when the occiput is anterior.

show   A discharge of mucus and blood at the onset of labour when the cervix dilates and the operculum (cervical mucus plug) falls out.

spurious or false labour   Painful uterine contractions without cervical effacement or dilation.

stages of labour:
   The *first stage* is dilation of the cervix which is finished when the uterine cavity and vagina are no longer separated by a rim of cervix.
   The *second stage* is expulsion of the fetus.
   The *third stage* is expulsion of the placenta and membranes.

stillbirth   An infant born after 24 weeks of pregnancy who did not breathe after birth or show any signs of life.

supine hypotensive syndrome   In late pregnancy 10% of patients experience faintness when lying supine owing to inferior vena caval obstruction causing reduced return and a fall in cardiac output, there being an inadequate collateral circulation via the paravertebral veins.

tachycardia   A fetal heart rate above 160 beats per minute and a maternal heart rate above 100 beats per minute; in each case indicative of distress.

term   From 37 to 42 completed weeks' gestation (259–293 days); neither premature delivery (<37 weeks) nor prolonged pregnancy (>42 weeks). Full term is 40 weeks – the due date of confinement (often mistakenly referred to as "term" in contradistinction to the above definition).

third-degree tear   A perineal laceration passing through the anal sphincter and laying open the anal canal.

threatened abortion   Any bleeding from the birth canal before 24 weeks gestation, with or without uterine pains, signifies a threat to abort.

trophoblast   That part of the blastocyst that invades the uterine wall.

umbilical cord   The connecting lifeline between the fetus and placenta; it contains two umbilical arteries and one umbilical vein encased in Wharton's jelly.

uterine inertia   May be primary (inefficient uterine activity) or secondary (uterine exhaustion). Occurs usually in the late first or second stage when uterine action becomes poor or ceases. The most common cause is obstruction due to a tight perineum in a nullipara.

vacuum extraction   Operation to deliver the fetal head by traction on a suction cup placed on the scalp (usually the occipital region).

varicose veins   Dilation of the veins of the lower half of the body. Usually occur for the first time or worsen in pregnancy.

weight gain   The average weight gain in pregnancy is about 12.5 kg. A weight gain of more than 0.5 kg per week in late pregnancy often precedes generalized oedema and thus preeclampsia.

Wharton's jelly   The mucoid connective tissue supporting the umbilical cord vessels.

Appendix C

Radio communications

Each ambulance service operates its own, unique radio communications network. This will consist of a central control room and a number of mobile (ambulance or other vehicle-based) radio users, portable (hand-held) radio sets, and fixed users based at ambulance stations, accident and emergency departments and occasionally coronary care units. The control room and all radios operating on the same frequency comprise the *radio net*. The radio frequencies used by an ambulance service, in keeping with other emergency services, are issued under licence by the Department of Trade and Industry Radio Regulatory Department (DTI/RRD) and their use is governed by statutory regulation. Improper use of radio communications may constitute a criminal offence.

It would not be unusual for an ambulance service to have access to more than one frequency (or *channel*). One channel may be used by a service's patient transport vehicles, non-urgent services, outpatient transport or perhaps a doctor's answering service (where the doctors have hand-held radios), while the second channel would be used for all communications by front-line emergency vehicles. A third channel, the emergency reserve channel (ERC), is a common frequency available to all ambulance services (including voluntary aid societies) which can be utilized during major incidents.

In addition, an ambulance service may also use other methods of communication including pagers, mobile telephones and of course conventional telephone systems (*land lines*).

THE RADIO NETWORK

Radio communications are central to the functioning of any emergency service and the control room is the focus of the ambulance service, without which it would be impossible for it to function. The control room is usually based at the ambulance service's headquarters and is manned 24 hours a day, 365 days a year. Control room staff will receive all requests for ambulances whether via 999 calls, general practitioner requests or hospital requests for emergency or urgent ambulances. The control room staff will then deploy vehicles and personnel in response to these requests via the radio net. Communication between the control room and users of the radio net must be conducted according to strict *radio procedure* in order to avoid errors and misunderstanding. The potential for errors can be compounded depending on the operating system in use.

SINGLE-FREQUENCY SIMPLEX SYSTEM

In the single-frequency system all users, including control, transmit and receive on the same frequency. All users can hear each other and can speak to each other; simultaneous transmission by any two users will therefore result in a garbled transmission. Strict radio procedure via the control is essential when using this operating system.

TWO-FREQUENCY DUPLEX SYSTEMS

In the two-frequency system, control transmits on one frequency and other members of the net transmit on a second frequency. Each user can communicate with control only, unless control allows "talk through" which allows one user to speak directly to another user. When the system is switched to "talk through", both sides of the conversation can be heard by all users (e.g. one unit giving directions to another). Normally, although control can be heard by all users, the user can only be heard by control. Other users usually hear a pulsed tone when a user transmits to control, which signifies that the channel is busy.

Each radio will be a two-way set capable of communicating with the control room staff on a number of preset radio channels. Each unit will be assigned a unique call sign which is used in all transmissions, for example *Mike Lima One, Medic Three, Quebec Two Zero One*.

RADIO VOICE PROCEDURE

The essentials of good radio voice procedure are *clarity, accuracy* and *brevity*. These are important in order to minimize transmission times, as radio networks can be very busy, and while you are speaking to control no-one else can.

It is important to pay particular attention to the way in which you speak. The *rhythm* should be regular (avoid long pauses between words or running words into each other); the *speed* should be slightly slower than normal conversational speech (words should be pronounced distinctly and at a rate of about 40–60 words per minute); the *volume* should be slightly louder than normal conversational speech (avoid shouting or whispering); the *pitch* is best aimed at that of a female voice which usually appears clearer over the radio; deeper, gruff voices are less clearly heard.

Remember RSVP	Rhythm
	Speed
	Volume
	Pitch

FORMULATING A MESSAGE

It is important to *listen* before transmitting to ensure that the frequency is clear and to avoid interrupting other transmissions. If a conversation is already taking place and your radio is on an open setting, the voice of control will be heard while the other users' conversation may be represented by a beeping tone. The radio may have a light-emitting diode (LED), which flickers when radio transmissions are occurring; looking at this will establish whether the channel is free before beginning to speak. (On some radios the same LED may also serve as a "battery low" indicator and will flash at a different rate to normal when the battery is failing.)

It is vital to think through what you wish to say before you transmit a message, and to consider whether it really needs to be transmitted at all. The radio should not be used for trivial conversations or messages that could be better passed by another method or at another time. Inexperienced personnel are advised to write the message down before transmitting.

Commencing a message

Before calling, you need to know:

- control's call sign (Leeds Control; Mid-Glamorgan Control; MIDAM Control). Normally, these will be abbreviated in everyday use to a shorter alternative or simply to "control"
- your own call sign (Oscar One; Mike Lima One Zero One)
- what you wish to say.

A typical conversation may be like this.

Oscar One:	Control from Oscar One, over.
Control:	Oscar One, go ahead, over.
Oscar One:	Oscar One, I have arrived at seventeen, one, seven, Birchgrove, acknowledge, over.

[Always identify yourself at the beginning of each message, giving *your* call sign and not that to which you are speaking. Acknowledge = confirm you have received my message. Give numbers in full, then separately: seventeen, one, seven.]

Control:	Control, message received [or Roger], over.
Oscar One:	Oscar One, there are three casualties and I require paramedic support, over.
Control:	Control, Roger, say again number of casualties, over.

["Say again" is used when a message is not received or the message is not understood. It can be used specifically, as in the above example, or refer to the whole of the preceding message when used alone.]

| *Oscar One*: | Oscar One, I say again three casualties, over. |
| *Control*: | Control, message received, three casualties, confirmed, paramedic support is on its way; ETA one zero minutes, out. |

[Do not acknowledge a message ending in "out". Some controls like to have the last word and "out" is reserved for their use only. The expression "over and out" is meaningless and should not be used.]

| *Oscar One*: | Oscar One, there are four casualties, wrong, three casualties, over. |

[*If you make a mistake, say "wrong" and give the correct message.*]

RADIO CHECK AND SIGNAL STRENGTH

When receiving a radio or assuming responsibility for radio equipment at the start of duty, it is important to check that the equipment is working properly and a good signal strength exists between you and control. This is established by the *radio check* and involves a brief conversation with control; an example is given below. It will confirm that you are able to communicate clearly with control and vice versa or will identify problems in transmission. If it is your first contact with the control room the conversation should also establish and confirm your call sign and present situation. When first contacting control you should establish the following.

- Who you are (e.g. for staff coming on duty)
- What your call sign is
- Your present location
- Your present status (e.g. taking charge of a vehicle and ready to respond to an incident if requested)
- Quality of radio reception, by control from you, and by you from control (radio check).

Table C1 Description of radio signal strength

Descriptive terms	Numerical scale
Loud and clear	5 Loud and clear
OK	4 Good but with background noise
Difficult	3 Weak, readable with difficulty
Broken	2 Very weak, rarely readable
Unworkable	1 Unreadable (fading, intermittent, interference)
Nothing heard	

The radio check will establish the signal strength (the quality of the transmission), which can be described either verbally or using a numbered scale (Table C1).

Numerical scale systems can be misinterpreted, but are still in use. Check the procedure used by your own control room.

Example of radio check procedure

Oscar One:	Control from Oscar One, radio check, over.
Control:	Oscar One from control, receiving loud and clear (strength five), over.
Oscar One:	Oscar One, receiving loud and clear (strength five), over.
Control:	Control out.

EQUIPMENT

Understand and familiarize yourself with any radio communication equipment you are expected to use. Radios differ in make and type and the features of operation of one radio may not be the same as another. Important features include the following.

- On/off button
- Volume control
- Channel selection
- Press to talk (PTT) button. This key is used to switch between receive and transmit modes. It normally needs to be pressed in order to transmit and is otherwise in the receive mode

- LED indicator. May have more than one function, indicating the radio is transmitting or the channel is busy, and may operate as a battery failure indicator
- Special features, for example Selcall.

GOLDEN RULES OF RADIO PROCEDURES

Know and follow correct radio procedure at all times.

- Know your control call sign
- Know your own or the radio's call sign
- Keep transmissions as brief as possible
- Think out your message before transmitting
- Do not transmit across others
- Do not speak too quickly; perfect your "radio voice"
- Where possible, avoid transmitting from noisy areas
- Do not hold the microphone too far from or too close to your mouth
- Remember confidentiality and avoid identifying full patient details, in addition to sensitive clinical information which may be linked to them.

Safety precautions

- Switch off radios when at petrol filling stations, as there is a potential risk of explosion
- Switch off radios when in the vicinity of explosive devices as there is potential for explosion if the devices are radio controlled.

TROUBLE-SHOOTING

If the equipment is dead, check:

- battery – is it (a) connected/fitted, (b) charged?
- radio – is it switched on?
- channel selector
- jack socket, ear piece, aerial
- fuses.

If there is background noise, weak sound transmission or distortion, check:

- channel switch
- aerial
- volume control
- mute control
- battery
- location
- verify problem with use of another set.

RADIO TERMINOLOGY

Over – used to signify the end of a message and that the speaker is awaiting an immediate reply

Out – the conversation is finished (may be reserved for use by the control operator)

Roger – message received and understood

OK – message received and understood

Willco – message received, understood and will be complied with

Wait – I am unable to receive your message or reply at this precise moment but will respond within the next 2 minutes

Wait out – as *Wait* but response may take longer, up to 5 minutes or more

Send – pass your message, I am ready to receive it

Go ahead – pass your message, I am ready to receive it

Say again – repeat what you said (requests caller to repeat all of the last message). This can be qualified, for example: *"Say again all after … over"* or *"Say again all before … over"*, *"Say again name"*, *"Say again address"*, etc.

Acknowledge – asks for confirmation that the message has been received

Stand by – stay alert and on open channel, there is further information to follow. This may be qualified by a time interval, (e.g.) *"Stand by one"* (1 minute), *"Stand by five"* (5 minutes)

Affirmative (yes), *Negative* (no) – although it is preferable to use simply "Yes" or "No", these terms are in common use

I spell – signifies a word or phrase is to be spelt phonetically

Priority, priority – (followed by the user's call sign) signifies an emergency situation serious enough to cut in on another transmission. Some radios have alarm buttons which alert the control in the same way

TERMS TO BE AVOIDED

Over and out – it is either *Over* OR *Out*
Negative, Positive – *Yes* or *No* will often suffice
Roger Dodger – slang
Ten Four – slang
Please, Thank you – unnecessary

It is important to avoid jargon that may not be understood. The use of obscene language and the passing of gambling information are expressly forbidden under the Radio Telephone Licensing Regulations.

Box C1 Common abbreviations

- ETA – estimated time of arrival
- ETD – estimated time of departure
- RTA – road traffic accident
- RTB – return to base

Box C2 Typical predesignated codes

Respond RED – 999 response requiring lights and sirens
Respond BLUE – urgent response, but not requiring the use of lights and sirens
Respond WHITE – non-urgent (often preplanned) response
Respond GREEN – available for call

CODED INFORMATION

Some ambulance and emergency services operate predesignated codes which are used to signify types of response. Examples are given in Box C2.

METHODS OF COMMUNICATION

PAGERS

A pager is a small radio receiver which when activated can respond in a number of ways depending on the type and model. Functions range from emitting a simple alert tone, usually accompanied by a flashing LED, to sophisticated models with a screen capable of displaying a message in alphanumerical form. Some modern pages may permit a reply to the sender via selection from a prepared list of responses.

MOBILE TELEPHONES

Mobile telephones are increasing in popularity but have their limitations. In particular, they may be unreliable in certain parts of the country (especially rural areas) and may not always be secure from the view-point of confidentiality. In addition, the mobile telephone network can be subject to system overload when many telephones are in simultaneous use in the same locality. This problem may occur during a major incident, but can be alleviated by using access control overload control (ACCOLC) which denies access to all mobile telephones other than those registered by the Home Office for emergency purposes.

Table C2 The phonetic alphabet

Letter	Phonetic equivalent	Letter	Phonetic equivalent
A	Alpha	N	November
B	Bravo	O	Oscar
C	Charlie	P	Papa
D	Delta	Q	Quebec
E	Echo	R	Romeo
F	Foxtrot	S	Sierra
G	Golf	T	Tango
H	Hotel	U	Uniform
I	India	V	Victor
J	Juliet	W	Whisky
K	Kilo	X	X-ray
L	Lima	Y	Yankee
M	Mike	Z	Zulu

Table C3 Numbers pronunciation

Number	Pronunciation
0	"ZERO"
1	"WUN" – emphasis on "N"
2	"TOO" – sharp "T", long "OO"
3	"TH–R–EE" – slightly full "R"
4	"FOUR" – long "O" as in "foe"
5	"FIFE" – emphasizing second consonant "F"
6	"SIX" – emphasizing "X"
7	"SEV–EN" – two distinct syllables: "EN" as in "hen"
8	"ATE" – long "A" and emphasizing "T"
9	"NINER" – long "I" and emphasizing each "N"

SELCALL

Selcall is a signalling system available on some radio networks with appropriate network and radio equipment. It uses a sequence of audible tones to identify individual radios or groups of radios. Selcall allows the pre-programming of radio sets with transmission codes (status codes) that can be signalled to control without having to engage in conversation. This allows transmission of standard information, for example, "mobile to incident", "arrival at incident", "mobile to hospital", etc., without taking up air time. The message will appear in alphanumeric form on the control operator's control screen, usually with the user's call sign and time of transmission displayed automatically.

THE NATO PHONETIC ALPHABET

The phonetic alphabet accepted for use by NATO assigns each letter of the alphabet a symbolic word with a distinct sound; these are listed in Table C2. Similarly, there are recommended ways of pronouncing numbers (Table C3).

Appendix D

Trauma scoring

The principal objective of trauma scoring is to relate a numerical scale of injury severity to the probability of survival. This can be done *prospectively* at the time of injury, when the results may be used by an ambulance officer to decide to which hospital the patient should be transported or whether the trauma team at the hospital should be alerted in advance. Trauma scoring is also performed *retrospectively* when the patient has been treated in hospital and has died or been discharged, when the scoring may involve complex mathematical calculations. This information is used to review an individual patient's treatment (*audit*) and to compare the expected outcome against a nationally agreed standard. In general, the retrospective scores will be a more sensitive indicator of probability of survival.

In prehospital care the objective of trauma scoring is to identify patients whose cases are "time critical" and whose outcome may be adversely affected if they do not receive rapid assessment and treatment at a hospital with appropriate trauma service facilities. Prehospital trauma scoring is therefore a triage tool (see Chapter 59). The aim is to deliver *the right patient to the right hospital at the right time.*

METHODS OF TRAUMA SCORING

There are two methods of assessing the severity of injury. One is to relate changes in the patient's physiology to the probability of survival; the other is to directly relate the anatomical injuries to survival.

PHYSIOLOGICAL SCORING SYSTEMS

The first scoring system was physiological and was introduced by Champion in the USA in 1981 as a triage tool for paramedics. This trauma score has five parameters.

- Systolic blood pressure
- Respiratory rate
- Respiratory effort
- Glasgow Coma Scale score
- Capillary return.

The maximum score is 16, which indicates "normal" physiology. A trauma score below 13 indicates a mortality rate of over 10% and has been used in the USA as an indication to transfer the patient directly to a regional trauma centre. Two problems were encountered with this scoring system:

- there is a lack of consistency in the interpretation of respiratory effort
- capillary return cannot be reliably measured in the dark or in the cold.

In 1989 Champion produced a *revised trauma score* (RTS), which relied solely on systolic blood pressure, respiratory rate and the Glasgow Coma Scale (GCS) score. He recognized that statistically GCS is more important than respiratory rate. Therefore each parameter is scored out of 4, then multiplied by a weighting coefficient to take account of the parameter's relative importance. The maximum total score is 7.84. It would be impractical to perform such a mathematical calculation at the roadside and this score is only used as a retrospective audit tool.

What can be used at the roadside is a modification of the RTS known as the *triage revised trauma score* (TRTS) (Table D1). The same three parameters as the RTS are again scored from 0 to 4. The scores are then added, with a maximum score of 12 which is physiologically "normal". If there is a fall of 1 point in any one parameter this is considered significant and in the USA the patient is deemed to require the services of a trauma centre. The probability of survival for each score is shown in Table D2.

Physiological scoring systems have the following disadvantages.

- The system may overestimate trauma in the very young (a systolic blood pressure of 80 mmHg in an infant is physiologically normal for that age).
- The system may underestimate trauma in the elderly (a systolic blood pressure of 100 mmHg in an 80-year-old is physiologically abnormally low for that age).

Table D1 Coded values for the TRTS (and RTS)

Parameter	Score	Coded value
Respiratory rate (breaths/min)	10–29	4
	>29	3
	6–9	2
	1–5	1
	0	0
Systolic blood pressure (mmHg)	>89	4
	76–89	3
	50–75	2
	1–49	1
	0	0
Glasgow Coma Scale	13–15	4
	9–12	3
	6–8	2
	4–5	1
	3	0

Table D2 The relationship of the TRTS with probability of survival

TRTS	Probability of survival (%)
12	99.5
11	96.9
10	87.9
9	76.7
8	66.7
7	63.6
6	63.0
5	45.5
4	33.3
3	30.3
2	28.6
1	25.0
0	3.7

ANATOMICAL SCORING SYSTEMS

Survival can also be retrospectively related to the severity of anatomical injury. The standard method is to use the *abbreviated injury scale* where the body is divided into six regions and injuries coded from "mild" (scores 1 point) to "untreatable" (scores 6 points) within each region. The highest scoring injuries from up to three body regions are taken, squared and added together to produce the *injury severity score* (ISS), which closely reflects the probability of survival. An "untreatable" (6 points) injury in any region is automatically awarded the highest total score, which becomes $5^2 + 5^2 + 5^2$ (i.e. 75). The term "major trauma" is used for casualties who have an ISS greater than 16.

COMBINED ANATOMICAL AND PHYSIOLOGICAL SCORING SYSTEMS

In the UK, the audit tool most commonly used to evaluate trauma care retrospectively is the Triage Revised Trauma Score and Injury Severity Score (TRISS) methodology. This combines the RTS (physiological score) with the ISS (anatomical score) and also takes into account the patient's age and whether the trauma was blunt or penetrating. Results are used nationally to compare a hospital's performance against an agreed norm and to see how a hospital performs in relation to others (although all other hospitals remain anonymous). This Trauma Audit Research Network (TARN, formerly Major Trauma Outcome Survey (MTOS)) programme is coordinated nationally from Manchester.

HOW CAN TRAUMA SCORING BE USED IN THE UK?

There is no integrated network of trauma services in the UK. In many areas the ambulance service will take a patient to the nearest hospital, without consideration for the resources of that hospital. A trauma scoring system can be used as a triage tool to allow ambulances to bypass small hospitals, but the following conditions are prerequisites.

- The ambulance service personnel must be taught the system and the application of the system must be monitored.
- The receiving hospitals must understand the system and the significance of an altered score.
- Paramedics may require extended protocols (procedures, and drugs) to sustain a patient over the longer primary road transfers.

In the absence of such a trauma system, physiological trauma scoring can still be used in prehospital care to identify patients at risk. This information can be used to inform the hospital in advance and the ambulance crew can then expect to have a suitably trained trauma team waiting in the accident and emergency department to receive the patient.

Abbreviations

AC	alternating current
ACLS	advanced cardiac life support
ACTH	adrenocorticotrophic hormone
ADH	antidiuretic hormone
AED	automated external defibrillator
AF	atrial fibrillation
AIDS	acquired immunodeficiency syndrome
APH	antepartum haemorrhage
ALS	advanced life support
AMI	acute myocardial infarction
AMPDS	advanced medical priority despatch system
ARDS	adult (or acute) respiratory distress syndrome
AST	aspartate aminotransferase
ATLS	advanced trauma life support
AV	atrioventricular
AVPU	Alert response to Vocal stimulation, response to Painful stimulation, Unresponsive
BASICS	British Association for Immediate Care
BLS	basic life support
BP	blood pressure
BSA	body surface area
CAA	Civil Aviation Authority
CBD	criteria-based despatch
CHD	coronary heart disease
CNS	central nervous system
COPD	chronic obstructive pulmonary disease
CPR	cardiopulmonary resuscitation
CRF	chronic renal failure
CSF	cerebrospinal fluid
CT	computed tomography (a specialized form of X-ray)
CVA	cerebrovascular accident
CVP	central venous pressure
DC	direct current
DM	diabetes mellitus
DNA	deoxyribonucleic acid

ECG	electrocardiogram
ECT	electroconvulsive therapy
EDD	estimated date of delivery
EMD	electromechanical dissociation
ERC	emergency reserve channel
FEV	forced expiratory volume (normally measured over a period of 1 second)
FHR	fetal heart rate
FVC	forced vital capacity
GCS	Glasgow Coma Scale
GTN	glyceryl trinitrate
Hb	haemoglobin
HEMS	helicopter emergency medical service
Hep	one of the forms of viral hepatitis normally followed by a letter such as A, B or C (e.g. Hep B)
HIV	human immunodeficiency virus
HPPF	human plasma protein fraction
IDD	insulin-dependent diabetes
IHD	ischaemic heart disease
ILM	intubating laryngeal mask
IM	intramuscular
IO	intraosseous
IV	intravenous
J	joule, a unit of energy usually used to measure the amount of electricity discharged from a defibrillator
JVP	jugular venous pulse/pressure
KED	Kendrick extrication device
LBBB	left bundle branch block (finding on a 12-lead ECG)
LMA	laryngeal mask airway
LMP	last menstrual period
LSD	lysergic acid diethylamide
LVF	left ventricular failure

MAST	military antishock trousers
MDMA	3,4-methylenedioxymethamphetamine (ecstasy)
mmHg	millimetres of mercury
MMR	measles, mumps and rubella (vaccine)
MOI	mechanism of injury
MRI	magnetic resonance imaging (a form of imaging of the body)
NIDD	non-insulin dependent diabetes
NSAID	non-steroidal antiinflammatory drug
PAC	premature atrial contraction
PASG	pneumatic antishock garment
PEA	pulseless electrical activity (EMD)
PEEP	positive end-expiratory pressure
PEFR	peak expiratory flow rate
PERLA	pupils equal reaction to light and accomodating
PET	preeclamptic toxaemia
PF	peak flow (same as PEFR)
pH	negative log of hydrogen ions – a measure of the acidity of a fluid
POM	prescription-only medicine
PPH	postpartum haemorrhage

PTLA	pharyngeal tracheal lumen airway
PTSD	posttraumatic stress disorder
PVC	premature ventricular contraction
RBBB	right bundle branch block
RED	Russell extrication device
RTA	road traffic accident
RTS	revised trauma score
SA	sinoatrial
SAD	semi-automatic defribrillator
SaO_2	saturation of a substance with oxygen
SCUBA	self-contained underwater breathing apparatus
SIDS	sudden infant death syndrome
SOCO	scenes of crime officer
SVT	supraventricular tachycardia
TIA	transient ischaemic attack
TRTS	triage revised trauma score
UKHIS	United Kingdom hazard information system
VF	ventricular fibrillation
VT	ventricular tachycardia

Notes: Page numbers in *italics* refer to figures, tables or boxed material. *vs.* indicates a comparison or differential diagnosis.